Management of Colorectal Cancer

Edited by

HARRY BLEIBERG, MD, PhD
Department of Gastroenterology
Institut Jules Bordet
B-1000 Brussels
BELGIUM

PHILIPPE ROUGIER, MD, PhD
Gastrointestinal Unit
Institut Gustave Roussy
F-94800 Villejuif
FRANCE

HANS-JOACHIM WILKE, MD
Department of Internal Medicine
University Hospital of Essen
D-45122 Essen
GERMANY

Provided as a professional courtesy by
Pharmacia & Upjohn Company

MARTIN DUNITZ

Although every effort has been made to ensure that drug doses and other information are presented accurately in this publication, the ultimate responsibility rests with the prescribing physician. Neither the publishers nor the authors can be held responsible for any consequences arising from the use of information contained herein.

© Martin Dunitz Ltd 1998

First published in the United Kingdom in 1998 by
Martin Dunitz Ltd
The Livery House
7–9 Pratt Street
London NW1 0AE

Reprinted 1999

A CIP catalogue record for this book is available from the British Library

ISBN 1-85317-377-0

Composition by Wearset, Boldon, Tyne and Wear
Printed and bound in the USA

Contents

Contributors

Enrique Aranda, MD, PhD
Medical Oncology Unit
Hospital Clinic Universitario
Avda Menendez Pidal sn
14004 Cordoba
SPAIN

Yves Bécouarn, MD
Department of Digestive Oncology and
Gastroenterology
Institut Bergonié
180 rue de Saint-Gènes
33076 Bordeaux
FRANCE

Harry Bleiberg, MD, PhD
Department of Gastroenterology
Institut Jules Bordet
Rue Héger-Bordet 1
B-1000 Brussels
BELGIUM

Geert H Blijham, MD
Section of Medical Oncology
Academisch Ziekenhuis Utrecht
Heidelberglaan, 100
3508 GA Utrecht
THE NETHERLANDS

Michele Boisdron-Celle, PharmD, PhD
Centre Paul Papin
2, rue Moll
49033 Angers Cedex 01
FRANCE

Fred T Bosman, MD, PhD
Institut Universitaire de Pathologie
Rue du Bugnon 25
CH-1011 Lausanne
SWITZERLAND

Jean-François Bosset, MD
Radiotherapy Department
Besançon University Hospital
25030 Besançon Cedex
FRANCE

Jean Bourhis, MD, PhD
Department of Radiotherapy
Institut Gustave-Roussy
39 rue Camille Desmoulins
94805 Villejuif Cedex
FRANCE

Peter Boyle, PhD
Division of Epidemiology and Biostatistics
European Institute of Oncology
Via Ripamonti 435
20141 Milano
ITALY

Thomas Büchele, MD
Department of Haematology/Oncology
Martin-Luther-Universität Halle
Ernst-Grube-Strasse, 40
06120 Halle (Saale)
GERMANY

Marc Buyse
Department of Oncology
International Institute for Drug
Development
430 avenue Louise Btc 14
B-1050 Brussels
FRANCE

Guy-Bernard Cadière, MD, PhD
Department of Surgery
University Hospital Saint Pierre
Free University of Brussels (ULB)
322 Hoogstraat
B-1000 Brussels
BELGIUM

Shousong Cao, PhD
Department of Experimental Therapeutics
Roswell Park Cancer Institute
Elm and Carlton Streets
Buffalo
New York 14263
USA

Andrés Cervantes, MD, PhD
Departments of Haematology and
Medical Oncology
Hospital Clinic Universitari
Avda. Vicente Blasco Ibáñez 17
46010 Valencia
SPAIN

Thierry Conroy, MD
Department of Medical Oncology
Centre Alexis Vautrin
Avenue de Bourgogne
Brabois
54511 Vandoeuvre-lès-Nancy Cedex
FRANCE

David Cunningham, MD, FRCP
Head: GI & Lymphoma Units
The Royal Marsden NHS Trust
Downs Road
Sutton
Surrey SM2 5PT
UK

Pierpaolo Da Pian, MD
Department of Surgery
Università di Padova
Via Giustiniani 2
35128 Padova
ITALY

Eduardo Díaz-Rubio, MD, PhD
Department of Medical Oncology
Hospital Clinico San Carlos
Calle Dr Martin Lagos sn
28040 Madrid
SPAIN

Pierre Dubé, MD
Department of Surgery
Institut Gustave-Roussy
39, rue Camille Desmoulins
94805 Villejuif Cedex
FRANCE

Michel Ducreux, MD
Gastrointestinal Unit
Institut Gustave Roussy
94800 Villejuif Cedex
FRANCE

François Echwège, MD
Chief, Department of Radiotherapy
Institut Gustave-Roussy
39 rue Camille Desmoulins
94805 Villejuif Cedex
FRANCE

Charles Erlichman, MD
Department of Oncology
Mayo Clinic
Rochester MN 55905
USA

John W Fielding, FRCS
University Department of Surgery
Queen Elizabeth Hospital
Birmingham B15 2TH
UK

Erick Gamelin, MD, PhD
Centre Paul Papin
2, rue Moll
49033 Angers Cedex 01
FRANCE

Sylvie Giacchetti, MD
Institut du Cancer et d'Immunogénétique
Hôpital Paul Brousse
12-16 Avenue Paul Vaillant-Couturier
94807 Villejuif Cedex
FRANCE

Richard M Goldberg, MD
Division of Medical Oncology
Department of Oncology
Mayo Clinic
Rochester MN 55905
USA

Gernot Hartung, MD
Centre for Oncology
Klinikum Mannheim
University of Heidelberg
68135 Mannheim
GERMANY

Paul Hermanek, MD, MDhc
Emeritus Professor of Surgical Pathology
Friedrich-Alexander-Universität
Krankenhausstrasse, 12
D-91054 Erlangen
GERMANY

Jacques M Himpens, MD
Department of Surgery
University Hospital Saint Pierre
Free University of Brussels (ULB)
322 Hoogstraat
B-1000 Brussels
BELGIUM

Jean-Claude Horiot, MD
Head, Radiotherapy Department
Centre Georges-François-Leclerc
F-21034 Dijon Cedex
FRANCE

Anders Jakobsen, MD
Department of Oncology
Vejle Sygehus
Kabbeltoft 25
DK-7100 Vejle
DENMARK

David J Kerr, MD, DSc, FRCP
CRC Institute for Cancer Studies
Department of Clinical Oncology
Clinical Research Block
The Medical School
Edgbaston
Birmingham B15 2TT
UK

Roberto Labianca, MD
Division of Medical Oncology
Azienda Ospedaliera San Carlo Borromeo
Via Pio Secondo, 3
20153 Milano
ITALY

Urban Th Laffer, MD
Chairman, Surgical Clinic
Regionalspital
Vogelsang 84
CH-2502 Biel
SWITZERLAND

Philippe Lasser, MD
Chief, Department of Surgery
Institut Gustave-Roussy
39, rue Camille Desmoulins
94805 Villejuif Cedex
FRANCE

Francis Lévi, MD, PhD
Institut du Cancer et d'Immunogénétique
Hôpital Paul Brousse
12-16 Avenue Paul Vaillant-Couturier
94807 Villejuif Cedex
FRANCE

Mario Lise, MD
Department of Surgery
Università di Padova
Via Giustiniani 2
35128 Padova
ITALY

Gino Luporini, MD
Division of Medical Oncology
Azienda Ospedaliera San Carlo Borromeo
Via Pio Secondo, 3
20153 Milano
ITALY

Antoine Lusinchi, MD
Department of Radiotherapy
Institut Gustave-Roussy
39 rue Camille Desmoulins
94805 Villejuif Cedex
FRANCE

Patrick Lynch, MD
Department of Gastrointestinal
Medical Oncology
UTMD Anderson Cancer Center
1515 Holcombe Boulevard
Houston TX 77030
USA

Alberto Marchet, MD
Department of Surgery
Università di Padova
Via Giustiniani 2
35128 Padova
ITALY

Urs Metzger, MD
Chief, Surgical Clinic
Birmensdorferstr 497
8063 Zürich
SWITZERLAND

Hans-Joachim Meyer, MD
Clinic for Abdominal and Transplant Surgery
Hannover Medical School
Carl-Neuberg-Strasse 1
D-30623 Hannover
GERMANY

Rachel Midgley, MRCP
CRC Institute for Cancer Studies
Department of Clinical Oncology
Clinical Research Block
The Medical School
Edgbaston
Birmingham B15 2TT
UK

Dion G Morton, FRCS
University Department of Surgery
Queen Elizabeth Hospital
Birmingham B15 2TH
UK

Donato Nitti, MD
Department of Surgery
Università di Padova
Via Giustiniani 2
35128 Padova
ITALY

Bernard Nordlinger, MD
Centre for Digestive Surgery
Hôpital Saint-Antoine
75571 Paris Cedex 12
FRANCE

Lars Påhlman, MD
Department of Surgery
Uppsala Universitet
S-751 85 Uppsala
SWEDEN

Gianfranco Pancera, MD
Division of Medical Oncology
Azienda Ospedaliera San Carlo Borromeo
Via Pio Secondo, 3
20153 Milano
ITALY

Jean-Jacques Pavy, MD
Radiotherapy Department
Besançon University Hospital
25030 Besançon Cedex
FRANCE

Christophe Penna, MD
Centre for Digestive Surgery
Hôpital Saint-Antoine
75571 Paris Cedex 12
FRANCE

M Adelaide Pessi, MD
Division of Medical Oncology
Azienda Ospedaliera San Carlo Borromeo
Via Pio Secondo, 3
20153 Milano
ITALY

Pascal Piedbois, MD
Department of Oncology
Hopital Henri Mondor
Av. du Maréchal de Lattre de Tassigny
94000 Creteil
FRANCE

Jean-Pierre Pignon, MD
Department of Oncology
Hopital Henri Mondor
Av. du Maréchal de Lattre de Tassigny
94000 Creteil
FRANCE

Pier Luigi Pilati, MD
Department of Surgery
Università di Padova
Via Giustiniani 2
35128 Padova
ITALY

Wolfgang Queißer, MD
Centre for Oncology
Klinikum Mannheim
University of Heidelberg
68135 Mannheim
GERMANY

Rudolf Raab, MD
Clinic for Abdominal and Transplant Surgery
Hannover Medical School
Carl-Neuberg-Strasse 1
D-30623 Hannover
GERMANY

Paul Ross, MRCP
GI & Lymphoma Units
The Royal Marsden NHS Trust
Downs Road
Sutton
Surrey SM2 5PT
UK

Philippe Rougier, MD, PhD
Gastrointestinal Unit
Institut Gustave Roussy
94800 Villejuif Cedex
FRANCE

Youcef M Rustum, PhD
Vice President for Scientific Affairs
Roswell Park Cancer Institute
Elm and Carlton Streets
Buffalo
New York 14263
USA

Werner Scheithauer, MD
Department of Oncology
Allgemeines Krankenhaus
Währinger Gürtel, 18-20
Vienna 1090
AUSTRIA

Hans-Joachim Schmoll, MD, PhD
Director
Department of Haematology/Oncology
Martin-Luther-Universität Halle
Ernst-Grube-Strasse, 40
06120 Halle (Saale)
GERMANY

Christoph Schöber, MD
Department of Haematology/Oncology
Martin-Luther-Universität Halle
Ernst-Grube-Strasse, 40
06120 Halle (Saale)
GERMANY

Alberto Sobrero, MD
Medical Oncology
Istituto Tumori
Largo Benzi 10
16132 Genoa
ITALY

Arvil D Stephens
Washington Hospital Center
Washington Cancer Institute
110 Irving St, NW
Washington DC 20010
USA

Paul H Sugarbaker, MD, FACS
Washington Hospital Center
Washington Cancer Institute
110 Irving St, NW
Washington DC 20010
USA

Eric Van Cutsem, MD, PhD
Department of Internal Medicine
University Hospital Gasthuisberg
Herestraat, 49
B-3000 Leuven
BELGIUM

Thierry Velu, MD
Department of Medical Oncology
Hôpital Erasme
Université Libre de Bruxelles
808 Route de Lennik
B-1070 Brussels
BELGIUM

Chris Verslype, MD
Department of Internal Medicine
University Hospital Gasthuisberg
Herestraat, 49
B-3000 Leuven
BELGIUM

Susan K White, RN, CNOR
Washington Hospital Center
Department of General Surgery/Shock-Trauma
Perioperative Clinical Nursing Division
110 Irving St, NW
Washington DC 20010
USA

1

Biology of colorectal cancer: An overview of genetic factors

Patrick Lynch

INTRODUCTION

Colorectal cancer (CRC) remains a leading malignancy, both in incidence and mortality. In 1997, more than 130 000 new cases will be diagnosed in the USA, with more than 40 000 afflicted patients dying of the disease.[1] It is universally accepted that the benign adenoma constitutes the precursor lesion to colorectal cancer. There is a typical transition from hyperproliferative epithelium, to focally dysplastic crypts, to macroscopically evident tubular adenoma, to progressively dysplastic and or villous adenoma, to invasive cancer. This process serves as an excellent model for the understanding of the biology of the carcinogenic process for solid tumors. There are excellent animal models involving both genetic predisposition, such as the 'MIN' (Multiple Intestinal Neoplasia) mouse,[2] modifiers of such predisposition, such as the 'Modifier of MIN' or 'MOM' gene,[3,4] and carcinogen induction that nicely demonstrate the adenoma–carcinoma transition, while offering opportunities for manipulation to provide a better understanding of colorectal carcinogenesis and potentially to prevent it.

The past ten years have seen an explosion in knowledge pertaining to the identification of genetic predisposition to cancer. At one level, genetic mutations accounting for susceptibility to common tumors such as those of the breast and colon now enables the characterization of carriers and noncarriers from families with widespread cancer over generations. At another level, the beginnings of an understanding of the relation between genotypes and phenotypes is providing further clues as to the pathogenesis of cancer in general, including common or nonfamilial adult-onset cancers.

Carcinogenesis comprises a progressive disorganization of architectural structure as well as a derangement of regulation of normal cell replication and differentiation. This transpires over a variable length of time at each biologic stage. Starting at the molecular level, inherited or acquired errors are associated with alterations in phenotype at successively higher levels of subcellular, cellular and architectural structure and function.[5,6] Thus the well-known 'Vogelgram' invokes as a unifying theme the presence of multiple, sequential, functional and structural genetic perturbations that in the aggregate cause a temporal progression in tumor formation. While these have commonly been thought of as 'steps' or 'stages' of initiation, promotion and progression, pathologically regarded as the dysplasia or adenoma–carcinoma sequence, a given series of tumors examined for these changes shows considerable variation in the nature of the genetic changes manifested. Thus progression toward invasive neoplasia is not inexorable, and is opposed by restorative factors that normally operate in healthy and even damaged tissues. Limited damage is recognized and repaired, while cells damaged beyond repair are culled and replaced. As might be expected, such restorative functions perform most effectively early in the mutagenic/carcinogenic process where relatively normal structure and function persist. The evolutionary conflict between these multiple opposing forces likely results in the multistep and multipath natures described in current models of carcinogenesis.

Colorectal cancer is an excellent model for 'field cancerization'.[7] While we shall see that inherited predisposition may be the best-understood process, other clear examples of the multifocality of genetic changes can be demonstrated, including even ostensibly inflammatory states such as ulcerative colitis and Crohn's disease.[8–10] In inflammatory bowel disease, careful mapping of resected, variably inflamed and dysplastic epithelium has been shown to express a complex geographic pattern of oncogene perturbations. As well understood as these events have become, they remain sufficiently poorly predictive of cancer localization as to have not yet entered into routine clinical use as an adjunct to cancer surveillance – much less provided a basis for pharmacologic intervention.

Establishment of biomarkers of carcinogenesis will continue to be a subject of critical importance to understanding mechanisms of disease. Whether such markers are actual participants in the biological processes or simply constitute epiphenomena, they will be necessary to carry investigation from an emphasis on secondary prevention through early detection to a mechanistically driven effort in chemoprevention. Such markers as epithelial crypt proliferation, while easily quantified with avail-

able techniques, have not been sufficiently predictive of clinical disease as to meaningfully further chemopreventive programs. Nevertheless, until better measures are developed, cellular population dynamics involving proliferation and apoptosis will, because they are modulable, serve as endpoints of clinical investigation.[11,12]

In this chapter, the role of genetic factors in colorectal cancer development will be reviewed, highlighting the study of inherited predisposing disorders, familial adenomatous polyposis (FAP) and hereditary nonpolyposis colorectal cancer (HNPCC).

FAMILIAL ADENOMATOUS POLYPOSIS

Familial adenomatosis polyposis (FAP) remains perhaps the best-known example of an inherited basis for the adenoma–carcinoma sequence.[13,14] Reports of diffuse colonic adenomatosis date from the 19th century,[15] with the colorectal cancer association and familial aggregation becoming apparent soon thereafter.[16] Inherited as a simple autosomal-dominant disorder,[17] there is no gender difference in frequency. Penetrance is high, with nearly all carriers of susceptibility becoming affected by age 50.[18] No significant variation in frequency exists between races, since worldwide reports have been published.[19–21] The gene frequency is 1 in 5000 to 1 in 25 000.[22] Because at least 30% of all patients lack a family history, the spontaneous mutation rate is thought to be high.[20]

What distinguishes the typical case of FAP from other conditions is the extraordinary number of adenomas that occur. Adenoma counts may reach the thousands in a given patient, while the histology of the adenoma is the same as that of the common adenoma. Symptoms of FAP include rectal bleeding, obstruction, anemia and malaise, and usually signal malignant transformation. The average onset of adenomas is 12–15 years. Symptoms due to polyps occur by about 25 years[23] and cancer at a mean age of 35–40.

When an immediate family history of poly-

Findings

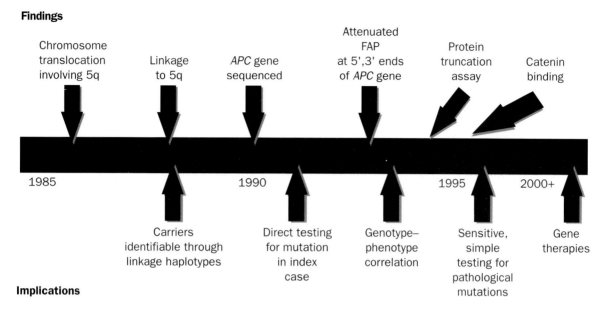

Figure 1.1 FAP molecular milestones.

posis is known for a young subject, surveillance should be initiated by age 15.[24] Endoscopic or X-ray contrast study may, in the earliest cases, reveal only scattered, flat lesions, though thousands of adenomas may be seen. These range from micro-adenomas, to sessile, pedunculated or cancer-containing polyps.[25] Involvement is usually greatest in the left colon, though the rectum may be relatively spared. If adenomas are found in the course of surveillance, it has traditionally been recommended that the patient undergo colectomy or proctocolectomy.

Molecular genetic advances in FAP

The newest and most exciting developments in FAP relate to molecular genetic advances[26–31] (Figure 1.1). The opportunity exists to identify carriers through sophisticated testing of samples of peripheral blood or any other normal tissue.[32–34] Such assays have been refined, and an in vitro synthesized protein assay is commercially available in the USA.[34] This RNA-based assay and sensitive DNA-based assays are commonly employed in research and clinical laboratories worldwide. Consistent with its history as a model for human carcinogenesis, studies of FAP germline mutations have been evaluated in the context of specific patterns of adenoma and other phenotypic expressions. Somatically acquired mutations in adenomas and carcinomas are adding to our understanding of the pathogenesis of FAP and colorectal malignancy in general.[5,35,36] For these reasons, an effort to understand the evolution of this work is critical.

In 1986, Herrera et al[37] had identified a patient with both FAP and severe mental retardation. Multiple developmental abnormalities, diffuse colonic adenomatosis, and a large abdominal desmoid tumor were all present. Cytogenetic studies with metaphase spreads of cultured leukocytes and G-banding revealed an interstitial deletion at chromosome 5q, occurring between 5q13 and 5q31. Utilizing this information, linkage analysis proceeded, using flanking polymorphic markers on 5q. With these probes, genetic linkage to the q21–22 region on this chromosome was soon established,[26,27] with confirmation of linkage and development of additional 'flanking markers' such as C11p11, YN5.48, YN5.64, D5S37 and EF5.44. With these markers came the opportunity to identify carrier or non-carrier status to a 95% level of confidence.[38]

Despite the potential ability to identify carriers, linkage analysis has many limitations when used in clinical predisposition testing. A given polymorphism may not be heterozygous in critical family members, and an insufficient number of family members may be affected or otherwise available for sampling. Fortunately, the gene responsible for FAP was cloned. It is called the *APC* gene (for *Adenomatous Polyposis of the Colon*).[28,29] Sequencing of the *APC* gene has led to opportunities for recognition of carrier status without the need to resort to evaluation of additional family members, as would be required if flanking markers were used.[33,34]

Knowledge of the FAP gene quickly led to the demonstration that mutations can occur throughout the gene.[39–41] Initially, there was no evidence that a given mutation was associated with a particular disease phenotype. However, important genotype–phenotype correlations have begun to emerge in the past several years. Congenital hypertrophy of the retinal pigment epithelium (CHRPE)[42–44] – a useful, early clinical marker of polyposis in a large subset of families – is absent in as many as 20% of adenoma-affected patients and families.[45]

It has been shown that patients and families with few or no CHRPE lesions have mutations 5' to exon 9 of the *APC* gene.[31,45] Families have been reported in which there is a much later age at disease onset, sometimes with only segmental distribution of adenomas, which may be far fewer in number than in 'typical' FAP.[46–50] Disease in such pedigrees has been linked to the *APC* gene.[49] It has also been demonstrated that mutations may be located in the 5' region of the gene in families with 'attenuated FAP'.[50] Interestingly, an attenuated phenotype has also been observed in association with very 3' mutations.[51–54] While the exact function of the *APC*

gene is still not known, the soluble protein product of the gene appears to become functional when forming insoluble oligomers with itself.[55] The markedly truncated protein that occurs in attenuated FAP may be unstable or readily degraded. By failing to produce a stable, albeit abnormal, complex with the wild-type parental allele, a relative abundance of normal protein may persist, perhaps accounting for the milder disease expression. Likewise, the presence of a near-normal-length protein, in the case of 5' mutations, may lead to near-normal oligomer conformations and thus account for the milder phenotype in subjects with mutations in this area.

In contrast to attenuated FAP, it is possible that a particularly heavy adenoma burden, particularly involving the rectum, may be associated with mutations in a particular part of the *APC* gene. Nagase et al[56] reported a 'profuse type' of FAP in which the APC protein was truncated in an area corresponding to a region in exon 15, between codons 1255 and 1467. Because exon 15 is so large, it has been subdivided into many segments designated alphabetically. Region 15G appears to be the location of mutations associated with a heavy rectal adenoma burden.[57] Truncating mutations in both the 5' or upstream and 3' or downstream direction were associated with a more sparse phenotype, although not as pronounced as in attenuated FAP. It is speculated that, depending on the length and conformation of the truncated APC protein, the wild-type allele forms a dimer with the mutated product that inactivates the normal protein complex to a greater or lesser extent.[58] Vasen et al[53] also concluded that relatively more 3' mutations (codon 1250 or more 3') were associated with greater adenoma burden, and recommended proctocolectomy – as opposed to more conservative subtotal colectomy with ileorectal anastomosis – in such subjects.

Davies et al[59] described severe Gardner syndrome phenotype (dental and osseous abnormalities on panorex radiographs) in affected individuals from families in which *APC* mutations occurred between codons 1444 and 1560. A higher proportion of desmoid tumor involvement was seen in the same group. Eccles et al[60] described desmoid disease in association with mutation at codon 1924 of the *APC* gene. In this report, polyp involvement was quite scant. Despite these reports, no consistent mutation cluster region in the *APC* gene has been conclusively shown to predict desmoid proneness.

As noted, mutations in the *APC* gene are typically associated with premature termination of translation and consequent 'truncation' of the corresponding protein product.[34,61] This phenomenon lends itself to application of a linked transcription–translation assay to identify mutations in the *APC* gene. Truncation assay is abnormal in from 70% to 85% of typical FAP cases. Because of the large size of the gene, the assay involves separate evaluation of about five overlapping segments. Once an abnormal band is identified, corresponding to a putative mutation, DNA sequencing within the involved region should be used to confirm and further characterize the mutation. One aspect of this protein truncation technique is that it will not identify missense mutations that do not result in a stop codon. While this increases the likelihood that any abnormality identified by a truncation assay will truly be pathologic, there may be cases in which a disease-associated or disease-causing mutation does not necessarily cause a truncated protein, and thus will be missed by such an assay. Typically, such alterations are detected by techniques like denaturing gradient gel electrophoresis (DGGE) and heteroduplex analysis. Interpretation of the significance of such non-truncating or missense mutations can be problematic. The abnormality may be no more than a harmless polymorphism in a given case, which may not change that codon's amino acid at all or may alter it in a fashion that does not affect protein structure or function. Thus, in a given case, the possibility that disease is associated with non-truncating mutations may necessitate segregation analysis within a given family, albeit utilizing the intragenic alteration itself as a marker. Databases of mutations are helpful in determining the genotype–phenotype significance of such variant sequences.

The precise function of the protein produced by the *APC* gene is not entirely known. It is known that it binds to β-catenin, among other proteins. β-Catenin itself binds to cadherins, which have cell-adhesion functions.[62] It may also be involved in activation of transcription when it complexes with T-cell transcription factors, such as Tcf-4.[63] By interacting with such proteins, the APC protein may block or slow transcription, the sort of function appropriate to the product of a tumor-suppressor gene.[64] In their excellent review, Kinzler and Vogelstein[65] stress the role of experiments utilizing infrahuman species to elucidate complex mechanisms of normal cellular housekeeping that provide clues to human disease.

In the future, development of assays for functional activity of the *APC* gene will be helpful in determining the presence and significance of *APC*-gene mutations. Such assays will advance knowledge of the role of the APC protein in the biology of colorectal cancer, both in FAP and in the general population, where both maternal and paternal copies of the *APC* gene become mutated or deleted in the cancers that form. Despite incomplete knowledge as to mechanisms by which the *APC* gene acts, a tremendous amount of study has been devoted to the possibility that medical treatment of prevention of adenomas might be possible, both in FAP and in sporadic adenomas. While such 'chemoprevention' is largely beyond the scope of this discussion, the opportunity may exist to exploit advances in the understanding of tumorigenesis – by designing and applying agents to block specific control steps in the adenoma–carcinoma pathway. Nonsteroidal anti-inflammatory drugs (NSAIDs), acting to block prostaglandin formation through inhibition of the arachidonic acid cascade, represent one promising category of agents.[66–68] Trials are underway with agents intended to selectively inhibit the inducible cyclooxygenase-2 enzyme.

HEREDITARY NONPOLYPOSIS COLORECTAL CANCER

It has been estimated that 2–5% of all cases of colon cancer occur in individuals from families with a specific inherited predisposition toward the disease.[69] While discovery of the family of mismatch repair (MMR) genes has begun to clarify the role of primary genetic factors in subjects lacking the striking adenomatosis of FAP, identifiable genetic aberrations have not been identified in the majority of individuals with a positive family history of the disease. There is no doubt, however, that family history of colorectal cancer (and likely even of adenoma) increases one's own risk of colorectal cancer.[70,71]

Hereditary nonpolyposis colon cancer (HNPCC) lacks a characteristic disease phenotype of the sort that exists in familial adenomatous polyposis.[72] Its recognition can thus be difficult. Conservative clinical criteria for HNPCC, the so-called 'Amsterdam criteria', were developed by the International Collaborative Group on HNPCC.[73] These include

(1) ≥3 relatives with documented CRC;
(2) one affected case is a first-degree relative of the other two;
(3) cases over ≥2 generations,
(4) one or more cases < age 50;
(5) FAP is excluded.

The need to exclude FAP is rarely mentioned, but the existence of the attenuated form of FAP can sometimes cause problems in differential diagnosis. As discussed further below, other clinical features of HNPCC include certain extracolonic neoplasms, and multiple or right-sided colon lesions.[74] None of these features were included in the Amsterdam criteria. Consequently, many attempts to modify the HNPCC criteria have been proposed, mainly in the interest of broadening the spectrum of families that could be regarded as having or probably having HNPCC. Until syndrome criteria are better refined, perhaps aided by molecular information, families that probably *do* have HNPCC would be excluded by the Amsterdam criteria, in the interest of specificity of clinical diagnosis.

In its typical presentation, HNPCC involves the clustering, in families, of colorectal cancer, with early onset of the disease, and an absence of adenomatosis of the colon and rectum.[72,75,76] It may be limited to the colorectum or it may coexist with a range of extracolonic tumors. Endometrial carcinoma is certainly the most frequent extraintestinal tumor, and in some families risk of endometrial cancer in women exceeds their risk of colorectal cancer.[77] Other extracolonic malignancies involve the stomach, small bowel, hepato-pancreato-biliary tract, ovary and uroepithelium, including transitional cell carcinomas of the bladder, ureter and renal pelvis.[78] Otherwise-uncommon skin tumors may occur in a subset of HNPCC patients. These include tumors of the sebaceous glands and keratoacanthomas, and comprise the so-called 'Muir–Torre' variant of HNPCC.[79] Whether or not breast cancer is a component tumor in the HNPCC spectrum remains controversial. Along with lung cancer, its overall frequency in HNPCC families has actually been reported to be *lower* than in comparison groups.[74] While it may occur at an early age in subjects with other HNPCC tumors, the possibility of phenocopy must be considered. Inheritance of HNPCC is autosomal-dominant.[80] An excess involvement of the right colon occurs in most, but not all, families.[81] Adenomas are a precursor,[82] though some concern exists that cancers may arise de novo and/or follow an accelerated growth phase.[83] In any case, it is unusual to have more than two or three adenomas in the colon at the time of cancer diagnosis or in the course of surveillance. Recall that part of the definition of HNPCC is the exclusion of FAP. If there are more than perhaps three to five adenomas, one should consider the possibility of APC gene mutations, particularly at the 5' end of the gene.

Finally, at the microscopic level, some characteristic features may be starting to emerge. Previously, adenomas and cancer in HNPCC were regarded as indistinguishable from those in the general population. Recall that even in FAP the tumors are individually unremarkable – it is the sheer number of lesions that is unique. In HNPCC, tumors are more likely to be grossly mucinous and poorly differentiated for their degree of invasion.[84] There may be a chronic, pericryptic inflammatory infiltrate.

Findings

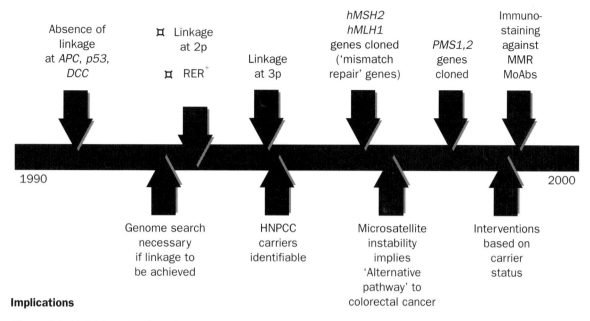

Implications

Figure 1.2 HNPCC molecular milestones.

This so-called 'Crohn's-like' reaction presumably arises against the tumor itself, though this has not been proven. Benign adenomas may be unremarkable and pedunculated, but they are often flat and villous-appearing, with advanced degrees of dysplasia not expected in otherwise innocent-appearing polyps.[83,84]

Molecular progress in HNPCC

Although utilizing the same molecular biology tools, and despite certain similarities in the sequence followed in characterizing responsible genes, unlocking of the molecular puzzle in HNPCC has differed somewhat from that involved in FAP (Figure 1.2). In FAP, linkage analysis was aided by the unique phenotype of diffuse colorectal adenomatosis, so that misclassification of subjects' phenotype occurred much

less often. In an HNPCC family, a given case of colorectal cancer could simply be a phenocopy – disease clinically identical to that prevalent in the family but occurring in a genotypically normal individual. Linkage in FAP was further facilitated by the case of gross karyotype abnormality involving 5q, as noted above. Without such help, linkage analysis in HNPCC started with evaluation of 'candidate' tumor-suppressor genes such as *APC*, *DCC* and *p53*, all of which failed to be linked to HNPCC.[85,86]

Failure to establish genetic linkage to candidate loci in HNPCC was followed by a systematic search through the human genome. This search was aided by new molecular genetic techniques and the resultant increase in polymorphic markers that had been mapped, and was facilitated to a significant degree by the Human Genome Project. In early 1993, a thoroughly international collaborative effort led to the establishment of highly significant linkage in Canadian and New Zealand HNPCC families.[87] Disease was linked to a locus on chromosome 2. This breakthrough by Peltomaki et al led to a series of important discoveries by this same Finnish group and other investigators.

Subsequent studies have shown that at least one-third of HNPCC families who meet Amsterdam criteria link or have mutations in this gene.[88,89] The polymorphic marker D2S123 shows strongest linkage, and nearby polymorphisms show varying degrees of linkage. Genetic heterogeneity was concluded to account for the fact that not all HNPCC families showed linkage to these markers. The gene responsible for this fraction of HNPCC has been cloned.[90,91] This required less time than did the sequencing of the *APC* gene in the case of FAP. The *hMSH2* gene (for *human Mut S Homolog*), was so named because of its homology to bacterial and yeast genes involved in repair of mismatched DNA.[90,92] Degenerate primers consisting of conserved oligonucleotide sequences were taken from the yeast *Saccharomyces cerevisia.* This primer was then used along with human cDNA as a template for replication. The human gene was of the expected length, and showed a high degree of homology to its fungal counterpart. The human sequence was then incorporated into an *E. coli* plasmid. When expressed, this was associated with a 10-fold increase in non-lethal mutations. This *hMSH2* gene was then localized to chromosome 2 by means of a chromosome-specific cell hybrid DNA, by means of Southern blot analysis. Mouse loci known to be homologous to long stretches of human DNA were then evaluated, and a region was found to show homology to band 21 of human chromosome 2, near the 2p16–15 location assigned by Peltomaki et al by linkage analysis.

Shortly after the report of linkage to the locus of the eventually characterized *hMSH2* gene, a group of Swedish investigators[93] identified a second likely HNPCC locus, located on chromosome 3 at 3p21–23. The LOD scores were not as high as they had been for the initial reports of the *hMSH2* gene, but microsatellite instability was demonstrated in tumors from affected

individuals from these newly linked families as well. This gene has also been sequenced, and, like the *hMSH2* gene, shows homology to a mismatch repair gene in prokaryotes.[94–96] This is referred to as the *human Mut L Homolog 1* or *hMLH1* gene. Linkage and/or mutations have been corroborated in many additional families. Initially, the *hMLH1* gene was thought to be less common than the *hMSH2* gene, but further studies indicate that it accounts for at least as many, if not more, families with HNPCC worldwide. Significant founder effects exist for the *hMLH1* gene, with many Finnish families found to have identical *hMLH1* mutations, traceable to a common ancestor more than 500 years ago.[97,98] In a recent series from Finland, this single mutation was observed in nearly half of all mutations that were identified in a consecutive series of cases subjected to mutational testing. Aaltonen et al[98a] initially performed a stepwise analysis of tumors for microsatellite instability, followed by testing of positive cases for HNPCC mutations.[97,99] About 500 consecutive (i.e. not selected for family history) colorectal cancers were evaluated for evidence of microsatellite instability. Of these, 12% showed positivity at multiple loci, and, on this basis, warranted testing for the presence of germline mutations in the *hMSH2* and *hMLH1* genes. Ten cases (2% of the total and 20% of the RER⁺ – see below) yielded such mutations. Five of these mutations were examples of the *hMLH1* 'founder mutation', while the remaining mutations involved other regions of the *hMLH1* and *hMSH2* genes. The authors recommended initially targeting certain patients, such as those below age 50 at diagnosis, those with any other colorectal cancer in the family, or those with additional personal history of colorectal or endometrial cancer. Once so screened, testing for microsatellite instability would carry an even higher yield in selecting cases for the always expensive and often difficult process of mutational testing. No germline mutations were identified in subjects lacking microsatellite instability.

As in the case of the *hMSH2* gene, only a subset of families showed linkage to or germline mutation in the *hMLH1* gene, leaving many

HNPCC families unaccounted for. Since HNPCC gene mutations were now known to involve mismatch repair, linkage to and mutations in other members of the mismatch repair family were identified quickly. The two other HNPCC-linked genes have been identified: the *hPMS1* and *hPMS2* genes on chromosomes 2q and 7p.[100] In a series of kindreds with Amsterdam criteria for HNPCC, *hMSH2* and *hMLH1* genes accounted for approximately 50% and 25% of identified mutations, with the *hPMS1* and *hPMS2* genes accounting for another 5–10% each.[99] Best efforts to date indicate that 30–50% of families meeting Amsterdam criteria cannot be linked to known genes. If the Amsterdam criteria are relaxed, mutations can only be identified in 10–25% of cases. While efforts continue to explore the possibility that still other genetic loci are associated with HNPCC, no such linkage has yet been established to another important member of the mismatch repair family, the guanine–thymine binding protein (GTBP).

Replication errors in HNPCC and sporadic tumors

While ostensibly looking for loss of heterozygosity in HNPCC tumors, Aaltonen et al[101] observed a phenomenon called replication error phenotype (RER⁺). Tumors that are RER⁺ display shifts in the electrophoretic mobility of microsatellite repeat fragments as a result of replication errors that have occurred in these sequences during tumor development, as measured against normal, germline tissue from the same subject. In DNA from 11 of 14 tumors from Amsterdam-criteria patients, Aaltonen et al[101] showed shifts in at least two of seven microsatellite markers from four different chromosomes. More recently, Liu et al[102] reported that 8% of 72 HNPCC kindreds studied did not display RER. Aaltonen et al[101] also examined 46 sporadic tumors for evidence of the RER phenotype. Of these, six tumors displayed band shifts for two or more of the seven markers. Like the typically right-sided and diploid HNPCC tumors, all six of the RER⁺ sporadic

tumors were on the right side, whereas only 17 of the 40 RER⁻ tumors were. Aneuploidy was also more common in the RER⁻ tumors than in the RER⁺ tumors. Thibodeau et al[103] also observed that these RER⁺-related mutations were correlated with overall better survival, and occurred most frequently in the proximal colon. Samowitz et al,[104] in a series of 188 population-based cases of CRC, found microsatellite instability in 16% of cases, but no correlation with family history was identified. However, mutational testing was not performed, leaving open the issue of a possible association between RER⁺ phenotype and mutation risk (see below). Peltomaki[105] has suggested that if HNPCC is similar to FAP in having a fairly high spontaneous mutation rate then this would account for the presence of FH⁻ cases having MMR mutations – a hypothesis that would only be testable in a representative population series in which thorough mutational testing is performed.

As in the case of FAP, a variety of methods have been utilized to detect HNPCC mutations. The in vitro transcription–translation or protein truncation assay is one such test. While this assay is now being used commercially in testing for APC mutations, its use in HNPCC is still investigational. Luce et al[88] reported on the use of the in vitro synthesized protein or IVSP (referred to by the authors as IVTT, for in vitro transcription–translation) in 19 families, 12 of which met Amsterdam criteria and 7 of which did not. Six of the 12 'Amsterdam families' had mutations (four *hMLH1* and two *hMSH2*), while none of the less clinically striking families had mutations. Mutations in the *hPMS1* and *hPMS2* genes were not sought. Similar findings were reported by Kohonen-Corish et al.[106] These investigators did express some concern over some of the limitations of the RNA-based testing. In the case of *hMLH1* mutations, a high frequency of alternatively transcribed protein fragments was reported. The presence of multiple transcripts made difficult the interpretation of *which* fragment corresponded to the actual germline event. Such events occurred more frequently when analysis involved whole blood as opposed to lymphoblastoid cell lines. Overall, the yield of HNPCC mutations using an in vitro transcription–translation assay is in the range of 50–70%.[88,102,106] However, the ability to achieve such high rates of mutation detection depends on the care with which families are selected. There will necessarily be a higher yield for well-characterized, extended, Amsterdam-criteria families in which linkage has already been established. The experience of the investigator and the care with which the method is carried out will influence outcome as well. At present, the absence of detectable abnormalities by the protein truncation test should not be interpreted as implying the absence of a mutation. Rather, the test may be best regarded as a straightforward way of screening for the presence of pathologic mutations. The laboratory and clinician must be aware of its limitations and be prepared to utilize other or additional complementary methods when attempting to identify mutations in a given family.

As noted previously, the likely yield of pre-disposition testing with available molecular genetic technology depends on the circumstances of the patient and family under consideration. Up to 70% of Amsterdam-criteria HNPCC families link to one of the known mismatch repair genes. But these families are rather exceptional. The typical patient who is concerned about his or her family history of colorectal cancer will likely present with a much less dramatic family history. In these more common but less compelling circumstances, testing may or may not be appropriate, but the rationale and yield clearly differ. An indirect, but simpler and perhaps more satisfactory screening test for the possible presence of HNPCC is the use of assays for microsatellite instability.[102] It is known that in definite HNPCC families, nearly all colorectal cancers show evidence of microsatellite instability. It is also known that 10–15% of sporadic colorectal cancers have microsatellite instability.[107] While early efforts to identify germline mutations in such cases were disappointing, the use of microsatellite testing in conjunction with clinical features such as age at onset may improve the overall yield. Utilizing age at onset as a screening tool, Liu et al[107] found instability in

18/31 (58%) of CRC patients under age 35, compared with 19/158 (12%) of those over 35. Of 12 young subjects who were evaluable for germline mutations, five were found to have them (three *hMSH2* and two *hMLH1*). Another possible clinical basis for choosing cases for microsatellite assessment is the presence of multiple primary cancers. Horii et al[108] found instability in 34 of 38 (89%) of cases with multiple primaries, compared with only 19 of 174 (11%) with solitary tumors. Germline testing for MMR mutations was not performed, but would be expected to carry a high yield. Jass et al[109] compared families meeting Amsterdam criteria with those falling short of this standard. Six microsatellites were evaluated, and instability of any was considered a positive. Families meeting Amsterdam criteria were, as might be expected, more likely to have other features usually associated with HNPCC, including early age at onset, multiple primaries, proximal localization, mucinous and poorly differentiated histology, and tumor DNA diploidy. Amsterdam-criteria-positive families were more likely to have microsatellite instability at multiple loci. Mutational testing to confirm the predictive power of microsatellite instability was not performed. Another series of otherwise-sporadic tumors was evaluated for microsatellite instability, in relation to various clinicopathologic correlates.[110] Among 137 sporadic stage II and III colorectal cancers, 13% showed instability. These patients were younger and had more proximally located lesions. There was no increase in family history positivity in the RER⁺ group. Pathologically, the RER⁺ tumors were more likely to be large, exophytic, poorly differentiated and mucinous, and to show a peritumoral lymphocytic infiltrate. They were less likely to have *p53* overexpression than the RER⁻ tumors. While germline mutational testing was not carried out, all of these features are typical of HNPCC. In each of the above studies, the possibility of directly confirming an HNPCC diagnosis by predisposition testing may render moot the distinctions between 'possible', 'probable' and 'definite' HNPCC, regardless of reported family history. Our own group has identified cases with MMR-gene mutations and no immediate family history of colorectal cancer.[111]

At least one study has urged reconsideration of the use of microsatellite instability as a clinical indicator of HNPCC. Samowitz et al[104] tested up to 10 microsatellite markers in colon (but not rectal) tumors from 170 subjects between age 30 and 79 and with no previous cancer diagnosis. Cases were not selected on the basis of family history, though a detailed family history was obtained retrospectively. Tumors were considered positive for instability if ≥30% of tested microsatellites showed new bands in tumors, relative to normal mucosa. As expected, the vast majority of cases showed no instability or instability at 20% or fewer tested loci. Instability was significantly associated with tumor location in the right colon and early age at onset. However, it did not predict a positive family history of colorectal cancer to any level of significance, though borderline significance existed for men with the strongest family histories. Testing for germline mutations was not carried out in any of the cases, with or without microsatellite instability. Recalling Liu's data showing a high rate of such mutations (regardless of family history) in young patients whose tumors showed instability, similar evaluation of cases from the Samowitz series might have been illuminating.

Besides screening tumors for evidence of microsatellite instability, immunohistochemical approaches are on the horizon.[103,112] Given that a carrier of an MMR germline mutation already carries one allelic 'hit', the occurrence of a second mutation or deletion in the remaining parental allele, occurring in the process of carcinogenesis, would leave no functional protein. In principle, a tagged monoclonal antibody against conserved sequences within the protein should bind to normal tissue, which expresses normal protein, but should fail to bind to tumor tissue, which lacks such protein, because of the resultant loss of both alleles. Thibodeau et al[103] have examined the protein expression pattern of hMSH2 and hMLH1 by immunohistochemistry studies of paraffin-embedded tumors. Specifically, they examined 7 patients with microsatellite unstable sporadic colorectal cancers, 13 patients with 'familial' colorectal cancer, and 12 patients who met the strict Amsterdam criteria for HNPCC. Expression of the gene products of hMSH2 and hMLH1 was examined, with attention given to the presence of germ line or somatic mutations in addition to the presence of tumor microsatellite instability. Findings disclosed that 19 of the 28 tumors studied demonstrated instability. Mutations in hMLH1 and hMSH2 were detected in 6 and 2 patients respectively. Of the eight MIN+/MMR− gene mutation+ cases, an absence of protein expression was observed for the corresponding gene product in all but one case (missense mutation in hMLH1). Furthermore, seven cases with microsatellite instability and demonstrable germline mutation showed absence of hMLH1 or hMSH2, while four cases with instability but no mutation showed normal protein expression. This further supports the notion that there are important differences in the significance that may be attached to microsatellite instability, depending on whether or not it is actually associated with HNPCC. As a 'negative control', no case lacking microsatellite instability and lacking an MMR-gene mutation showed any protein expression abnormalities. It was concluded that examination of protein expression employing immunohistochemistry may provide a rapid test to aid in the prescreening of HNPCC tumors for the identification of mutations in the MMR genes.

As noted above, the endpoint of microsatellite instability is a consistent feature in HNPCC. However, the mechanism by which mismatch repair deficits lead to cancer, and colon cancer susceptibility in particular, remain elusive. However, clues are appearing in this area of great basic scientific inquiry. That HNPCC genes indeed act by a mechanism of mismatch repair has been demonstrated in experiments in which mismatch repair deficits in human cancer cell lines with hMLH1 mutations have been corrected by addition of the normal hMLH1 gene.[113]

Other work has been performed evaluating possible targets of mismatch repair deficiency. Grady et al[114] describe TGF-β as a family of three highly homologous peptides, namely TGF-β1,

TGF-β2, and TGF-β3, whose role is to inhibit growth of most epithelial tissues, including colonic epithelium. These peptides can directly induce apoptotic cell death,[115] and for this reason are important in mediating differentiation and cell death. Consequently, Markowitz et al[116] have suggested that the TGF-β receptor (RII) acts as a tumor-suppressor gene in human colon cells. In their review of the subject, Grady et al[114] note that mutation in RII is strongly associated with, and is present in more than 90% of patients with, colon cancers showing microsatellite instability. Parsons et al[117] found that RII is somatically altered in HNPCC. Akiyama et al[118] studied the role of RII alterations in HNPCC tumorigenesis with particular attention to adenomas, identifying alterations of the TGF-β RII gene at a short poly A repeat in 8 (57%) of adenomas and in 11 (85%) of colon cancers. These alterations were identified at an earlier stage of adenomas, with two of the adenomas showing two-hit inactivation of mismatch repair genes. Replication errors were found in 13 (93%) of the adenomas, and mutations in *K-ras* codon 12 were identified in 50% of the adenomas. These investigators concluded that there was a strong association between TGF-β RII gene alterations and adenoma–carcinoma progression in HNPCC.

CONCLUSIONS

The molecular genetic events that characterize the vast bulk of sporadic colorectal cancers are fundamentally similar to those involving the two conditions, FAP and HNPCC, that have been the focus of this overview. If the general model of carcinogenesis indeed involves a requirement of gain, loss or alteration in function of both copies of critical regulatory genes then these disease models provide a relatively simple starting point in evaluating the complex processes. Since every cell carries the same susceptibility mutations, the investigation of second, somatic events can be investigated in the context of a rather homogeneous substrate.

It is now technically possible to test virtually everyone for the presence of genetic mutations that predispose to several of the most common cancers in the Western world. However, because such mutations are rare and the mutational assays imperfect, the cost and yield of routinely carrying out such testing cannot be justified at this time. In addition, it is becoming apparent that significant social considerations will limit the widespread application of susceptibility testing for the foreseeable future. Improvements will have to be made in the clinical benefit that proceeds from the labeling of individuals with such susceptibilities. Stigmas associated with such status will need to be addressed forthrightly. Appropriate attention must be devoted to prevention of unfair discrimination against those at risk.

Available surveillance measures and prophylactic surgery constitute useful interventions to reduce the risk of actually developing inherited colorectal cancer. As additional preventive measures become available, including chemopreventive agents and gene therapies, there will be added incentive for the development of more accurate means of recognizing those carrying such inherited susceptibilities.

Efforts will continue to characterize the similarities and differences between familial and sporadic colorectal cancers. In the case of sporadic tumors, there continues to be conflicting data over molecular genetic issues that should be amenable to conclusive study. Whether loss of a given tumor-suppressor gene predicts outcome independent of TNM stage remains to be seen, since existing reports are not in agreement.[5,119–122] Such disagreement may relate to the heterogeneity that exists among sporadic colorectal cancers. Each new piece of information obtained regarding familial tumors contributes to better categorization of apparently sporadic tumors.

REFERENCES

1. Parker SL, Tong T, Bolden S, Wingo PA, Cancer statistics, 1997. *CA: Cancer J* 1997; **47:** 5–27.
2. Moser AR, Pitot HC, Dove WF, A dominant mutation that predisposes to multiple intestinal neoplasia in the mouse. *Science* 1990; **247:** 322–4.
3. Dietrich WF, Lander ES, Smith JS et al, Genetic identification of Mom-1, a major modifier locus affecting Min-induced intestinal neoplasia in the mouse. *Cell* 1993; **75:** 631–9.
4. MacPhee M, Chepenik KP, Liddell RA et al, The secretary phospholipase A2 gene is a candidate for the MOM1 locus, a major modifier of APC^{Min}-induced intestinal neoplasia. *Cell* 1995; **81:** 957–66.
5. Vogelstein B, Fearon ER, Hamilton SR et al, Genetic alterations during colorectal tumor development. *N Engl J Med* 1988; **319:** 525–32.
6. Vogelstein B, Kinzler K, The multistep nature of cancer. *Trends Genet* 1993; **9:** 138–41.
7. Slaughter DP, Southwick HW, Smejkal W, Field cancerization in oral statified squamous epithelium: clinical implication of multicentric origin. *Cancer* 1953; **6:** 963–8.
8. Burmer GC, Levine DS, Kulander BG et al, c-Ki-ras mutations in chronic ulcerative colitis and sporadic colon carcinoma. *Gastroenterology* 1990; **99:** 416–20.
9. Chen J, Compton C, Cheng E et al, c-Ki-ras mutations in dysplastic fields and cancers in ulcerative colitis. *Gastroenterology* 1992; **102:** 1983–7.
10. Loefberg R, Brostrom O, Karlen P et al, DNA aneuploidy in ulcerative colitis: reproducibility, topographic distribution, and relation to dysplasia. *Gastroenterology* 1992; **102:** 1149–54.
11. Koike M, Significance of spontaneous apoptosis during colorectal tumorigenesis. *J Surg Oncol* 1996; **62:** 97–108.
12. Greenwald P, Kelloff GJ, Boone CW et al, Genetic and cellular changes in colorectal cancer: proposed targets of chemopreventive agents. *Cancer Epidemiol Biomark Prev* 1995; **4:** 691–702.
13. Bussey HJR, *Familial Polyposis Coli: Family Studies, Histopathology, Differential Diagnosis, and Results of Treatment.* Baltimore: Johns Hopkins University Press, 1975.
14. Bussey HJR, Historical developments in familial adenomatous polyposis. In: *Familial Adenomatous Polyposis* (Herrera L, ed). New York: Alan R Liss, 1990; 1–7.
15. Cripps WH, Two cases of disseminated polyps of the rectum. *Trans Pathol Soc Lond* 1882; **33:** 165–8.
16. Handford H, Disseminated polypi of the large intestine becoming malignant. *Trans Pathol Soc Lond* 1890; **41:** 133–4.
17. Alm T, Licznerski G, The intestinal polyposes. *Clin Gastroenterol* 1973; **2:** 577–602.
18. Murday V, Slack J, Inherited disorders associated with colorectal cancer. *Cancer Surv* 1989; **8:** 139–57.
19. Ponz de Leon M, Sassatelli R, Zanghieri G et al, Hereditary adenomatosis of the colon and rectum: clinical features of eight families from northern Italy. *Am J Gastroenterol* 1989; **84:** 906–16.
20. Ushio K, Genetic and familial patterns in colorectal cancer. *Jpn J Clin Oncol* 1985; **15**(Suppl): 281–98.
21. Krokowicz P, Management of familial polyposis in Poland. In: *Hereditary Colorectal Cancer* (Utsunomiya J, Lynch HT, eds). Tokyo: Springer-Verlag, 1990; 71–7.
22. Reed TE, Neel JV, A genetic study of multiple polyposis of the colon. *Am J Human Genet* 1955; **7:** 236–63.
23. Lockhart-Mummery P, Cancer and heredity. *Lancet* 1925; **i:** 427–9.
24. Jagelman DG, Clinical management of familial adenomatous polyposis. *Cancer Surv* 1989; **8:** 159–67.
25. Muto T, Bussey HJR, Morson BC, The evolution of cancer of the colon and rectum. *Cancer* 1975; **36:** 2251–70.
26. Bodmer WF, Bailey CJ, Bodmer J et al, Localization of the gene for familial adenomatous polyposis on chromosome 5. *Nature* 1987; **328:** 614–16.
27. Leppert M, Dobbs M, Scambler P et al, The gene to familial polyposis coli maps to the long arm of chromosome 5. *Science* 1987; **238:** 1411–13.
28. Groden J, Thliveris A, Samowitz W et al, Identification and characterization of the familial adenomatous polyposis coli gene. *Cell* 1991; **66:** 589–600.
29. Nishisho I, Nakamura Y, Miyoshi Y et al, Mutations of chromosome 5q21 genes in FAP and colorectal cancer patients. *Science* 1991; **253:** 665–9.
30. Burn J, Delhanty J, Wood C et al, The UK Northern Region genetic register for familial

adenomatous polyposis: use of age of onset, congenital hypertrophy of the retinal pigment epithelium, and DNA markers in risk calculations. *J Med Genet* 1991; **28;** 289–96.

31. Bunyan DJ, Shea-Simonds J, Reck AC et al, Genotype–phenotype correlations of new causative APC gene mutations in patients with familial adenomatous polyposis. *J Med Genet* 1995; **32:** 729–31.

32. Morton DG, Macdonald F, Cachon-Gonzales MB et al, The use of DNA from paraffin wax preserved tissue for predictive diagnosis in familial adenomatous polyposis. *J Med Genet* 1992; **29:** 571–3.

33. Groden J, Gelbert L, Thliveris A et al, Mutational analysis of patients with adenomatous polyposis: identical inactivating mutations in unrelated individuals. *Am J Hum Genet* 1993; **52:** 263–72.

34. Powell SM, Petersen GM, Krush AJ et al, Molecular diagnosis of familial adenomatous polyposis. *N Engl J Med* 1993; **329:** 1982–7.

35. de Benedetti L, Sciallero S, Gismondi V et al, Association of *APC* gene mutations and histological characteristics of colorectal adenomas. *Cancer Res* 1994; **54:** 3553–6.

36. Ichii S, Takeda S, Horii A et al, Detailed analysis of genetic alterations in colorectal tumors from patients with and without familial adenomatous polyposis (FAP). *Oncogene* 1993; **8:** 2399–405.

37. Herrera L, Kakati S, Gibas L et al, Gardner syndrome in a man with an interstitial deletion of 5q. *Am J Med Genet* 1986; **25:** 473–6.

38. Meera-Khan P, Tops CMJ, Brock M et al, Close linkage of a highly polymorphic marker (D5S37) to familial polyposis and confirmation of FAP localization on chromosome 5q-21-q22. *Hum Genet* 1988; **79:** 183–5.

39. Ando H, Miyoshi Y, Nagase H et al, Detection of 12 germ-line mutations in the adenomatous polyposis coli gene by polymerase chain reaction. *Gastroenterology* 1993; **104:** 989–93.

40. Fodde R, van der Luijt R, Wijnen J et al, Eight novel inactivating germ line mutations at the APC gene identified by denaturing gradient gel electrophoresis. *Genomics* 1992; **13:** 1162–8.

41. Joslyn G, Carlson M, Thliveris A et al, Identification of deletion mutations and three new genes at the familial polyposis locus. *Cell* 1991; **66:** 601–13.

42. Traboulsi EI, Krush AJ, Gardner EJ et al, Prevalence and importance of pigmented ocular fundus lesions in Gardner's syndrome. *N Engl J Med* 1987; **316:** 661–7.

43. Llopis D, Menozo JL, Congenital hypertrophy of the retinal pigment epithelium and familial polyposis of the colon. *Am J Ophth* 1987; **103:** 235–6.

44. Baba S, Tsuchiya M, Watanabe I, Machida H, Importance of retinal pigmentation as a subclinical marker in familial adenomatous polyposis. *Dis Colon Rectum* 1990; **33:** 660–5.

45. Olschwang S, Tiret A, Laurent-Puig P et al, Restriction of ocular fundus lesions to a specific subgroup of APC mutations in adenomatous polyposis coli patients. *Cell* 1993; **75:** 959–68.

46. Lynch HT, Lynch PM, Follett KL, Harris RE, Familial polyposis coli: heterogeneous polyp expression in two kindreds. *J Med Genet* 1979; **16:** 1–7.

47. Lynch HT, Smyrk T, Lanspa SJ et al, Flat adenomas in a colon cancer-prone kindred. *J Natl Cancer Inst* 1988; **80:** 278–82.

48. Leppert M, Burt R, Hughes JP et al, Genetic analysis of an inherited predisposition to colon cancer in a family with a variable number of adenomatous polyps. *N Engl J Med* 1990; **322:** 904–8.

49. Spiro L, Otterud B, Stauffer D et al, Linkage of a variant or attenuated form of adenomatous polyposis coli to the adenomatous polyposis coli (APC) locus. *Am J Hum Genet* 1992; **51:** 92–100.

50. Spirio L, Olschwang S, Groden J et al, Alleles of the *APC* gene: an attenuated form of familial polyposis. *Cell* 1993; **75:** 951–7.

51. Scott RJ, van der Luijt R, Spycher M et al, Novel germline APC mutation in a large familial adenomatous polyposis kindred displaying variable phenotypes. *Gut* 1995; **36:** 731–6.

52. van der Luijt RB, Meera Khan P, Vasen HFA et al, Germline mutations in the 3' part of APC exon 15 do not result in truncated proteins and are associated with attenuated adenomatous polyposis coli. *Hum Genet* 1996; **98:** 727–34.

53. Vasen HFA, van der Luijt RB, Slors JF et al, Molecular genetic gests as a guide to surgical management of familial adenomatous polyposis. *Lancet* 1996; **348:** 43–5.

54. McKinlay RJ, Kool D, Edkins E et al, The clinical correlates of a 3' truncating mutation (codons 1982–1983) in the adenomatous polyposis coli gene. *Gastroenterology* 1997; **113:** 326–31.

55. Su L-K, Vogelstein B, Kinzler KW, Association

of the APC tumor suppressor protein with catenins. *Science* 1993; **262**: 1734–7.

56. Nagase H, Miyoshi Y, Horii A et al, Correlation between the location of germ-line mutations in the *APC* gene and the number of colorectal polyps in familial adenomatous polyposis patients. *Cancer Res* 1992; **52**: 4055–7.

57. Gayther SA, Wells D, SenGupta SB et al, Regionally clustered APC mutations are associated with a severe phenotype and occur at a high frequency in new mutation cases of adenomaous polyposis coli. *Hum Mol Genet* 1994; **3**: 53–6.

58. Friedl W, Meuschel S, Caspari R et al, Attenuated familial adenomatous polyposis due to a mutation in the 3' part of the APC gene. A clue for understanding the function of the APC protein. *Hum Genet* 1996; **97**: 579–84.

59. Davies D, Armstrong J, Thakker N et al, Severe Gardner syndrome in families with mutations restricted to a specific region of the APC gene. *Am J Hum Genet* 1995; **57**: 1151–8.

60. Eccles DM, van der Luijt R, Breukel C et al, Hereditary desmoid disease due to a frameshift mutation at codon 1924 of the *APC* gene. *Am J Hum Genet* 1996; **59**: 1193–201.

61. van der Luijt R, Meera Khan P, Vasen H et al, Rapid detection of translation-terminating mutations at the adenomatous polyposis coli (APC) gene by direct protein truncation test *Genomics* 1994; **20**: 1–4.

62. Kemler R, From cadherins to catenins: cytolasmic protein interactions and regulation of cell adhesion. *Trends Genet* 1993; **9**: 317–21.

63. Molinaar M, van de Wetering M, Oosterwegel M et al, XTcf-3 transcription factor mediates beta-catenin-induced axis formation in *Xenopus* embryos. *Cell* 1996; **86**: 391–9.

64. Morin PJ, Sparks AB, Korinek V et al, Activation of beta-catenin-Tcf signaling in colon cancer by mutations in beta-catenin or APC. *Science* 1997; **275**: 1787–90.

65. Kinzler KW, Vogelstein B, Lessons from hereditary colorectal cancer. *Cell* 1996; **87**: 159–70.

66. Waddell WR, Loughry RW, Sulindac for polyposis of the colon. *J Surg Oncol* 1983; **24**: 83–7.

67. Giardiello FM, Hamilton SR, Krush AJ et al, Treatment of colonic and rectal adenomas with sulindac in familial adenomatous polyposis. *N Engl J Med* **328**: 1313–16.

68. Eberhart CE, DuBois RN, Eicosanoids and the gastrointestinal tract. *Gastroenterology* 1995; **109**: 285–301.

69. Mecklin J-P, Frequency of hereditary nonpolyposis colorectal carcinoma. *Gastroenterology* 1987 **93**: 1021–5.

70. Fuchs CS, Giovannucci EL, Colditz GA et al, A prospective study of family history and the risk of colorectal cancer. *N Engl J Med* 1994; **331**: 1669–74.

71. Winawer SJ, Zauber AG, Gerdes H et al, Risk of colorectal cancer in the families of patients with adenomatous polys. *N Engl J Med* 1996; **334**: 82–7.

72. Lynch HT, Smyrk TC, Watson P et al, Genetics, natural history, tumor spectrum, and pathology of hereditary nonpolyposis colorectal cancer: an updated review. *Gastroenterology* 1993; **104**: 1535–49.

73. Vasen HFA, Mecklin J-P, Meera Khan P, Lynch HT, The international collaborative group on hereditary nonpolyposis colorectal cancer (ICG-HNPCC). *Dis Colon Rectum* 1991; **34**: 424–5.

74. Watson P, Lynch HT, Extracolonic cancer in hereditary nonpolyposis colon cancer. *Cancer* 1993; **71**: 677–85.

75. Mecklin J-P, Jarvinen H, Clinical features of colorectal carcinoma in cancer family syndrome. *Dis Colon Rectum* 1986; **29**: 160–4.

76. Rustgi AK, Hereditary gastrointestinal polyposis and nonpolyposis syndromes. *N Engl J Med* 1994; **331**: 1694–702.

77. Vasen HFA, Wijnen JT, Menko FH et al, Cancer risk in families with hereditary nonpolyposis colorectal cancer diagnosed by mutation analysis. *Gastroenterology* 1996; **110**: 1020–7.

78. Vasen HFA, Offerhaus GJA, den Hartog Jager FCA et al, The tumor spectrum in hereditary nonpolyposis colorectal cancer: a study of 24 kindreds in the Netherlands. *Int J Cancer* 1990; **46**: 31–4.

79. Cohen PR, Kohn SR, Kurzrock R, Association of sebaceous gland tumors and internal malignancy: the Muir–Torre syndrome. *Am J Med* 1991; **90**: 606–13.

80. Lynch P, Lynch HT, *Colon Cancer Genetics*. New York: Van Nostrand Reinhold, 1985; 313.

81. Lynch P, Lynch HT, Harris RE, Hereditary proximal colonic cancer. *Dis Colon Rectum* 1977; **20**: 661–8.

82. Love RR, Adenomas are precursor lesions for malignant growth in nonpolyposis hereditary carcinoma of the colon and rectum. *Surg Gyn Obstet* 1988; **102**: 8–12.

83. Jass J, Smyrk TC, Stewart SM et al, Pathology of hereditary nonpolyposis colorectal cancer.

Anticancer Res 1994; **14**: 1631–4.

84. Jass JR, Stewart SM, Stewart J et al, Hereditary nonpolyposis colorectal cancer – morphologies, and mutations. *Mutat Res* 1994; **310**: 125–33.

85. Peltomaki P, Sistonen P, Mecklin JP et al, Evidence supporting exclusion of the DCC gene and portion of chromosome 18q as the locus for susceptibility to hereditary nonpolyposis colorectal carcinoma in five kindreds. *Cancer Res* 1991; **51**: 4135–40.

86. Peltomaki P, Sistonen P, Mecklin JP et al, Evidence that the MCC–APC gene region in 5q21 is not the site for susceptibility to hereditary nonpolyposis colorectal carcinoma. *Cancer Res* 1992; **52**: 4530–3.

87. Peltomaki P, Aaltonen LA, Sistonen P et al, Genetic mapping of a locus predisposing to human colorectal cancer. *Science* 1993; **290**: 610–12.

88. Luce MC, Marra G, Chauman DP et al, In vitro transcription/translation assay for the screening of *hMLH1* and *hMSH2* mutations in familial colon cancer. *Gastroenterology* 1995; **109**: 1368–74.

89. Piepoli A, Santoro R, Cristofaro G et al, Linkage analysis identifies gene carriers among members of families with hereditary nonpolyposis colorectal cancer. *Gastroenterology* 1996; **110**: 1404–9.

90. Fishel R, Lescoe MK, Rao MRS et al, The human mutator gene homolog MSH2 and its association with hereditary nonpolyposis colon cancer. *Cell* 1993; **75**: 1027–38.

91. Leach FS, Nicolaides NC, Papadopoulos N et al, Mutations of a mutS homolog in hereditary nonpolyposis colon cancer. *Cell* 1993; **75**: 1215–25.

92. Strand M, Prolla TA, Liskay RM et al, Destabilization of tracts of simple repetitive DNA in yeast by mutations affecting DNA mismatch repair. *Nature* 1993; **365**: 274–6.

93. Lindblom A, Tannergard P, Werelius B, Nordenskjold M, Genetic mapping of a second locus predisposing to hereditary non-polyposis colon cancer. *Nature Genet* 1993; **5**: 279–82.

94. Bronner CE, Baker SM, Morrison PT et al, Mutation in the DNA mismatch repair gene homologue hMLH1 is associated with hereditary non-polyposis colon cancer. *Nature* 1994; **368**: 258–61.

95. Kolodner RD, Hall NR, Lipford J et al, Structure of the human MLH1 locus and analysis of a large hereditary colorectal carcinoma kindred

for m1h1 mutations. *Cancer Res* 1995; **55**: 242–8.

96. Papadopoulos N, Nicolaides NC, Wei Y-F et al, Mutation of a mutL homolog in hereditary colon cancer. *Science* 1994; **263**: 1625–8.

97. Nystrom-Lahti M, Sistonen P, Mecklin J-P et al, Close linkage to chromosome 3p and conservation of ancestral founding haplotype in hereditary nonpolyposis colorectal cancer families. *Proc Natl Acad Sci USA* 1994; **91**: 6054–8.

98. Moisio A-L, Sistonen P, Weissenbach J et al, Age and origin of two common MLH1 mutations predisposing to hereditary colon cancer. *Am J Hum Genet* 1996; **59**: 1243–51.

98a. Aaltonen LA, Sankila R, Mecklin JP et al, A novel approach to estimate the proportion of hereditary nonpolyposis colorectal cancer of total colorectal cancer burden. *Cancer Detect Prev* 1994; **18**: 57–63.

99. Nystrom-Lahti M, Parsons R, Sistonen P et al, Mismatch repair genes on chromosomes 2p and 3p account for a major share of hereditary nonpolyposis colorectal cancer families evaluable by linkage. *Am J Hum Genet* 1994; **55**: 659–65.

100. Nicolaides NC, Papadopoulos N, Liu B et al, Mutations of two PMS homologues in hereditary nonpolyposis colon cancer. *Nature* 1994; **371**: 75–80.

101. Aaltonen LA, Peltomaki P, Leach FS et al, Clues to the pathogenesis of familial colorectal cancer. *Science* 1993; **260**: 812–16.

102. Liu B, Parsons R, Papadopoulos N et al, Analysis of mismatch repair genes in hereditary nonpolyposis colorectal cancer patients. *Nature Med* 1996; **2**: 169–74.

103. Thibodeau SN, French AJ, Roche PC et al, Altered expression of hMSH2 and hMLH1 in tumors with microsatellite instability and genetic alterations in mismatch repair. *Cancer Res* 1996; **56**: 4836–40.

104. Samowitz W, Slattery ML, Kerber RA, Microsatellite instability in human colonic cancer is not a useful clinical indicator of familial colorectal cancer. *Gastroenterology* 1995; **109**: 1765–71.

105. de la Chapelle A, Peltomaki P, Genetics of hereditary colon cancer. *Ann Rev Genet* 1995; **29**: 329–48.

106. Kohonen-Corish M, Ross VL, Doe WF et al, RNA-based mutation screening in hereditary nonpolyposis colorectal cancer. *Am J Hum Genet* 1996; **59**: 818–24.

107. Liu B, Nicolaides NC, Markowitz S et al,

Mismatch repair gene defects in sporadic colo-rectal cancers with microsatellite instability. *Nature Genet* 1995; **9:** 48–55.

108 Horii A, Han H-J, Shimada M et al, Frequent replication errors at microsatellite loci in tumors of patients with multiple primary cancers. *Cancer Res* 1994; **54:** 3373–5.

109. Jass   JR, Cottier DS, Jeevaratnam P et al, Diagnostic use of microsatellite instability in hereditary non-polyposis colorectal cancer. *Lancet* 1995; **346:** 1200–1.

110. Kim H, Jen J, Vogelstein B, Hamilton SR, Clinical and pathologic characteristics of spo-radic colorectal carcinomas with DNA replica-tion errors in microsatellite sequences. *Am J Path* 1994; **145:** 148–56.

111. Jeon HM, Lynch PM, Howard L et al, Mutation of the hMSH2 gene in two families with heredi-tary nonpolyposis colorectal cancer. *Hum Mutat* 1966; **7:** 327–33.

112. Leach FS, Polyak K, Burrell M et al, Expression of the human mismatch repair gene hMSH2 in normal and neoplastic tissues. *Cancer Res* 1996; **56:** 235–40.

113. Koi M, Umar A, Chauhan DP et al, Human chromosome 3 corrects mismatch repair deficiency and microsatellite instability and reduces N-methyl-N'-nitro-N-nitrosoguanidine tolerance in colon tumor cells with homozygous *hMLH1* mutation. *Cancer Res* 1994; **54:** 4308–12.

114. Grady W, Rajput A, Myeroff L et al, What's new with RII? *Gastroenterology* 1997; **112:** 297.

115. Wang CY, Eshleman JR, Willson JKV, Markowitz S, TGF-beta and substrate release are both inducers of apoptosis in a human colon adenoma cell line. *Cancer Res* 1995; **55:** 5101–5.

116. Markowitz S, Wang J, Myeroff L et al, Inactivation of the type II TGF-beta receptor in colon cancer cells with microsatellite instability. *Science* 1995; **268:** 1336–8.

117. Parsons R, Myeroff L, Liu B et al, Microsatellite instability and mutations of the transforming growth factor beta type II receptor gene in colo-rectal cancer. *Cancer Res* 1995; **55:** 5548–50.

118. AkiyamaY, Iwanaga R, Saitoh K et al, Transforming growth factor B Type II receptor gene mutations in adenomas from hereditary nonpolyposis colorectal cancer. *Gastroenterology* 1997; **112:** 33.

119. Kern SE, Fearon ER, Tersmette KW et al, Allelic loss in colorectal cancer. *J Am Med Assoc* 1989; **261:** 3099–103.

120. Jen J, Kim H, Piantadosi S et al, Allelic loss of chromosome 18q and prognosis in colorectal cancer. *N Engl J Med* 1994; **331:** 213–21.

121. Grewel H, Guillem JG, Klimstra DS et al, p53 nuclear overexpression may not be an indepen-dent prognostic marker in early colorectal can-cer. *Dis Colon Rectum* 1995; **38:** 1176–81.

122. Cohn KH, Ornstein DL, Wang F et al, The sig-nificance of allelic deletions and aneuploidy in colorectal carcinoma. *Cancer* 1997; **79:** 233–44.

123. Church J, Data presented at 1995 Leeds Castle Polyposis Group Meeting, Toronto, 1995.

124. Miyoshi Y, Nagase H, Ando H et al, Somatic mutations of the APC gene in colorectal tumors: mutation cluster region in the APC gene. *Hum Mol Genet* 1992; **1:** 229–33.

125. Nugent FW, Haggit RC, Gilpin PA et al, Cancer surveillance in ulcerative colitis. *Gastroenterology* 1991; **100:** 1241–8.

2

Some recent developments in the epidemiology of colorectal cancer

Peter Boyle

CONTENTS • **Introduction** • **Descriptive epidemiology of cancer of the colon and rectum** • **Temporal trends in colorectal cancer mortality (ICD9 153 and 154)** • **Analytical epidemiology** • **Physical activity, body mass index and energy intake** • **Dietary and nutritional practices** • **Hormone replacement therapy** • **Non-steroidal anti-inflammatory drugs** • **Summary and conclusions**

INTRODUCTION

Colorectal cancer is the fourth commonest form of cancer that occurs worldwide with an estimated 678 000 new cases diagnosed in 1985.[1] It affects men and women almost equally, with approximately one-third of a million new cases diagnosed in each gender group each year. The disease is most frequent in occidental countries, and particularly so in North America, Australia, New Zealand and parts of Europe. The diseases of colon and rectal cancer appear to be distinct, but unfortunately there are recognized difficulties in distinguishing between them in mortality statistics for a variety of reasons.[2] Wherever possible, the distinction between colon and rectum will be preserved.

Colon cancer is a disease of economically 'developed' countries. Before 60 years of age, the disease is slightly more common in women, whereas it is more frequent in men thereafter.[3] In men, nine of the ten highest incidence rates of colon cancer are recorded in population groups in the USA with the tenth highest in neighbouring Canada (Table 2.1). It is of potentially considerable significance that these high rates are to be found in a variety of population groups, including Japanese in Hawaii (37.2 per 100 000) and Los Angeles (33.1), Whites in Connecticut (35.9) and Iowa (32.6), and Blacks in Alameda County (35.7) and Los Angeles (33.6). In men, the lowest incidence rates are found in a variety of population groups in the developing countries, with the lowest rate reported in The Gambia (0.67 per 100 000). In women, the group of highest incidence rates includes population groups in North America, with the lowest rates recorded in a similar group of populations as in men (Table 2.1). In each sex, a number of low-rate regions are found in India.

Ethnic and racial differences in colon cancer as well as studies on migrants suggest that environmental factors play a major role in the aetiology of the disease. In Israel, male Jews born in Europe or America are at higher risk for colon cancer than those born in Africa or Asia, and a change in risk in the offspring of Japanese having migrated to the USA heralded by Haenszel and Kurihara[4] has now taken place, the incidence rates approaching or surpassing those in whites in the same population, and being three or four times higher than among Japanese in Japan.

In a long-term perspective, incidence rates of

Table 2.1 Ten highest and ten lowest average, annual, all ages, age-standardized, incidence rates for colon cancer in men and women worldwide around the mid-1980s (data are abstracted from reference 1)

Colon, male ICD9 153 Registry	Cases	Rate per 100 000	Colon, female ICD9 153 Registry	Cases	Rate per 100 000
US, Hawaii: Japanese	414	37.2	Bermuda: Black	31	34.4
US, Connecticut: White	3 749	35.9	Canada, Newfoundland	499	30.7
US, Alameda: Black	187	35.8	New Zealand: Non-Maori	3 398	30.5
US, NY State (less City)	11 860	33.7	US, New Orleans: Black	330	30.3
US, Los Angeles: Black	708	33.6	US, Bay Area: Black	388	29.6
US, Detroit: Black	756	33.5	US, Alameda: Black	206	29.5
US, Los Angeles: Japanese	110	33.1	US, Los Angeles: Japanese	120	28.9
US, New York City	7 958	32.9	US, Los Angeles: Black	857	28.8
US, Iowa	3 419	32.6	US, Iowa	4 343	28.3
Canada, Newfoundland	473	32.5	US, Detroit: Black	802	26.6
Peru, Trujillo	17	3.6	Poland, Nowy Sacz	43	3.7
India, Bombay	428	3.2	Kuwait: Kuwaitis	22	3.4
Mali, Bamako	12	2.9	India, Bombay	284	2.6
India, Bangalore	123	2.3	China, Qidong	70	2.2
China, Qidong	52	2.0	Mali, Bamako	8	1.8
Kuwait, Kuwaitis	13	1.9	India, Bangalore	81	1.8
India, Ahmedabad	91	1.8	India, Madras	79	1.5
India, Madras	94	1.5	India, Ahmedabad	42	1.0
Algeria, Setif	12	1.0	Algeria, Setif	10	0.9
The Gambia	3	0.7	The Gambia	0	–

colon cancer are rising slowly, in particular in areas formerly at low risk, left-sided tumours having shown larger increases.[5] In Australia, between 1973 and 1993, colorectal cancer occurred most frequently in the sigmoid colon and the rectum. In the right colon, cancer occurred most commonly in the caecum. From 1973 to 1993, incidence rates increased in the right colon (by 2.8% per annum in men and 2.0% per annum in women) and in the left colon (1.6% in men and 0.7% in women). Incidence rates also increased from cancer of the rectum, by 2.0% per annum in men and by 0.7% per annum in women.[6] More complex patterns are seen in high-risk countries.

While mortality rates are increasing in US Blacks for both sexes, in Whites the increase is confined to older men and rates are decreasing in women. In the USA, incidence is rising slowly in women. Increasing rates are observed in the Nordic countries, while in England and Wales mortality rates are declining in both sexes.

DESCRIPTIVE EPIDEMIOLOGY OF CANCER OF THE COLON AND RECTUM

Although somewhat less frequent than colon cancer, rectal cancer shows many features of colon cancer in geographic distribution. In contrast to colon cancer, rectal cancer is more common in men, with a sex ratio of 1.5–2.0. Little difference exists in the incidence rates between western countries of North America, Europe and Australia, with rates in the range of 15–20 for men and 8–12 for women. In contrast, the mortality rates in the USA are among the lowest in developed countries, with large declines in mortality rates in Blacks and Whites for both sexes and very little change in incidence. This is believed to be artefactual, since half the patients diagnosed with rectal cancer have their deaths certified to colon cancer.[7,8] Elsewhere, time trends are not consistent with rising rates in Japan and declining rates in Denmark and England and Wales.

The highest incidence rate of rectal cancer in men is found in Bohemia and Moravia in the Czech Republic (22.9 per 100 000). There is little geographic pattern to the highest-rate regions, which contain a diversity of populations in the USA, Hungary, Italy, France, Australia, Canada and Israel (Table 2.2). An unexpected feature of these data is the high incidence rates found in Japanese men in Los Angeles (21.4) and Hawaii (20.3). In women, the highest rates are lower than those in men, and there is a variety of population groups among the highest incidence rates. In each sex, there is a variety of population groups from the developing world among the regions with the lowest rates (Table 2.2).

Unlike colon cancer, mortality from rectal cancer did not rise much in Japanese migrants to the USA.[4] Polish migrants have shown an increased risk for both sites.[9]

TEMPORAL TRENDS IN COLORECTAL CANCER MORTALITY (ICD9 153 AND 154)

The major problem in comparison of death rates from colon and rectal cancer separately between populations is the problem of attribu-tion of 'vaguely' defined cancer on the death certificate. The root of the problem was the habit of any death ascribed by the certifying physician as 'cancer of the large intestine' being given the three-digit code for colon: this of course could have been a rectal cancer. For this and several other reasons, it is preferable to investigate mortality from colon and rectal cancer together as a single entity. However, there is a recognized loss of information that could be available if mortality data were of a higher quality.

In Canada, the truncated and overall age-adjusted mortality rates remained relatively stable in men until earlier 1970s, and have been decreasing ever since. In women, both the truncated and overall age-adjusted mortality rates have been decreasing since 1955. Birth cohort examination shows that the rates have been stable or decreasing in successive birth cohorts in men and women for age groups examined, although the decrease in rates was more pronounced in women. Canada is one of the few countries outside the Nordic countries where national incidence and mortality data are available.[10] Colorectal cancer incidence and mortality rates are higher by about 50% in men compared with women. In each gender group, the incidence and mortality rates increased to a peak in the mid-1980s, and the all-ages rates have subsequently declined (Figure 2.1).

In Japan, both the truncated and overall age-adjusted mortality rates have been increasing in both men and women since 1955. Examination of rate by birth cohorts suggests a consistent increase in rates in successive birth cohorts born before 1940 in both sexes. For cohorts born after, the rates seem to have levelled off, and may have even declined in either sex.[11]

In Czechoslovakia, both the truncated and overall age-adjusted mortality rates have been increasing in both men and women since 1955. Birth-cohort examination indicates an increase in rates in successive birth cohorts in both sexes, although the rates in younger age groups seem to be levelling off.

In Poland, both the truncated and overall age-adjusted mortality rates have been increasing since 1959 in both men and women.

Table 2.2 Ten highest and ten lowest average, annual, all ages, age-standardized, incidence rates for rectal cancer in men and women worldwide around the mid-1980s (data are abstracted from reference 1)

Rectum, male ICD9 154 Registry	Cases	Rate per 100 000	Rectum, female ICD9 154 Registry	Cases	Rate per 100 000
Czech: Bohemia and Moravia	7 496	22.9	Israel: Born Europe or America	1 114	16.1
US, Los Angeles: Japanese	70	21.4	Israel: All Jews	1 519	13.6
Hungary, Vas	205	20.5	New Zealand: Non-Maori	1 374	12.3
New Zealand: Non-Maori	1 815	20.4	Hungary, Vas	161	12.0
US, Hawaii: Japanese	216	20.3	US, Hawaii: Chinese	30	11.8
Italy, Trieste	111	20.1	Canada, British Columbia	1 339	11.7
France, Bas Rhin	558	20.0	Canada, Quebec	2 776	11.7
Australian Capital Territory	88	19.9	Czech: Bohemia and Moravia	5 546	11.7
Canada, Quebec	3 501	19.4	Canada, New Brunswick	236	11.7
Israel: Born Europe or America	1 259	19.0	US, Alameda: White	383	11.4
India, Bangalore	161	3.0	India, Bangalore	125	2.7
Thailand, Khon Kaen	27	2.8	India, Bombay	273	2.5
Mali, Bamako	12	2.6	Bermuda: White and Other	5	2.5
Paraguay, Asuncion	27	2.5	India, Ahmedabad	104	2.5
Peru, Trujillo	12	2.5	India, Madras	112	1.9
India, Madras	140	2.4	Thailand, Khon Kaen	16	1.5
Kuwait: Kuwaitis	17	2.4	Algeria, Setif	17	1.3
Kuwait: Non-Kuwaitis	28	1.3	Mali, Bamako	6	1.2
Algeria, Setif	11	1.0	Kuwait: Kuwaitis	10	1.1
The Gambia	5	0.7	The Gambia	3	0.6

Examination by birth cohorts suggests an increase in rates in successive birth cohorts for almost all age groups examined, and in both sexes.

In Germany, both the truncated and overall age-adjusted mortality rates increased between 1955 and 1979. Thereafter, the rates in women have been decreasing – more so in the truncated rates. In men, after a brief and slight decrease between 1980 and 1983, the rates seem to increase again in the last few years. Birth-cohort examination shows an increase in rates for earlier birth cohort and a decrease in recent birth cohorts at all age groups examined, and in both men and women.

In the UK, the overall age-adjusted mortality rates experienced a slight decrease in men since 1955, although the truncated rates remain relatively unchanged. In women, both the truncated and overall age-adjusted mortality rates have been decreasing during the entire study period. Birth-cohort examination shows similar

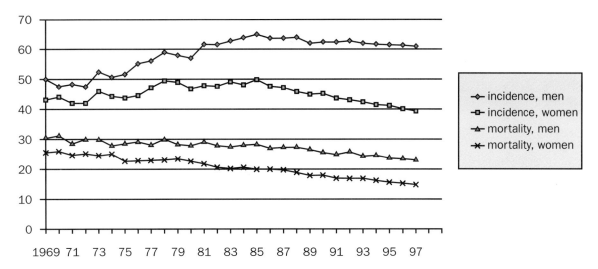

Figure 2.1 Colorectal cancer incidence and mortality rates (per 100 000) in men and women in Canada.

rates in successive birth cohorts born before 1930 and a slight decrease born after. In women, the rates have been decreasing in successive birth cohorts for all the age groups examined.

In Denmark, there is no clear overall time trend for either truncated or overall age-adjusted mortality rates in men since 1955. In women, however, a slight decrease was observed for both truncated and overall age-adjusted mortality rates during the entire study period. Birth-cohort examination suggests that the rates are similar in men and decreasing in women in successive birth cohorts.

In Australia, both the truncated and overall age-adjusted mortality rates have been increasing in men since 1955, although the increase in the overall age-adjusted mortality rates seems to have slowed down over the last few years. In women, a slight decrease was observed for both truncated and overall age-adjusted mortality rates since the early 1970s. Birth-cohort examination shows an increase in rates in successive birth cohorts born before 1935 in men and a decrease in rates born after. In women, the rates

are similar or have been decreasing in successive birth cohorts for most of the age groups examined, except for the age groups between 40 and 49, where a slight increase in rates in successive birth cohorts was observed. There have been interesting data published recently regarding a comprehensive analysis of the descriptive epidemiology of colorectal cancer in New South Wales.[6]

Colorectal cancer was the second most common cancer reported in men and women in New South Wales in 1993.[6] The age-standardized incidence rates in men and women in 1993 were 46.1 and 31.0 per 100 000 respectively: this is considerably lower than the incidence rates in Canada (Figure 2.1). From 1973 to 1993, the incidence rates rose by an average of 1.9% per annum in men and 0.9% in women, while mortality was steady in men and fell by 0.9% in women. These increases in incidence in men occurred over the age of 45 and in women between the ages of 45 and 74. The overall mortality rate in men remained stable despite a fall in rates in younger men. In women, the fall in mortality of 0.9% per annum

Table 2.3 Ten highest and ten lowest average, annual, all ages, age-standardized, incidence rates for colon and rectum cancer in men and women worldwide around the mid-1980s (data are abstracted from reference 1)

Colorectum, male ICD9 153–154 Registry	Cases	Rate per 100 000	Colorectum, female ICD9 153–154 Registry	Cases	Rate per 100 000
US, Hawaii: Japanese	630	57.4	New Zealand: Non-Maori	4 772	42.8
US, Los Angeles: Japanese	180	54.5	Bermuda: Black	38	42.0
US, Connecticut: White	5 473	53.1	Canada, Newfoundland	642	39.9
Italy, Trieste	286	51.5	US, Los Angeles: Japanese	166	39.5
New Zealand: Non-Maori	4 602	51.3	US, Alameda: Black	274	39.3
US, NY State (less City)	17 596	50.5	US, Bay Area: Black	511	39.1
US, Detroit: White	4 596	48.8	US, New Orleans: Black	417	38.1
US, New York City	11 433	48.0	US, Los Angeles: Black	1 110	37.5
US, Iowa	4 951	47.9	US, Iowa	5 626	37.3
US, Bay Area: White	4 089	47.9	US, Detroit: Black	1 086	36.5
Kuwait: Non-Kuwaitis	86	7.3	Israel: Non-Jews	65	7.5
India, Ahmedabad	297	6.4	Thailand, Khon Kaen	57	5.7
India, Bombay	843	6.4	India, Bombay	557	5.1
Peru, Trujillo	29	6.0	Kuwait: Kuwaitis	32	4.5
Mali, Bamako	24	5.4	India, Bangalore	206	4.5
India, Bangalore	284	5.3	India, Ahmedabad	146	3.5
Kuwait: Kuwaitis	30	4.3	India, Madras	191	3.4
India, Madras	234	3.9	Mali, Bamako	14	3.0
Algeria, Setif	23	2.0	Algeria, Setif	27	2.3
The Gambia	8	1.3	The Gambia	3	0.7

could be attributed to falls in the very youngest and oldest age groups.[6]

In Italy, the mortality rate of colorectal cancer in both men and women have been increasing steadily since 1955. Since 1980, there has been a levelling-off in rates in women, particularly in the truncated age range.

For comparison purposes, incidence data from colon and rectal cancer have been combined (Table 2.3): this serves to help realize more clearly the impact of colorectal cancer on communities worldwide. For colorectal cancer, the highest incidence rates in men are reported from Japanese communities in Los Angeles (54.5 per 100 000) and Hawaii (57.4), and the highest rates are dominated by populations in North America. The lowest rates are found in various developing countries, with the range between the lowest rate (1.3 in The Gambia) and the highest (57.4 in Hawaiian Japanese) being considerable. Similar patterns and differences exist in women (Table 2.3).

ANALYTICAL EPIDEMIOLOGY

As already mentioned, colorectal cancer is the fourth commonest form of cancer that occurs worldwide (an estimated 678 000 new cases diagnosed in 1985).[1] High incidence rates are found in Western Europe and North America, and intermediate rates in Eastern Europe, with the lowest rates to be found in sub-Saharan Africa.[3] Most colorectal cancers, between 67% and 90%, arise from benign, adenomatous polyps lining the wall of the bowel, with those that grow to a large size and have a villous appearance or contain dysplastic cells being most likely to progress to cancer.[12] The development of colorectal cancer is a multistep process, involving genetic mutations in mucosal cells, the activation of tumour-promoting genes and the loss of genes that suppress tumour formation.[13] The natural history and the role of several risk factors in the aetiology of colorectal cancer are becoming more clearly understood,[14,15] and the genetic events involved in colorectal cancer susceptibility are being uncovered with increasing frequency:[16,17] the recent rate of progress in our understanding of the genetics of colorectal cancer is impressive.[18,19] Few specific risk factors of a non-dietary origin have been established for colorectal cancer; inflammatory bowel diseases and familial polyposis syndromes produce a high risk of colorectal cancer in affected individuals, but account for only a small proportion of the overall incidence of colorectal cancer.[20,21]

PHYSICAL ACTIVITY, BODY MASS INDEX AND ENERGY INTAKE

Evidence from epidemiological studies appears strong that men with high occupational or recreational physical activity appear to be at a lower risk of colon cancer.[22] Such evidence comes from follow-up studies of cohorts who are physically active or who have physically demanding jobs, as well as case-control studies that have assessed physical activity, by, for example, measurement of resting heart rate, or by questionnaire. The association remains, even after control for potential confounding factors such as diet and body mass index. The risk of colorectal cancer and self-reported occupational and recreational physical activity was investigated recently in a population-based cohort in Norway.[23] Physical activity at a level equivalent to brisk walking four hours per week was associated with a decreased risk of colon cancer among women when compared with the (referent) sedentary group (RR = 0.62, 95% CI (0.40, 0.97)): this was particularly marked in the proximal colon (RR = 0.51, 95% CI (0.28, 0.93)). The trend in reducing risk with increased physical activity was similar in women and in men aged over 45.[23]

It has been a fairly consistent finding in studies that have examined the issue that energy intake is higher in cases of colorectal cancer than in the comparison group: the mechanism is, however, complex.[24] Physically active individuals are likely to consume more energy, but recent studies suggest that physical activity reduces colorectal cancer risk.[25–27] There has been some recent attention given to the study of such factors in the development of adenomas, the benign lesions from which the majority of colorectal cancers develop. A case-control study was conducted among patients seen at three colonoscopy practices in New York City: all patients had a history of adenomas.[28] Men in the upper quarters of body mass index (BMI) were found to have an increased risk of recurrent adenomas: the odds ratios were found to be 2.2, 1.9 and 1.9 respectively in the second, third and fourth quarters of BMI compared with the lowest quarter. However, no effect was found in women. This either detracts from the findings given the lack of internal consistency or indicates that there is a true biological interaction: in any event, this issue deserves further study.

A case-control study of new adenoma cases and adenoma-free controls demonstrated that physical activity in leisure protected women against colorectal adenomas. There was no evidence of a protective effect of work activity among either women or men, although men who participated in no sport were at an increased risk for adenomas (OR = 1.68, 95% CI (0.93, 3.20)).[29]

Giovannucci et al[30] took the opportunity to examine the role of physical activity, body mass index and the pattern of adipose distribution with the risk of colorectal adenomas. Within the Nurses' Health study, 13 057 female nurses, aged 40–65 years in 1986, had an endoscopy between 1986 and 1992. During this period, 439 were newly diagnosed with adenomas of the distal colorectum. After controlling for age, prior endoscopy, parental history of colorectal cancer, smoking, aspirin use and dietary intakes, physical activity was associated inversely with the risk of large adenomas (greater or equal to 1 cm) in the distal colon (RR = 0.57, 95% CI (0.30, 1.08)), comparing high and low quintiles of average weekly energy expenditure from leisure activities. Much of this benefit came from activities of moderate intensity such as brisk walking.

Additionally, body mass index was associated directly with risk of large adenomas in the distal colon (RR = 2.21, 95% CI (1.18, 4.16)), for BMI 29 kg/m^2 or over compared with BMI values less than 21 kg/m^2. The relationships between BMI or physical activity were considerably weaker for rectal adenomas.[30] This study indicates a similar association between physical activity and occurrence of adenomas in many respects similar to that for colorectal cancer. Exercise appears to protect against adenomas and colorectal cancer, as does increasing body mass index serve to increase the risk of both.

The reason for such an inverse association has not been identified, but has been postulated as being due to the effect of exercise on bowel transit time,[31] the immune system,[32] or serum cholesterol and bile acid metabolism.[33] The same consistent results have not been reported until recently on studies in women, but one possible explanation is that the lower variation in, for example, occupational activity among women may make such an association more difficult to detect.

The available data, however, show no consistent association between obesity and colorectal cancer risk (although analysis and interpretation of this factor is difficult in retrospective studies, where weight loss may be a sign of the disease), although there is now evidence that there may be an association with adenomas. This positive effect of energy does not appear to be merely the result of overeating, therefore, and may reflect differences in metabolic efficiency. (If the possibility that the association with energy intake is a methodological artefact is excluded, since it seems unlikely that such a consistent finding would emerge from such a variety of study designs in a diversity of population groups, it would imply that individuals who utilize energy more efficiently may be at a lower risk of colorectal cancer.)

DIETARY AND NUTRITIONAL PRACTICES

There appears to be consistent evidence from epidemiological studies that intake of dietary fat and meat is positively related to colorectal cancer risk: this evidence is obtained from ecological studies, animal experiments, case-control and cohort studies. Many of these studies have failed to demonstrate that the association observed with fat intake is independent of energy intake. Willett et al[34] published the results obtained from the United States Nurses Health study (a prospective design) involving follow-up of 88 751 women aged 34–59 who were without cancer or inflammatory bowel diseases at recruitment. After adjustment for total energy intake, consumption of animal fat was found to be associated with increased colon cancer risk. The trend in risk was highly significant ($p = 0.01$), with the relative risk in the highest compared with the lowest quintile of intake being 1.89 (95% CI (1.13, 3.15)). No association was found with vegetable fat. The relative risk of colon cancer in women who ate beef, pork or lamb as a main dish every day was 2.49 (95% CI (1.24, 5.03)) as compared with those women reporting consumption less than once per month. The authors interpreted their data as providing evidence for the hypothesis that a high intake of animal fat increases the risk of colon cancer, and they support existing recommendations to substitute fish and chicken for meats high in fat.[34]

This study provides the best epidemiological evidence to date identifying increased meat consumption as a risk factor for colon cancer independently of its contribution to fat intake and total caloric intake. Laboratory evidence is available that strongly suggests that cooked meats may be carcinogenic, particularly with regard to aminoimidazoazarenes (AIAs) that are produced when meats are cooked.[35,36] As well as being highly mutagenic in bacterial assays, there is now evidence that AIAs are mammalian carcinogens: feeding experiments in mice have produced tumours in various anatomic sites.[37] However, the situation is not entirely straightforward: for example, it has been shown that anticarcinogenic compounds are produced in fried ground beef.[38] Thus in the same food the potential exists to have mixtures of potentially carcinogenic and anticarcinogenic substances.

Whittemore et al[27] performed a case-control study of Chinese in North America and China, thus ingeniously utilizing the large difference in risk of colorectal cancer that exists between the two continents. Colorectal cancer risk in both continents was increased with increasing intake of total intake of energy, and specifically by saturated fat: however, no relationship was found with other sources of energy in the diet. Colon cancer risk was elevated among men employed in sedentary occupations, and, in both continents and in each sex, the risks for cancer of the colon and rectum increased with increased time spent sitting: the association between colorectal cancer risk and saturated fat was stronger among the sedentary than the active. Risk among sedentary Chinese Americans of either sex increased more than fourfold from the lowest to the highest category of saturated-fat intake. Among migrants to North America, risk increased with increasing time spent in North America. Attributable risk calculations suggest that, if these associations are causal, saturated-fat intakes exceeding 10 g/day, particularly in combination with physical inactivity, could account for 60% of colorectal cancer incidence among Chinese-American men and 40% among Chinese-American women.[27]

The specific fatty acids in the diet may also be important: animal experiments suggest that linoleic acid (an N-6 polyunsaturated fatty acid) promotes colorectal carcinogenesis[39,40] and that a low-fat diet rich in eicopentaenoic acid (an N-3 polyunsaturated fatty acid) has an inhibitory effect on colon cancer.[41] However, there have been no epidemiological studies conducted to date regarding N-3 and N-6 fatty acids and colorectal cancer risk.

The original hypothesis of the protective effect of dietary fibre was based on a clinical/pathological observation and a hypothesized mechanism whereby increasing intake of dietary fibre increases faecal bulk and reduces transit time: more recent thinking suggests that this mechanism may not be as relevant to colorectal carcinogenesis as previously thought.[42] The term 'fibre' encompasses many components, each of which has specific physiological functions. The commonest classification is into the insoluble, non-degradable constituents (mainly present in cereal fibre) and into soluble, degradable constituents like pectin and plant gums, which are mainly present in fruits and vegetables. Epidemiological studies have reported differences in the effect of these components. For example, Tuyns et al[43] and Kune et al[44] found a protective effect for total dietary fibre intake in case-control studies, and the same was found in one prospective study.[45] However a large number of studies could find no such protective effect (for a review see reference 24). The large majority of studies in humans have found no protective effect of fibre from cereals, but have consistently found a protective effect of fibre from vegetable and, perhaps, fruit sources,[24,46] and dietary diversity has been shown to be an important element in this protection.[47] This could conceivably reflect an association with other components of fruits and vegetables, with 'fibre' intake acting merely as an indicator of consumption.

A potential pathway for this association was recently investigated in a novel epidemiological study design.[48] Cruciferous vegetable intake exhibited a significant inverse association with colorectal cancer risk (OR = 0.59, 95% CI (0.34, 1.02)). When tumours were characterized by p53 overexpression (*p53 positive*), aetiological heterogeneity was suggested for family history of colorectal cancer (OR = 0.39, 95% CI (0.16, 0.93)), intake of cruciferous vegetables (test for trend, $p = 0.12$) and beef consumption (test for trend, $p = 0.08$). Cruciferous-vegetable consumption exhibited a significant association when p53-positive cases were compared with controls (OR = 0.37, 95% CI (0.17, 0.82)). When p53-negative cases were compared with controls, a significant increase in risk was observed for family history of cancer (OR = 4.46, 95% CI (2.36, 8.43)) and beef consumption (OR = 3.17, 95% CI (1.83, 11.28)). The authors concluded that the p53 (positive)-dependent pathway was characterized by an inverse association with cruciferous-vegetable intake, and p53-independent tumours were characterized by family history and beef consumption.[48]

Although calcium has been proposed as potentially having a modifying role in colorectal carcinogenesis,[49] little supporting evidence is forthcoming from epidemiological studies.[50] These studies in humans are of limited value because of questionable study design or the inadequacy of the estimation of diet. A number of studies have reported positive associations with alcohol consumption,[51] but it remains to be proven whether the putative association is with alcohol per se and not with the calorie contribution of alcohol or due to influences in the components of diet in alcohol drinkers. There is some experimental evidence that vitamin E and selenium may be protective against colon tumours,[39] and there is support for the hypothesis that beta-carotene is also protective.[24] Lactobacilli, found in some dairy products, may have a favourable effect on the intestine.[52] Twelve case-control studies of sufficient quality have addressed the issue of coffee consumption and the risk of colorectal cancer, and 11 of these have indicated inverse (protective) associations.[53] No association has been found with tea drinking or caffeine intake from all sources considered.

HORMONE REPLACEMENT THERAPY

There is increasing evidence supporting (an originally unexpected) association between hormone replacement therapy (HRT) use and a reduced risk of colorectal cancer. A Medline search was used to identify observational studies published between January 1974 and December 1993 for a meta-analysis.[54] The overall risk for colorectal cancer and oestrogen replacement therapy was 0.92 (95% CI (0.74, 1.5)). There was no separate effect when colon and rectal cancer were considered as separate entities.[54] Subsequent to this report, further studies have been published.

A case-control study from Seattle, USA among 193 women aged 30–62 with colon cancer and an equal number of controls was conducted to examine the relationship between colon cancer and female hormone use.[55] Use of non-contraceptive hormones after age 40 was associated with a reduced risk of colon cancer (OR = 0.60, 95% CI (0.35, 101)). The risk among women with five or more years of use was 0.47 (0.24, 0.91).[55]

Colorectal cancer mortality was examined in some detail in the American Cancer Society Prospective Study. With the risk set to 1.0 among women who reported to be never users of HRT (the referent group), the risk associated with ever use was 0.69 (95% CI (0.60, 0.79)).[56] Relative to the risk in never users, the risk associated with less than 1 year of use was 0.81 (0.63, 1.03), with between 2 and 5 years of use it was 0.76 (0.61, 0.95), for between 6 and 10 years of use it was 0.55 (0.39, 0.77), and for 11 or more years of use it was 0.54 (0.39, 0.76).

Of 19 published studies of HRT and colorectal cancer risk, 10 support an inverse association, and the remaining five show a significant reduction in risk. The risk seems lowest among long-term users. Although there are still some contradictions in the available literature, it appears likely that use of HRT reduces the risk of colorectal cancer in women. The risk appears to halve with 5–10 years of such use. The role of unopposed as compared with combination HRT is an open issue for colorectal cancer.

NON-STEROIDAL ANTI-INFLAMMATORY DRUGS

Non-steroidal anti-inflammatory drugs (NSAIDs) have recently been implicated as potential protective agents against colorectal cancer and adenomatous polyps. Initial anecdotal reports noting regression of adenomas in patients with familial adenomatous polyps have been followed by substantial epidemiological studies. There is a general level of agreement in the finding of a protective effect from such studies. There are randomized trials of familial adenomatous polyps demonstrating the regression of adenomas by NSAIDs. For example, there was complete regression of rectal polyps in 6 or 9 patients taking sulindac and partial regression in three others: in the placebo group, polyps increased in 5, remained unchanged in 2 and decreased in the remaining 2.[57] In laboratory rodents, piroxicam, sulindac and aspirin have all been shown to reduce the frequency of development of colorectal neoplasia.[58] The mechanism of any effect remains obscure, as does the dose required, and it is disappointing that the randomized intervention trial of low-dose aspirin in US physicians was null, although this may represent a situation where the dose given was too low or the period of use too short to achieve the protective effect.[59] However, there is a very good case for a controlled trial of NSAIDs, probably using aspirin, in the prevention of colorectal cancer.[60]

SUMMARY AND CONCLUSIONS

Colorectal cancer is the fourth commonest form of cancer worldwide, with an estimated 678 000 new cases diagnosed in 1985.[1] High incidence rates are found in Western Europe, North America and Australasia, and intermediate rates in Eastern Europe, with the lowest rates found in sub-Saharan Africa.[3] The disease is not uniformly fatal, although there are large differences in survival according to stage of disease. In advanced colorectal cancer in which curative resection is possible, five-year survival in Dukes B is 45%, which drops to 30% in Dukes C.[61] Five-year survival in resected Dukes A is around 80%, and survival following simple resection of an adenomatous pedunculated polyp containing carcinoma in situ (or severe dysplasia) or intramucosal carcinoma is generally close to 100%. It is estimated that there are, however, still 394 000 deaths from colorectal cancer worldwide annually.[62]

The large differences in survival between early- and late-stage disease clearly indicate the advantage of detecting colorectal cancer at an early age. The simplest advice is to ensure that any change in bowel habits or unexpected presence of blood in the stool should be investigated. Faecal occult blood testing (FOBT) is aimed at the detection of early asymptomatic cancer, and is based on the assumption that such cancers will bleed and that small quantities of blood lost in the stool may be detected chemically, or immunologically. A significant reduction in colorectal cancer mortality with annual testing using haemocult has been reported.[63] The cumulative annual mortality rate in the group screened annually was 5.88 per 1000, compared with 8.83 in the control group and 8.33 in the group screened biennially. The results are of considerable importance, but it is difficult to ignore the observation that 38% of those screened annually and 28% of those screened biennially underwent at least one colonoscopy during the study period, although it is somewhat reassuring that the incidence of colorectal cancer was so similar in the three groups (23, 23 and 26 per 1000 for those screened annually, those screened biennially and those in the control group respectively). The authors considered that the likely effect of colonoscopy, in removing polyps, had not yet affected the incidence and mortality from colorectal cancer.

Faecal occult blood (FOB) testing has been reported from case-control studies to reduce colorectal cancer mortality rates by 31%,[64] and 57% in women.[65] In a non-randomized study, it was shown that annual rigid sigmoidoscopy and FOB testing, rather than sigmoidoscopy alone, was associated with a reduction in colorectal cancer mortality.[66] There have now been three randomized trials of FOB testing, each demonstrating a reduction in colorectal cancer mortality. Mandel et al[63] reported a reduction of 33% in colorectal cancer mortality after 13 years in subjects who were offered annual screening with FOB tests, but a non-significant reduction (of 6%) in those who were offered biennial screening. In two more-recent studies, from Nottingham, UK[66] and Denmark,[67] the colorectal cancer mortality rates in the group offered biennial FOB testing were respectively 0.85 and 0.82 times the rate in the control population. An (approximate) combined analysis of these latter studies produces a relative risk of colorectal cancer death of 0.84 (95% CI, 0.75–0.94).[68]

These findings are important confirmation that haemocult screening may be effective in the prevention of death from colorectal cancer. There are both advantages and disadvantages to FOBT. On the one hand, it is of low cost, although the investigation of false positives (around 1–3% per test) certainly increases the cost, and it 'examines' the entire colon and rectum. However, FOBT is currently characterized by a low sensitivity (with around 40% of cancers and 80% of adenomas missed by the test[69,70]), and the fact that it detects colorectal cancers at the later stages in the natural history at which lesions bleed implies a short lead time and the requirement for frequent testing. Rehydration of slides results in increased positivity, but also an increased number of colonoscopies and a decreased specificity of the test. The costs must be weighed against the benefits before public health policy on this topic is formulated.[63]

Until a randomized controlled trial is undertaken and reported, the efficacy of flexible sigmoidoscopy as a screening test for preventing death from colorectal cancer will remain unproved. However, there is now a good deal of evidence supporting infrequent sigmoidoscopy as a potentially effective screening modality for colorectal cancer. Impressive reductions in rectal cancer and cancer of the proximal colon have been reported from demonstration studies: 85% reduction in 21 000 subjects undergoing 'clearing' proctosigmoidoscopy followed by annual proctosigmoidoscopy with removal of all lesions detected;[71]

70% reduction in risk of colorectal cancer for 10 years following sigmoidoscopy;[72] 80% reduction in incidence following examination, mostly performed by flexible sigmoidoscopy;[73] and an 85% reduction of rectal cancers achieved by the removal of adenomas.[74] Although the initial examination may be expensive, there is an advantage that polyps may be removed at the time of the initial procedure, and no follow-up visits will be required. Use of a 65 cm flexible sigmoidoscope appears to be the most effective proposition at the present time, since this avoids the more complicated colonoscopy and yet still covers.

There are currently some extremely important issues to address in the area of colorectal cancer screening.

- *Should FOB testing now be recommended as a population screening method?* This decision depends on many factors, including the value placed on the magnitude of the mortality reduction, the false-positive rate associated with haemocult testing, the acceptance of the test to the general population and the economic costs involved.

- *Should consideration be given to other screening modalities for colorectal cancer?* Screening with sigmoidoscopy has been demonstrated in case-control and non-randomized studies to reduce the incidence and mortality from colorectal cancer by over 50%:[72,75,76] FOB testing does not appear to reduce the incidence of colorectal cancer.

- *Since a large proportion of individuals tested for FOB have positive tests and are referred for colonoscopy, could it prove effective to bypass FOB testing and go directly to a screening colonoscopy or to flexible sigmoidoscopy?* This latter strategy is currently being assessed in a large, randomized trial, and it is a clear reflection of the tremendous potential for colorectal cancer early detection by screening, which is clearly outlined in detail elsewhere.[77] This should continue to be a priority research activity at present.

Risk of colorectal cancer appears to be increased by increasing consumption of fat, protein and meat, and to be reduced by increased consumption of fruits and vegetables.[78] It has been hypothesized that alterations to serum triglycerides and/or plasma glucose could be one possible vehicle for the effects of various aetiological factors.[79] Thus there are prospects for primary prevention, although it is difficult to know how to successfully bring about such large-scale alterations to the diets of large proportions of populations. The large bowel is not generally considered as a site where the risk of cancer is linked to cigarette smoking,[80] although it has been recently suggested that it may be an independent risk factor that may be specifically associated with the early stages of colorectal epidemiology.[81,82] However, there is also interesting evidence suggesting that specific chemo-preventive strategies could prove useful in the prevention of colorectal cancer. While there are many questions to be resolved, it is apparent that colorectal cancer is increasingly understood and prospects for prevention are becoming apparent: this is a great success for epidemiology.

ACKNOWLEDGEMENT

It is a pleasure to acknowledge that this work was conducted within the framework of support by the Italian Association for Cancer Research (Associazone Italiana per la Ricerca sul Cancro).

REFERENCES

1. Parkin DM, Pisani P, Ferlay J, Estimates of the worldwide incidence of eighteen major cancers in 1985. *Int J Cancer* 1993; **55**: 594–606.
2. Boyle, P, Relative value of incidence and mortality data in cancer research. *Recent Results Cancer Res* 1989; **114**: 41–63.
3. Boyle P, Zaridze DG, Smans M, Descriptive epidemiology of colorectal cancer. *Int J Cancer* 1985; **36**: 9–18.
4. Haenszel W, Kurihara M, Studies of Japanese migrants I. Mortality from cancer and other diseases among Japanese in the United States. *J Natl Cancer Inst* 1968; **40**: 43–68.
5. Haenszel N, Correa P, Cancer of the colon and rectum and adenomatous polyps. A review of epidemiologic findings. *Cancer* 1971; **28**: 14–24.
6. Bell J, Coates M, Day P, Armstrong BK, *Colorectal Cancer in New South Wales in 1972 to 1993.* Sydney: Cancer Council, New South Wales Health Department, 1996.
7. Sondik E, Young JL, Horm JW et al (eds), *1985 Annual Cancer Statistics Review.* Bethesda, MD: NIH Publication 86-2789, NCI, 1986.
8. National Cancer Institute, *1987 Annual Cancer Statistics Review Including Cancer Trends 1950–1985.* Bethesda, MD: NIH Publication No. 88-2789, NCI, 1988.
9. Staszewski J, Migrant studies in alimentary tract cancer. *Recent Results Cancer Res* 1972; **39**: 85–97.
10. National Cancer Institute of Canada, *Canadian National Cancer Statistics 1997.* Toronto: National Cancer Institute of Canada, 1997.
11. Boyle P, La Vecchia C, Negri E et al, Trends in diet-related cancers in Japan: a conundrum? *Lancet* 1993; **342**: 752.
12. Peipens LA, Sandler RS, Epidemiology of colorectal adenomas. *Epidemiol Rev* 1994; **16**: 273–97.
13. Vogelstein B, Fearon ER, Hamilton SR et al, Genetic alterations during colorectal-tumour development. *N Engl J Med* 1988; **319**: 525–32.
14. Fearon ER, Vogelstein B, A genetic model for colorectal tumorigenesis. *Cell* 1990; **61**: 759–67.
15. Morotomi M, Guillem J, LoGerfo P, Weinstein IB, Production of diacylglycerol, an activator of protein kinase C, by human intestinal microflora. *Cancer Res* 1990; **50**: 3595–9.
16. Bodmer WF, Balley CJ, Bodmer J et al, Localization of the gene for familial adenomatous polyposis on chromosome 5. *Nature* 1987; **328**: 614–18.
17. Hall NR, Murday VA, Chapman P et al, Genetic linkage in Muir–Torre syndome to the same chromosomal region as cancer family syndrome. *Eur J Cancer* 1994; **30**: 180–2.
18. Bishop DT, Thomas HJW, The genetics of colorectal cancer. *Cancer Surv* 1990; **9**: 585–604.
19. Bishop DT, Hall NR, The genetics of colorectal cancer. *Eur J Cancer* 1990; **30**: 1946–56.
20. Cohen AM, Minsky BD, Schilsky RL, Colon cancer. In: *Principles and Practice of Oncology* (de Vita

VT, Hellman S, Rosenberg SA, eds). Philadelphia: JB Lippincott, 1993.

21. McMichael AJ, Giles GG, Colorectal cancer. In: *Cancer Surveys: Trends in Incidence and Mortality* (Doll R, Fraumeni JF, Muir CS, eds). Cold Spring Harbor, NY: Cold Spring Habor Press, 1994.

22. Shephard RJ, Exercise in the prevention and treatment of cancer – an update. *Sports Med* 1993; **15:** 258–80.

23. Thune I, Lund E, Physical activity and risk of colorectal cancer in men and women. *Br J Cancer* 1996; **73:** 1134–40.

24. Willett WC, The search for the causes of breast and colon cancer. *Nature* 1989; **338:** 389–94.

25. Vena JE, Graham S, Zielezny M et al, Occupational exercise and risk of cancer. *Am J Clin Nutr* 1987; **45:** 318–27.

26. Slattery ML, Schumacher ML, Smith KR et al, Physical activity, diet and role of colon cancer in Utah. *Am J Epidemiol* 1988; **128:** 989–99.

27. Whittemore AS, Wu-Williams AH, Lee M et al, Diet, physical activity and colorectal cancer among Chinese in North America and China. *J Natl Cancer Inst* 1990; **82:** 915–26.

28. Davidow AL, Neugut AL, Jacobsen JS et al, Recurrent adenomatous polyps and body mass index. *Cancer Epidemiol Biomarkers Prev* 1996; **5:** 313–15.

29. Sandler RS, Pritchard MI, Bangiwala SI, Physical activity and the risk of colorectal adenomas. *Epidemiology* 1995; **6:** 602–6.

30. Giovannucci E, Colditz GA, Stampfer MJ, Willett WC, Physical activity, obesity and risk of colorectal cancer in women (United States). *Cancer Causes Control* 1996; **7:** 253–63.

31. Holdstock DJ, Misiewicz JJ, Smith T et al, Propulsion (mass movements) in the human colon and its relationship to meals and somatic activity. *Gut* 1970; **11:** 91–9.

32. Simon HB, The immunology of exercise. *J Am Med Assoc* 1984; **252:** 2735–8.

33. Bartram HP, Wynder EL, Physical activity and colon cancer risk? Physiological consideration. *Am J Gastroenterol* 1989; **84:** 109–12.

34. Willett WC, Stampfer MJ, Colditz GA et al, Relation of meat, fat, and fiber intake to the risk of colon cancer in a prospective study among women. *N Engl J Med* 1990; **323:** 1664–72.

35. Sugimura T, Past, present and future of mutagens in cooked foods. *Environ Health Perspect* 1986; **67:** 5–10.

36. Felton, JS, Knize MG, Shen NH et al, Identification of the mutagens in cooked beef. *Environ Health Perspect* 1986; **67:** 17–24.

37. Schiffman MH, Felton JS, Fried foods and the risk of colon cancer. *Am J Epidemiol* 1990; **131:** 376–8.

38. Ha WI, Grim NK, Periza MW, Anticarcinogenics from fried ground beef: heat-altered derivatives of linoleic acid. *Carcinogenesis* 1987; **8:** 1881–7.

39. Zaridze DG, Environmental etiology of large-bowel cancer. *J Natl Cancer Inst* 1983; **70:** 389–400.

40. Sakaguchi M, Hiramatsu Y, Takada H et al, Effect of dietary unsaturated and saturated fats on azoxymethane-induced colon carcinogenesis in rats. *Cancer Res* 1984; **44:** 1472–7.

41. Minoura YT, Takata T, Sakaguchi M et al, Effect of dietary eicopentaenoic acid on azoxymethane induced colon carcinogenesis in rats. *Cancer Res* 1988; **46:** 4790–4.

42. Kritchevsky D, Diet, nutrition and cancer: the role of fibre. *Cancer* 1986; **58:** 1830–6.

43. Tuyns AJ, Haeltermann M, Kaaks R, Colorectal cancer and the intake of nutrients: oliogosaccharides are a risk factor, fats are not. A case-control study in Belgium. *Nutr Cancer* 1987; **10:** 181–96.

44. Kune S, Kune GA, Watson LF, Case-control study of dietary aetiological factors: the Melbourne colorectal cancer study. *Nutr Cancer* 1987; **9:** 21–42.

45. Heilbrun LK, Hankin JH, Nomura AMY et al, Colon cancer and dietary fat, phosphorous and calcium in Hawaiian–Japanese men. *Am J Clin Nutr* 1986; **43:** 306–9.

46. Steinmetz KA, Potter JD, Vegetable, fruit, and cancer I. Epidemiology. *Cancer Causes Control* 1991; **2:** 325–58.

47. Fernandez E, d'Avanzo B, Negri E et al, Diet diversity and the risk of colorectal cancer in northern Italy. *Cancer Epidemiol Biomarkers Prev* 1996; **5:** 433–6.

48. Freedman AN, Michalek AM, Marshall JR et al, Familial and nutritional risk factors for p53 over-expression in colorectal cancer. *Cancer Epidemiol Biomarkers Prev* 1996; **5:** 285–91.

49. Newmark HL, Wargovich MJ, Bruce WR, Colon cancer and dietary fat, phosphate and calcium: a hypothesis. *J Natl Cancer Inst* 1984; **72:** 1323–5.

50. Sorenson AW, Slattery ML, Food MH, Calcium and colon cancer: a review. *Nutr Cancer* 1988; **11:** 135–45.

51. Longnecker MP, Orza MJ, Adams ME et al, A meta-analysis of alcoholic beverage consumption in relation to risk of colorectal cancer. *Cancer Causes Control* 1990; **1:** 59–68.

52. Goldin BR, Gorbach SL, The effect of milk and lactobacillus feeding on human intestinal bacterial enzyme activity. *Am J Clin Nutr* 1984; **39:** 756–61.
53. IARC (International Agency for Research on Cancer), *Monographs on the Evaluation of the Carconogenic Risk of Chemicals to Man.* Vol 44. *Coffee, Tea, Mate, Methylxanthines (Caffeine, Theophylline, Theobromine) and Methylglyoxal.* Lyon: IARC, 1988.
54. MacLennan SC, MacLennan AH, Ryan P, Colorectal cancer and oestrogen replacement therapy: a meta-analysis of epidemiological studies. *Med J Austr* 1994; **162:** 491–3.
55. Jacobs EJ, White E, Weiss NS, Exogenous hormones, reproductive history and colon cancer. *Cancer Causes Control* 1994; **5:** 359–66.
56. Calle EE, Miracle-McMahill HL, Thun MJ, Heath CW, Estrogen replacement therapy and risk of fatal colon cancer in a prospective cohort of postmenopausal women. *J Natl Cancer Inst* 1995; **87:** 517–23.
57. Labayle D, Fischer D, Vielh P et al, Sulindac causes regression of rectal polyps in familial adenomatous polyposis. *Gastroenterology* 1991; **101:** 307–11.
58. Skinner SA, Penny AG, O'Brien PE, Sulindac inhibits the rate of growth and appearance of colon tumours in rats. *Arch Surg* 1991; **126:** 1094–6.
59. Gann PH, Manson J, Glynn RJ et al, Low-dose aspirin and incidence of colorectal tumours in a randomised trial. *J Natl Cancer Inst* 1993; **85:** 1220–4.
60. Farmer KC, Goulston K, Macrae F, Aspirin and non-steroidal anti-inflammatory drugs in the chemoprevention of colorectal cancer. *Med J Austr* 1993; **159:** 649–50.
61. Morson BC, *Gastrointestinal Pathology.* Oxford: Blackwell, 1979.
62. Pisani P, Parkin DM, Ferlay J, Estimates of the worldwide mortality rate from 18 major cancers in 1985. Implications for prevention and projections of future burden. *Int J Cancer* 1993; **55:** 891–903.
63. Mandel JS, Bond JH, Church TR et al, Reducing mortality from colorectal cancer by screening for fecal occult blood. *N Engl J Med* 1993; **328:** 1365–71.
64. Selby JV, Friedman GD, Quesenberry CP, Weiss NS, Effect of fecal occult blood testing on mortality from colorectal cancer: a case-control study. *Ann Intern Med* 1993; **118:** 1294–7.
65. Wahrendorf J, Robra BP, Wiebelt H et al, Effectiveness of colorectal cancer screening: a population-based case-control study in Saarland, Germany. *Eur J Cancer Prev* 1993; **1:** 221–7.
66. Hardcastle JD, Chamberlain JO, Robinson MHE et al, Randomised controlled trial of faecal-occult-blood screening for colorectal cancer. *Lancet* 1996; **348:** 1472–7.
66. Winawer SJ, Flehinger BJ, Schottenfeld D, Miller DG, Screening for colorectal cancer by screening with fecal occult blood testing and sigmoidoscopy. *J Natl Cancer Inst* 1993; **85:** 1311–18.
67. Kronberg O, Fenger C, Olsen J et al, Randomised study of screening for colorectal cancer with faecal-occult-blood test. *Lancet* 1996; **348:** 1467–71.
68. Hardcastle JD, Screening for colorectal cancer. *Lancet* 1997; **349:** 358.
69. Rozen P, Ron E, Fireman Z et al, The relative value of fecal occult blood tests and flexible sigmoidoscopy in screening for large bowel neoplasia. *Cancer* 1987; **60:** 2553–8.
70. Allison J, Feldman R, Tekawa I, Hemocult screening in detecting colorectal neoplasm. *Ann Intern Med* 1990; **112:** 328–33.
71. Gilbertson VA, Nelms JM, The prevention of invasive cancer of the rectum. *Cancer* 1978; **41:** 1137–9.
72. Selby JV, Friedman GD, Quesenberry CP et al, A case-control study of screening sigmoidoscopy and mortality from colorectal cancer. *N Engl J Med* 1992; **26:** 653–7.
73. Newcomb PA, Norfleet RG, Storer BE et al, Screening sigmoidoscopy and colorectal cancer mortality. *J Natl Cancer Inst* 1992; **84:** 1572–5.
74. Atkin WS, Morson BC, Cuzick J, Long-term risk of colorectal cancer after excision of rectosigmoid adenomas. *N Engl J Med* 1992; **326:** 658–62.
75. Greenberg R, Baron J, Prospects for preventing colorectal cancer death. *J Natl Cancer Inst* 1993; **85:** 1182–4.
76. Boyle P, Progress in preventing death from colorectal cancer. *Br J Cancer* 1995; **72:** 528–30.
77. Mandel J, Colon and rectal cancer. In: *Cancer Screening* (Reintgen DS, Clark RA, eds). St Louis: Mosby, 1996; 55–96.
78. Potter JD, Slattery ML, Bostwick RM, Gapstur SM, Colon cancer: a review of the epidemiology. *Epidemiol Rev* 1993; **15:** 499–545.
79. McKeown-Eyssen G, Epidemiology of colorectal cancer revisited: are serum triglycerides and/or plasma glucose associated with risk. *Cancer Epidem Biom Prev* 1994; **3:** 687–95.
80. IARC (International Agency for Research on

Cancer), *Monographs on the Evaluation of the Carconogenic Risk of Chemicals to Man.* Vol 38. *Tobacco Smoking.* Lyon: IARC, 1986.

81. Giovannucci E, Rimm EB, Strampfer MJ et al, A prospective study of cigarette smoking and risk of colorectal adenoma and colorectal cancer in US men. *J Natl Cancer Inst* 1994; **86:** 183–91.

82. Giovannucci E, Colditz GA, Strampfer MJ et al, A prospective study of cigarette smoking and risk of colorectal adenoma and colorectal cancer in US women. *J Natl Cancer Inst* 1994; **86:** 192–9.

3

Pathology of colorectal cancer

Paul Hermanek

INTRODUCTION

In this chapter, we shall deal only with those areas of pathology that are relevant for treatment decisions, analysis of treatment results and quality management. Thus we do not include diagnosis and differential diagnosis, epidemiology, genetics, precancerous conditions and lesions, causal and formal pathogenesis, and the dysplasia–carcinoma sequence. Because 95% of all malignant tumors of the colon and rectum are carcinomas, predominantly the pathology of carcinomas will be discussed, and only in the last section will a short overview be given of the other, very uncommon, malignant tumors (endocrine, mesenchymal and lymphoid).

DEFINITION OF CARCINOMA IN THE COLON AND RECTUM

In contrast to the stomach or the small intestine, a neoplasm in the colon and rectum has metastatic potential only after invasion of at least the submucosa. Thus, for the colorectum in the biological and clinical sense, carcinoma is present only after the submucosa has been invaded. Such lesions are termed *invasive carcinomas*.

Between dysplasia in the general definition of an intraepithelial lesion and an invasive carcinoma as defined above, we find an intermediate step of malignant progression, namely a neoplastic lesion that shows invasive growth into the lamina propria or between the fibers of the muscularis mucosae, but does not reach the submucosa. According to clinical experience, lymph-node metastasis is not to be expected in these 'mucosal' or 'intramucosal' lesions.[1] Thus Morson[2] recommended that the use of the word 'carcinoma' should be restricted to that stage of the dysplasia–carcinoma sequence that has crossed the line of the muscularis mucosae with invasion of the submucosa. We use this nomenclature in the following.

Unfortunately, outside the United Kingdom and the German-speaking countries, the term 'carcinoma' is not used uniformly. Thus, in any cancer statistics and in any treatment results report, one has to make sure whether the data relate to invasive carcinoma only or include high-grade dysplasia (non-invasive carcinoma) too.

SITE DISTRIBUTION

The pathologies of carcinoma of the colon and rectum are essentially the same, although there are differences in epidemiology and etiology. In the literature, the definitions of colon and rectum vary. This renders comparisons difficult and explains some differences among data. According to the International Documentation System of Colorectal Cancer (IDS for CRC),[3] carcinomas that have a lower border of the tumor 16 cm or less from the anal verge (measured by a rigid rectosigmoidoscope) are classified as rectal carcinomas. Using this definition, in high-incidence areas about 50% of all colorectal carcinomas are located in the rectum, 25% in the sigmoid colon and 25% in the remaining parts of the colon. However, in the past two decades a slow change in the distribution, with a shift to the right, has been reported in some but not all high-incidence countries. In this context, it is interesting that in low-incidence countries the proportion of carcinomas of the right colon is relatively high.

GROSS MORPHOLOGY

Early carcinomas of the colon and rectum, i.e. tumors limited to the submucosa, present in most cases as polypoid (exophytic) lesions, pedunculated, semipedunculated or sessile. Sometimes flat lesions are observed with no or only slight elevation (not more than twice the height of mucosa). In such flat lesions a slight central depression may also be present.

Advanced carcinomas (invading beyond the submucosa) present in four types, similar to the Borrmann categories of gastric carcinoma:

- polypoid (protuberant);
- ulcerated, with sharply demarcated margins;
- ulcerated, without definite borders;
- diffusely infiltrating.

In contrast to gastric carcinoma, the latter two types are uncommon, the ulcerated tumor with sharply demarcated margins is by far the most common type, followed by the polypoid type as second.

HISTOMORPHOLOGY

Histological typing

The present WHO classification is shown in Table 3.1. Adenocarcinoma and mucinous adenocarcinoma (sometimes still termed mucoid or colloid adenocarcinoma) account for 90–95% of carcinomas; all other types are uncommon. Mucinous adenocarcinomas are more frequently observed in the colon (about 15%) than in the rectum (about 10%).

Some adenocarcinomas show areas with abundant mucus production. However, unless mucus contributes to more than 50% of the tumor bulk, the tumor should still be classified as adenocarcinoma. Also, the presence of scattered Paneth cells and endocrine cells or of small foci of squamous differentiation does not influence the classification. Signet-ring cells may be present in mucinous adenocarcinomas. However, more than 50% of the tumor should comprise signet-ring cells before it is classified as signet-ring-cell carcinoma. The uncommon undifferentiated carcinoma (former designations: carcinoma simplex, anaplastic, medullary, trabecular carcinoma) should be distinguished from poorly differentiated adenocarcinoma, small-cell carcinoma, lymphoma and leukemic deposits by use of mucin stains and immunohistochemistry.

Extremely uncommon carcinomas not listed in the WHO classification, and reported in only a few cases, include clear-cell (hypernephroid) carcinoma, spindle-cell carcinoma, choriocarcinoma, melanotic adenocarcinoma, carcinomas arising in endometriosis, calcified adenocarcinoma, giant-cell carcinoma and Paneth-cell-rich papillary adenocarcinoma.

Histological grading

Histopathological grading of tumors is performed to provide some indication of their aggressiveness, which may in turn relate to prognosis and/or treatment choice.

The traditional system of grading distinguishes four grades:

Table 3.1 Histological typing and grading: WHO classification[4]

Type	Definition	Grading system (G1–4)	Low/high (L/H)
Adenocarcinoma	Glandular epithelium, tubular and/or villous	1–3	L/H
Mucinous adenocarcinoma	More than 50% extracellular mucin	1–3	L/H
Signet-ring-cell carcinoma	More than 50% signet-ring cells (intracytoplasmatic mucin)	3	H
Squamous-cell carcinoma	Exclusively squamous differentiation	1–3	L/H
Adenosquamous carcinoma	Adenocarcinoma plus squamous-cell carcinoma	1–3	L/H
Small-cell carcinoma (oat-cell carcinoma)	Similar to small-cell carcinoma of the lung (with neuroendocrine differentiation)	4	H
Undifferentiated carcinoma	No glandular structure or other features to indicate definite differentiation	4	H

- G1 well-differentiated: a carcinoma with histological and cellular features that closely resemble normal epithelium;
- G2 moderately differentiated: a carcinoma intermediate between G1 and G3;
- G3 poorly differentiated: a carcinoma with histological or cellular features that only barely resemble normal epithelium (there must be at least some gland formation or mucus production);
- G4 undifferentiated: no glandular or squamous differentiation at all (thus G4 applies in the colon and rectum to small-cell and undifferentiated carcinoma only, see Table 3.1).

The WHO classification[4] also provides a grading system with two classes:

- low-grade, encompassing G1 and G2;
- high-grade, including G3 and G4.

This grading system fulfils all clinical requirements, and can be performed with higher reproducibility. Thus, we prefer grading with only two categories.

When a carcinoma shows different grades of differentiation, the higher grade should determine the final categorization. Thus a carcinoma that shows both low- and high-grade areas should be classified as high-grade. However, the disorganized glands seen commonly at the advancing edge of the carcinoma should not be considered as high-grade malignancy. High-grade carcinomas account for 20–25% of resected carcinomas.

Additional histological parameters

For describing the histomorphology of an individual colorectal carcinoma, there are some further parameters to be considered:

- the character of the invasive margin (expanding or well-circumscribed versus diffusely infiltrating);[5]
- peritumoral inflammation;[5,6]
- the presence of peritumorous lymphoid aggregates;[6]
- fibroblastic stromal reaction (desmoplasia);[6]
- invasion of lymphatics – L classification:[7] L0, no lymphatic invasion; L1, lymphatic invasion; LX, lymphatic invasion cannot be assessed;
- venous invasion – V classification:[7] V0, no venous invasion; V1, microscopic venous invasion; V2, macroscopic venous invasion; VX, venous invasion cannot be assessed; in the case of microscopic venous invasion, it is important to distinguish between involvement of intramural veins (submucosa, muscularis propria) and that of extramural veins (beyond muscularis propria);
- invasion of perineural spaces.

In addition, the type of lymph-node reactions may be recorded, because it reflects the host reactions. There may be follicular hyperplasia (in more than 50% or in 50% or less of regional nodes) or paracortical hyperplasia or both.[8]

SPECIAL CLINICAL TYPES OF COLORECTAL CARCINOMA

Hereditary non-polyposis colon cancer (HNPCC)

Carcinomas in this hereditary syndrome have a tendency to occur primarily in the right colon and at a much younger age (most cases between 35 and 45 years) than the usual sporadic carcinoma (preferred age 55–65 years). Mucinous adenocarcinomas and high-grade tumors are observed relatively often. There is an increased incidence of metachronous multiple primary tumors. HNPCC accounts for 4–6% of all colorectal carcinoma.[9,10]

Carcinoma arising in familial adenomatous polyposis (FAP)

Less than 1% of colorectal carcinomas arise in FAP and in the 'hereditary flat adenoma syndrome' (HFAS), a variant of FAP, usually with fewer than 100 adenomas, mostly of flat type. The histological features are similar to those of sporadic cancers; however, there is a high proportion of multiple synchronous primary tumors in symptomatic cases (up to a third of cases).

Carcinoma developing in inflammatory bowel disease

Carcinomas in inflammatory bowel disease arise predominantly in extensive ulcerous colitis with a history of 10 years or longer. There are often synchronous multiple carcinomas. The incidence of flat and diffusely infiltrating carcinomas, high-grade tumors, mucinous adenocarcinomas and signet-ring-cell carcinomas is higher than in ordinary colorectal carcinomas. Less than 1% of all colorectal carcinomas arise in inflammatory bowel disease.

TUMOR SPREAD

Knowledge of tumor spread is of paramount importance for surgical procedure in treating colorectal carcinoma. The possible routes of tumor spread are shown in Figure 3.1.

Local spread

The different types of local spread determine the extent of surgical resection, and lead to the demand for avoidance of local tumor spillage.

(a) Extent of resection

In colon carcinoma the extent of resection is determined by the extent of lymph-node dissection and the vascular supply. However, in rectal carcinoma the distal margin of clearance may be critical, especially in tumors located in the lower rectum. In this context, it is important

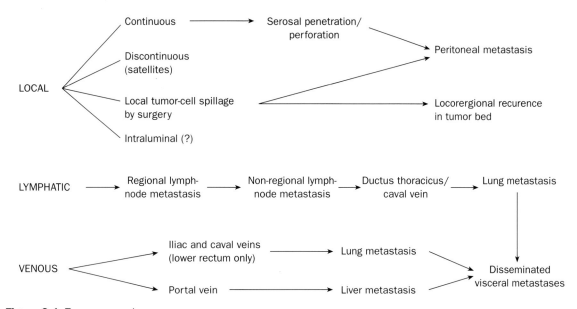

Figure 3.1 Tumor spread.

that histological examination of rectal carcinomas in curable stages demonstrates that the continuous distal local spread usually extends no more than some millimeters beyond the grossly recognizable margin of the tumor. However, in the perimuscular tissue discontinuous spread in the form of so-called satellites must be considered. Such microscopic tumor nodules, without residua of lymph-node tissue and not more than 2–3 mm in diameter, are found in the mesorectum, predominantly in the radial direction, but also distal, some centimeters from the lower tumor margin. Thus low anterior resection for tumors of the middle and lower rectal third has to include total mesorectal excision down to the pelvic floor,[11] while the margin of clearance within the proper wall of the rectum (muscularis propria, submucosa, mucosa) may be limited to 1 cm in situ except in cases of high-grade tumors, which require 2 cm distal margin.[12]

(b) Avoidance of local spillage of tumor cells
A local spillage of tumor cells results in a signif-

icantly increased incidence of loco-regional recurrence.[13] This is observed in rectal carcinoma after iatrogenic tumor perforation during mobilization or in cases of two-step low anterior resection (first resection with tumor in the distal resection line, further resection with tumor-free resection line) with transsection of tumor tissue. Adherence of a tumor to adjacent organs may be caused by peritumorous inflammation or by tumorous invasion. A respective discrimination by gross inspection of palpation is not possible. In such cases a primary multivisceral resection is indicated if a curative operation is intended. Any biopsy from the adherence should be avoided, because in cases of tumor invasion biopsy results in local tumor spillage.[14]

The basis of local therapy

The classical concept for curative oncological surgery is the so-called radical resection, which includes wide resection of the primary together with formal (systematic) regional lymphadenectomy. For selected carcinomas without lymph-node metastases, local procedures such as endoscopic polypectomy or surgical local excision can also be used with curative intention.[15,16] The indication for such procedures is determined by the risk of lymph-node metastasis already present compared with the increased risk of surgical mortality from radical procedures.

The probability of regional lymph-node metastasis depends primarily on histological features of the primary tumor such as depth of invasion, histological grade and absence or presence of lymphatic invasion. This is shown in Table 3.2, which is based on the careful histological examination of 2720 radical tumor resections for cure (R0). It shows that the risk of lymph-node metastasis already present is minimal in pT1 tumors with so-called low-risk histology, i.e. low grade of malignancy (G1, G2) *and* no demonstrable lymphatic invasion (L0). Thus local therapy in curative intention can be considered predominantly for carcinomas of low-risk histology invading the submucosa only. In patients with increased surgical risk, it may also be used for carcinomas invading the inner muscularis propria if low-risk histology is present.

Lymph-node dissection for colon carcinoma

The extent of lymph-node dissection in radical surgery is determined by the lymph drainage. While most parts of the colon drain into one direction, for both flexures and the right and left third of the transverse colon a bidirectional

Table 3.2 Frequency of regional lymph-node metastasis in colorectal carcinoma. Pathological findings in radical resection specimens – only cases with resection for cure (R0). (Department of Surgery, University of Erlangen, 1969–1993.)

Depth of invasion	Frequency of regional lymph-node metastasis	
	Low-risk histology[a]	High-risk histology[b]
pT1 Submucosa	5/172 = 2.9%	12/71 = 17%
pT2 Muscularis propria:		
inner (circular) layer	19/212 = 9.0%	34/93 = 37%
outer (longitudinal) layer	58/299 = 19.4%	39/97 = 40%
pT3 Subserosa/pericolic/ perirectal tissue; extension beyond muscularis propria:		
≤5 mm	82/432 = 19.0%	337/522 = 64.6%
>5 mm	38/142 = 26.8%	290/346 = 83.8%
pT4 Serosa/adjacent structures	36/126 = 28.6%	149/208 = 71.6%

[a] Low-risk: low grade (G1,2) *and* no histologically detectable invasion of lymphatics (L0).
[b] High-risk: high grade (G3,4) *or* histologically detected invasion of lymphatics (L1).

lymph drainage exists.[17,18] Tumors of the hepatic flexure and the right third of the transverse colon drain into nodes along the right as well as the middle colic artery. Therefore radical resection should be performed as extended right hemicolectomy (right and transverse colectomy), with removal of the nodes along the ileocolic, right and middle colic arteries. The bidirectional lymph drainage of tumors of the splenic flexure and the adjacent left third of the transverse colon and upper third of the descending colon requires an extended left hemicolectomy (left and transverse colectomy) for radical resection.

Lymphatic spread of rectal carcinoma

The main lymph drainage of rectal carcinoma occurs upwards to the nodes along the superior rectal and inferior mesenteric vessels. Skipping of nodes is uncommon, and occurs in about 3% of cases with node metastasis (9/234 = 2.8%).[17] In curable cases, retrograde lymph-node metastasis (along the inferior rectal arteries to inguinal nodes) is exceptional. The reports on the incidence of lateral lymphatic spread are controversial. If lateral metastasis is defined as metastasis along the iliac vessels outside the mesorectum, involvement of these nodes in curable cases is obviously rare. Thus an indication for additional lateral dissection of the iliac nodes is at least questionable, in particular when considering the significant morbidity of this procedure.[19]

The extent of dissection upwards is still under discussion (low or high ligature of the inferior mesenteric artery). The analysis of 821 curative radical resections with high ligature revealed involvement of high nodes in about 3% (Department of Surgery, University of Erlangen: 18/590 = 3.1%; multicenter study of the German Study Group on Colo-Rectal Carcinoma (SGCRC): 8/231 = 3.4%). Between 10% and 20% of these patients survive 5 years;[20] thus high ligature presents a benefit to only about 0.5% of all patients operated on. This explains why in clinical studies an advantage cannot yet be proved.

TUMOR COMPLICATIONS

Colorectal carcinoma may cause severe acute complications with the need for urgent or emergency surgery, for example acute ileus and/or free perforation or massive bleeding. Ileus and perforation are predominantly observed in colon carcinoma. Patients with such complications have a high surgical risk; in addition, the long-term prognosis is poor. In treatment statistics, these patients should be separated from those with elective surgery.

Other complications, such as fistulas or peritumorous abscesses, are of minor influence on prognosis, but may lead to extended surgery.

CLASSIFICATION OF ANATOMIC EXTENT BEFORE TREATMENT

In the history of staging, the introduction of a pathological stage classification for rectal carcinoma by Cuthbert Dukes[21] in 1930 was an important step. However, in the following years the Dukes system was repeatedly modified, indicating that the original system no longer fulfilled modern requirements and led to considerable confusion.[22] In particular, the Dukes classification does not take into consideration distant metastasis, does not allow the recognition of early carcinomas (limited to the submucosa) and does not consider the number of regional lymph nodes involved. Thus today the anatomic extent of colorectal carcinoma should be classified according to the TNM system.

Until May 1997, the 4th edition, 2nd revision (1992)[7,23] was valid. Recently, the 5th edition,[23a] approved by all national TNM Committees, has been published. The TNM system was recommended for daily use and clinical trials by the NIH Consensus Conference on Adjuvant Treatment[24] and introduced in Germany and the USA for general use in cancer hospitals. The system is shown in Table 3.3. To classify a tumor according to pTNM (pathological classification), some requirements must be met (Table 3.4). The stage grouping of the TNM system is shown in Table 3.5.

Table 3.3 TNM/pTNM classification[7,23,23a]

The definitions of the clinical classification (TNM) correspond to those of the pathological classification (pTNM).

T/pT – Primary tumor

TX/pTX	Primary tumor cannot be assessed
T0/pT0	No evidence of primary tumor
Tis/pTis	Carcinoma in situ: intraepithelial or invasion of lamina propria[a]
T1/pT1	Tumor invades submucosa
T2/pT2	Tumor invades muscularis propria
T3/pT3	Tumor invades through muscularis propria into subserosa or into non-peritonealized pericolic or perirectal tissues
T4/pT4	Tumor invades other organs or structures directly[b] and/or perforates visceral peritoneum

Notes: [a] This includes cancer cells confined within the glandular basement membrane (intraepithelial) or lamina propria (intramucosal), with no extension through the muscularis mucosae into the submucosa.
[b] Direct invasion in T4/pT4 includes invasion of other segments of the colorectum by way of the serosa, e.g. invasion of the sigmoid colon by a carcinoma of the cecum.

N/pN – Regional lymph nodes

NX/pNX	Regional lymph nodes cannot be assessed
N0/pN0	No regional lymph-node metastasis
N1/pN1	Metastasis in 1–3 pericolic or perirectal lymph nodes
N2/pN2	Metastasis in 4 or more pericolic or perirectal lymph nodes
N3/pN3	Metastasis in any lymph node along the course of a named vascular trunk and/or metastasis to apical node(s) (when marked by the surgeon)

Note: For the 5th edition of the TNM classification, published in 1997,[23a] the category N3/pN3 will be omitted, thus limiting consideration to the number of involved regional nodes only. The definitions of N1/pN1 and N2/pN2 will be as follows:
N1/pN1   Metastasis in 1–3 regional lymph nodes
N2/pN2   Metastasis in 4 or more regional lymph nodes

M/pM – Distant metastasis

MX/pMX	Presence of distant metastasis cannot be assessed
M0/pM0	No distant metastasis
M1/pM1	Distant metastasis

Regional lymph nodes

Regional lymph nodes are the pericolic and perirectal and the nodes along the named vascular trunks supporting the various anatomic subsites:

Appendix	ileocolic
Cecum	ileocolic and right colic
Ascending colon	ileocolic, right colic and middle colic
Hepatic flexure	middle colic and right colic
Transverse colon	right colic, middle colic, left colic and inferior mesenteric
Splenic flexure	middle colic, left colic and inferior mesenteric
Descending colon	middle colic, left colic and inferior mesenteric

Table 3.3 cont

Sigmoid colon ⎫ left colic, superior rectal (hemorrhoidal) and
Rectosigmoid ⎬ inferior mesenteric
Rectum   superior rectal (hemorrhoidal), inferior mesenteric and internal iliac

The nodes along the sigmoid arteries are considered pericolic.

Perirectal nodes include the mesorectal (paraproctal), lateral sacral, presacral, sacral promotory (Gerota), middle rectal (hemorrhoidal) and inferior rectal (hemorrhoidal) nodes. Metastasis in the external iliac or common iliac nodes is classified as distant metastasis.

Ramifications (i.e. optional subdivisions of existing TNM/pTNM categories) and **optional specifications**[25]

pT3   pT3a   Minimal: tumor invades through the muscularis propria into the subserosa or into nonperitonealized pericolic or perirectal tissues, not more than 1 mm beyond the outer border of the muscularis propria

     pT3b   Slight: tumor invades through the muscularis propria into the subserosa or into nonperitonealized pericolic or perirectal tissues, more than 1 mm but not more than 5 mm beyond the outer border of the muscularis propria

     pT3c   Moderate: tumor invades through the muscularis propria into the subserosa or into nonperitonealized pericolic or perirectal tissues, more than 5 mm but not more than 15 mm beyond the outer border of the muscularis propria

     pT3d   Extensive: tumor invades through the muscularis propria into the subserosa or into nonperitonealized pericolic or perirectal tissues, more than 15 mm beyond outer border of the muscularis propria

pT4   pT4a   Invasion of adjacent organs or structures, without perforation of visceral peritoneum
     pT4b   Perforation of visceral peritoneum

(mi)   The addition of '(mi)' is applied to cases with micrometastasis only (i.e. no metastasis larger than 2 mm), e.g. pN1(mi) or pM1(mi)

(i)   The addition of '(i)' indicates the finding of isolated (disseminated) tumor cells in bone marrow, which is classified as M1(i). Such cases have to be distinguished from those with micro- or macrometastasis and must be analyzed separately from other M1 and pM1 cases.
     '(i)' can also be applied to the findings of isolated tumor cells in the sinus of lymph nodes, e.g. N1. These findings must also be distinguished from micrometastasis, which is classified as pN1(mi) or pN2(mi)

HISTOPATHOLOGICAL ASSESSMENT OF TREATMENT

While TNM and pTNM describe the anatomical extent of cancer before treatment, the residual tumor (R) classification deals with tumor status after treatment. It reflects the effects of therapy, influences further therapeutic procedures and is the strongest predictor of outcome.[27] Thus, following tumor resection, first of all, the patholo-

---

Table 3.4 Requirements for pT, pN, and pM classification[7,23a,25]

pT3 or less

Pathological examination of the primary carcinoma removed by short segment (limited) or radical resection *with no gross tumor* at the deep (radial, lateral), proximal and distal margins of resection (with or without microscopic involvement), *or* pathological examination of the primary carcinoma removed by endoscopic polypectomy or local excision with histologically tumor-free margins of resection

pT4

Pathological confirmation of perforation of the visceral peritoneum, *or* microscopic confirmation of invasion of adjacent organs or structures

Note: Pathological confirmation may be achieved from biopsies or resection specimens or by cytology or specimens obtained from the serosa overlying the primary tumor.

pN0

Histological examination of a regional lymphadenectomy specimen, which will ordinarily include 12 regional lymph nodes

pN1/2

If the pathology report does not indicate the number of involved nodes or their localization, classify as pN1

pN3

Microscopic confirmation of a metastasis in a node along the course of a named vascular trunk. The 'apical node' in radical resection specimens can be considered the equivalent of one on a named vascular trunk

Note: For colorectal carcinoma, the International Documentation System[3] contains the following recommendation: 'Before deeming a radical resection to be without lymph node metastasis, it is recommended that at least 12 lymph nodes be examined . . . The Working Party recognized, however, that not all specimens will contain this number of lymph nodes, and this is particularly true of the patients who have received preoperative irradiation.' This recommendation is based on data of Scott and Grace[26] and of the German Study Group on Colo-Rectal Carcinoma (SGCRC).[25]

pM1 Microscopic (histologic or cytologic) confirmation

---

gist has to examine the resection lines to obtain the R classification, which is based on clinical as well as histopathological findings (Figure 3.2). In this regard, the main problem is the examination of the lateral (circumferential), i.e. mesorectal and mesocolon, resection margins. In general, at least two conventional blocks or a large-area (giant) block have to be submitted for histology (for detailed methodic recommendations see reference 28).

In addition to the R classification, the surgi-

cal pathology report on resection specimens includes some statements that reflect the oncological quality of surgery (see below).

In cases of neoadjuvant (preoperative) radio- and/or chemotherapy the pathologist has to assess the tumor response. Unfortunately, there are not yet any internationally agreed systems for describing the regressive changes and staging methods in such cases. Complete regression is possible, but, from our experience, it is very uncommon, provided that the tumor region is

Table 3.5 Stage grouping[7,23,23a]			
	(p)M0		pM1
	pN0	pN1,2[23a] (pN1–3)[7,23]	
pT1 pT2	I		
		III	IV
pT3 pT4	II		

carefully worked-up. Thus, for regression grading, detailed statements on work-up should be given to enable estimation of the reliability of findings.

PROGNOSTIC FACTORS

Prognostic factors are variables (covariates) with independent influence on outcome. They may differ according to the various ways of measuring outcome (various endpoints) (e.g. overall survival, disease-free survival, relapse rate, and response to treatment) and also for different patient subgroups.[29] The identification of prognostic factors, in particular the acceptance of new prognostic factors, should follow certain rules.[27,30]

Table 3.6 shows the prognostic factors for patients with residual tumor and those with complete resection of the tumor. They are divided into proven and probable. For rectal carcinomas of the middle and lower third, complete excision of the mesorectum has to be added as at least a probable prognostic factor.[31–33]

It should be emphasized that the independent prognostic significance of all biological and molecular factors (factors of the so-called new pathology) remains to be proven.[27]

Proven as well as probable prognostic factors

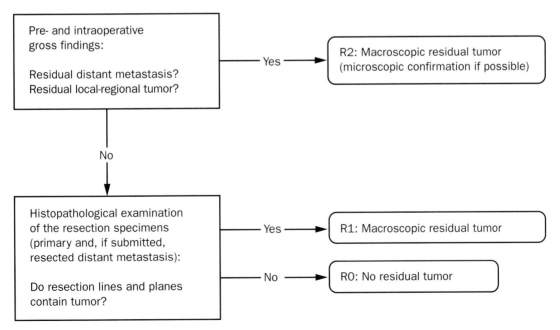

Figure 3.2 Residual tumor (R) classification.[25]

Table 3.6 Prognostic factors in colorectal carcinoma[27] (unfavorable level of covariates is shown in parentheses)

A.   Patients with residual tumor (R1, R2)
Proven prognostic factors
Distant metastasis (present)
Localization of residual tumor (distant)
For patients with multiple distant metastases: performance status (increasing ECOG grade, decreasing Karnofsky)

B.   Patients with complete resection of tumor (no residual tumor, R0)

	Proven prognostic factors	Probable prognostic factors
Tumor-related	Anatomic extent: pTNM and stage grouping (higher category) Histologic grade (high-grade) Venous invasion (present, predominantly extramural)	Anatomic site of primary (lower rectum) Tumor perforation/obstruction (present) Lymphatic and perineural invasion (present) Histological pattern of tumor margin (infiltrative) Peritumoral lymphoid cells/ lymphoid aggregates (non-conspicious/absent)
Patient-related	—	Gender (male) CEA serum level (more than 5 mg/l)
Treatment-related	Surgeon	Technique of tumor mobilization (other than 'no-touch') Local spillage of tumor cells (iatrogenic perforation or incision into tumor)

have to be included in analyses of clinical trials and also in retrospective studies; otherwise the results cannot be accepted without doubt.

THE HISTOPATHOLOGICAL REPORT

The histopathological report has to include all possible information important in relation to tumor classification, description or surgical procedure, and prognostic factors. This enables diagnosis, treatment decisions, estimation of prognosis, and analysis of treatment results and of the quality of diagnosis and treatment.

Specific recommendations for the content of surgical pathology reports were published in the 1980s.[34–37] In 1991 an International Documentation System for Colorectal

Table 3.7 International Documentation System for Colorectal Carcinoma (IDS for CRC)[3]

Information type	Clinical features	Pathological features
Basic information	Country Hospital (name/code) Patient identification (name/code) Patient race Past tumor history	Number of primary tumors Tumor measurements Appearance of serosal surface Associated pathology Tumor type

Variables of proven prognostic significance	Surgeon (name/code)
	Patient gender and age
	Presentation
	Anatomic extent of
	  tumor
	Residual tumor
		Extent of direct spread
		Regional nodal status
		  Site and number of involved
		  nodes/number of examined
		  nodes
		Distant metastasis status
		Venous involvement
		Histology of infiltrating margins
		Tumor grade

Information of probable prognostic significance	Pre-operative treatment
	Anatomic site of primary
	Tumor mobility
	Technique of tumor
	  mobilization
	Tumor perforation
	Surgical procedure
	Resection of distant
	  metastases
	Postoperative treatment
		Tumor perforation
		Inflammatory cell infiltrate
		Lymphoid aggregates

Carcinoma (IDS for CRC) was developed by an International Working Group[3] (Table 3.7). It was the principal basis of further recommendations for reporting pathology findings.[38–42]

The German Cancer Society[43] introduced in Germany a so-called minimal program for surgical pathology reporting (Figure 3.3), which should be used in each institution. It may be extended (extended program) in specialized institutions and in clinical studies. This extended program[40] includes all features with proven or probable prognostic significance and those included in the IDS for CRC (see Tables 3.6 and 3.7).

QUALITY MANAGEMENT AND PATHOLOGY

Quality management is a requirement for diagnostic activities in pathology departments as well as for treatment of cancer and for clinical studies.

1. Information on R classification

(a) Findings on resection lines

	F = Free of tumor	T = With tumor	X = Not examined	
Oral	☐	☐	☐	☐
Aboral	☐	☐	☐	☐
Mesocolon/mesorectum	☐	☐	☐	☐
Adjacent organs	☐	☐	☐	☐

(b) In case of binding statements on clinical R classification:
Definite R classification
0 = No residual tumor (R0); 1 = Microscopic residual tumor (R1)
2 = Macroscopic residual tumor, not microscopically confirmed (R2a)
3 = Macroscopic residual tumor, microscopically confirmed (R2b)   ☐

If residual tumor, localization	N = No	Y = Yes	
Locoregional	☐	☐	☐
Distant metastasis	☐	☐	☐

2. Tumor perforation
N = No; S = Spontaneous; I = Iatrogenic

3. Minimal distance between tumor border and oral or aboral resection line, macroscopically measured (mm) _____

Method of measurement: ☐ fresh specimen, without tension
☐ fixed specimen, pinned ☐ fixed specimen, unpinned   ☐

4. pTNM classification

(y) _____ pT _____ (m) ____ pN _____ (mi) ____

☐	☐☐	☐	
y	pT	m	

(pM) _____ (mi) ____ (i) ____

☐☐	☐	☐☐	☐	☐
pN	mi	pM	mi	i

Number of examined lymph nodes _____

Number of involved lymph nodes _____

☐☐	☐☐
exam	invols

5. Histological type (Who) ICD–O

Adenocarcinoma	8140/3	Mucinous adenocarcinoma	8480/3	☐☐☐☐ [3]
Signet-ring-cell		Squamous-cell carcinoma	8070/3	
carcinoma	8490/3	Undifferentiated carcinoma	8020/3	
Adenosquamous		Small-cell carcinoma	8041/3	
carcinoma	8560/3	Other type: _____		

6. Histological grade of differentiation
1 = G1; 2 = G2; 3 = G3; 4 = G4
L = Low-grade (G1,2), H = High-grade (G3,4), X = GX   ☐

7. Associated lesions

	N = No	Y = Yes	
Familial adenomatous polyposis	☐	☐	☐
Ulcerous colitis	☐	☐	☐
Other chronic inflammatory disease	☐	☐	☐
Adenoma(s)	☐	Number _____	☐☐

Figure 3.3 Surgical pathology report on colorectal carcinoma resection specimens: minimal program (translation of the form recommended by the German Cancer Society[43]).

Quality management within pathology departments

The methods of quality management within pathology departments have recently been described and summarized by Rosai.[42] In this context, we must emphasize that pathological reports have to include all features of proven and probable prognostic significance as listed in the IDS for CRC (Table 3.7) and also features that indicate the oncological quality of the surgical procedure (see below).

There are indicators of the quality of histopathological assessment and work-up (Table 3.8). In all pathology departments, the respective data should currently be collected and analysed. Any deviation from the usual values (ranges) and changes in frequencies should lead to careful analysis and response.

Special attention should be directed to careful examination of the circumferential resection margin[28,44] and lymph nodes because of the crucial prognostic significance of the respective findings. In regard to lymph-node examination, Lewin et al[38] stated: 'Evidence of a good nodal dissection is the finding of lymphoid tissue in the 1- to 3-mm range, with a sprinkling of pieces of fibrofatty tissue and small vessels ... Conversely, inadequate sampling is characterized by the finding of only few nodes measuring 1 cm or more.'

Pathology findings in resection specimens indicative of oncological quality of surgery

The most important goal of surgical treatment is to achieve complete tumor resection (R0 resection). Thus the rate of R0 resections related to all patients is an important intermediate indicator of quality. However, there also some pathological findings on resection specimens that give further information on the oncological quality of surgery:

1. Evidence of local spillage of tumor cells: iatrogenic tumor perforation or tumor resection not en bloc with transsection of tumor tissue? (see page 39).
2. Length of resected bowel: limited (segmental) resection or radical resection with ligature of the trunk of the supplying vessels?
3. In cases of colon carcinomas with multidirectional lymph drainage: dissection of one or two lymph drainage areas?
4. Number of removed lymph nodes (provided there is an adequate node-examination technique)?
5. In rectal carcinoma of the upper third: distal margin of clearance in muscular wall as well as in mesorectum (no coning) not less than 5 cm in situ corresponding to 3 cm measured on the fresh resection specimen without tension?
6. In rectal carcinoma of the middle and lower third:
   • Careful gross inspection of the surface of the specimen: bilobed appearance of the correctly mobilized mesorectum with intact smooth surface?[11]
   • Distal margin of clearance in muscular wall not less than 1 cm measured on the fresh resection specimen without tension?

Data on all these parameters are needed for a reasonable assessment of the oncological quality of surgical treatment.[45]

Quality assurance of clinical trials on adjuvant and neoadjuvant therapy: the surgical pathologist's point of view

From the point of view of a surgical pathologist who has spent many years directing a tumor registry and has intensively investigated prognostic factors in colorectal carcinoma, it is remarkable how many of the protocols on adjuvant or neoadjuvant therapy have failed to adequately consider quality assurance in regard of pathology and surgical treatment.[46]

In adjuvant treatment, the quality of pathological examination of resection specimens influences the *selection of patients* and thus the results. Therefore data indicating the quality of pathology (Table 3.8) must always be included in reports on respective clinical trials. The frequency of all tumor resections, of resections without and with microscopic residual tumor

Table 3.8 Quality indicators for pathological diagnosis (modified from reference 43)

Parameter	Range		Indicative of
	Colon	**Rectum**	
Tumor type:			
Mucinous adneocarcinoma/frequency	~15%	~10%	Adherence to WHO classification
Tumor grade:			
High-grade/frequency	20–25%		
R classification:			
Frequency of R1 related to resections considered as complete by the surgeon	0–5%	5–10 (–20%)	Carefulness of histological examination of resection lines[a]
Regional lymph nodes:			
• Frequency of node-positive cases related to radical resections for cure (R0 resections)	40–50%		Carefulness of histological examination of regional lymph-node drainage area[a]
• Number of examined nodes in radical standard resections for cure (R0)[b,c]/mean	20–30		
• Frequency of cases with fewer than 12 nodes[c]	<5%		

[a] Also influenced by the surgeon.
[b] Radical standard resection is defined as bowel resection with formal dissection of a single lymph-drainage area.
[c] Except cases with neoadjuvant therapy.

(R0, R1), and the pN classification for *all* patients seen at the institution(s) during the study period must be stated. This information indicates the general surgical attitude as well as the quality of pathologic examination.

Tumor classification according to international recommendations is an important indicator of the quality of oncological studies. Any comparison of results will be made impossible by authors who do not classify their tumors according to the generally accepted international systems.

In presentation of results, a pooling of substages with different prognosis should be avoided. For stage III, a subdivision into the prognostically different subgroups pN1 versus pN2,3 is necessary: the 5-year survival rates are significantly different: for rectal carcinoma, observed 47% versus 34%, relative 59% versus 41% ($p < 0.05$); for colon carcinoma, observed 50% versus 34%, relative 68% versus 44% ($p < 0.01$).[47] Therefore, in studies with a limited number of patients, different treatment results for stage III may be explainable by different proportions of the substages.

In each report on results, the distribution of proven and probable *independent prognostic factors* (Table 3.6) is mandatory. Only recently have sufficient data become available to demonstrate that surgical treatment and the individual surgeon are independent prognostic factors in colorectal cancer.[27,48,49] This is extremely important in multicenter studies on adjuvant and neoadjuvant treatment. In such studies, quality assessment of surgery is crucial. However, in the most recent studies, surgery is still inadequately described, and thus the results of such studies are doubtful. Therefore, for adjuvant and neoadjuvant treatment trials, the surgical treatment has to be described in detail; the individual surgeon should be documented, of course by local code,[3] and stratification according to institution and individual surgeon should be considered.[46]

MALIGNANT TUMORS OTHER THAN CARCINOMAS

Traditionally, *carcinoid tumors* have been separated from epithelial tumors and considered as tumors in which a differentiation between benign and malignant behavior may not be possible on histological grounds alone. A revised classification of neuroendocrine tumors, including small-cell carcinoma, was proposed in 1995 (Table 3.9).[50] Classes 1–3 include well-differentiated tumors, and correspond to the traditional carcinoid tumors. Most cases are observed in the rectum and belong to classes 1 and 2. The most useful indicators for behavior are size and anatomic extent. Tumors less than 1–2 cm and limited to mucosa and submucosa are usually treated and cured by local excision, while in larger tumors and those invading beyond the submucosa, radical resection as in carcinomas is indicated. Colonic carcinoid tumors are usually larger and therefore more frequently malignant than those of the rectum. In about 5%, multiple primary tumors are present. The course in the case of distant metastasis is often surprisingly prolonged; thus surgical treatment should be considered for patients with distant metastasis too.

About 1% of all malignant colorectal tumors are *leiomyosarcomas* or so-called *gastrointestinal stromal tumors* (GIST). The latter term is a collective name for tumors in which an assignment as myogenic or neurogenic is not reliably possible.

Kaposi sarcoma in the colon and rectum is usually observed in patients with AIDS and Kaposi sarcoma of the skin or lymph nodes. In most cases, the involvement of the large intestine is clinically silent. Other malignant mesenchymal tumors are extremely rare.

Some *malignant melanomas* in the rectum (without involvement of the anal region) have been reported.

Primary colorectal lymphomas (no evidence of liver, spleen, non-mesenteric lymph node and bone marrow involvement at the time of presentation) are very rare, most cases involving the ileocecal region and the rectum. Sometimes an association with ulcerous colitis or Crohn's disease has been observed. Grossly, a nodular or polypoid mass or a diffuse infiltrate may be present. The classification is not yet standardized.

For further details on non-carcinomatous malignant tumors see reference 38.

Table 3.9 Classification of colorectal neuroendocrine tumors according to Capella et al[50]

Class	Function	Differentiation	Subtype[a]	Size	Extent	Angioinvasion
1. Benign	Non-functioning	Well-differentiated	L-cell or EC-cell	<2 cm	Mucosa, submucosa	Absent
2. Benign or low-grade malignant	Non-functioning	Well-differentiated	L-cell or EC-cell	<2 cm	Mucosa, submucosa	Present
3. Low-grade malignant[b]	(a) Non-functioning (b) Functioning (carcinoid syndrome)[c]	Well-differentiated	EC-cell	>2 cm and/or beyond submucosa	Any	Any
4. High-grade malignant	Functioning or Non-functioning	Poorly differentiated	Intermediate or small cell carcinoma	Any	Any	Any

[a] L-cell tumors: trabecular pattern, produce enteroglucagon, usually in the rectum, only rarely in the colon; EC-cell tumors: insular pattern, produce serotonin, usually in the colon (prevalence of cecum), extremely rare in the rectum.

[b] If metastases or gross invasion are present, the tumor should be called a 'low-grade neuroendocrine carcinoma'.

[c] As serotonin is metabolized and inactivated by the liver, serotonin-secreting tumors of the gut only produce a carcinoid syndrome if liver metastases are present.

REFERENCES

1. Fenoglio-Preiser CM, The distribution of large intestine lymphatics: relationship to risk of metastasis from carcinomas of the large intestine. In: *Adenomas and Adenomas Containing Carcinoma of the Large Bowel: Advances in Diagnosis and Therapy* (Fenoglio-Preiser CM, Rossini FP, eds). New York/Verona: Raven Cortina International, 1985.

2. Morson BC, *The Pathogenesis of Colorectal Cancer.* Philadelphia: WB Saunders, 1978.

3. Fielding LP, Arsenault PA, Chapuis PH et al, Clinicopathological staging for colorectal cancer: An International Documentation System (IDS) and an International Comprehensive Anatomical Terminology (ICAT). *J Gastroenterol Hepatol* 1991; **6**: 325–44.

4. Jass JR, Sobin LH, *Histological Typing of Intestinal Tumours*, 2nd edn. Berlin: Springer-Verlag, 1989.

5. Jass JR, Atkins WS, Cuzick J et al, The grading of rectal cancer: historical perspectives and a multivariate analysis of 447 cases. *Histopathology* 1986; **10**: 437–59.

6. Halvorsen T, Seim E, Association between invasiveness, inflammatory reaction, desmoplasia and survival in colorectal cancer. *J Clin Pathol* 1989; **42**: 162–6.

7. UICC, *TNM Classification of Malignant Tumours*, 4th edn, 2nd revision (Hermanek P, Sobin LH, eds). Berlin: Springer-Verlag, 1992.

8. Dworak O, Morphology of lymph nodes in the resected rectum of patients with rectal carcinoma. *Pathol Res Pract* 1991; **187**: 1020–4.

9. Lynch HT, Smyrk TC, Watson P et al, Genetics, natural history, tumor spectrum, and pathology of hereditary nonpolyposis colorectal cancer: an updated review. *Gastroenterology* 1993; **104**: 1535–48.

10. Ponz de Leon M, Sassotelli R, Benatti P, Roncucci L, Identification of hereditary nonpolyposis colorectal cancer in the general population. *Cancer* 1993; **71**: 3493–501.

11. Heald RJ, Ryall RD, Husband E, The mesorectum in rectal cancer surgery: clue to pelvic recurrence. *Br J Surg* 1982; **69**: 613–16.

12. Hohenberger W, Hermanek Jr P, Hermanek P, Gall FP, Decision-making in curative rectum carcinoma surgery. *Onkologie* 1992; **15**: 209–20.

13. Zirngibl H, Husemann B, Hermanek P, Intraoperative spillage of tumor cells in surgery for rectal cancer. *Dis Colon Rectum* 1990; **33**: 610–14.

14. Hermanek P Jr, Multiviscerale Resektion beim kolorektalen Karzinom – Erfahrungen der SGKRK-Studie. *Langenbecks Arch Chir* 1992; Suppl II (Kongreßber): 95–100.

15. Gall FP, Hermanek P, Update of the German experience with local excision of rectal cancer. *Surg Oncol Clinics N Am* 1992; **1**: 99–109.

16. Hermanek P, Marzoli GP (eds), *Lokale Therapie des Rektumkarzinoms. Verfahren in kurativer Intention.* Berlin: Springer-Verlag, 1994.

17. Hermanek P, Giedl J, Neues aus der chirurgischen Pathologie des kolorektalen Karzinoms. *Wien med Wschr* 1988; **138**: 292–6.

18. Jatzko G, Lisberg P, Wette V, Improving survival rates for patients with colorectal cancer. *Br J Surg* 1992; **79**: 588–91.

19. Scholefield JH, Northover JMA, Surgical management of rectal cancer. *Br J Surg* 1995; **82**: 745–8.

20. Pezim ME, Nicholls RJ, Survival after high or low ligation of the inferior mesenteric artery during curative surgery for rectal cancer. *Ann Surg* 1984; **200**: 729–33.

21. Dukes CE, The spread of cancer of the rectum. *Br J Surg* 1930; **12**: 643–8.

22. Kyriakos M, The President's cancer, the Dukes classification, and confusion. *Arch Path Labor Med* 1985; **109**: 1063–6.

23. American Joint Committee on Cancer (AJCC), *Manual for Staging of Cancer*, 4th edn (Beahrs OH, Henson DE, Hutter RVP, Kennedy JB, eds). Philadelphia: Lippincott, 1992.

23a. UICC, *TNM Classification of Malignant Tumours*, 5th edn (Sobin LH, Wittekind Ch, eds). New York: Wiley, 1997.

24. NIH Consensus Conference, Adjuvant therapy for patients with colon and rectal cancer. *J Am Med Assoc* 1990; **264**: 1444–50.

25. UICC, *TNM Supplement 1993. A Commentary on Uniform Use* (Hermanek P, Henson DE, Hutter RVP, Sobin LH, eds). Berlin: Springer-Verlag, 1993.

26. Scott KWM, Grace RH, Detection of lymph node metastases in colorectal carcinoma before and after fat clearance. *Br J Surg* 1989; **76**: 1165–7.

27. Hermanek P, Gospodarowicz MK, Henson DE et al (eds), *Prognostic Factors in Cancer.* Berlin: Springer-Verlag, 1995.

28. Hermanek P, Wittekind Ch, The pathologist and the residual tumor (R) classification. *Pathol Res Pract* 1994; **190**: 115–23.

29. Hermanek P, Hutter RVP, Sobin LH, Prognostic grouping; the next step in tumor classification. *J Cancer Res Clin Oncol* 1990; **116:** 513–16.

30. Hermanek P, Evaluation of new prognostic factors in oncology. *Virch Arch Pathol* 1995; **427:** 335–6.

31. MacFarlane JK, Ryall RDH, Heald RJ, Mesorectal excision for rectal cancer. *Lancet* 1993; **341:** 457–60.

32. Heald RJ, Rectal cancer: the surgical options. *Eur J Cancer* 1995; **31A:** 1189–92.

33. Arbman G, Nilsson E, Hollböök O, Sjödahl R, Local recurrence following total mesorectal excision for rectal cancer. *Br J Surg* 1996; **83:** 375–9.

34. Hermanek P, *Pathologische Begutachtung von Tumoren.* Erlangen: Perimed, 1983.

35. Japanese Research Society for Cancer of the Colon and Rectum, General rules for clinical and pathological studies on cancer of the colon, rectum and anus. *Jpn J Surg* 1983; **13:** 557–73.

36. UKCCCR (United Kingdom Co-ordinating Committee on Cancer Research), *Handbook for the Clinico-Pathological Assessment and Staging of Colorectal Cancer.* London: UKCCCR, 1989.

37. Rosai J, *Ackerman's Surgical Pathology*, 7th edn. St Louis, MO: Mosby, 1989.

38. Lewin KJ, Riddell RH, Weinstein WM, *Gastrointestinal Pathology and its Clinical Implications.* Tokyo: Igaku-Shoin, 1992.

39. Henson DE, Hutter RVP, Sobin LH, Bowman HE, for the members of the Cancer Committee, College of American Pathologists, and the Task Force for Protocols on the Examination of Specimens from Patients with Colorectal Cancer, Protocol for the examination of specimens removed from patients with colorectal carcinoma. *Arch Pathol Lab Med* 1994; **118:** 122–5.

40. Wagner G, Hermanek P, *Organspezifische Tumordokumentation.* Berlin: Springer-Verlag, 1995.

41. Association of Directors of Anatomical and Surgical Pathology, Recommendations for the reporting of resected large intestinal carcinomas. *Hum Pathol* 1996; **27:** 5–8.

42. Rosai J, *Ackerman's Surgical Pathology*, 8th edn. St Louis, MO: Mosby, 1996.

43. Hermanek P (ed), *Diagnostische Standards. Lungen-, Magen-, Pankreas- und kolorektales Karzinom.* München: W Zuckschwerdt, 1995.

44. Adam IJ, Mohamdee MO, Martin IG et al, Role of circumferential margin involvement in the local recurrence of rectal cancer. *Lancet* 1994; **334:** 707–11.

45. Hermanek P, Qualitätsmanagement bei Diagnose und Therapie kolorektaler Karzinome. *Leber Magen Darm* 1996; **26:** 20–4.

46. Hermanek P, Data collection aspects for the design of adjuvant treatment protocols in colorectal carcinoma. *Onkologie* 1991; **14:** 491–7.

47. Hermanek P, Long-term results of a German prospective multicenter study on colo-rectal cancer. In: *Recent Advances in Management of Digestive Cancer* (Takahashi T, ed). Tokyo: Springer-Verlag, 1993.

48. Hermanek P, Wiebelt H, Staimmer D, Riedl St, and the German Study Group Colo-Rectal Carcinoma (SGCRC), Prognostic factors of rectum carcinoma – experience of the German multicentre study SGCRC. *Tumori* 1995; **81**(Suppl): 60–4.

49. Hermanek P Jr, Wiebelt H, Riedl St et al, und die Studiengruppe Kolorektales Karzinom (SGKRK), Langzeitergebnisse der chirurgischen Therapie des Coloncarcinoms. Ergebnisse der Studiengruppe Kolorektales Karzinom (SGKRK). *Chirurg* 1994; **65:** 287–97.

50. Capella C, Heitz PhU, Höfler H et al, Revised classification of neuroendocrine tumours of the lung, pancreas and gut. *Virchows Arch* 1995; **425:** 547–60.

4

Surgery for rectal cancer

Rudolf Raab, Hans-Joachim Meyer

INTRODUCTION

Rectal carcinoma is still one of the most frequent cancers in so-called developed countries.[1,2] Complete tumour removal is the only measure that gives prospects of cure for the patient. During the last 25 years, a better survival of all afflicted has been achieved by an increase in curative (i.e. R0) resections and by a decrease in perioperative mortality. Apart from this, in the opinion of many authors,[3–6] no substantial improvement of prognosis could be attained. The most important prognostic factor is the tumour stage according to UICC or Dukes. Next to this, the individual surgeon performing the operation is of decisive importance.[7,8] There is great variability between institutions and surgeons with regard to local recurrence rates and overall results of surgery.[9] Thus the comments of one of the pioneers in abdominal surgery, the famous German surgeon Johann von Mikulicz, dating from the year 1903 is still valid:[10] *'Wenn wir auch heute schon sagen können, dass das Darmcarcinom eines der dankbarsten Gebiete der Abdominalchirurgie abgiebt, so lassen unsere Resultate doch manches zu wünschen übrig. Sie müssen durch eine Vervollkommnung der Technik besser werden.'* ('Although even today we may say that bowel cancer is one of the most satisfactory fields in abdominal surgery, our results leave much to be desired. They must be improved by a perfection of technique.')

Radical resection of rectal cancer is the rule. In our opinion, technical irresectability does not really exist, because there is no neighbouring structure that cannot be resected en bloc with the tumour. Therefore the only reasons for leaving the tumour in place are the very rare situations of general inoperability, and the judgement that resection is of no value for the patient because of widespread formation of irresectable metastases. Cases in which local R0 resection is not feasible are very infrequent. Furthermore, this can generally only be recognized after crossing the 'point of no return' during the course of the operation. Radical resection can be done safely even in the ninth or tenth decade of life. Old age alone is not a contraindication.

Nowadays, in general, the resection rate should be above 90% and the operative mortality should be below 5%.[11–14] The first essentials for operative success are good preparation of the bowel and prophylactic antibiotics. Postoperatively, a close-meshed follow-up is necessary, because early recognized metastases or local recurrences can be reoperated upon in some cases with curative intention, and because in 2–3% of cases a second metachronous carcinoma occurs.[15] Treatment of recurrences and metastases depends on the individual situation. In these cases interdisciplinary concepts will probably gain more importance in the future.

PREOPERATIVE DIAGNOSTICS

Obligatory examinations

Besides the common preparatory measures for the operation, the following examinations should routinely be done in patients with rectal cancer:

- *Tumour marker carcinoembryonic antigen (CEA), possibly Ca 19-9 as well.* The main purpose of the determination of tumour markers is to get an initial value for the postoperative follow-up examinations.[16] Immediate therapeutic consequences may arise if the initial CEA value is very high. Values above 25 µg/l give reasonable suspicion of distant spread; values above 50 µg/l are as good as a proof of blood-borne metastases.
- *Abdominal ultrasonography* is the most important measure to exclude liver metastases and ureteral dilatation. With improvements in this method, intravenous pyelography is no longer obligatory but only indicated if there is suspicion of ureteral obstruction.
- *Chest X-ray in two planes.* The radiographic examination of the chest is generally sufficient to exclude lung metastases.
- *Complete colonoscopy with examination of the entire rectum and colon up to the caecum.* Endoscopy is the most important measure to localize the tumour and to exclude synchronous adenomas (frequency 25–50%) as well as synchronous carcinomas (frequency about 4%). During endoscopy, a tumour

biopsy should be taken to prove the diagnosis. If preoperatively a complete colonoscopy is impossible because of a stenosing tumour, it should be done postoperatively – and in case of any doubt even intraoperatively. To determine the exact distance of the lower edge of the tumour from the anal verge, it is always recommended that the surgeon himself perform an endoscopy with a rigid rectoscope in addition to the colonoscopy. This is because the distance is not infrequently overestimated during examinations with the flexible instrument.

- *A double-contrast barium enema* is only the second-best method for bowel examination, because no biopsy can be taken. In addition, evacuation of the contrast medium may be delayed or incomplete, especially if there is a stenosis due to the tumour. Remaining barium at the time of the operation might be harmful to the patient if it spills into the abdominal cavity.

Optional examinations

There are some complementary examinations in rectal cancer. Some of them are not yet (e.g. endorectal ultrasound) or are no longer (e.g. intravenous pyelography) part of the routine diagnostic measures:

- It is possible by endorectal ultrasonography to determine the depth of infiltration of the bowel wall (T-classification) with an accuracy of about 90%.[17-19] This method serves for preoperative T-classification if in early stages (uT1) an operation of limited radicality or in advanced stages (uT3/uT4) neoadjuvant therapy is considered.
- A computed tomography of the abdomen and the small pelvis may be helpful for planning the operation if there is any suspicion of distant metastases or infiltration of neighbouring organs or structures. However, this is seldom absolutely necessary. A CT scan of the chest is indicated if lung metastases are suspected – but only if

therapeutic consequences would result from the findings (e.g. a lung resection or a limited radical resection of the bowel).

- A cystoscopy is always indicated if there is suspicion of an entero-vesical fistula or direct tumour infiltration to the urinary bladder. Both occur only rarely.
- Nuclear magnetic resonance tomography might give additional information in the case of a T4 tumour, a local recurrence, or metastases. A definitive assessment of its relative importance is not yet possible.

Methods under clinical evaluation

- *Positron emission tomography.* PET examination allows a differentiation between scar and tumour tissue on the basis of different metabolic activities.[20] This may be of clinical importance, especially if a local recurrence is suspected after extirpation of the rectum.
- *Immunoscintigraphy.* This method is used to localize local recurrences or metastases.[19,21] So far, it has not gained any clinical importance – primarily because of its lack of sensitivity. Moreover, if murine antibodies are used, there is a risk of HAMA formation, which may limit the possible therapeutic use of antibodies in the later course of the disease.

Histological examination

As pointed out above, a histological confirmation of the diagnosis should be aimed at. In the lower third of the rectum the differentiation between adenocarcinomas and squamous cell carcinomas is of importance because of different therapeutic approaches towards the two entities. If local excision is considered, a preoperative grading is necessary, because operations of limited radicality are contraindicated in high-grade malignancy (G3/G4). In general, the same applies for tumours that show invasion of veins or lymphatic vessels.

SPECIFIC PREOPERATIVE MEASURES

Cleansing of the bowel

The measures for preoperative cleansing of the bowel mainly depend on the degree of stenosis of the bowel lumen. The method of choice is an orthograde lavage,[22,23] which is always possible if there is a flat or ulcerated tumour without significant stenosis. The patient should drink a solution of polyethylene glycol (PEG), which is not absorbable. Thus absorption of greater amounts of water can be prevented by an osmotic effect. If the patient is not able to drink the necessary 3–4 litres of fluid, it may also be given by a feeding tube placed in the duodenum. In this case greater amounts of the solution are needed (6–8 litres or more). The fluid should always be at body temperature, and the lavage should be continued until nearly clean liquid is discharged. If cardiac symptoms or crampy pain in the abdomen arise, the lavage should be stopped. Although PEG has no or only negligible side-effects on the cardiovascular system, in cases of severely impaired cardiac or renal function orthograde lavage should be considered contraindicated. If moderate stenosis exists, an attempt with orthograde lavage (possibly fractionated) is justified. Alternatively, the patient is given a fully absorbable diet and daily high enemas for 5–7 days. If there is severe stenosis, the preparation consists of complete parenteral nutrition and repeated high enemas for 1–2 weeks. In addition, intraoperative lavage might be required. The rare cases with a complete ileus necessitate an immediate operation, with intraoperative lavage. If this is not possible or not sufficient, a subtotal or total colectomy must be considered.

Antibiotics

Prophylactic administration of antibiotics is now a routine measure in colorectal surgery.[24] A broad-spectrum antibiotic that is also effective on anaerobes is given as a single shot at the beginning of anaesthesia. Antibiotic treatment should only be continued if there is an ileus, a perforation, or a similar situation with high risk of postoperative infection.

Colostomy

With the patient lying on the operating table, the determination of the best localization for a preternatural anus might be impossible. Therefore, if a temporary or definite colostomy is being considered, the exact possible positions must be marked preoperatively with waterproof ink after examining the patient in the sitting and upright positions.

PRINCIPLES OF SURGICAL MANAGEMENT

The operative removal of the primary tumour with its draining lymphatic vessels is the basis of the surgical therapy of colorectal cancer. Surgical technique and radicality are of greatest importance.[25–28] No adjuvant therapy can ever make good what was not done surgically. Spacious access is required for a safe and radical operation. We recommend a long median laparotomy. This allows exact exploration of the entire abdomen and the performance of all interventions on colon and rectum, including extension of the resection to other organs. Opening the abdomen is followed by palpation and inspection of the abdominal organs. Intraoperative ultrasound of the liver is always desirable. In no case can decisions be based on the presence of liver metastases that are diagnosed by palpation only. In judging the R0-resectability of a tumour, it should be kept in mind that infiltration of surrounding tissues or organs might be mimicked by concomitant inflammation. Only 50–60% of all supposed T4 tumours, in fact, show a crossing of the organ borders histologically. Nevertheless, just the suspicion of infiltration mandates the inclusion of the respective organs or border layers in the resection. As a general rule, a monobloc resection should be possible. The worst possible incident during an operation for colorectal cancer is a tear or cut of the tumour. In such a case the chance of cure decreases rapidly.

A negative influence of perioperative blood or plasma substitution on survival is possible.[29] Even if this has not yet been definitively proved, unnecessary transfusions should be avoided by a strict blood-saving operative technique.

CURATIVE SURGICAL INTERVENTIONS FOR PRIMARY RECTAL CANCER

All rectal carcinomas can be removed by one of the two standard procedures: anterior resection or abdominoperineal extirpation. Sphincter-saving resections are increasingly used. Provided the entire mesorectum is removed, this is as good as or even better than those operations sacrificing the anus.[30–32] The definitive decision on sphincter preservation is only possible intraoperatively. It depends on the individual situation and the extent of the tumour. If the tumour is not too big and the sphincter function is normal, there should be a minimum distance of 1 cm between the lower edge of the tumour and the dentate line – the lowest possible level of resection. Thus the distance from the anal verge should be at least 3.5–4 cm. If the level of resection is higher than the dentate line, a greater safety margin of approximately 3 cm is necessary.

Anterior resection of the rectum

The surgical procedure is now well standardized.[33–35] This is due not least to Bill Heald and Warren Enker.[27,36–38] With the patient in a lithotomy position, the operation starts with a midline incision, abdominal exploration, and intraoperative ultrasound examination of the liver. In all operations with curative intent the inferior mesenteric vessels are divided centrally – the artery at the level of its offspring from the aorta, and the vein at the level of the lower edge of the pancreas. For this purpose, mobilization of the duodenum with dissection of the ligament of Treitz is required as a first step. After severing the vessels, the sigmoid colon, the descending colon and the splenic flexure are detached. If this is done keeping strictly within the right plane, there is no need to identify or even snare the left ureter. The colon is divided in the region of the descending or upper sigmoid part. The mobilization of the rectum from the small pelvis requires meticulous care, exactness and attention in order to combine the greatest possible oncological radicality with the greatest possible preservation of sexual and voiding functions. The mesorectum must always be removed completely – at least if the tumour is located in the lower or middle third of the rectum. At the same time, particular care should be taken of the autonomic nerve system, which consists of the superior hypogastric plexus, the right and left hypogastric nerves, the inferior hypogastric plexuses, and subplexuses supplying the different pelvic organs.[39,40] These requirements cannot be fulfilled by mobilizing the rectum in the traditional way dorsally with the surgeon's bare hands and laterally by means of clamps and ligatures or even staplers. Instead of this, only scissors and retractors should be used, and the hypogastric nerves should be identified and preserved unless they are directly infiltrated by the tumour. Dorsally the dissection follows a plane right above the fascia of Waldeyer. Lateral to the rectum, the tissue is sharply dissected along the roughly sagittal layer of the internal iliac vessels and the inferior hypogastric plexuses respectively. Along this way, the only bleeding vessels worth mentioning are the middle rectal arteries. Mostly these can be stanched by bipolar coagulation – undersewing is seldom necessary. Only after the dorsal and lateral mobilization has been completed down to the pelvic floor is the bowel detached anteriorly. In doing this, care should be taken not to injure the dorsal wall of the vagina or the seminal vesicles and the prostate respectively. Nevertheless, if a T4 tumour is suspected, all the respective organs should be included in the monobloc resection.

At the end of the pelvic part of the operation, a definitive decision is made about whether an anterior resection is possible or an abdomino-intersphincteric resection or even an abdomino-perineal extirpation of the rectum is necessary. If the resection can be done anteriorly, a right-angled clamp is positioned below the tumour, and the bowel wall is divided below this clamp.

We rinse the pelvis after the tumour removal with distilled water. This is followed by re-establishment of bowel continuity by a termino-terminal anastomosis. In the case of a very deep resection, we prefer the formation of a short (5–6 cm) J-pouch of the colon with a pouch–rectal or a pouch–anal anastomosis. In both instances it is of secondary importance whether the anastomosis is hand-sewn or done with a circular stapler. The use of staplers presupposes mastery of the standard technique to cope with all possible complications. The double-stapling technique is especially controversial. The increased risk of anastomotic leakage probably outweighs the possible advantage of the technique that it may be time-saving. The formation of a double-barrelled transverse colostomy (or ileostomy) is always up to the surgeon's discretion. From our point of view, it has proved to be wise to decide for a protective stoma in all cases of doubt.

Abdomino-intersphincteric resection

For most tumours in the lower third of the rectum, a standard anterior resection is not possible. If the lower edge of the tumour is at least 1 cm above the dentate line and there is no direct infiltration of the levator ani, an intersphincteric resection may be considered.[41–43] The abdominal part of the operation is identical to that described above. However, no right-angled clamp is positioned, and the bowel wall is divided not from above but transanally. After exposing the situs by means of one or two anal retractors (we use two Gelpi retractors positioned crosswise), the mucosa and the internal anal sphincter are divided at the level of the dentate line. The remains of the rectum are released intersphincterically, and the specimen is removed anteriorly. In our opinion, a colo-anal pouch formation is obligatory in these cases. But, despite such a re-creation of a presphincteric reservoir, disturbances in continence may occur. Thus only patients with an unaltered sphincter function are eligible for this procedure. A transanally hand-sewn anastomosis is obligatory, because there is no material left that can be used for a purse-string suture.

Abdomino-perineal extirpation of the rectum

In about 5–10% of tumours of the middle third and about 30–40% of tumours of the lower third of the rectum, the anal sphincter cannot be preserved. Nevertheless, the abdominal part of the operation is again identical to the anterior resection (see above). Following complete anterior mobilization of the rectum, the operation is continued from a perineal approach, whereas a simultaneous operation with two teams from above and below is incompatible with the demands for oncologically and functionally sufficient surgery as described above. The anus is closed with a purse-string suture. After dividing the skin and the subcutaneous fat, the levator ani is dissected cranio-laterally as far as possible. The preparation begins dorsally with the division of the ano-coccygeal ligament, and is continued laterally. Again the ventral dissection is the last part, because there is the highest risk of damaging the prostatic plexus, the corpora cavernosa-plexus or the urethra. The specimen may be removed in either direction, and the perineal wound is closed primarily.

If postoperative radiotherapy is considered or at least possible, care should be taken to keep the small bowel out of the small pelvis. The best measure to achieve this goal is anterior resection, because the pelvis is filled with parts of the large bowel, which is not so sensitive to radiation. In the case of an abdomino-perineal resection, a pedicled omental graft may be used.[44] Only if this is not possible is an absorbable mesh inserted and fixed between the symphysis and the promontory to prevent the small bowel from descending into the pelvis.[45] However, with this method, a hollow space is left behind in the pelvis, which carries the risk of infection.

RESULTS OF TREATMENT

At Hannover Medical School we have operated upon 966 patients with primary rectal cancer in the 20-year period from 1971 to 1990. Follow-up was complete until 1995. The median age was 64 years (18–87 years). Figure 4.1 shows the

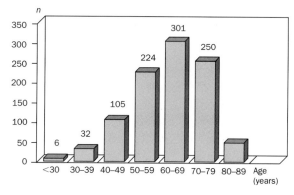

Figure 4.1 Distribution of age in patients with primary rectal cancer.

Table 4.1 Relative frequency of cancer in the different parts of the rectum

Period of time	Upper third	Middle third	Lower third
1971–75 ($n = 191$)	27.7%	53.9%	18.3%
1976–80 ($n = 313$)	37.1%	39.6%	23.3%
1981–85 ($n = 268$)	28.7%	38.8%	32.5%
1986–90 ($n = 194$)	19.6%	32.0%	48.5%
1971–90 ($n = 966$)	29.4%	40.7%	29.9%

frequency in the different age groups. Overall, most of the tumours were located in the middle third of the rectum, but the proportion of lower tumours was increasing rapidly. In the last 5-year period we saw nearly 50% of the tumours in the lower third (Table 4.1). Likewise, an increase in the number of the more advanced stages, especially UICC IV, could be observed. Overall, the distribution of the stages was 29.4%, 29.5%, 24.4% and 16.7% for UICC stages I, II, III and IV respectively.

Sphincter-saving resections were performed with increasing frequency. Figure 4.2 shows the development for the different parts of the rectum during the 1970s and 1980s. In the last 5 years (1991–96), only 4% of the patients with tumours of the middle rectum and only 38% of those with tumours of the lower rectum underwent an abdomino-perineal resection. In 78% R0 resections were possible, whereas in 21.2% only an R2 resection was possible. This was mostly because of irresectable distant metastases (see Table 4.2). Microscopic residual tumour, i.e. R1 resection, was a rare exception (0.8%). The total complication rate was rather high (41%), but most of the complications were minor ones like urinary-tract or wound infections. Anastomotic leakage occurred in 7.3% and adverse cardio-respiratory events were seen in 8.6%. Operative mortality could be lowered from 9.9% in the early 1970s to 3.6% in the second half of the 1980s. The remaining deaths were due to cardio-circulatory complications.

The observed overall 5-year survival rate was 47.2% (mortality included). After R0 resection, nearly 60% of all patients survived 5 years, while the rate for non-radical resection was only 3.3% (see Figure 4.3). Besides the R-classification, the tumour stage according to UICC was the most important prognostic factor. As shown in Table 4.3, survival rates could be improved significantly over time for stage I and II tumours, but not for stage III lesions. Most impressive was the progress in the cases with distant metastases, i.e. UICC IV. While 25 years ago none of such patients survived, at the end of the 1980s the 5-year survival rate was 8.1%, and now it is 13.2%. This is an impressive reflection of the success of surgery for liver (and

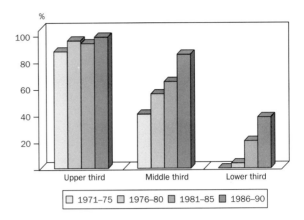

Figure 4.2 Development of the proportion of sphincter-saving resections according to the different parts of the rectum.

Table 4.2 R-classification of the operation in relation to the UICC-stage classification

Stage	R0 resection	R1/2 resection
UICC I	98.9%	1.1%
UICC II	96.0%	4.0%
UICC III	92.0%	8.0%
UICC IV	5.8%	94.2%

lung) metastases. Thus estimates that only around 5% of all patients with liver metastases may profit from liver resection appear clearly to be too conservative. Nonetheless, much is left to future efforts in adjuvant, additive and palliative treatment.

PROCEDURES WITH LIMITED RADICALITY

In some cases of rectal cancer a limited radical approach is sufficient, either with curative intent in early invasive tumours or with palliative intent if there are already irresectable metastases or the patient is inoperable for major abdominal surgery.

Table 4.3 Observed 5-year survival rates following R0 resection of primary rectal cancer according to UICC-stage classification (operative mortality included)

Stage	1971–75	1976–80	1981–85	1986–90	1971–90
UICC I	67.7%	74.3%	83.9%	81.4%	75.7%
UICC II	51.0%	57.7%	60.0%	80.0%	59.4%
UICC III	40.5%	41.5%	40.3%	39.4%	40.4%

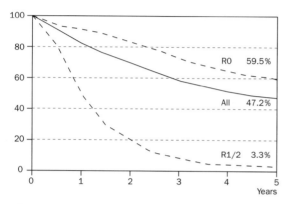

Figure 4.3 Observed overall survival following resection of primary rectal cancer (operative mortality included, not corrected for age).

Table 4.4 pN-category in relation to pT-category and grading in primary rectal cancer

pT-category and grading	Positive lymph nodes (pN1–4)
pT1, G1	3.0%
pT1, G2	3.4%
pT1, G3	(n = 0)
pT2, G1	17.8%
pT2, G2	26.4%
pT2, G3	40.0%

Curative intent

Early invasive tumours of the lower and middle third of the rectum may be treated by a local excision. A prerequisite is a preoperative endoanal ultrasound to determine the T-category and a histological examination of a tumour biopsy. In uT1 tumours the risk of lymph-node metastases is around 3%, and therefore within the range of the operative mortality of anterior or abdomino-perineal resections. In uT2 tumours positive nodes are found already in about 20% (see Table 4.4). The situation is analogous for G3/G4 tumours (high-grade malignancy) and for tumours with a histologically proven invasion of lymph vessels or veins. Postoperative radiation therapy cannot improve the results in patients with T2 or T3 tumours.[46,47] Thus only patients with good or moderately differentiated uT1 tumours without infiltration into lymph vessels or veins are eligible for a limited excision with curative intent.[48]

The access is transanally, either by a normal anal retractor or by the transanal endoscopic microsurgery (TEM) system according to Buess.[49–51] The tumour is removed by a full-thickness excision of the rectal wall with a portion of perirectal fat and a safety margin of 0.5–1 cm. The defect in the bowel wall is closed by a running or interrupted suture with absorbable material. If the definite histological examination of the specimen shows a different result from the initial examination of the biopsy (e.g. a higher T-category or a perirectal lymph-node metastasis) then a radical re-operation should be carried out unless there are severe contraindications. An alternative to the transanal approach is the Kraske technique.[52] The tumour is then removed via a parasacral incision and a posterior rectotomy. This approach even allows for segmental resections of the low or middle rectum.

Palliative intent

As has been pointed out, it is very seldom indicated to leave the tumour in place. If a radical operation gives no prospects of cure or at least good palliation, procedures with local destruction or partial ablation of the tumour might be justified. In our institution the rate of such interventions is less than 2% of all rectal cancers. Several techniques are described in the literature, including treatment modalities with heat or cryosurgery. We prefer well-aimed local tumour reduction under sight by means of a resectoscope, which is normally used to treat benign prostate hyperplasia. This has several advantages: it is available in all hospitals with a urological department, it is easy to handle, it yields material for a histological examination, the lumen of the rectum can be modelled up to the desired diameter, the method is safe, and it might be repeated under regional anaesthesia as often as necessary.[53]

SURGICAL TREATMENT OF LOCOREGIONAL RECURRENCE

In most instances, early anastomotic recurrence can be treated sufficiently by a repeated anterior resection. The planes of oncologically correct rectal surgery are very often found untouched during the re-operation. In many of the advanced cases with broad extraluminal growth, R0 re-resection is still possible. In our experience, this gave a renewed chance of cure for about 30% of the patients. But such operations are mostly multivisceral resections. Therefore they should be reserved for specialized centres. Sometimes a complete pelvic exenteration or a sacral resection is needed. These are often desperate interventions that are only justified by the desperate situation of the patient. Thus it is always the patient's sole decision whether he or she is willing to undergo extended surgery of such a kind.

Nearly all cases of anastomotic recurrence and many cases of local recurrence of rectal cancer are caused by the initial procedure, although this cannot be proved for an individual case. Actually, it can be stated that the variability of local recurrence rates between surgeons is in the range of 5–50%. Therefore the surgeon is one of the most important prognostic factors in colorectal cancer, and by far the best method to deal with locoregional recurrence is to avoid it by an adequate technique during the primary operation.

REFERENCES

1. Haenszel W, Correa P, Epidemiology of large bowel cancer. In: *Epidemiology of Cancer of the Digestive Tract* (Correa P, Haenszel W, eds). The Hague: Martinus Nijhoff, 1982; 85–126.
2. Schatzkin A, Schiffman MH, Etiology and prevention: the epidemiologic perspective. In: *Colorectal Cancer* (Wanebo HJ, ed). St Louis, MO: Mosby–Year Book, 1993; 3–19.
3. Enblad P, Adami H-O, Bergström R et al, Improved survival of patients with cancers of the colon and rectum. *J Natl Cancer Inst* 1988; **80:** 568–91.
4. Hawley PR, Rectal carcinoma: surgical progress. *Ann R Coll Surg Engl* 1990; **72:** 168–9.
5. Herfarth Ch, Magen- und kolorektale Tumouren – Stagnation? *Schweiz Med Wschr* 1983; **113:** 1272–9.
6. Williams NS, Changing patterns in the treatment of rectal cancer. *Br J Surg* 1989; **76:** 5–6.
7. Fielding LP, Steward-Brown S, Dudley HA, Surgeon-related variables and the clinical trial. *Lancet* 1978; **i:** 778–9.
8. McArdle CS, Hole D, Impact of variability among surgeons on postoperative morbidity and

mortality and ultimate survival. *Br Med J* 1991; **302**: 1501–5.

9. Hermanek Jr P, Wiebelt H, Riedl S et al, and Studiengruppe Kolorektales Karzinom (SGKRK), Langzeitergebnisse der chirurgischen Therapie des Coloncarcinoms. Ergebnisse der Studiengruppe Kolorektales Karzinom (SGKRK). *Chirurg* 1994; **65**: 287–97.

10. von Mikulicz J, Chirurgische Erfahrungen über das Darmcarcinom. *Arch f Klin Chir* 1903; **69**: 28–47.

11. Hermanek P, Wiebelt H, Staimmer D, Riedl S, Prognostic factors of rectum carcinoma – experience of the German Multicenter Study SGCRC. German Study Group Colorectal Carcinoma. *Tumori* 1995; **81**(Suppl 3): 60–4.

12. McDermott FT, Hughes ESR, Pihl E et al, Comparative results of surgical management of single carcinomas of the colon and rectum: a series of 1939 patients managed by one surgeon. *Br J Surg* 1981; **68**: 850–5.

13. Moreaux J, Catala M, Carcinoma of the colon: long-term survival and prognosis after surgical treatment in a series of 798 patients. *World J Surg* 1987; **11**: 804–9.

14. Northover JMA, Results of curative surgery for colorectal cancer. *Scand J Gastroenterol* 1988; **23**(Suppl 149): 155–8.

15. Raab R, Werner U, Löhlein D, Colorectale Mehrfachcarcinome: Eigenschaften und Langzeitprognose. *Chirurg* 1988; **59**: 96–100.

16. Moore M, Jones DJ, Schofield PF, Harden DG, Current status of tumor markers in large bowel cancer. *World J Surg* 1989; **13**: 52–9.

17. Beynon J, McC Mortensen NJ, Channer JL, Rigby H, Rectal endosonography accurately predicts depth of penetration in rectal cancer. *Int J Colorect Dis* 1992; **7**: 4–7.

18. Glaser F, Schlag P, Herfarth Ch, Endorectal ultrasonography for the assessment of invasion of rectal tumours and lymph node involvement. *Br J Surg* 1990; **77**: 883–7.

19. Feifel G, Hildebrandt U, New diagnostic imaging in rectal cancer: endosonography and immunoscintigraphy. *World J Surg* 1992; **16**: 841–7.

20. Lehner B, Schlag P, Strauss L et al, Die Wertigkeit der Positronen-Emmissions-Tomographie für die Diagnostik des Rektumkarzinomrezidivs. *Zentralbl Chir* 1990; **115**: 813–17.

21. Hölting T, Schlag P, Steinbächer M et al, The value of immunoszintigraphy for the operative retreatment of colorectal cancer. *Cancer* 1989; **64**: 830–3.

22. DiPalma JA, Brady CE, Colon cleansing for diagnostic and surgical procedures: polyethylene glycol–electrolyte lavage solution. *Am J Gastroenterol* 1989; **84**: 1008–16.

23. Hewitt J, Reeve J, Rigby J, Cox AG, Whole-gut irrigation in preparation for large-bowel surgery. *Lancet* 1973; **ii**: 337–40.

24. Menaker GJ, The use of antibiotics in surgical treatment of the colon. *Surg Gynecol Obstet* 1987; **164**: 581–6.

25. Hermanek P, Sobin LH, Colorectal carcinoma. In: *Prognostic Factors in Cancer* (Hermanek P, Gospodarowicz MK, Henson DE et al, eds). Berlin: Springer-Verlag, 1995; 64–79.

26. Hermanek P, Hohenberger W, The importance of volume in colorectal cancer surgery. *Eur J Surg Oncol* 1996; **22**: 213–15.

27. MacFarlane JK, Ryall RDH, Heald RJ, Mesorectal excision for rectal cancer. *Lancet* 1993; **341**: 457–60.

28. Sugarbaker PH, Corlew S, Influence of surgical techniques on survival in patients with colorectal cancer. *Dis Colon Rectum* 1982; **25**: 545–57.

29. Francis DMA, Relationship between blood transfusion and tumour behaviour. *Br J Surg* 1991; **78**: 1420–8.

30. Bozetti F, Mariani L, Miceli R et al, Cancer of the low and middle rectum: local and distant recurrences, and survival in 350 radically resected patients. *J Surg Oncol* 1996; **62**: 207–13.

31. Husemann B, Löw R, Panhans W et al, Überlebenszeit und Lebensqualität beim operierten Dickdarmkarzinom. *Zentralbl Chir* 1977; **102**: 1549–58.

32. Jatzko G, Lisborg P, Wette V, Improving survival rates for patients with colorectal cancer. *Br J Surg* 1992; **79**: 588–91.

33. Köckerling F, Gall FP, Chirurgische Standards beim Rektumkarzinom. *Chirurg* 1994; **65**: 593–603.

34. Rosen HR, Schiessel R, Die vordere Rectumresection. *Chirurg* 1996; **67**: 99–109.

35. Stelzner F, Begründung, Technik und Ergebnisse der knappen Kontinenzresektion beim Rektumkarzinom. *Zentralbl Chir* 1992; **117**: 63–6.

36. Enker WE, Designing the optimal surgery for rectal carcinoma. *Cancer* 1996; **78**: 1847–50.

37. Heald RJ, Ryall RDH, Husband E, The mesorectum in rectal cancer surgery: clue to pelvic recurrence. *Br J Surg* 1982; **69**: 613–16.

38. Heald RJ, The 'holy plane' of rectal surgery. *J R Soc Med* 1988; **81**: 503–8.

39. Lepor H, Gregermann M, Crosby R et al, Precise localization of the autonomic nerves from the pelvis plexus to the corpora cavernosa: a detailed anatomical study of the adult male pelvis. *J Urol* 1985; **133:** 207–12.

40. Walsh PC, Schlegel PN, Radical pelvic surgery with preservation of sexual function. *Ann Surg* 1988; **208:** 391–400.

41. Parks AG, Per-anal anastomosis. *World J Surg* 1982; **6:** 531–8.

42. Parks AG, Percy JP, Resection and sutured colo-anal anastomosis for rectal carcinoma. *Br J Surg* 1982; **69:** 301–4.

43. Schumpelick V, Braun J, Die intersphinctäre Rectumresektion mit radikaler Mesorectum-excision und coloanaler Anastomose. *Chirurg* 1996; **67:** 110–20.

44. DeLuca FR, Ragins H, Construction of an omental envelope as a method of excluding the small intestine from the field of postoperative irradiation to the pelvis. *Surg Gynecol Obstet* 1985; **160:** 365–6.

45. Kavanah MT, Feldmann MI, Devereux DF, Kondi ES, New surgical approach to minimize radiation-associated small bowel injury in patients with pelvic malignancies requiring surgery and high-dose irradiation. *Cancer* 1985; **56:** 1300–4.

46. Minsky BD, Cohen AM, Enker WE, Mies C, Sphincter preservation in rectal cancer by local excision and local radiation therapy. *Cancer* 1991; **67:** 908–14.

47. Willet CG, Tepper JE, Donnelly S et al, Patterns of failure following local excision and local excision and postoperative radiation therapy for invasive rectal adenocarcinoma. *J Clin Oncol* 1989; **7:** 1003–8.

48. Hermanek P, Guggenmoos-Holzmann I, Gall FP, Prognostic factors in rectal carcinoma. A contribution to the further development of tumor classification. *Dis Colon Rectum* 1989; **32:** 593–9.

49. Berry AR, Souter RG, Campbell WB et al, Endoscopic transanal resection of rectal tumours – a preliminary report of its use. *Br J Surg* 1990; **77:** 134–7.

50. Buess G, Mentges B, Manncke K et al, Technique and results of transanal endoscopic micro-surgery in early rectal cancer. *Am J Surg* 1992; **163:** 63–70.

51. Buess G, Kayser J, Technik und Indikation zur sphinctererhaltenden transanalen Resektion beim Rectumcarcinom. *Chirurg* 1996; **67:** 121–8.

52. Schildberg FW, Wenk H, Der posteriore Zugang zum Rectum. *Chirurg* 1986; **57:** 779–91.

53. Boeminghaus F, Coburg AJ, Transanale Resektion von obstruierenden Rektumtumoren mittels TUR-Technik (TAR). *Fortschr Gastroenterol Endosk* 1986; **15:** 172–6.

5

Conservative treatment in rectal cancer

Philippe Lasser, Pierre Dubé

CONTENTS • **Introduction** • **Local resection** • **Contactherapy** • **Electrocoagulation** • **Conclusions**

INTRODUCTION

Local curative treatments for rectal cancer run up against the dogmas of classical cancer surgery, which consider the best treatment to be the excision of the affected organ and of the various ganglionic relays dependent on that organ. Effectively, these treatments apply only to the tumor, totally disregarding the ganglionic problem. They overlook a possible ganglionic invasion.

They have a double advantage over classic resection surgery, in that they are less mutilating, especially for low cancer (avoiding a definitive colostomy), and they are less shocking. On the other hand, they are subject to local recurrences, which may appear at the tumor site if the resection was incomplete, or on an undetected and untreated invaded mesorectal ganglion. Indications for these local treatments must be rigorous. Several types of local treatment can be applied.

- *Local excision or resection of the tumor.* This has a great advantage over the other techniques, in that it supplies a specimen for examination by the anatomopathologist, who will be in a position to evaluate the

chance of a possible ganglionic invasion, based on a certain number of histopathological prognostic factors.

- *Destruction of the tumor by radiotherapy (contactherapy), electrocoagulation, laser or cryosurgery.* These techniques merely destroy the tumor; therefore one cannot accurately assess its in-depth infiltration and make any predictions as to the risk of ganglionic invasion.

LOCAL RESECTION

Surgical techniques

Several approaches can be used for local resection.

The endoanal or transanal approach
Two types of local excisions can be performed.[1-4]

- *Submucous excision.* After infiltrating the submucosa with an adrenalized saline solution, the mucosa and submucosa are incised with the scalpel 1 cm from the lower pole of the tumor, until the muscularis is reached.

The resection will thus be performed from bottom to top, by gradually lifting the tumor and freeing it from the muscular plan. On the periphery, resection limits must allow for a safety margin of 1 cm. Hemostasis is achieved with an electric scalpel. The surgical wound can be sutured with separate stitches or left open without any risk.

- *Transmural excision (entire rectal wall).* The principle of the resection is the same as above, but it is deeper, affecting the entire thickness of the rectal wall. The perirectal fat is exposed and the rectal muscularis is totally resected. The rectal tumor on its base is referred to the anatomopathologist. Closing the surgical wound is recommended by numerous surgeons, to avoid infection and secondary hemorrhage, but it is not always feasible. Some surgeons[5-7] electrocoagulate the tumor site extensively to complete hemostasis and to destroy a possible tumoral residuum.

This excision of the entire rectal wall can only apply to lower located subdouglasian tumors to avoid peritoneal perforation, and to tumors located on the posterior and lateral surfaces. When the lesion is located on the anterior surface, there is effectively a risk of perforation of the rectovaginal wall in women and a risk of ureteral lesions in men.

Other approaches

- *Kraske's retroanal or transsacral route.*[8] The patient is placed in the prone position after section of the anococcygeal body, the coccyx and eventually the last sacral pieces, and the rectum is approached on its posterior face. Incision of the mesorectum and of the rectal wall provides an excellent opening on the anterior and lateral faces.
- The same applies to *York Masson's posterior transsphincteral route*[9] (*posterior anorectomy*), which involves the total section of the sphincter.
- The *anterior anorectotomy* technique, as described by Toupet,[10] gives an excellent

opening on posterior tumors.

Posterior approach routes are preferable, since they allow exploration of the mesorectum, and the discovery of adenopathies undetected by preoperative examinations. However, they are subject to rectal fistulas (20% of cases), and a temporary colostomy is advisable to avoid them. As to Kraske's route, it does not provide an adequate opening for tumors located rather high (6–10 cm). The endoanal route, then, appears preferable to us.

Operating mortality is practically nil as reported in the various series of publications. Morbidity essentially consists of the falling off of eschars (around postoperative day 5 or 6), which sometimes necessitates repeat surgery. In the Gall and Hermanek series,[1] out of 69 local resections (16 submucous excisions, 31 excisions of the entire wall and 22 excisions by the transsphincteral route), there were 13 complications necessitating new operations (9%). One might occasionally note the remote development of a variously extensive arc-shaped adhesion, the importance of which depends on the extent of the local resection. It rarely hinders the transit, and may be sectioned if too extensive.

The tumor, resting on its base, is totally resected, preferably without fragmentation, and is then placed on cork before it is referred to the anatomopathologist, who will evaluate a certain number of prognostic factors, as described by Morson:[11]

- *degree of parietal infiltration,* using the UICC pTNM classification, which is more precise than Dukes or Aster–Coller: T1 is a tumor invading the mucosa and the submucosa;
- *degree of malignancy* of the tumor, as initially evaluated on preoperative biopsies;
- safety margins, by making several cuts.

Prognostic factors

What criteria can be used to determine whether a rectal cancer can benefit from local treatment? These criteria are clinical and chiefly anatomopathological. The basic objective is to avoid overlooking an underlying ganglionic invasion.

Clinical criteria

Size of tumor

Is there a maximum diameter above which local resection is inconceivable? What is the risk of a ganglion being attacked according to the size of the tumor? Of course, a smaller tumor will be more amenable to local resection. But the diameter of the tumor is no indication of its in-depth extension. The 'small-cancer' concept relates to its size, and not to its in-depth extension. UK and US writers call 'early carcinomas' those cancers limited to the submucosa.

Killingback,[12] in studying the local recurrence rate according to tumor diameter, notes in 36 patients 12.5% of local recurrence with a tumor diameter of less than 3.5 cm, as opposed to 33% when the diameter is larger than 3.5 cm. This difference, however, is not statistically significant. Most writers reporting on local resections estimate that the maximum tumor diameter is 3 cm.

It may be concluded that tumor size is not a major prognostic factor, but a diameter of less than 3 cm seems to be the maximum reasonable size when considering a local resection, since if a 1 cm safety margin is to be preserved around the tumor, the diameter of the surgical wound will be 5 cm. If a larger tumor is involved, the chances are that the minimal safety margin will not be adhered to, which might account for a higher percentage of local recurrence.

The macroscopic features of the tumor

Exophytic tumors are only lightly penetrating, as opposed to ulcerated tumors, which show faster in-depth extension. The ganglionic invasion rate is higher when the tumor is ulcerated than when it is budding.[12,13] However, the ulcerated character of a tumor is not a contraindication to local treatment.[14]

Anatomopathological criteria

Degree of in-depth infiltration of the tumor

This is one of the basic prognostic factors for considering local treatment. This treatment cannot be evaluated correctly unless the tumor is totally excised. The excision must then remain limited to the wall and not go beyond the muscularis. The risk of ganglionic invasion is closely related to parietal invasion. What is the risk of ganglionic invasion in relation to the penetration of the cancer through the rectal wall? The risk is present as soon as the cancer goes beyond the muscularis mucosae.

Two recent studies (Table 5.1) have attempted to evaluate the ganglionic invasion

Table 5.1 Lymph-node invasion when the tumor is limited to the bowel wall

Ref	Level of invasion	Lymph nodes invaded (no. of patients)	Lymph nodes not invaded (no. of patients)	Total
15	Submucosae	3 (11%)	24	27
	Muscularis propriae	19 (23%)	63	82
		22 (30%)	87	109
16	Mucosae	0	10	10
	Submucosae	4 (25%)	12	16
	Muscularis propriae	16 (16%)	81	97
		20 (16%)	103	123

risk in relation of parietal invasion. Huddy et al,[15] in a study of 454 resected rectal cancers, evaluated the ganglionic invasion rate for the 109 tumors that were limited to the rectal wall. Of 27 cancers limited to the submucosa, 3 (11%) showed ganglionic invasion; and of the 82 cancers limited to the muscularis, 9 (23%) showed ganglionic invasion. The ganglionic invasion rate, then, is 20% when tumors are limited to the wall (Dukes A). We conducted an identical study at l'Institut Gustave Roussy on 400 resected rectal cancers:[16] in 123 instances, the tumor was limited to the rectal wall. Of 16 patients with a tumor classified as T1, there was ganglionic invasion in 4 instances; and of 97 patients with a tumor classified as T2, there was ganglionic invasion in 16 instances (16%). It appears from these two studies that when a local resection is performed for a tumor limited to the wall (submucous T1 and muscular T2), the risk of overlooking a ganglionic invasion is 16–20%. These figures are slightly higher than those of Morson et al,[7] which were respectively 11% ganglionic invasion for T1 tumors and 12% for T2 tumors. Hojo et al[17] found slightly higher ganglionic invasion rates: 18% for T1 and 38% for T2. Hager et al[2] found 8% for T1 and 17% for T2.

Histopathological differentiation
Tumors are classified into three grades of malignancy according to their degree of differentiation: well-differentiated tumors (grade 1),

moderately differentiated (grade 2) and poorly differentiated (grade 3). Some writers add a fourth grade for undifferentiated tumors. The less differentiated the tumor, the higher is the risk of a ganglionic invasion. Morson[18] shows a risk of ganglionic invasion of 25% for grade 1 tumors, 50% for grade 2 and 80% for grade 3. This does not take into account the in-depth extension of the tumor.

Morson[18] states that the poorly differentiated character of the tumor is a formal contraindication to local treatment, whatever its size and in-depth penetration. Locke et al[19] have published a study of the prognostic value of histological differentiation in local resection. This study involved 152 patients who had been treated with local resection at St Mark's Hospital from 1948 to 1984. Table 5.2 summarizes the results in this series: it is shown that 17 patients out of 152 (11%) died from their cancer following local treatment. In the light of this study, Lock is of the opinion that local resection is perfectly justified for low-grade malignancy tumors. This technique, however, is inadvisable when the tumor is of intermediate grade or worse.

It may be concluded that one must take into account the histological differentiation of the tumor before considering local resection. All writers agree to eliminate poorly differentiated (grade 3) or undifferentiated (grade 4) tumors. There is no consensus concerning moderately differentiated tumors (grade 2). Serious prob-

Table 5.2 Risk of cancer-related death versus histopathological grade[19]

Histopathological grade	No. of patients	Cancer-related deaths	Death after surgery for recurrence	Total
Low	56	1	0	1
Intermediate	81	8	2	10
High	15	5	1	6
Total	152	14	3	17 (11%)

lems are set by this type of classification and by the different interpretations by anatomopathologists. Seventy percent of the tumors show different differentiation characteristics according to location, and although it is easy to classify tumors in extreme groups (grades 1 and 4), the same does not apply to intermediate groups. Finally, it must be emphasized that the limitations of tumor biopsies do not permit predictions as to the exact histological type. For tumors with a high grade of malignancy, there is only 40% concordance between biopsy data and thorough examination of the tumor. This shows the importance of a meticulous anatomopathological examination of the *entire* resection piece for a precise classification.

Other anatomopathological factors

Several writers[1,5,18] have emphasized the negative prognosis of mucinous cancers, which account for 10–20% of rectal cancers, but the series only report a few cases, and it is rather hard to draw definite conclusions.

More recently, anatomopathologists have emphasized the presence or absence of tumoral emboli in the lymphatics or vessels. The prognostic significance of such emboli in contact with the tumor is little known, and it is often difficult to determine their exact location: lymphatic vessels or blood vessels. According to Gall and Hermanek,[1] detection of such emboli

implies classification of the patient in the high-risk lymphatic-invasion group just as with grades 3 and 4, and they advise against local treatment for such patients.

The same goes for perinervous tumoral sheathing, which is a much more important prognostic factor. It is an independent prognostic factor, both in terms of five-year survival (28% of cases of positive perinervous tumoral sheathing versus 62% with negative perinervous tumoral sheathing) and of local recurrence (81% versus 30%).

Importance of resection margin

Local excision of rectal cancer is acceptable only when tumor resection can be complete and when the risk of ganglionic invasion is minimal.[1] Morson[7] has demonstrated well the prognostic importance of the resection margin following local resection. He singles out three different types of resection: complete resection, incomplete resection (resection margin invaded by the tumor), and dubious or uncertain resection (when the anatomopathologist detects tumoral cells inside the coagulated peripheral tissues).

In the series of 119 patients treated with local resection at St Marks Hospital, Morson et al[7] studied the local recurrence rate and the survival rate in relation to the type of resection (Table 5.3). The evolution in patients who had

Table 5.3 Risk of recurrence and survival versus resection quality[7]

Quality of local resection	No. of patients	No. of recurrences	Overall 5-year survival (%)	Corrected 5-year survival (%)
Complete	91	3 (3%)	82	100
Doubtful	14	2 (14%)	64	96
Incomplete	14	5 (36%)	57	83
Total	119	10	—	—

had a dubious resection is noteworthy. Of 14 patients who had a local resection complemented by electrocoagulation of the tumor site, Morson et al noted 2 recurrences (1 local, and 1 metastatic). Of the 4 patients who had salvage surgery, 2 had no tumoral residue, and 2 had intraparietal residue.

Wille et al[20] noted 33% of local recurrence when the margin was invaded, 15% when the margin was free of tumor, and 9% when resection limits could not be evaluated. Graham et al[21] found 6% of recurrence when resection was complete, against 52% when resection was incomplete. One cannot overlook the problems that anatomopathologists face in evaluating the character of the resection, given the secondary artefacts secondary to electrocoagulation. Only highly trained anatomopathologists can adequately classify the resection in the uncertain or dubious group.

Local resection of rectal cancer must be considered only when excision of the tumor can be complete and when the risk of ganglionic invasion is minimal. As demonstrated, the ganglionic risk depends on two factors: the degree of penetration of the tumor through the wall, and the histological differentiation grade. These factors can be evaluated adequately only after complete anatomopathological examination of the resected piece.

Results described in the literature

The risk of performing local resection of a rectal cancer basically refers to local recurrence. This local recurrence may be diagnosed early by adequate follow-up. It can benefit from salvage surgery, the frequency of which is variously estimated. Graham et al[21] show an 89% five-year survival rate and a total local recurrence rate of 24%, of which only 42% were salvaged by major surgery (22–100%, depending on the series). This low percentage of salvage surgery is due either to inadequate follow-up or to the type of recurrence (ganglionic in the mesorectum, developing unobtrusively, belatedly diagnosed, rapidly settling posteriorly and thus ineradicable in terms of cure). Gall and Hermanek[1] were able to perform curative salvage surgery in only 5 cases out of 9 (50%) (Table 5.4).

Table 5.4 Literature review: results regarding local resections

Ref	No. of patients	Level of invasion			Local recurrence rates (%)	Disease-free survival at 5 years (%)
		T1[a]	T2[b]	T3[c]		
2	59	39	20	0	10	84
7	142	115	20	7	10	93
14	33	12	16	5	12	88
9	12	—	14	—	14	100
22	31	15	14	2	26	90
12	34	0	28	6	23	82
20	29	20	5	4	15	77
5	57	25	29	3	—	83
6	44	28	15	1	7.5	88

[a] Mucosae, submucosae.
[b] Muscularis propriae.
[c] Serosae.

It is more interesting to study survival and frequency of local recurrences according to the T classification and the histopathological differentiation grade; this makes it possible to define therapeutic indications.

When the tumor is limited to the submucosa (pT1) – grade 1 or 2 – we note from 0% to 13% local recurrence, and a five-year survival rate of 90–100%. When the tumor invades the muscularis without going beyond (pT2) – grade 1 or 2 – we note from 17% to 44% local recurrence, and a five-year survival rate of 78–82%. The series of Hager et al[2] is shown in Table 5.5. It clearly shows the importance of in-depth invasion when the tumor is well or moderately differentiated. When the resection is complete, the local recurrence rate is 8% for T1 tumors and 17% for T2 tumors. The metastasis rate is 3% for T1 tumors and 6% for T2 tumors. The mortality rate from cancer is 0% for T1 and 6% for T2. The five-year survival rate is 89.6% for T1 and 78% for T2. In this series, 36 patients had a T3 tumor, or a grade 3 or 4 tumor, or an invaded margin, or lymphatic or vascular emboli; Hager et al noted 24% local recurrences, 39% deaths from cancer, and 15% metastases.

Most authors agree in singling out grade pT1 tumors of grades 1 or 2 as the ideal indication for local resection: and in formally contraindicating local resection in pT3 tumors, or in pT1 and pT2 tumors with a high malignancy grade. The discussion remains open regarding pT2 tumors with a low malignancy grade in total resection.

Indications for local resection

This technique applies to few patients. At St Mark's Hospital, from 1948 to 1972, 3999 rectal cancers were treated, and only 143 patients (3.6%) had total local resection. The indications for this technique have gradually increased; the technique was used in only 1.4% of all cases from 1948 to 1952, but this rate went up to 7.5% of all cases from 1968 to 1972. In all the other series in the literature, local resection was performed in less than 10% of all treated rectal cancers.[5,6,23]

Local resection of rectal cancer is performed in two steps. First, tumors suitable for local treatment are selected, and then the rationale for this treatment is confirmed after resection and by complete anatomopathological examination of the piece. Justification for local treatment is effectively based on the quality of resection, the in-depth extension of the tumor, and the degree of histological differentiation.

Selection of tumors

- *Digital rectal examination:* local resection must apply to tumors that are easily accessible through digital rectal examination. This is the best way to select tumors. It makes it possible to evaluate the tumor site, the macroscopic character, and the mobility in relation to adjacent structures, and to look for suspicious adenopathies in the mesorectum.[24] Digital examination, however, does not permit differentiation between submucous invasion and muscularis invasion. As far as the presence of ganglionic invasion is concerned, digital examination is reliable only half of the time. It may be performed under anesthesia when examination of the patient proves difficult.
- *Endorectal echography* makes it possible to eliminate any tumors that have extended beyond the muscularis (T3), and any other

Table 5.5 The series of Hager et al[2]		
Details	**Group I (T1)**[a]	**Group II (T2)**[b]
Number of patients	39	20
Local recurrence	3 (8%)	3 (17%)
Metastasis	1 (3%)	1 (6%)
Cancer-related deaths	—	2 (11%)
5-year survival	89.6%	78%

[a] Mucosae, submucosae.
[b] Muscularis propriae.

tumors associated with suspicious adenopathies in the mesorectum.

- Preoperative biopsy makes it possible to accurately evaluate the histological type and degree of differentiation of the tumor; since an accurate classification can only be achieved through examination of the resected part.

Neither the pelvic scanner nor nuclear magnetic resonance are of use for tumor selection. Lymphoscintigraphy has not yet demonstrated its usefulness. *Digital rectal examination, endoscopy with biopsy, and endorectal echography allow the selection of tumors for local resection:*

- mobile cancers of York Masson stages I or II, located at the lower third of the rectum, and with a diameter less than or equal to 3 cm without any palpable or suspicious ganglion;
- cancers that do not go beyond the rectal muscularis, well or moderately differentiated, and ideally located on the posterior or lateral faces.

Local resection is then performed, and the surgeon waits for anatomopathological findings; the patient is advised of the possibility of new surgery should conditions for local resection prove unsatisfactory. This rate of complementary surgery following resection varies according to writers and to initial selection criteria (9–17%). This complementary surgery will be performed in the event of unfavorable prognostic factors (grades 3 or 4, lymphatic or vascular emboli, perinervous sheathing), whatever the degree of parietal invasion. Of course, this surgery must be performed only if a pT3 tumor reaching beyond the rectal muscularis is involved. Finally, it must be performed only if resection is incomplete in pT2 tumors whatever the degree of histological differentiation (rf organigram).

Local resection and radiotherapy

Over the last few years, a number of writers[25] have associated local resection with postoperative radiotherapy (RT) to reduce and even avoid local recurrences and eventually to sterilize metastatic adenopathies. The usual doses are around 45 Gy on the entire pelvis, associated with an overdose at the tumor-site level (a total of 60 Gy).

Bailey et al[26] get 8% local recurrence with systematic irradiation of tumors. These figures are identical to those obtained with only local resection for this type of tumor. Willett et al[20] found 18% local recurrence with T2 tumors postoperatively irradiated; they conclude that this RT might be indicated when resection margins are invaded. They compared two groups of patients – 40 without RT and 26 with postoperative RT – and reported, when the margin was invaded, 33% local recurrence in the first group and 0% in the second group (but the latter included only 6 patients).

This postoperative RT is not free from complications. For doses of 53 Gy, McCready et al[27] observed 29% of postoperative complications. These consisted of fistulas in 17% of cases (local excision was performed by the posterior route), and local infection in 12%. Rich et al[28] report 50% of hemorrhagic rectitis with doses above 60 Gy, and only 6% with doses below 60 Gy. Finally, Coco et al[23] report radic proctitis necesitating a colostomy. Other surgeons used RT postoperatively or 'sandwiched' without reducing the local recurrence rate.

It may be concluded that the role of postoperative RT is not yet clearly defined and that it should be possible to effect randomized therapeutic trials, but this seems hard to achieve, in view of the low number of patients who could benefit from local resection. It might be indicated in certain T2 tumors when their resection is incomplete (invaded margins), or when they have lymphatic emboli, especially when complementary surgery is risky, or when an abdominoperineal amputation is turned down.

Follow-up

Local resection of a rectal cancer can only be considered if patients submit to strict follow-up. Salvage surgery following local recurrence will be possible only following an early diagnosis. Patients must be examined every 3 months in the first 2 years, and then every 6 months for the next 5 years. In addition to digital rectal examination and complete clinical examination, an endoscopy, an endorectal echography and a thoracic radiography should be performed. Should there be the slightest doubt, an examination under anesthesia should be performed, with deep biopsies. Patients who cannot be adequately followed up will not benefit from local treatment.

CONTACTHERAPY

This technique, which was described at Montpellier in 1940 by Lamarque and Gros, has chiefly been developed and used at Lyon by Papillon at Centre Léon-Bérard since 1951.[29,30]

Technique

This technique is applied with a Philips RT50 (50 kV, 12 mA) instrument. The localizer has a 30 mm diameter at its distal end, and can slide in a rectoscope. The patient is placed in a genupectoral position, and local anesthesia of the sphincter is sufficient. The rectoscopy permits exact localization of the tumor, following which the contactherapy tube is introduced into the rectoscope after checking the technical conditions of the irradiation, which may then begin. The treatment is applied by the radiotherapist alone, or by the radiotherapist assisted by a gastroenterologist, to avoid tube displacement during the treatment. Irradiation time is brief: 1–3 minutes for an output of 20–40 Gy[29] or 50 Gy.[31]

Papillon gives 4 sessions, spread over 4 weeks with ambulatory patients. The time between sessions makes it possible to assess tumor development during the first 3 weeks, that is, after 2 radiotherapy sessions. Some tumors on day 21 are not altered by radiotherapy; they remain indurated and ulcerated, indicating extensive parietal infiltration. In such cases, they cannot be treated by radiotherapy alone, and radical surgery must be performed. It is the third-week test that shows the radiosensitivity of the cancer. Eschwege, on the other hand, gives 3 sessions at 8-day intervals, for a total dose of 100–150 Gy, each session lasting 15–30 minutes. Papillon makes an iridium implantation with a two-tined fork, one month after termination of contactherapy, delivering an additional 20–30 Gy at the tumor-site level. Complications associated with this technique are nil.

Results

Papillon's outstanding series is reported in Table 5.6. Of the 233 patients cured at year 5, 228 (97%) had a normal anal function. There

Table 5.6 Intraluminal radiotherapy results (Papillon's series)

No. of patients	Disease-free at 5 years	Cancer-related deaths	Deaths unrelated to cancer	Post-operative deaths	Local recurrence
312	233 (75%)	25 (8%)	50 (16%)	4 (1.2%)	26 (8.3%)

were 14 cases (4.5%) of local recurrence, and 12 cases (3.8%) of ganglionic failures. Of these 26 patients, 7 were saved by salvage therapy (5 abdominoperineal amputations and 2 perirectal lymphadenectomies). A total of 15 patients had a rectal amputation; 4 of them died at the post-operative stage.

Among the other series in literature, we may quote Sischy et al[32] (Rochester, NY); after treating 192 patients with contactherapy, with a follow-up of 1–14 years, they show a local recurrence level of 6%, and their five-year survival rate is identical to Papillon's. Horiot, at Dijon, treated 72 patients, with a five-year survival rate of 78% and a local recurrence rate of 15%.[33] Finally, Eschwege shows a five-year survival rate of 72% and a local recurrence rate of 20%.[31]

Indications

As with local resection, radiotherapists insist on strict selection of patients, and on the importance of close follow-up. This technique applies to T1 or small T2 tumors. According to Eschwege, tumor size must be less than or equal to 3 cm, which is consistent with the diameter of the rectoscope to which the Philips instrument is connected. Papillon states that the tumor must be above 4–5 cm long (two superimposed irradiation aprons) by 2 cm wide – that is, one-quarter of the circumference of the rectal ampulla. In his series, he notes that when the diameter is less than 3 cm, five-year survival is 80%, and goes down to 58% with tumors exceeding 3 cm in diameter. Local recurrence rates are respectively 9% and 17.5%.

Tumors must be well or moderately differentiated (grades 1 or 2), without any adenopathy palpable by digital rectal examination or suspected at endorectal echography. In height, they may be located up to 12–14 cm from the anal margin. Anterior-location tumors seem to be an excellent indication for contactherapy (as opposed to local resection or to electrocoagulation).

Some juxtasphincteral posterior-seat tumors are not easily accessible for contactherapy. In fact, the rectoscope is hindered by sphincter tonus and canal angulation, and its beam will not entirely reach these tumors.

ELECTROCOAGULATION

Electrocoagulation and fulguration are two features of surgical diathermy, a method that involves destruction of tissues by heat, by means of an electric current running through them. EC has long been used as palliative treatment of inoperable rectal cancers, Strauss et al[34] and Poirier et al[35] advocated it as curative treatment.

Technique

The object of this technique is to destroy the tumor completely if possible, in a single surgical session. 'Seeing adequately, exposing adequately, cleaning adequately' (Poirier). The operation is performed with the point of the scalpel[36] or with sharp-edged curettes, to gradually eliminate carbonized and necrotic tissues.[37,38] First, the healthy mucosa is coagulated at 1 cm at the circumference of the tumor, thus delimiting the EC area. Effectively, once this is initiated, digital rectal examination is inadequate to appreciate the external limits of the tumor, since the coagulated tissues give an impression of rigidity and pseudotumoral infiltration. Destruction of the tumor is done from the surface into the depth, and the perirectal fat must be reached. Mean duration of the operation is from 1 to 2 hours.

Postoperative care

The residual eschar falls off around day 8 to 10; an endoscopic checkup is then done, and the patient leaves the department. Some writers advocate a new EC session around day 10. This is justifiable only if the operator feels that the tumor has not been totally destroyed. Madden and Kandalaft[36] give approximately 34 EC sessions per patient.

Complications

Operative death is nil in the series of Crile and Turnbull[37] and Madden and Kandalaft.[36] It is 2% in the Institut Gustave-Roussy series. Complications are infrequent (2–25%). They may consist of hemorrhage when eschars fall out, of perforation of the Douglas pouch when the tumor is located too high, of the ischiorectal fossa necessitating drainage by a low route, or of transitory sphincteral incontinence when the coagulated tumor was low (juxtasphincteral). Sequelae basically consist of cicatricial stenosis (2% of cases), especially with voluminous tumors.

Indications for electrocoagulation[39]

The tumor must not be located too high – because of risk of perforation of the Douglas pouch – or too low – because of risk of sphincteral incontinence. It must be on the posterior or lateral faces, since, as with local resection, anterior-seat tumors are prone to rectovaginal fistulas in women and to ureteral lesions in men.

CONCLUSIONS

Local excision has the great advantage of providing the anatomopathologist with an item for analysis, as opposed to local destruction techniques (contactherapy and electrocoagulation). Contactherapy has the great advantage of being performed under local anesthesia on ambulatory patients and without any complications. The other two techniques necessitate hospitalization, and complications have been experienced. When patients are strictly selected (budding tumor with a diameter of less than 3 cm, mobile, of grades 1 or 2, without ganglionic invasion (T1 or T2)), findings are approximately identical, whether with local resection or contactherapy (8% versus 10%). But local resection provides the only way to evaluate the exact degree of parietal infiltration. Finally, contactherapy, especially when associated with radiotherapy, can only be administered by highly trained teams.

Local resection would seem advisable, whenever possible. Contactherapy should be restricted to anterior or high-location tumors in elderly patients who do not easily tolerate anesthesia or hospitalization. The indications for EC have gradually diminished, and they are merely the contraindications for other techniques.

Whatever the local treatment used for curative purposes, to quote Papillon, 'the surgeon or radiotherapist must be aware of the responsibility he assumes when agreeing to local treatment of a patient who could be cured by traditional radical surgery'. Here, more than anywhere else, the therapist is not entitled to errors.

REFERENCES

1. Gall FP, Hermanek P, Cancer of the rectum. Local excision. *Sur Clin N Am* 1988; **68**: 1353–65.
2. Hager TH, Gall FP, Hermanek P, Local excision of cancer of the rectum. *Dis Col Rectum* 1983; **26**: 149–51.
3. Mann CV, Transphincteric approach to rectal lesions. *Ann Surg* 1977; **9**: 171–94.
4. Nivatvongs S, Wolff B, Technique of per anal excision for carcinoma of the low rectum. *Sur Gynecol Obst* 1992; **13**: 447–50.
5. Decosse JJ, Wong RJ, Quan SHQ et al, Conservative treatment of distal rectal cancer by local excision. *Cancer* 1989; **63**: 219–23.
6. Lasser Ph, Padilla R, Bognel C et al, Traitement conservateur des cancers du bas rectum par tumorectomie et électrocoagulation. A propos de 44 observations. *Cahiers Cancer* 1990; **2**: 8–12.
7. Morson BC, Bussey HJR, Samoorian S, Policy of local excision for early cancer of the colo-rectum. *Gut* 1977; **18**: 1045–50.
8. O'Brian PH, Kraske's approach to the rectum. *Sur Gynecol Obst* 1976; **142**: 412–14.

9. Masson Y, Transphincteric approach to rectal lesion. *Ann Surg* 1977; **9**: 171–94.

10. Toupet A, Une nouvelle voie d'abord périnéale des tumeurs du rectum. L'anorectomie antérieure avec section des sphinctères de l'anus. *J Chir* 1980; **117**: 705–12.

11. Morson BC. Histological criteria for local excision. *Br J Surg* 1985; **72**(Suppl): 53–4.

12. Killingback MJ. Indications for local excision of rectal cancer. *Br J Surg* 1985; **72**(Suppl): 54–6.

13. Greaney RA, Garnsey L, Milburn-Jessup J, Local excision of rectal carcinoma. *Dis Col Rectum* 1977; **20**: 463–6.

14. Whiteway J, Nicholls RJ, Morson BC, The role of surgical local excision in the treatment of rectal cancer. *Br J Surg* 1985: **72**: 694–7.

15. Huddy SPJ, Husband EM, Cook MG et al, Lymph node metastasis in rectal cancer. *Br J Surg* 1993; **80**: 1457–8.

16. Lasser Ph, Bognel C, Elias D et al, Le risque ganglionnaire en cas de cancers du rectum limités à la paroie – les limites des exérèses locales. *Gastroenterol Clin Biol* 1993; **17**: A180.

17. Hojo K, Koyama Y, Moriya Y, Lymphatic spread and its prognostic value in patients with rectal cancer. *Am J Surg* 1982; **144**: 350–4.

18. Morson BC, Factors influencing the prognosis of early cancer of the rectum. *Proc R Soc Med* 1966; **59**: 607–8.

19. Lock MR, Ritchie JK, Hawley PR, Reappraisal of radical local excision for carcinoma of the rectum. *Br J Surg* 1993; **80**: 928–9.

20. Willett C, Tepper JE, Donelly S et al, Patterns of failure following local excision and local excision and post-operative radiation therapy for invasive rectal carcinoma. *J Clin Oncol* 1989; **7**: 1003–8.

21. Graham RA, Garnsey L, Milburn-Jessup J, Local excision of rectal carcinoma. *Am J Surg* 1990; **160**: 306–12.

22. Stearns MW, Sternberg SS, Decosse JJ, Treatment alternatives: localized rectal cancer. *Cancer* 1984; **54**: 2691–4.

23. Coco C, Magistrelli P, Cranone P et al, Conservative surgery for early cancer of the distal rectum. *Dis Col Rectum* 1992; **35**: 131–6.

24. Nicholls RJ, York-Mason A, Morson BG et al, The clinical staging of rectal cancer. *Br J Surg* 1982; **69**: 404–9.

25. Billingham RP, Conservative treatment of rectal cancer. Extending the indications. *Cancer* 1992; **70**: 1355–63.

26. Bailey HR, Huval WV, Max E et al, Local excision of carcinoma of the rectum for cure. *Surgery* 1992; **111**: 555–61.

27. McCready DR, Ota DM, Rich TA et al, Prospective phase I trial of conservative management of low rectal lesions. *Arch Surg* 1989; **124**: 67–70.

28. Rich TA, Weis DR, Mies RS et al, Sphincter preservation in patients with low rectal cancer treated with radiation therapy with or without local excision or fulguration. *Radiology* 1985; **56**: 527–31.

29. Papillon J, *Rectal and Anal Cancers. Conservative Treatment by Irradiation: An Alternative to Radical Surgery.* New York: Springer-Verlag, 1982.

30. Papillon J, Berard Ph, Endocavitary irradiation in the conservative treatment of adenocarcinoma of the low rectum. *World J Surg* 1992; **16**: 451–7.

31. Lasser Ph, Eschwege F, Lacour J et al, Traitement conservateur à but curatif des cancers du rectum. (A propos de 93 observations). In: *Actualités Carcinologiques de l'Institut Gustave-Roussy.* Paris: Masson, 1983; 35–46.

32. Sischy B, Hinsone EJ, Wilkinson DB, Definitive radiation therapy for selected cancers of the rectum. *Br J Surg* 1988; **75**: 901–3.

33. Roth S, Horiot JC, Calais C et al, Prognostic factors in limited rectal cancer treated with intra cavitar irradiation. *Int J Radiat Oncol Biol Phys* 1989; **16**: 1445–51.

34. Strauss A, Appel M, Saphir O, Rabinoviz AJ, Immunologic resistance to carcinoma produced by electrocoagulation. *Surg Gynecol Obstet* 1965; **121**: 989–95.

35. Poirier A, Poirier JP, Payrard J, Traitement de certains cancers par diathermocoagulation. *Rev Med* 1970; **12**: 680–7.

36. Madden JL, Kandalaft S, Clinical evaluation of electrocoagulation in the treatment of cancer of the rectum. *Am J Surg* 1971; **122**: 347–52.

37. Crile G, Turnbull RB, The role of electrocoagulation in the treatment of carcinoma of the rectum. *Surg Gynecol Obstet* 1972; **135**: 391–6.

38. Lasser Ph, Michel G, Lacour J, Electrocoagulation des cancers du rectum. *EMC Instantanés Medicaux* 1982; **53**: 45–6.

39. Lasser Ph, Lacour J, Gadenne C, The place of electrocoagulation in the treatment of cancer of the rectum. *J Exp Clin Cancer Res* 1983; **4**: 427–9.

6

Surgery for colonic cancer

Dion G Morton, John W Fielding

INTRODUCTION

Surgical treatment of colonic cancer has progressed considerably since the first resection and anastomosis performed by Reybard in 1833. Despite recent advances in modern multidisciplinary treatment, there has been little or no improvement in 5-year survival in the last 30 years. Radical surgery still remains the only potentially curative treatment for this common cancer.

The principles for colonic resection in the treatment of colorectal cancer have changed little in recent history. Major improvements in resuscitation, antibiotic treatment and anaesthesia have, however, allowed the surgeon to be more radical, particularly in the emergency setting. These improvements in supportive care have at the same time increased the prominence of surgical morbidity. As mortality has fallen, so surgeons have increasingly looked at morbidity, in particular at the necessity for stoma formation. Stomas are most often required for emergency patients who present with peritonitis or obstruction. On-table lavage or subtotal colectomy can now provide 'stoma-free' alternatives for selected patients, even in the emergency setting.

The key outcome measures in the treatment of colonic cancer are still 5-year survival and 2-year local recurrence rates. The stage of disease at the time of presentation remains the most influential factor affecting 5-year survival. Conversely, the local recurrence rate is greatly influenced by obstruction/perforation at the time of presentation. Surgical technique has also been implicated in influencing the local recurrence rate,[1] particularly for the resection of rectal tumours.[2]

Our ability to assess the likely success of surgical treatment at the time of operation remains limited, but new intraoperative investigations such as radioimmune-guided surgery (RIGS) and intraoperative ultrasound (IOUS) may prove to be suitably sensitive tools with which to assess tumour clearance and help to guide adjuvant therapy.

The frequency of emergency presentation in many series remains over 30%, and is a disappointingly high figure. It is to be hoped that increased public awareness, and perhaps screening, could reduce the frequency of emergency presentation and so reduce the associated morbidity and mortality.

This chapter sets out to address the issues

concerning safe radical surgery for curative treatment of colorectal cancer in both the elective and emergency settings, and discusses some of the new developments that may influence its management in forthcoming years.

ELECTIVE SURGERY

Elective surgery for colorectal cancer is undertaken in 65–85% of operative cases, with the remaining cases presenting as emergencies. Surgery may be carried out with either curative or palliative intent. Palliative resection is usually considered for the treatment of advanced colonic cancer, even in the presence of metastases, in order to prevent the later complications of obstruction and perforation. Palliative surgery may involve a local resection of the primary tumour, or occasionally bypass of a locally advanced lesion.

Outcome is considerably influenced by the mode of presentation and the nature of the surgery. Radical surgery in the elective setting results in a 5-year survival more than twice that for emergency surgery (Table 6.1). Further improvements in outcome for colorectal cancer will depend upon maximizing the number of patients on whom elective radical resection can be performed.

In the absence of distant metastases or diffuse peritoneal spread, which is relatively rare, radical resection should be considered, since it offers the only curative therapeutic option. The overall 5-year survival in patients undergoing attempted curative surgery is over 50% in most series. Even in locally advanced lesions, in which adjacent structures are invaded, a 5 year survival approaching 30% can be achieved.[6]

The main focus of the following section will be on radical elective surgery.

Preoperative assessment

Effective treatment requires a multidisciplinary care team. The gastroenterologist, medical oncologist and stomatherapist may all need to be involved in the planning of treatment. The management plan should also be discussed with the general practitioner, the community nurse, and in selected cases the social services and the palliative-care team so that adequate support can be provided once the patient is discharged from hospital.

Preoperative evaluation must include evaluation of any co-morbid medical factors, as well as determining the extent of disease. Co-morbid medical illness rarely precludes surgical treatment, since local resection provides the most

Table 6.1 Presentation and outcome in patients with colorectal cancer (data adapted from references 3–5)

Mode of presentation	% of all patients	Resection performed (%)	In-hospital mortality (%)	5-year survival (%)
Elective surgery	60	>95	5	50
Emergency	25	70	20	25
Non-operative	15	—	40	<5

effective symptomatic control. Elective surgery can be delayed for treatment of reversible conditions and for stabilizing chronic disease.

Preoperatively, it is advised that patients undergo either a double-contrast barium enema or a total colonoscopy in order to exclude proximal synchronous tumours. These have been estimated to occur in up to 6% of cases, of which 50% lie outside the range of resection.[7] Colonoscopy has the advantage over barium enema of providing access for biopsy and histological confirmation of any tumour. It is also more effective in detecting small adenomas. This is most important in the small group of young patients with familial predisposition in whom the presence of satellite adenomas can be an indication for an extended colectomy to facilitate subsequent control of metatachronous disease.

Preoperative staging of the primary tumour in colonic cancer is less likely to influence management than in the case of rectal cancer. However, CT scanning of the liver to look for metastases should be performed as an adjunct to intraoperative assessment. Intraoperative palpation of the liver has been repeatedly shown to underestimate the presence of metastases. This is of particular importance in colorectal cancer, since >50% of distant metastases first present in the liver.[8] Accurate staging of liver metastases is becoming increasingly important with the development of locoregional intrahepatic arterial chemotherapy and hepatic resection as adjuvant therapeutic options following primary resection. Intraoperative ultrasonography has been reported as being more specific than preoperative CT scanning for the detection of liver metastases,[9] and is being more widely used in an attempt to improve perioperative staging. Preoperative serum carcinoembryonic antigen (CEA) estimation has also been advocated, since a subsequent postoperative rise in this level can be the first sign of early recurrence. A recent report found elevated CEA levels in patients with recurrent tumour in whom preoperative serum levels had been normal, suggesting that this follow-up investigation can be useful regardless of the preoperative serum level.[10]

Resection technique

In the elective setting, where preoperative bowel preparation has been performed, primary anastomosis should be feasible, and a protecting temporary stoma is rarely required for colonic lesions.

The principles of radical surgical resection for colonic cancer remain the same regardless of the site of the primary tumour, namely ligation of the major vascular pedicle, obtaining tumour-free margins, and resection of any contiguous organs involved by tumour. Ligation of the major vascular pedicle allows for wide excision of the lymph nodes draining the tumour. In a formal hemicolectomy the proximal resection margin is usually determined by the level of the major vascular ligation (Figure 6.1). In a left hemicolectomy, ligation of the inferior mesenteric artery flush with the aortic origin has been strongly advocated.[11] No resultant increase in survival has been shown, and notably no long-term survivors in patients with apical node metastases have been reported.[12] A wide resection, including the vascular pedicle, will, however, provide the maximum number of lymph nodes and so help in accurate tumour staging.

More recently, subtotal colectomy has been advocated for young patients (<50 years) and for those patients with synchronous tumours (Figure 6.2), in order to reduce the risk of developing metachronous cancer later in life. Except for those patients with a known inherited syndrome, this approach, as yet, has no proven benefit in terms of reduced cancer recurrence rates and prolonged survival. It may, in fact, be the case that regular colonoscopic follow-up, with polypectomy where required, is as effective in preventing metachronous tumours, and could have a lower resultant morbidity, particularly in terms of subsequent frequency of bowel action.

For over 40 years, surgeons have been concerned that tumour mobilization and manipulation could cause metachronous tumours by local tumour-cell seeding and also cause distant metastatic spread.[13,14] These early reports encouraged the development of the 'no-touch

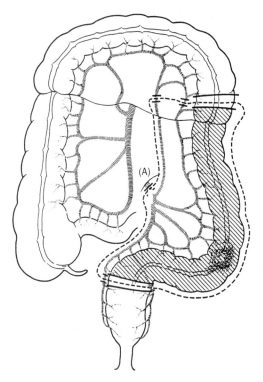

Figure 6.1 Left hemicolectomy. The diagram shows the limits of resection for a sigmoid carcinoma. High ligation of the inferior mesenteric artery (A) is performed in order to remove the lymphatics draining the tumour. The blood supply to the colon is maintained via the marginal artery. Reproduced with permission from Keighley MRB, Williams NS, *Surgery of the Anus, Rectum and Colon*. WB Saunders Company Ltd, 1993.[72]

technique', in which the vascular supply to the colon is ligated and the colonic lumen occluded by tapes prior to mobilization of the tumour. One early report showed an increased disease-free interval compared with historic controls.[15] A more recent prospective randomized trial found a trend towards a reduced number and greater time to the development of liver metastases in a no-touch isolation group, but these differences did not reach statistical significance.[16] The findings from these studies suggest a limited benefit from this approach. Although many surgeons would advocate intrarectal irrigation with cytotoxic agent during a low anterior resection, in colonic resections, where the distal resection margin is

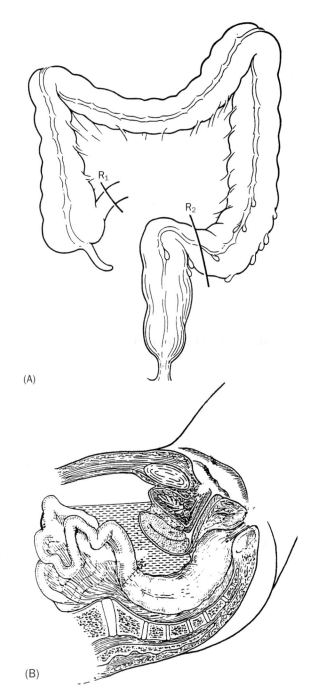

Figure 6.2 A subtotal colectomy and ileorectal anastomosis. The limits of resections are shown in (A): R_1–R_2. An end-to-end ileorectal anastomosis is shown in (B). Retaining the rectum preserves the reservoir and reduces problems with postoperative diarrhoea. Reproduced with permission of WB Saunders Company Ltd.[72]

usually further away from the tumour, the potential benefits are unclear. Recurrent tumour at the site of the colonic anastomosis is rarely seen following curative resection for colonic tumours. The main focus of attention in colonic resections for cancer is in obtaining node clearance.

It has been argued that lymph-node invasion occurs in a stepwise fashion, involving first the para-colic nodes before spreading to the mesenteric vessel nodes and so to the para-aortic nodes. Skip lesions are now recognized,[17] re-emphasizing the importance of multiple node sampling by the histopathologist, for accurate staging of the tumours. Radical resection is therefore required not only for tumour clearance, but also to provide adequate lymph-node samples for histology. This is now influencing patient selection for adjuvant chemotherapy, and so, although high arterial ligation may confer little survival benefit to the patient from primary surgery, its benefit in the future is likely to be seen in more appropriate selection for adjuvant treatment. A similar myth – that distant metastases will only occur after lymph-node involvement – has also been dispelled,[18] re-emphasizing the importance of optimal perioperative assessment for liver metastases.

Prophylactic colectomy

Prophylactic colectomy has been well established in the treatment of longstanding total colitis, and familial adenomatous polyposis. The development of restorative proctocolectomy has provided a continent option for the treatment of these patients (Figure 6.3). Advances in our understanding of the molecular genetics of other inherited cancer syndromes, most notably hereditary non-polyposis colorectal cancer (HNPCC),[19] have considerably increased the number of patients for whom prophylactic colectomy can be considered.[20] In HNPCC families the tumours are predominantly right-sided, and so rectal resection is not usually required. The therapeutic options are colonoscopic surveillance and polypectomy or subtotal colectomy and ileorectal anastomosis,

with subsequent follow-up surveillance of the rectal stump. Because of the high risk of colorectal cancer (>80% lifetime risk) and the significant risk of interval cancer development during colonoscopic surveillance,[21] increasing numbers of known gene carriers are likely to request prophylactic colectomy. Other tumours are also commonly seen in HNPCC families,

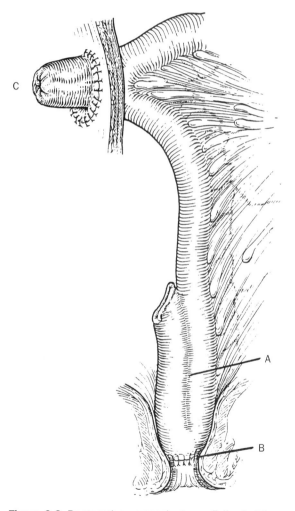

Figure 6.3 Restorative protocolectomy. Following the removal of the whole colon and rectum, a neo-reservoir is fashioned from the terminal ileum (A). Continuity is restored by anastomosis to the anal canal (B). The anastomosis is usually protected by a temporary loop ileostomy (C). Reproduced with permission of WB Saunders Company Ltd.[72]

notably ovarian and endometrial carcinoma. The benefits of synchronous prophylactic hysterectomy and oophorectomy in post-menopausal female family members are uncertain, and further work is required in HNPCC families to clarify these issues.

Laparoscopy

The development of new laparoscopic instruments has encouraged their application in colorectal cancer surgery. Prior to 1993, more than 1500 laparoscopic colectomies had been reported in the literature, about half of which were for colorectal cancer. The enthusiasm for this approach lay in the perceived reduced early morbidity associated with a colectomy. There remains considerable concern about the ability to achieve wide tumour clearance with this technique. It seems likely that such technical problems will be overcome.

A second area of concern is that of port-site recurrence, which has been reported in up to 4% of cases.[22] This problem appears to be directly related to the laparoscopic approach, and has been reported even in association with early-stage disease. The site of recurrence is independent of the site of removal of the resected specimen. The phenomenon may prove to be an aerosol effect, but at the present time the mechanism is not known. For these reasons, it is generally agreed that laparoscopic colectomy for neoplastic disease should be restricted to clinical trials.

Surgery in the elderly

Major efforts to reduce colorectal cancer-related mortality are being undertaken by health services worldwide. These currently focus on the implementation of presymptomatic diagnosis in order to downstage disease at the time of presentation and the development of adjuvant chemotherapeutic regimes to increase long-term survival in patients who have undergone attempted curative surgery for locally advanced disease. These two approaches have both been shown to be of proven efficacy in randomized controlled trials. It must be remembered, however, that elderly patients are largely excluded from screening and adjuvant chemotherapy, and in an increasingly elderly population the benefits of these advances will be diluted in the total patient population.

The incidence of colorectal cancer approximately doubles with each decade from 40 to 80 years, and two-thirds of colorectal cancer patients are now over 65 years at the time of diagnosis. In an ageing population this figure can be expected to rise.[23] Guidelines for the treatment of elderly patients are clearly required. In a multicentre review, Samet et al[24] found that as few as 54% of patients over 75 years of age received definitive surgery for colorectal cancer. A large number of studies in elderly patients have been reported.[25] Co-morbid disease and emergency presentation have been shown to significantly influence survival,[26] but these studies have failed to show any relationship between age at presentation and perioperative mortality or age-adjusted 5-year survival. These findings support the use of radical surgery in elderly patients. The high incidence of co-morbid disease requires that these patients be carefully assessed prior to surgery. Reversible risk factors have been identified in up to 60% of elderly patients presenting with colorectal cancer,[26] highlighting the importance of preoperative assessment. In five series reported from the British Isles between 1982 and 1994, a considerable reduction in perioperative mortality (Table 6.2) and a resultant rise in the 5-year survival is seen over the 13 years. These figures appear to reflect the impact of careful preoperative assessment and improved perioperative patient care over the 20-year period. Inadequate primary surgery in the elderly population is likely to result in increased morbidity and an increase in subsequent emergency treatment, with resulting higher costs to the health services. Adequate primary surgery for elderly patients is required, even if they are excluded from the potential benefits of screening and adjuvant therapy programmes.

Table 6.2 Surgery in the elderly. Five series from the British Isles reviewing the outcome of surgery for colorectal cancer in elderly patients (all patients were 70 years of age or older)

Ref	Year of publication	Median year of diagnosis	No. of patients	Perioperative mortality (%)	5-year survival (%)
27	1984	1972	327	29	26
28	1984	1977	288	19	—
29	1989	1978	1147	12	—
30	1988	1982	171	6	48
31	1994	1984	225	5	52

EMERGENCY SURGERY

Between 16% and 35% of patients with colorectal cancer present as emergencies. The early mortality in this group of patients is three times that of elective cases, and the overall 5-year survival rate is little over 10%.[32,33] As a consequence, the main emphasis in the treatment of these patients is aimed at minimizing early mortality. Achieving long-term cure is necessarily of secondary importance. The poor outcome for these patients has stimulated a wide range of therapeutic options. There remains a lack of consensus as to the optimal surgical management. It is clear, however, that minimizing the number of patients presenting as emergencies could produce a profound improvement in survival for patients with colorectal cancer, and should be a focus of attention for health care services in the future.

The commonest reasons for emergency presentation are obstruction or perforation of the colon. Massive rectal bleeding is an unusual event in colorectal cancer, being more commonly associated with bleeding from diverticular disease or angiodysplasia.

In the presence of free peritonitis, primary resection with colonic anastomosis is associated with a high risk of anastomotic dehiscence and potentially lethal consequences.[34] In such a situation, formation of an end-stoma, usually with resection of the tumour and perforated bowel, is the accepted therapeutic option.

Aggressive preoperative resuscitation with intravenous fluids and antibiotics is of paramount importance in the emergency setting. Because this is often an elderly population, the requirement of a postoperative intensive-care bed should be sought. In the frailer patient, preoperative resuscitation with central pressure monitoring in a high-dependency unit may be required.

The optimal treatment for patients with a localized perforation, or a left colonic obstruction, is more controversial. Some form of large-bowel decompression should be considered for all obstructed patients, since, even in extremis, it provides the only effective palliative option.

Confirmation of obstruction should be obtained preoperatively by a single-contrast enema in order to exclude pseudo-obstruction.

Traditionally, a three-stage surgical approach

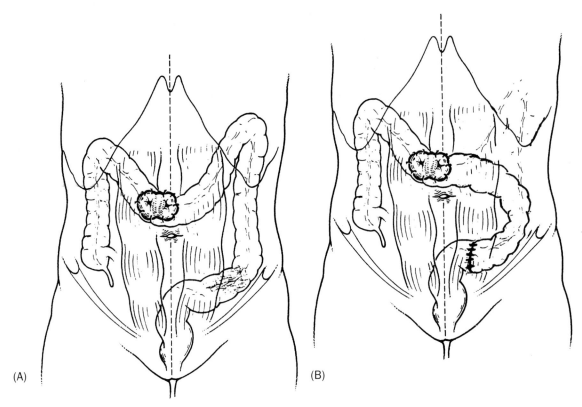

(A) (B)

Figure 6.4 Three-stage procedure. An obstructing carcinoma in the sigmoid colon is shown. The colon is decompressed by fashioning a transverse loop colostomy (A). In the second procedure, the tumor is resected and a primary anastomosis fashioned (B). In the third stage, the loop colostomy is closed (not shown). Reproduced with permission from Keighley MRB, Williams NS, *Surgery of the Anus, Rectum and Colon.* WB Saunders Company Ltd, 1993.[72]

(Figure 6.4) has been used, despite a reported cumulative postoperative mortality as high as 30%,[35] and a correspondingly high surgical morbidity. These poor results have cast doubt on the advisability of delayed resection. An initial temporary loop colostomy has a reported mortality of over 5%,[36] and has an associated morbidity of at least 20%. The major complication rate is in excess of 10% for subsequent closure of these colostomies, and less serious complications, notably prolapse and retraction, are not uncommon events. The cumulative morbidity and mortality following subsequent resection and closure of the stoma has prompted surgeons to attempt primary resection at the time of initial operations.[37]

A 'blowhole' caecostomy has also been advocated for the management of obstruction.[38] It provides a minimally invasive option that can be carried out under local anaesthetic for high-risk patients in order to stabilize them prior to more major surgery. This had previously lost favour because of incomplete decompression and leakage resulting in peritonitis. The use of a large-gauge Foley catheter with regular irrigation every few hours to prevent blockage, combined with careful suturing of the caecum to the abdominal wall, makes this option safer. It is, however, generally considered an unreliable method of decompression, and has associated heavy demands on nursing attention.

The poor long-term survival figures associ-

Table 6.3 Outcome after emergency surgery for obstructed colorectal cancer

Procedure	No. of patients (No. of series)	Overall mortality (%)	Permanent stoma rate (%)	Length of hospital stay (days)	References
Three-stage resection	195 (5)	11	25	34[a]	36, 40, 42–44
Hartmann's resection	295 (5)	11	30	30[a]	37, 40, 45–47
Primary anastomosis	42 (6)	5	—	16	45, 46, 48–51

[a] In those undergoing reversal of their stoma.

There is a notable fall in the length of hospital stay between two- and three-stage procedures, and one-stage resection and anastomosis.

The number of cases in the one-stage series is considerably smaller, indicating a higher degree of case selection for these more major procedures.

ated with the three-stage procedure resulted in primary resection of obstructing tumours, with formation of an end colostomy, being more frequently performed during the 1970s. This is known as Hartmann's procedure (Figure 6.5).[39] This procedure combines the advantages of resection of the disease at the time of first operation with an overall shorter hospital stay than a three-stage procedure.[37,40] Retrospective series have reported comparable perioperative morbidity and mortality between the two- and three-stage procedures (Table 6.3).[41]

The major perceived disadvantage of Hartmann's resection is the relatively low rate of stoma closure (60%) in the secondary procedure.[55] The technical feasibility of laparoscopic reversal of Hartmann's procedure is now established,[56] and it seems possible that this could reduce the perioperative morbidity associated with the secondary stoma closure.

In addition to the high mortality from emergency surgery for colorectal cancer, surgeons have been concerned about the high rates of stoma formation and the associated morbidity both in terms of complications from the stoma and in terms of the psychological and functional

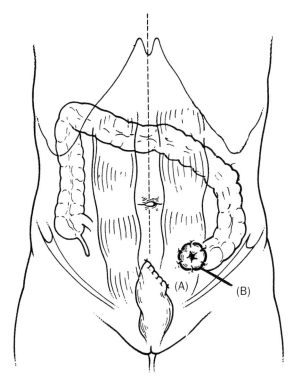

Figure 6.5 Hartmann's procedure. An obstructing carcinoma of the sigmoid colon has been resected. The rectal stump is closed (A) and an end colostomy fashioned (B). Reproduced with permission of WB Saunders Company Ltd.[72]

impact upon this largely elderly patient population. These factors have pushed surgeons towards performing primary anastomosis and avoidance of a stoma. The description of on-table colonic lavage prior to anastomosis of previously unprepared bowel[57,58] resulted in a resurgence of this approach (Figure 6.6).[59] It is now recognized that this is a major procedure that cannot be undertaken lightly, particularly in elderly unfit patients.[46] It is of interest that the importance of mechanical bowel preparation to protect a colonic anastomosis is not

entirely proven,[60] but the consensus remains that a clean prepared bowel is likely to confer an additional measure of safety and perhaps reduce intraoperative contamination. Reported leak rates following on-table lavage are less than 5%,[61,62] but are generally from retrospective studies in selected patients and are unlikely to reflect the overall leak rate were this procedure more widely performed. The duration of hospital stay is reduced by this technique, and the crude 5-year survival rate is acceptable.[44]

An alternative to on-table lavage is subtotal colectomy and ileo-sigmoid anastomosis.[49,63] This procedure has the advantage of removing the distended bowel, and is particularly suitable for cases in which the bowel wall has been compromised by distension. The operative mortality rate is reported as less than 10%, and the reported anastomotic leakage rate is considerably less than 5%.[54,64] One prospective study has compared on-table lavage with subtotal colectomy,[65] and no difference in mortality has been identified in the two groups. The main concern about subtotal colectomy is the technical demands of the operation, but with an experienced surgeon, in selected patients, this does not appear to be a clinical problem. One area of concern is that of uncontrollable diarrhoea as a consequence of the extensive resection. Most reports suggest this is not a major clinical problem, with patients having a bowel frequency of no more than three times a day.[65] The literature would suggest that good results from these more aggressive procedures are likely to result from careful patient selection.

SURGERY FOR EXTRAHEPATIC RECURRENCE

The commonest site for recurrent colonic cancer is the liver (Figure 6.7). Locoregional recurrence is seen in little over 10% of cases. Diffuse peritoneal disease is seen in a further 10% of cases, but is clearly not amenable to salvage surgery. Cohort series suggest that only about 10% of cases with locoregional recurrence are potentially resectable at the time of symptomatic presentation. Early diagnosis of asymptomatic

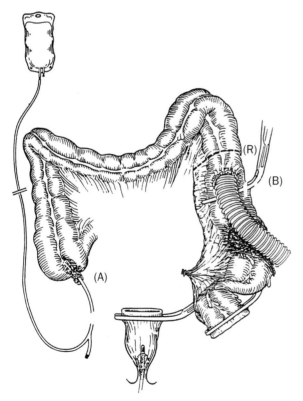

(R)

(B)

(A)

Figure 6.6 On-table lavage. An obstructing carcinoma of the descending colon is being resected. The proximal bowel is washed out by antegrade lavage. A catheter is placed in the caecum via the appendix stump (A). The effluent is collected via plastic tubing as shown (B). Following lavage, the left colon is resected as shown (R), and primary anastomosis fashioned. Reproduced with permission of WB Saunders Company Ltd.[72]

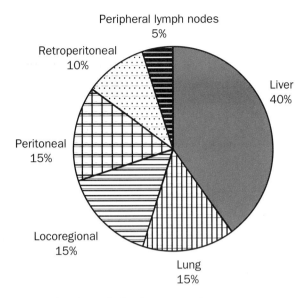

Peripheral lymph nodes
5%

Retroperitoneal
10%

Liver
40%

Peritoneal
15%

Locoregional
15%

Lung
15%

Figure 6.7 The relative frequency of recurrence at different sites following attempted curative resection for colon cancer.

recurrence has therefore been explored in order to increase the potential for attempted curative surgery. Unfortunately, no study has yet been completed that shows a survival benefit for patients treated in this way.

Early studies in this field were based on a second-look laparotomy.[66] In an early series from Minnesota of 377 patients undergoing potentially curative surgery, 110 patients underwent relook laparotomy, of whom 40 were found to have residual/recurrent cancer. Seven patients with recurrent disease ultimately were rendered disease-free for more than 5 years. However, six patients died as a result of their surgery, and no benefit could be demonstrated from this approach.

A more selective approach to second-look surgery has subsequently been advocated. Intensive follow-up by colonoscopy, CT scanning and serum carcinoembryonic antigen (CEA) testing is widely employed. For patients who are then found to have evidence of recurrence, a second-look laparotomy has been advocated.

Serum CEA levels have been investigated for the early diagnosis of asymptomatic recurrence. Schneebaum et al[67] reported a relationship between the CEA level and the resectability of the recurrent tumour at subsequent operation. A separate study found that the resection rate was not improved for asymptomatic patients, identified by elevated CEA or CT scan findings,[68] suggesting that these tests are insufficiently sensitive to identify 'early' locoregional recurrence. Preliminary reports using follow-up magnetic resonance imaging (MRI) and positron emission tomography (PET) scanning are also inconclusive, but warrant further investigation.[69]

Radioimmuno-guided surgery (RIGS) provides a novel method of intraoperative assessment of tumour spread,[70] and it could complement preoperative staging. The principal of this technique is to use a gamma-detecting probe in order to detect the presence and location of a radioisotope-labelled tumour-associated antibody. One potential use of this approach is in identifying, at the time of operation, the limit of involvement of the draining lymphatics and so help to define the small group of patients who may benefit from salvage surgery for recurrent tumour.

Follow-up surveillance of the liver for recurrent disease can be justified outside clinical trials. At the present time there is no proven benefit in intensive surveillance for extrahepatic recurrence. There is one ongoing trial of follow-up being carried out in Denmark, and the results from this study are awaited.[71] There is clearly a need for further work in the field of follow-up and surveillance in colorectal cancer management.

CONCLUSIONS

Although there has been little recent change in surgical technique in the treatment of colon cancer, there has been increased clarity in terms of optimal surgical management. Radical surgery has been demonstrated to provide the optimal treatment, even in an elderly population; and, provided that the patient's preoperative condition is stabilized, such surgery can be safely undertaken, even in the presence of significant co-morbid disease. The importance of radical surgery lies in providing accurate disease staging as well as providing local control of disease. The importance of accurate staging will increase in the foreseeable future as novel adjuvant therapeutic regimens become available.

There will be an increase in the number of prophylactic colectomies performed, particularly in patients carrying mutations in the genes causing hereditary non-polyposis colorectal cancer. Such prophylactic surgery will be suitable for laparoscopic resection, particularly as improved instrumentation becomes available. One area that has been under-investigated is how the health services will cope with an increasingly elderly population, for whom presymptomatic diagnosis and aggressive adjuvant therapy may not be appropriate or feasible.

Preoperative investigation has, as yet, had little impact upon colon cancer management. Novel intraoperative assessment by ultrasound scanning, and radioimmune-guided surgery, may result in some changes in practice. They may facilitate more accurate intraoperative staging of disease and help to select for locoregional therapy, such as the placement of peritoneal catheters, hepatic artery and portal vein cannulae, or intraoperative radiotherapy.

There remains a considerable proportion of patients for whom current therapeutic options are either unsuccessful or inappropriate. Twenty-five percent of patients present as emergencies, and a further 15% are deemed unfit for any surgical intervention. In order to make any sizeable impact on overall morbidity and mortality, earlier diagnosis is required for these patients. It is hoped that increased public awareness, combined with presymptomatic diagnosis by surveillance of high-risk groups, and screening of defined age groups in the community, will go some way towards addressing this problem.

REFERENCES

1. McArdle CS, Hole D, Impact of variability among surgeons on postoperative morbidity and mortality and ultimate survival. *Br Med J* 1991; **302:** 1501–5.
2. Heald RJ, Ryall RDH, Recurrence and survival after total mesorectal excision for rectal cancer. *Lancet* 1986; **ii:** 1479–82.
3. Allum WH, Slaney G, McConkey CC, Powell J, Cancer of the colon and rectum in the West Midlands 1957–1987. *Br J Surg* 1994; **81:** 1060–3.
4. McArdle CS, Hole D, Hansell B et al, Prospective study of colorectal cancer in the West of Scotland: 10 year follow-up. *Br J Surg* 1990; **77:** 280–2.
5. Scott NA, Jeacock J, Kingston RD, Risk factors in patients presenting as an emergency with colorectal cancer. *Br J Surg* 1995; **82:** 321–3.
6. Durdey P, Williams NS, The effect of malignant and inflammatory fixation of rectal carcinoma on prognosis after rectal excision. *Br J Surg* 1984; **71:** 787–90.
7. Barillari P, Ramacciato G, De Angelis R et al, Effect of preoperative colonscopy on the incidence of synchronous and metachronous neoplasms. *Acta Chir Scand* 1990; **156:** 163–6.
8. Baer HU, Matthews JB, Blumgart LH, Hepatic secondaries from colorectal cancer: results of surgery. *Curr Pract Surg* 1989; **I:** 81–6.
9. Paul MA, Siblinga Mulder L, Cuesta MA et al, Impact of intraoperative ultrasonography on treatment strategy for colorectal cancer. *Br J Surg* 1994; **81:** 1660–3.
10. Zeng Z, Cohen AM, Urmacher C, Usefulness of carcinoembryonic antigen monitoring despite normal preoperative values in node-positive colon cancer patients. *Dis Colon Rectum* 1993; **36:** 1063–8.
11. Bacon HE, Kubchandani I, The rationale of aortico-pelvic lymphadenectomy and high ligation of the inferior mesenteric artery for carcinoma of the left half of the colon and rectum. *Surg Gynecol Obstet* 1964; **118:** 503–9.
12. Grinnell RS, Results of ligation of inferior mesenteric artery at the aorta in resection of carcinoma of the descending and sigmoid colon and rectum. *Surg Gynecol Obstet* 1965; **121:** 1031–5.

13. Cole WH, Packard D, Southwick HW, Cancer of the colon and special reference to prevention of recurrence. *J Am Med Assoc* 1954; **155:** 1549–55.

14. McGraw EA, Lars JP, Cole WH, Free malignant cells in relation to recurrence of cancer of the colon. *J Am Med Assoc* 1964; **154:** 1251–4.

15. Turnbull RB, Kyle K, Wilson FR, Spratt J, Cancer of the colon: the influence of the no-touch isolation technique in survival rate. *Ann Surg* 1967; **166:** 420–6.

16. Wiggers T, Jeekel J, Arends JW et al, No-touch isolation technique in colon cancer: a controlled prospective trial. *Br J Surg* 1988; **75:** 409–15.

17. Jinnai D, Quoted in *Surgery of the Anus, Rectum and Colon*, 4th edn (Goligher JC, ed). London: Bailliere Tindall, 1984; 447.

18. Finlay IG, Meek DR, Gray HW et al, Incidence and detection of occult hepatic metastases in colorectal carcinoma. *Br Med J* 1982; **284:** 803–5.

19. Mecklin J-P, Jarvinen HJ, Hakkiluoto A et al, Frequency of hereditary nonpolyposis colorectal cancer. *Dis Colon Rectum* 1995; **38:** 588–93.

20. Lynch HT, Is there a role for prophylactic subtotal colectomy among hereditary non-polyposis colorectal cancer germline mutation carriers? *Dis Colon Rectum* 1996; **39:** 109–10.

21. Vasen HFA, Taal BG, Nagengast FM et al, Hereditary nonpolyposis colorectal cancer: Results of long-term surveillance in 50 families. *Eur J Cancer* 1995; **31A:** 1145–8.

22. Wexner SD, Cohen SM, Port site metastases after laparoscopic colorectal surgery for cure of malignancy. *Br J Surg* 1995; **82:** 295–8.

23. Decosse J, Ptioulias GJ, Jacobson JS, Colorectal cancer, detection, treatment and rehabilitation. *CA Cancer J Clin* 1994; **44:** 27–42.

24. Samet J, Hunt WC, Key C et al, Choice of cancer therapy varies with age of patient. *J Am Med Assoc* 1986; **255:** 3385–90.

25. LaMar S, McGinnis MD, Surgical treatment options for colorectal cancer. *Cancer* 1994; **74**(Suppl): 2147–50.

26. Fitzgerald SD, Longo WE, Daniel GL et al, Advanced colorectal neoplasia in the high risk elderly patient: is surgical resection justified? *Dis Colon Rectum* 1993; **36:** 161–6.

27. Umpleby HC, Bristol JB, Rainey JB et al, Survival of 727 patients with single carcinomas of the large bowel. *Dis Colon Rectum* 1984; **27:** 803–10.

28. Edwards RT, Bransom CJ, Crosby DL, Pathy MS, Colorectal carcinoma in the elderly: a geriatric and surgical practice compared. *Age Ageing* 1984; **12:** 256–62.

29. Fielding LP, Phillips RK, Hittinger R, Factors influencing mortality after curative resection for large bowel cancer in elderly patients. *Lancet* 1989; **i:** 595–7.

30. Irvin TT, Prognosis of colorectal cancer in the elderly. *Br J Surg* 1988; **75:** 419–21.

31. Mulcahy HE, Parchett SE, Daly L, O'Donoghue DP, Prognosis of elderly patients with large bowel cancer. *Br J Surg* 1994; **81:** 736–8.

32. Aldridge MC, Phillips RK, Hittinger R et al, Influence of tumor site on presentation, management and subsequent outcome in large bowel cancer. *Br J Surg* 1986; **73:** 663–70.

33. Fielding LP, Wells BW, Survival after primary and staged resection for large bowel obstruction caused by cancer. *Br J Surg* 1974; **61:** 16–18.

34. Irvin TT, Greaney MG, The treatment of colonic cancer presenting with intestinal obstruction. *Br J Surg* 1977; **64:** 741–4.

35. Clark J, Hjall AW, Moosa AR, Treatment of obstructing cancer of the left colon and rectum. *Surg Gynecol Obstet* 1975; **141:** 541–4.

36. Gutman M, Kaplan O, Skornick Y et al, Proximal colostomy: still an effective emergency measure in obstructing carcinoma of the large bowel. *J Surg Oncol* 1989; **41:** 210–12.

37. Dixon AR, Holmes JT, Hartmann's procedure for carcinoma of rectum and distal sigmoid colon: 5 year audit. *J R Coll Surg Edinb* 1990; **35:** 166–8.

38. Salim AS. Percutaneous decompression and irrigation for large bowel obstruction. New approach. *Dis Colon Rectum* 1991; **34:** 973–80.

39. Adams WJ, Mann LJ, Bokey EL et al, Hartmann's procedure for carcinoma of the rectum and sigmoid colon. *Aust NZ J Surg* 1992; **62:** 200–3.

40. Gandrup P, Lund L, Balslev I, Surgical treatment of acute malignant large bowel obstruction. *Eur J Surg* 1992; **158:** 427–30.

41. Mileski WJ, Rege RV, Joehl RJ, Jahrwold DL, Rates of morbidity and mortality after closure of loop and end colostomy. *Surg Gynecol Obstet* 1990; **171:** 117–21.

42. De Almeida AM, Gracias CW, dos Santos NM, Aldeia FJ, Surgical management of acute, malignant obstruction of the left colon with colostomy. *Acta Med Port* 1991; **4:** 257–62.

43. Malafosse M, Goujard F, Gallot D, Sezeur A, Traitement des occlusions aigues par cancer du colon gauche. *Chirurgie* 1989; **115**(Suppl 2): 125–5.

44. Sjodahl R, Franzen T, Nystrom PO, Primary versus staged resection for acute obstructing colorectal carcinoma. *Br J Surg* 1992; **79:** 685–8.

45. Ambrosetti P, Borst F, Robert J et al, L'excrese-anastomose en un temps dans les occlusions coliques gauche operees en urgence. *Chirurgie* 1989; **115**(Suppl 2): IVII.

46. Koruth NM, Krukowski ZH, Youngson GG et al, Intra-operative colonic irrigation in the management of left-sided large bowel emergencies. *Br J Surg* 1985; **72**: 708–11.

47. Pearce NW, Scott SD, Karran SJ, Timing and method of reversal of Hartmann's procedure. *Br J Surg* 1992; **79**: 839–41.

48. Amsterdam E, Krispin M, Primary resection with colostomy for obstructive carcinoma of the left side of the colon. *Am J Surg* 1985; **150**: 558–60.

49. Dorudi S, Wilson NM, Heddle RM. Primary restorative colectomy in malignant left-sided large bowel obstruction. *Ann R Coll Surg Engl* 1990; **72**: 393–5.

50. Hong JC, Hwang DM, Wang YH, Intraoperative antegrade colon irrigation – in the management of obstructing left-sided colon cancer. *Jao Hsiun I Hsueh Ko Ksueh Tsa Chih* 1989; **5**: 309–13.

51. Murray JJ, Schoetz DJ Jr, Coller JA et al, Intraoperative colonic lavage and primary anastomosis in non-elective colon resection. *Dis Colon Rectum* 1991; **34**: 527–31.

52. Brief DK, Brener BJ, Goldenkranz R et al, Defining the role of subtotal colectomy in the treatment of carcinoma of the colon. *Ann Surg* 1991; **213**: 248–52.

53. Slors JF, Taat CW, Mallonga ET, Brummelkamp WH, One-stage colectomy and ileorectal anastomosis for complete left-sided obstruction of the colon. *Neth J Surg* 1989; **41**: 1–4.

54. Wilson RG, Gollock JM, Obstructing carcinoma of the left colon managed by subtotal colectomy. *J R Coll Surg Edinb* 1989; **34**: 25–6.

55. Koruth NM, Hunter DC, Krukowski ZH, Matheson NA, Immediate resection in emergency large bowel surgery: a 7 year audit. *Br J Surg* 1985; **72**: 703–7.

56. Gorey TF, O'Connell PR, Waldron D et al, Laparoscopically assisted reversal of Hartmann's procedure. *Br J Surg* 1993; **80**: 109.

57. Radcliff AG, Dudley HA, Intraoperative antegrade irrigation of the large intestine. *Surg Gynecol Obstet* 1983; **156**: 721–3.

58. Dudley HAF, Radcliff AG, McGeehan D, Intraoperative irrigation of the colon to permit primary anastomosis. *Br J Surg* 1980; **67**: 80–1.

59. White CM, MacFie J, Immediate colectomy and primary anastomosis for acute obstruction due to carcinoma of the left colon and rectum. *Dis Colon Rectum* 1985; **28**: 155–7.

60. Duthie GS, Foster ME, Price-Thomas JM, Leaper DJ, Bowel preparation or not for elective colorectal surgery. *J R Coll Surg Edinb* 1990; **35**: 169–71.

61. Yu BM, Surgical treatment of acute intestinal obstruction caused by large bowel carcinoma. *Chung Hua Wai Ko Tsa Chih* 1989; **27**: 285–6.

62. Konishi F, Muto T, Kanazawa K, Morioka Y, Intraoperative irrigation and primary resection for obstructing lesions of the left colon. *Int J Colorectal Dis* 1988; **3**: 204–6.

63. Hughes ESR, McDermott FT, Polglase AL, Nottle P, Total and subtotal colectomy for colonic obstruction. *Dis Colon Rectum* 1985; **28**: 162–3.

64. Stephenson BM, Shandall AA, Farouk R, Griffith G, Malignant left-sided large bowel obstruction managed by subtotal/total colectomy. *Br J Surg* 1990; **77**: 1098–102.

65. Arnaud J-P, Bergamaschi R, Emergency subtotal/total colectomy with anastomosis for acutely obstructed carcinoma of the left colon. *Dis Colon Rectum* 1994; **37**: 685–8.

66. Wangensteen OH, Sosin H, How can the outlook in alimentary tract cancer be improved? *Am J Surg* 1968; **115**: 7–16.

67. Schneebaum S, Arnold MW, Young D et al, Role of carcinoembryonic antigen in predicting resectability of recurrent colorectal cancer. *Dis Colon Rectum* 1993; **36**: 810–5.

68. Hida J-I, Yasutomi M, Shindoh K et al, Second-look operation for recurrent colorectal cancer based on carcinoembryonic antigen and imaging techniques. *Dis Colon Rectum* 1996; **39**: 74–9.

69. Beets G, Penninckx F, Schiepers C et al, Clinical value of whole-body positron emission tomography with [^{18}F]fluorodeoxyglucose in recurrent colorectal cancer. *Br J Surg* 1994; **81**: 1666–70.

70. Thurston MO, Majzisik CM, History and development of radioimmunoguided surgery. *Sem Colon Rectal Surg* 1995; **6**: 185–91.

71. Kronborg O, Fenger C, Deichgraeber E, Hansen L, Follow-up after radical surgery for colorectal cancer: design of a randomized study. *Scand J Gastroenterol* 1988; **149**(Suppl): 159–62.

72. Keighley MRB, Williams NS, *Surgery of the Anus, Rectum and Colon*. London: WB Saunders, 1993.

7

Left colectomy for cancer

Guy-Bernard Cadière, Jacques M Himpens

CONTENTS • **Introduction** • **Technique** • **Results** • **Conclusions**

INTRODUCTION

There have been reports of trocar-site recurrences as well as mini-laparotomy recurrences after laparoscopic colon resection for cancer. Hence the question arises of whether it is ethical to perform laparoscopic colon operations in cases of cancer. This question can actually be subdivided into two parts:

- Does laparoscopic surgery for colon cancer result in an increased number of recurrences?
- Is an oncologically correct resection feasible by laparoscopy?

The problem of abdominal wall recurrences

Background
Drouard (St-Quentin) was the first to report an abdominal wall recurrence after laparoscopic cholecystectomy in which the gallbladder unexpectedly appeared to contain adenocarcinoma.[1] Since then, as early as 1993, Fausco, Hork, Alexander, Mouiel and Boulez have all published cases of abdominal wall recurrences after laparoscopic colectomies for cancer.[2–4]

However, parietal metastasis after cancer colectomy is not a new finding, and is not specifically attributable to laparoscopy. In 1983, a multicenter study was published by Hughes[5] concerning the problem of parietal tumor recurrences after colectomy by laparotomy. This study collected 2439 colectomies, 1603 of which had been considered curative. Of these latter 1603, 16 patients presented parietal recurrences: 11 in the laparotomy incision itself, 3 on a drain site and 2 on the colostomy (1%).

Drouard reported the multicenter FDCL (Fondation pour le Developpement de la Chirurgie Laparascopique) study on laparoscopic colectomy (LCR).[6] The incidence of abdominal wall recurrences was 10 out of 545 colectomies (1.8%). Nine surgeons reported 10 parietal recurrences in 268 colectomies, whereas 14 other surgeons had no recurrences in 277 colectomies. In the recurrent cases, the original tumor was staged as Dukes A in 2, Dukes B in 1, Dukes C in 3 and Dukes D in 4.

The site of the original tumor was the right colon in 4, the sigmoid colon in 5 and the rectum in 1. The original treatment had been colectomy (8 cases), anterior resection (1 case), and colotomy and polypectomy (1 case). Pathological examination of the original tumor reported a maximal tumor diameter of 6.7 cm on average (range 2–11 cm). All original tumors were adenocarcinomas, well differentiated in 3 patients, moderately differentiated in 4 patients and poorly differentiated in 2 patients. The number of lymph nodes sampled varied between 0 and 20 (average 9). Vascular tumor permeation was reported in 2 patients.

The site of recurrence was the trocar insertion site on 9 occasions, the specimen extraction site in 1 patient and the drain site in 2.

There were multiple tumors in 4 cases, and a single location was reported in 6. The delay of appearance after the original case was 153 days on average (between 30 and 270 days). The most significant risk factor was an inexperienced surgeon (i.e. one who has performed fewer than 50 procedures). In all cases, bowel mobilization had occurred before vascular control. Accidental colon-wall disruption had occurred in 1 patient; only 2 patients had benefited from a wound-protector device for extraction of specimens. Anastomosis was mechanical in 8 patients and manual in 2. Specimen extraction had been performed via mini-laparotomy in 3 cases and via a trocar site in 1.

Pathogenesis

Many factors can contribute to tumor cells seeding[7]: type and stage of the tumor, immunological status, tumor manipulation, instruments used,[8] operative time, accidental opening of the gut lumen, blood transfusion, among others.[9]

Concerning abdominal wall recurrences, the implant mechanism is probably not hematogenous, since the venous blood coming from the colon preferentially goes to the lungs and liver. The abdominal wall blood supply represents only a small fraction of the total flow. Moreover, the early appearance of these recurrences (much faster than at other localizations), as well as the pathology of the lesions where cancer cells are mixed with fibromuscular cells and are on the abdominal wall, which is not invaded, suggest a mechanical cause for implantation.

Tumor cells are shed, and will preferentially settle in traumatized parietal tissue,[7] which constitutes an ideal feeding medium. The traumatized tissue reacts by inflammation. This, together with hematoma and ischemia, enhances neoangiogenesis. Cancer cells are trapped in these newly formed blood vessels. Since these sites are immunologically isolated, most defense mechanisms are impaired, and tumor growth ensues.

Specific risks related to laparotomy

Mini-laparotomy

This is a relatively unusual site of tumor recurrence (2 cases).[6] If this incision is not sufficiently wide, and if the wall remains unprotected, tumor grafting by local contact is possible.

Trocar sites

Trocar wiggling during the procedure usually causes considerable local trauma and hence ischemia. Moreover, the peritoneum at the trocar site is imperfectly – if at all – sutured, thereby providing an ischemic, ecchymotic deperitonized area, which seems to be an ideal feeding soil for tumor cells.[10]

Pneumoperitoneum

The continuous flow of CO_2 in a relatively humid environment is likely to disseminate viable exfoliated cancer cells, which will be expelled under pressure via the trocar opening during exsufflation at the end of the procedure.[11,12]

Instrumentation

Laparoscopic tools are long, rigid and traumatic, and prone to cause accidental perforation of the bowel wall, again causing dissemination of viable cancer cells. Additionally, lack of laparoscopic experience increases the number of instrument changes in the trocar, thereby reducing trocar stability and tending to cause gas leaks, which can carry live tumor cells.[11,12]

Surgeon inexperience

In the FDCL study, all tumor recurrences appeared early on in the surgeon's experience.

Rules for oncologically acceptable laparoscopic colon resection

In theory, an oncologically satisfactory colon resection should be conducted as follows:

(1) use of stable trocars, reducing local parietal trauma;
(2) minimal tumor mobilization (no-touch technique);
(3) vascular control first;
(4) tumor exclusion plus bowel lumen occlusion proximally as well as distally;
(5) protection of extraction site;
(6) radical lymph-node sampling;
(7) reduced peroperative lavage plus immediate aspiration of all lavage fluid.

Other more controversial rules are as follows:

(8) good parietal hemostasis;
(9) systematic suture of all peritoneal disruption (trocars, pelvis) sites;
(10) reduction of pneumoperitoneum pressure;
(11) use of cytotoxic agents for lavaging;
(12) use of an abdominal wall lifting device rather than pneumoperitoneum.

Three preliminary conditions, however, appear even more important:

(i) The surgeon must have good laparoscopic skills so as to be able to perform the laparoscopic state of the art procedure.
(ii) Patient selection has to be strict (obesity, multiple adhesions, extensive tumor bulk, and loss of planes of cleavage are contraindications). Tumor staging, however, does not intervene in the actual indication.
(iii) The surgeon's armamentarium has to be excellent, including camera, optical system, etc.

In 1995, numerous experimental studies were carried out to analyse the influence of CO_2 flow and of local site conditions in the diffusion of tumor cells. American clinical studies (Franklin, Fleischman, Wexner) presently mention a follow-up of less than 5 years, but so far there have been no significant differences as far as global survival and recurrence rate are concerned. It is, however, imperative that surgeons performing LCR do so in the context of a multicenter prospective trial.

TECHNIQUE

Patient position (Figure 7.1)

Figure 7.1 Patient position.

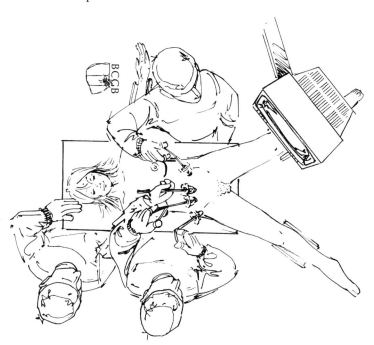

The patient is put in the lithotomy position. The surgeon stands to the patient's right. The first assistant is to the patient's left and the second assistant to his or her right. The TV monitor is located at the level of the patient's left thigh, so that surgeon, optical system and TV monitor are more or less on one line.

Placement of trocars and tools (Figure 7.2)

The first trocar (10 mm) is placed just proximal to the umbilicus, and will be used for the optical system. A second 10-mm trocar is located in the right lower quadrant, just medial to the anterosuperior iliac spine. This trocar opening can be enlarged if necessary in order to harbor a 12-mm trocar for an endostapler. A third 10-mm trocar is placed half-way between these latter two.

Finally, a fourth trocar, 5 mm in diameter, is introduced in the left flank. If necessary, a fifth 5-mm trocar can be inserted (suprapubically), located in the future minilap. The second trocar allows the introduction of the scissors (Ci-2), or the coagulating hook (CR-2) held by the surgeon. The third trocar will contain the grasping forceps (PF-3), in the surgeon's left hand. The fourth trocar in the left flank allows introduction of an atraumatic forceps (PAT-4) for grasp-ing the sigmoid, which needs to be pulled cranially and laterally to the left. The trocar has to be secured so as to minimize the movements in the skin opening. Instrument switching is kept to a minimum.

Inspection

After initial exploration of the abdominal cavity (peritoneum, viscera and liver), the tumor is localized. This can be performed in two ways (Urbain): by preoperative injection of methylene blue or Indian ink, or by peroperative colonoscopy. This latter technique has the double disadvantage of necessitating additional equipment in the OR and of reducing the intraperitoneal working space because of the insufflation of the bowel. In a female, exposure of the pelvis is greatly improved by transfixing the uterus with a suture and pulling it anteriorly by tying the suture on the abdominal wall.

Exposure of the left colon (Figure 7.3 A,B)

The patient is put in 30° Trendelenburg tilt, with a lateral roll of 20° to the right. The greater omentum is grasped and positioned in front of

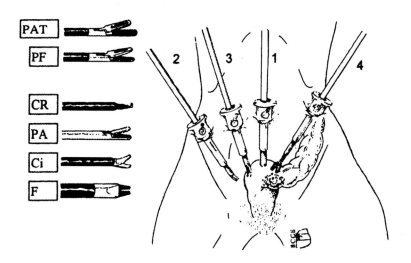

Figure 7.2 Placement of trocars and tools.

A B

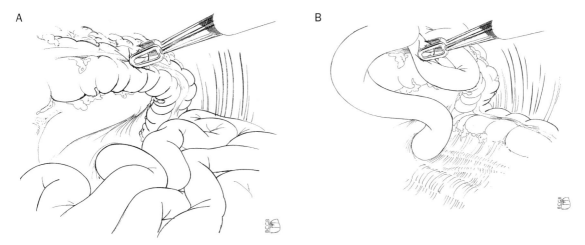

Figure 7.3 (A,B) The transverse colon and the small bowel are reclined cephalad.

the stomach and the left lobe of the liver, thereby exposing the transverse colon. The small bowel is reclined cephalad in a supramesocolic position. The angle of Treitz is exposed.

Ligation of inferior mesenteric artery and vein (IMA and IMV) (Figure 7.4)

The top of the sigmoid loop is grasped with a

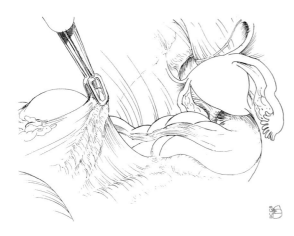

Figure 7.4 The sigmoid loop is grasped, and the vascular axis becomes visible.

grasper (PAT-4) introduced in the fourth trocar. The bowel itself is not touched, but rather the mesocolic peritoneum near its insertion on the bowel wall.

By pulling the bowel anteriorly, the vascular axis of the IMA becomes visible. The peritoneum is incised using scissors (Ci-2) starting 2 cm distal to the aortic bifurcation and orienting cranially along the anterior aspect of the aorta until the ligament of Treitz is reached, where the orientation of the incision is changed to lateral to the left up to the lower pole of the spleen. Usually, the emergence of the IMA is readily visible. In obese patients, however, additional hook dissection has to be performed in order to individualize the artery. In benign disease, when the splenic flexure does not need to be liberated, the artery is ligated distal to the bifurcation of the ascending colic artery (sigmoid artery).

Dissection to the left reveals the IMV, which is sometimes more than 1.5 cm away. Ligation is performed with a 2.0 absorbable suture introduced by a needle holder (PA-2) and tied with the help of a fine grasper in the third trocar (PF-3) in the surgeon's left hand. After suture ligation, additional clips can be placed for safety.

Dissection of Toldt's fascia (Figure 7.5)

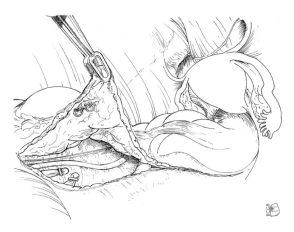

Figure 7.5 Ligation of artery and vein, and dissection of Toldt's fascia.

In classical surgery, dissection is initiated by freeing the left colon at Toldt's fascia, which is logical since the surgeon is standing to the patient's left. In laparoscopy, however, the surgeon views the operative field from the right. Moreover, once Toldt's fascia is incised, the colon loop has a tendency to drop to the right (this is even more the case since the patient is in a 20° lateral tilt), and the view is obscured. In order to avoid this problem, the mesocolon is grasped by the grasper PAT-4 right at the level where vascular control has been obtained. The mesocolon is dissected away from the posterior retroperitoneum from right to left. The gonadal vessels, the ureter and the perirenal fascia are all dissected posteriorly and left attached to the retroperitoneum. Hence, a cone is dissected with the PAT-4 grasper at the top and the left retroperitoneum at the base of the cone.

Dissection of the posterior mesorectum (Figure 7.6 A,B)

At the level of the promontorium, the 'holy' presacral plane is opened and dissected as far down as possible. Pneumodissection facilitates this step. The holy plane is limited by the presacral fascia posteriorly and by the mesorectum anteriorly.

Incision of the left paracolic gutter (Figure 7.7)

The PAT-4 grasper pulls the sigmoid loop toward the patient's right. PF-3 grasps the peritoneal reflexion (Toldt's line) and creates adequate counter-traction. Toldt's white line is then

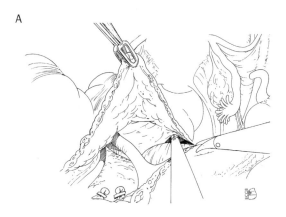
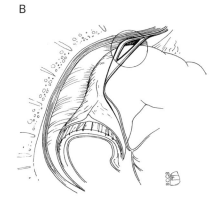

Figure 7.6 (A,B) Opening of the presacral plane.

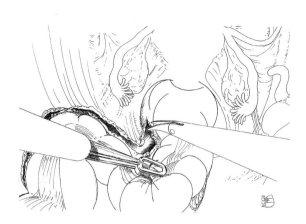

Figure 7.7 Incision of the left paracolic gutter.

incised from distal to proximal, starting at the level of the promontorium and ending at the already-divided peritoneum just distal to the spleen's lower pole.

Pelvic peritoneal incision (Figure 7.8 A,B)

Incision of Toldt's fascia is then carried out and taken to the pelvis to the left of the rectum, remaining shallow of the vessels and the left ureter. Finally, PAT-4 grasps the upper rectum and pulls it towards the patient's head. PT-3

grasps the prevesical peritoneum and pulls it anteriorly. The peritoneal reflexion is then sectioned in front of the rectum, and Denonvilliers' fascia is opened. The parietal peritoneal incision is then continued to the right until the original incision around the vessels is reached.

Dissection of mesorectum (Figure 7.9)

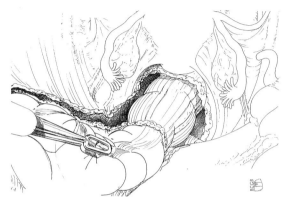

Figure 7.9 Dissection of the mesorectum until the muscular wall is freed.

At the limit set for rectal transsection, the mesorectum is dissected by hook or scissors until the muscular wall is freed along its entire circumference. Vascular control is usually

A

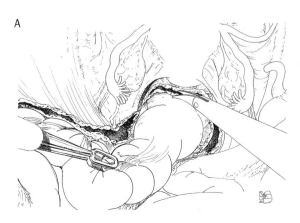

B

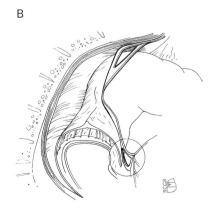

Figure 7.8 (A,B) Incision of Toldt's fascia.

obtained by coagulation, with the exception of the lateral ligaments, in which the mid-hemorroidal vascular pedicle can be controlled by clips. The rectum is then transsected by a stapler introduced by enlarging the trocar opening in the right lower quadrant or in the suprapubic position.

Incision of the mesocolic peritoneum

At the level chosen for proximal bowel transsection, the peritoneum is incised from posterior to anteriorly until the vascular arch is reached. Vessels are controlled by clips or by coagulation. Even though this step can be postponed until after extirpation of the colon and before final transsection, it is safer to control it intracorporeally in order to avoid traction lesions in an effort to exteriorize the bowel. Only the periserosal colonic dissection can safely be performed outside.

Transsection of the rectum (Figure 7.10)

The second 10-mm trocar in the right lower quadrant is replaced by a 12-mm one containing the linear stapling and cutting device. Since the axis of the colon and the stapling device are not perpendicular to each other, this step can actually be quite difficult. Usually, several firings of the stapler are needed.

Extraction and resection of the specimen (Figure 7.11)

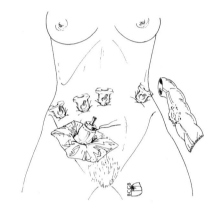

Figure 7.11 Resection of the specimen.

A mini-laparotomy is performed either in the right lower quadrant or suprapubically on the midline by enlarging the stapler orifice. A wound-protecting device (V drape) is used. The bowel is extirpated and transsected proximally. The anvil of the stapler is introduced inside the bowel, and a pursestring performed in the usual fashion. The proximal colon is now ready for anastomosis, and is reintroduced inside the abdomen. The mini-laparotomy incision is closed hermetically in layers.

Anastomosis (Figure 7.12)

The colon anastomosis is performed as usual after transanal introduction of the circular stapler. This step may be more difficult, since the distal colon stump is longer.

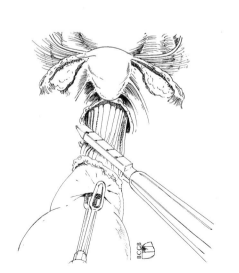

Figure 7.10 Transection of the rectum.

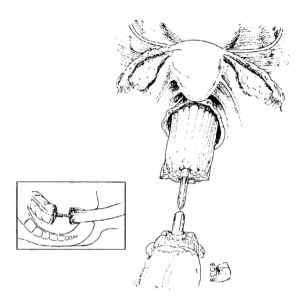

Figure 7.12 Anastomosis.

Early recurrences have been described. However, they are only case reports of surgeons with marginal experience. Presently, evaluation of large series after only a short follow-up show no difference.[13] The only series with 5-year follow-up is Franklin's, and this study also fails to show any difference in recurrence rate between laparoscopic and open surgery.

224 open and 192 laparoscopic patients have been compared in a prospective manner. Anastomotic recurrences seem fewer with the LCR, and are perhaps secondary to colonoscopic determination of the lower margin of resection. Lymph-node harvest, disease-free interval and margins of resection are essentially the same. Death rates and recurrence rates have been compared, and appear to be similar five years into the study. From the data in this study, it is clear that laparoscopic colon surgery for carcinoma does not harm patients, and offers many benefits in the hands of careful laparoscopic surgeons.

RESULTS

Reports on evaluation of LCR have become more frequent. Feasability has been demonstrated, and operative morbidity seems to go down as the surgeon gains experience – the now-classical learning curve in laparoscopic surgery.

Peroperative blood loss, delay of return of bowel function, and time off work diminish. Pathology reports usually show an identical number of lymph nodes harvested and safe resection margins.[6,13]

The main problem is the 5-year follow-up. In theory, laparoscopy could reduce immunological impairment[12,14–17] as compared with open surgery. Some studies,[18] however, have not corroborated these findings.

CONCLUSIONS

Laparoscopic left colectomy for cancer can only be performed on selected patients by well-trained surgeons, with respect for the rules of cancer surgery. The problem of parietal tumor grafts should not be overestimated, since the incidence of parietal malignant grafts after laparoscopic colectomy is not significantly different from conventional colectomy. The problem should not, however, be underestimated, since laparoscopy carries definite – albeit theoretical – risks of dissemination and parietal seeding for cancer cells.[19] Hence this type of surgery should only be done by experienced laparoscopists, in connection with a multicenter prospective trial.

REFERENCES

1. Drouard F, Delamarre J, Capron JP, Cutaneous seeding of gallbladder after laparoscopic cholecystectomy. *N Engl J Med* 1991; **325:** 1316.

2. Alexander RJT, Jacques BC, Mitchel KG, Laparoscopically assisted colectomy and wound recurrence. *Lancet* 1993; **341:** 249–50.

3. Fusco MA, Paluzzi MW, Abdominal wall recurrence after laparoscopic-assisted colectomy for adenocarcinoma of the colon: report of a case. *Dis Colon Rectum* 1993; **36:** 858–61.

4. Nduka CC, Monson JRT, Menzies-Gow N, Darzy A, Abdominal wall metastases following laparoscopy. *Br J Surg* 1994; **81:** 648–52.

5. Hughes ES, MacDermott FT, Polglase AL, Johnson WR, Tumor recurrence in the abdominal wall scar after large bowel cancer surgery. *Dis Colon Rectum* 1983; **6:** 571–2.

6. Cadière GB, Leroy J, Drouard F et al, Colectomie gauche pour cancer par voie laparoscopique. *J Coelio-Chirurgie* 1994; **12:** 17–22.

7. Gilliland R, Williamson KE, Wilson RH et al, Colorectal cell kinetics. *Br J Surg* 1996; **83:** 739–49.

8. Gertsch P, Baer HU, Kraft R et al, Malignant cells are collected on circular staplers. *Dis Colon Rectum* 1992; **35:** 238–41.

9. O'Rourken N, Price PM, Kelly S, Sikora K, Tumor inoculation during laparoscopy. *Lancet* 1993; **342:** 368.

10. Allardyce R, Morreau Ph, Bagshaw Ph, Tumor cell distribution following laparoscopic colectomy in a porcine model. *Off J Am Soc Colon Rectal Surg* 1996; **39**(10): s47–52.

11. Hewett PJ, Thomas WM, King G, Eaton M, Intraperitoneal cell movement during abdominal carbon dioxide insufflation and laparoscopy. *Off J Am Soc Colon Rectal Surg* 1996; **39**(10): s62–6.

12. Hubens G, Pauwels M, Hubens A et al, The influence of a pneumoperitoneum on the peritoneal implantation of free intraperitoneal colon cancer cells. *Surg Endosc* 1996; **10:** 809–12.

13. Fleshman JW, Nelson H, Peters WR et al, Early results of laparoscopic surgery for colorectal cancer. Retrospective analysis of 372 patients treated by clinical outcomes of surgical therapy (cost) study group. *Off J Am Soc Colon Rectal Surg* 1996; **39**(10): s53–8.

14. Allendorf JDF, Bessler M, Whelan RL et al, Better preservation of immune function after laparoscopic-assisted vs open bowel resection in a murine model. *Off J Am Soc Colon Rectal Surg* 1996; **39**(10): s67–72.

15. Jacobi CA, Ordemann J, Böhm B et al, Increased tumor growth after laparotomy and laparoscopy with air vs CO_2. *Fourth International Congress of the European Association for Endoscopic Surgery, Trondheim, 23–26 June 1996*; Abst 291.

16. Marthy SM, Goldschmidt RA, Rao LN et al, The influence of surgical trauma on experimental metastasis. *Cancer* 1989; **64:** 2035–44.

17. Morino M, Miglietta C, Garrone C et al, Oncologic laparoscopic colon resection and the immunity system: a randomized trial. *Fourth International Congress of the European Association for Endoscopic Surgery, Trondheim, 23–26 June 1996*; Abst 289.

18. Fukushima R, Kawamura YJ, Saito H et al, Interleukin-6 and stress hormone responses after uncomplicated gasless laparoscopic-assisted and open sigmoid colectomy. *Off J Am Soc Colon Rectal Surg* 1996; **39**(10): s29–34.

19. Laroy HM, Garcia-Valdecasas JC, Delgado S et al, Short-term outcome, port-site recurrence and cost analysis of a randomized study comparing laparoscopic vs open colectomy for colon cancer. *Fourth International Congress of the European Association for Endoscopic Surgery, Trondheim, 23–26 June 1996*; Abst 137.

8

Surgery of metastatic disease

Christophe Penna, Bernard Nordlinger

INTRODUCTION

Distant metastases, particularly liver deposits, represent the major cause of death of patients who have been treated for colorectal adenocarcinoma. Depending on the stage of the primary tumor, liver metastases occur in 20–70% of patients, and lung metastases in 10–20%. Brain and adrenal metastases are less frequent. Surgical resection remains the only treatment that can ensure long-term survival in some patients. However, selection criteria for surgical resection of metastases should be strict, and less than 10% of liver metastases and 4% of lung metastases are suitable for surgery. We shall successively discuss the preoperative assessment, surgical techniques and results of surgical resection for liver and lung metastases, and give some information on the few available data on the surgical treatment of brain metastases.

LIVER METASTASES

Spontaneous survival rates rarely exceed 3 years, but the natural history of hepatic metastases depends on numerous factors. In a large prospective study conducted from 1980 to 1990 and including 484 patients with untreated hepatic metastases from colorectal cancer, the median survival was 31% at 1 year, 7.9% at 2 years, 2.6% at 3 years and 0.9% at 4 years. Factors that independently influenced survival were the volume of the liver involvement, the presence of extrahepatic disease, metastatic lymph nodes in the mesentery, carcinoembryonic antigen (CEA) level and the age of the patient. According to the presence or the absence of these criteria, the median survival varied from 3.8 to 21 months.[1]

Surgical resection is to date the only therapeutic modality able to ensure 5-year survival rates of 25–30% and to ultimately cure some patients, and therefore should be discussed in every case.

Selection of patients for surgery

The decision and the extent of surgical resection for liver metastases is based upon the patient's condition and liver function. Surgical resection should only be performed with a curative intent, leaving no macroscopic residual disease.

Patient's condition

Standard clinical and anamnestic criteria, briefly summarized in the ASA score, should be used to determine if the patient is suitable for general anaesthesia and potentially hemorrhagic surgery. Particular attention is given to the cardiocirculatory status, since clamping manoeuvres of the hepatic pedicle and the vena cava may be used during the hepatic resection. The hemodynamic changes resulting from these temporary vascular occlusions are poorly tolerated in patients whose cardiac function is altered, and preoperative ultrasonographic assessment of cardiac function may be useful. It is important to assess coagulation profile, since major resections may be accompanied by a transient decrease in vitamin-K-dependent clotting factors and an increase in plasma fibrinogen concentration and fibrinogen degradation products.[2]

Liver function

The hepatic functional reserve should be sufficient to allow resection and to ensure that postoperative liver function will be sufficient. If remnant liver parenchyma is normal, up to 6 of the 8 anatomical segments (75% of the volume of the liver) can be resected without inducing postoperative liver failure. Such major resections cannot be performed safely if remnant liver parenchyma is abnormal. The functional capacity of the liver can be assessed by the classic Child–Turcotte classification modified by Pugh et al[3] and other hepatic biological blood tests (AST, ALT, alkaline phosphatases, gamma GT). The indocyanine green (ICG) or bromosulfophthalein retention tests are useful in evaluating the liver function preoperatively. For patients with an ICG 15-minute retention of greater than 30%, resections other than enucleation of small tumors are not advisable. In most cases, these tests are not necessary before resection. In metastatic disease, liver parenchyma is rarely fibrotic or cirrhotic, but can have been damaged by previous chemotherapy. Recent data have demonstrated that prolonged systemic chemotherapy could induce portal and periportal fibrosis and microvascular changes such as peliosis and sinusoidal congestion.

These vascular changes can be responsible for increased risk of bleeding during surgery. A transcutaneous needle biopsy of non-tumorous liver may be helpful to assess the status of liver parenchyma. In some selected cases, the amount of liver parenchyma of the segments that will be left in place after surgery can be increased by preoperative selective portal embolization of the lobe where the tumor is located.[4]

Control of primary and extrahepatic sites

Local control of the primary tumor

Metastases can be detected at the same time as the primary colorectal cancer (synchronous metastases) or several months after the treatment of the primary (metachronous metastases).[5] In cases of metastases discovered during the follow-up after resection of a colorectal cancer, adequate control of the site of the primary tumor should be assessed. This is usually done by rectal digital examination and colonoscopy to eliminate anastomotic recurrence or a new colonic cancer, and a CT scan to verify the absence of locoregional spread. Endorectal ultrasonography can be helpful after primary rectal cancer excision and low anterior anastomosis. Magnetic resonance imaging seems to be of value when local recurrence is suspected after abdominoperineal excision.

Control of other metastatic sites

A chest X-ray and thoracic CT scan are performed to rule out lung metastases; however, solitary lung metastasis does not constitute a contraindication to hepatic resection, provided that it can be entirely resected by a simultaneous or delayed resection (see below). Brain CT scan and bone scintigraphy are performed only if there is a clinical suspicion of brain or bone metastasis. Their presence usually contraindicates a liver resection.

Preoperative assessment of the hepatic involvement

Liver resections leaving behind intrahepatic metastases do not prolong survival[6,7] and should not be performed. It is therefore of major relevance to precisely localize all intrahepatic lesions before performing surgical resection. This is also important to plan an adequate type of resection. A wide range of imaging techniques is now available to delineate hepatic lesions. Ultrasonography is helpful to determine the relations between deposits and the intrahepatic vessels and the vena cava. Bolus-dynamic computed tomography has good sensitivity, and allows a good appreciation of the volume of the non-tumorous liver parenchyma – helpful information to decide which type of resection should be performed.[8,9] If a liver resection is planned, CT during arterial portography should be performed. Although its specificity is low, its strong sensitivity is helpful to detect small lesions (<5 mm) that could have been missed by other procedures.[10] The MRI is less invasive, and appears to be promising, but to date its sensitivity is inferior to that of arterial portography.[11]

Intraoperative assessment
The exact role of laparoscopy used alone or in combination with laparoscopic ultrasound has not yet been fully evaluated, but recent studies have suggested that it could be helpful in some cases – either to avoid unnecessary laparotomy or to adapt abdominal incision to the extent of resection.[12]

During laparotomy, a careful exploration of the abdominal cavity is performed. The gastrointestinal tract and the site of the primary tumor are examined. The diaphragm, the paracolic gutters and the Douglas pouch are palpated, looking for peritoneal deposits. The anatomical routes of lymphatic drainage of the primary tumor are exposed and palpated, as is the origin of the inferior mesenteric artery for a primary left colonic or rectal cancer. The coeliac axis and the hepatoduodenal ligament are explored. If enlarged or suspicious lymph nodes or peritoneal deposits are found, the specimens are examined intraoperatively by frozen sections. The presence of metastatic lymph nodes in the porta hepatis and the coeliac region considerably worsens the prognosis, but should not be considered as an absolute contraindication to resection, if they can be completely removed. Five-year recur-

rence-free surviving patients have been reported in such cases.[7] Assessment of the resectability is determined after incision of the lesser omentum and the division of the falciform, triangular and coronary ligaments.

Intraoperative ultrasound should be performed by the surgeon, eventually helped by a radiologist. Using high-frequency probes, it can detect small intraparenchymatous lesions, and can modify the extent of the initially planned operation.[13] It may guide the fine-needle biopsies that can be necessary to precisely determine the nature of the detected lesions, and gives a precise mapping of the anatomical relations of the metastases to the main intraparenchymatous vascular pedicles[14] in order to select the type of resection.

Surgical treatment

Surgical resection is the only potentially curative treatment of colorectal metastases. Liver transplantation has been withdrawn for this indication because of its disappointing results. In a collective review of 43 cases of orthotopic liver transplantation for metastases, the 2-year survival rate was 14% and there were no surviving patients at 5 years.[15]

Different types of liver resections
Liver resections can be divided into two groups: anatomical resections removing one or several segments according to Couinaud, and atypical or wedge resections removing a portion of liver parenchyma surrounding a hepatic lesion. Resections removing two or more continuous segments are defined as major hepatic resections. Four types of major liver resections are commonly performed: left lobectomy (segments II and III), right hepatectomy (segments V, VI, VII and VIII), left hepatectomy (segments II, III and IV) and right lobectomy (segments IV, V, VI, VII and VIII). Other types of anatomical resections can be performed: extended left hepatectomy (left trisegmentectomy) extending a left hepatectomy to segments V and VIII, central hepatectomy (segments IV, V, VIII) or bisegmentectomies V–VI, VII–VIII and VI–VII.[16–19]

Choice of operation

The goal of surgery for liver metastases is to remove all the metastatic sites with free margins of at least 1 cm. The type of liver resection is not by itself a prognostic factor. The extent of liver resection depends on the size, the number and the location of the metastases, on their relation to the main vascular and biliary pedicles and on the volume of the liver parenchyma that can be left in place after surgery. Small metastases located near the liver capsule can be resected by wedge resections; larger lesions often require segmental resections.

However, it is sometimes necessary to perform a major liver resection to remove a small solitary metastasis if it is located near a main vascular pedicle (hepatic vein) or in the center of the liver parenchyma. In some cases there can be some hesitation, with a choice between performing several wedge resections or a major liver resection removing all the deposits at once. The first solution preserves more healthy liver parenchyma, but the cut section of the liver may be larger, increasing the risk of postoperative hemorrhage or fluid collections. On the other hand, a major liver resection allows a better margin between tumor deposits and the cut section of the liver, better control of preoperative hemorrhage and recognition of main intrahepatic vessels, but removes more parenchyma, with a risk of post-resectional hepatic failure and the theoretical risk of promoting the development of dormant liver metastases by the mechanisms involved in liver regeneration.[20]

In cases of synchronous metastases discovered at the same time as the primary, a wedge resection of an isolated easily accessible metastase can be performed. In other cases, although combined resections of both primary and liver metastases have been reported without added morbidity,[5,6] most surgeons prefer to delay the hepatic resection for several reasons. The incision necessary to ensure good exposure is usually different for the colorectal and liver resections. Bowel section and subsequent peritoneal contamination can favor the infection of an intraabdominal or subphrenic fluid collection. Hemodynamic changes and portal hyper-

tension subsequent to vascular clamping can be detrimental to the viability of digestive sutures. Finally, a 2–4-month delay can be helpful to appreciate the natural behavior of the metastatic disease. In a large multicenter trial,[7] the postoperative morbidity was significantly increased when both resections were performed simultaneously (6.1% versus 2.4%). The most common attitude is therefore to resect small metastases simultaneously if they can be removed with 1 cm margin with a minor resection by the same incision. In the other cases, the liver resection is postponed and performed 2–4 months later. During this period, systemic chemotherapy is usually performed, but its results have not been, to date, prospectively assessed.

Operative technique

Incision can be either a right or bilateral subcostal incision or a transverse upper abdominal and median incision. In some cases of large tumors lying posteriorly in the right lobe and involving the vena cava, a thoracoabdominal approach may be necessary. Following complete abdominal exploration, the liver is fully mobilized by dissection of its ligaments.

Preoperative hemorrhage is associated with increases in postoperative mortality and morbidity.[21–24] In order to reduce blood losses, several methods of vascular clamping have been described and are increasingly used.[21,22,25–30] Normal liver can be subjected to the induced normothermic ischaemia for 90 minutes with good clinical and biological tolerance.[21,22,30]

To avoid blood loss due to backflow from the hepatic veins, a complete vascular exclusion of the liver, including clamping of the hepatic pedicle, the infrahepatic vena cava and the suprahepatic vena cava, can be performed.[21,31,32] This hepatic vascular exclusion is of importance in cases of large tumors involving the main hepatic veins or the vena cava. It induces a drop in cardiac output of about 50%, while the mean arterial pressure is usually maintained. The magnitude of these changes and their tolerance vary among patients, and a preliminary test of 5 minutes of vascular exclusion should be performed before starting the liver resection. In very selected cases necessitating complex vascular reconstructions, a resection 'ex situ, ex vivo' followed by an auto-transplantation[33] or an 'ex situ, in vivo' without resection of the hepatic pedicle[34] have been proposed.

Vascular pedicles can be divided either in the liver during the division of the parenchyma[35] or during the preliminary dissection of the porta hepatis. The liver tissue is crushed either between finger and thumb or using a Kelly forceps or similar instrument leaving the vessels intact. A vibrating ultrasonic instrument may also be used to divide the liver tissue and expose the vessels.[36] Once located, vessels and bile ducts are occluded by metal clips, ligated or stapled, according to their size. Hemostasis of the cut liver surface is secured by suture ligation and application of fibrin tissue-adhesive sealant, or argon laser-beam coagulation can be used.

At the end of the operation, a cholangiography can be performed to control the biliary pedicles. A drainage of the subdiaphragmatic space is generally left in place after major resections.[37]

Results of liver resection for colorectal metastases

Postoperative complications

In most recent studies, in-hospital mortality varies from 0% to 5% (Table 8.1), and is strongly influenced by preoperative blood loss,[38–42] preoperative liver function and extent of liver resection. Postoperative complications are observed in 25% of patients.[6,7,41,43–46] Morbidity after hepatic resection is usually due to transient liver failure, hemorrhage, subphrenic abcesses or biliary fistula. The mean hospital stay after liver surgery averages 12–15 days in the absence of complications.

Long-term results

Liver resection of colorectal metastases is associated with 3- and 5-year survival rates of 40% and 25% respectively (Table 8.1). Comparison with the natural history of unresected metastases is biased by the selection of patients having resectable lesions and whose general condition is good enough to allow resection. In

Table 8.1 Results of surgical resection of liver metastases from colorectal cancer

Study	Number of patients	Post-operative mortality (%)	Post-operative morbidity (%)	2-year survival (%)	3-year survival (%)	5-year survival (%)
Fortner et al (1984)[73]	65	9	27	71	57	30
Hugues et al (1986)[a,49]	859	—	—	—	—	33
Adson et al (1984)[74]	141	2.8	—	—	—	23
Iwatsuki et al (1986)[53]	60	0	13	72	53	45
Nordlinger et al (1987)[41]	80	5	13	51	40	25
Holm et al (1990)[39]	35	0	—	57	31	31
Scheele et al (1991)[6]	207	5	22	—	41	31
Doci et al (1991)[75]	100	5	39	—	—	30
AFC (1992)[a,7]	1818	2	24	—	41	26

[a] Multicenter trials.

a retrospective study, 3-year survival rates of patients with multiple or unique resectable metastases were respectively 0% and 20% in the absence of resection and 40% when resection was performed.[47]

After resection, recurrences are observed in two-thirds of the patients, and generally involve the liver.[7,48,49] In a large retrospective study, the 5-year survival rates were 28% in 1588 patients who had a resection of isolated colorectal liver metastases and 15% in 250 patients who had resected liver and extrahepatic metastases. None of the 77 patients who had a palliative resection survived 5 years.[7]

Prognostic factors
In order to improve prognosis and provide a better selection of patients before surgery, numerous studies have been directed towards

the search for factors influencing survival. These are summarized in Table 8.2. Age, sex and the site of the primary tumor do not influence the outcome. The stage of the primary tumor seems of major relevance, with 5-year survival rates after resection of hepatic metastases of 70% in stage I or II tumors and of 33% when lymph nodes were invaded.[7] The prognosis seems better in cases of metachronous metastases,[6,7,50,51] small lesions[7,38,46,50,52–54] and when there are fewer than four lesions,[7,46,50,52–54] but the involvement of one or both lobes does not seem to influence the outcome. CEA level is strongly correlated with recurrence-free survival.[6,7,54,55] Obtaining a free margin of at least 1 cm is one of the strongest prognostic factors.[6,7,39,43,46,50,56] In a retrospective study, the 5-year survival rates were 30% when the margin was more than 1 cm, 15% when it was less than

Table 8.2 Predictive factors associated with tumor recurrence and survival following surgical resection of liver metastases

Ref	Number of patients	Size of metastases	Number of metastases	Stage of primary	Synchronous versus metachronous	Free margin >1 cm
74	141	No	No	Yes	No	—
44	62	No	No	Yes	No	No
75	100	—	No	Yes	No	—
46	72	Yes	Yes	No	No	Yes
73	65	No	No	Yes	—	—
52	78	Yes	Yes	No	No	—
50[a]	859	Yes	Yes	Yes	Yes	Yes
41	80	No	No	No	No	—
6	207	No	No	Yes	Yes	Yes
54	116	Yes	Yes	No	No	—
7[a]	1818	Yes	Yes	Yes	No	Yes

[a] Multicenter.

1 cm and 0% when resection was incomplete. The type of resection does not seem to influence the prognosis, providing that a clear margin is obtained. Blood transfusions could be associated with an adverse outcome, but may reflect the surgical difficulties faced with large and numerous lesions.[54]

Repeat liver resections for metastases
Recurrences limited to the liver following previous hepatic resection are amenable to iterative resection.[7,57–60] Such recurrences occur in 25–53% of cases.[7,41,57,61] Postoperative mortality and morbidity do not differ from those reported after a first resection,[7] and the mean survival time approaches 2 years.[59–62] Hepatic recurrences should therefore be resected whenever possible.

Liver metastases: summary and conclusions

Resection should be considered when liver metastases can be totally resected with clear margins and when there is no extrahepatic disease. However, some patients can gain benefit from associated resection of lung or locoregional recurrence.

The best candidates for resection are those with fewer than four lesions, with lesions smaller than 5 cm, without extrahepatic disease, with lesions that appeared more than 2 years after the resection of a stage I or II colorectal cancer, and whose CEA level is lower than 5 mg/ml. The choice between anatomical or wedge resection depends on the number and location of the metastases; clamping methods limit blood loss. After the resection, a follow-up with ultrasonography of the liver every 3 months during 2 years and then every 6 months can detect hepatic recurrences eventually amenable to repeat hepatectomy.

LUNG METASTASES

Although lung metastases are less frequent than lever metastases, their indications for resection are similar. After complete resection,

significant improvements in survival and the numbers of long-term survivors can be observed. Indications for surgery have increased in the last decade, and resection is now proposed not only for patients with solitary deposits but also for some with multiple metastases or in whom liver metastases have been resected previously.

Selection criteria

As for liver secondaries, the primary tumor should be totally resected, and there should be no evidence of local recurrence or other extrapulmonary disease, although combined resection of liver and lung metastases can be discussed in selected cases. Surgery can be considered only when complete removal of all pulmonary metastases is possible. Preoperative evaluation should include a CT scan in order to detect small lesions of less than 5 mm, and a bronchoscopy to visualize any endobronchic lesion that would preclude a simple metastasectomy and indicate a segmental resection. Pulmonary function (gasometry and spirometric tests) as well as general status (ASA score) should be assessed.

Only 2–4% of patients with lung metastases are amenable to surgical resection.[63,64]

Surgical aspects

The incision is usually a postero-lateral thoracotomy in the 5th intercostal space. In cases of bilateral metastases, the choice is between a median sternotomy – allowing the treatment of all lesions in one session with less detrimental effects on pulmonary function[65] – or two thoracotomies at 7–12 days' interval – allowing better exploration of each lung.[66] As opposed to the liver, there is no regeneration after pulmonary resection. Therefore surgery should be conservative whenever possible,[66–69] and wedge resections are preferred in most cases. Anatomical resections (lobectomy, bi-lobectomy or pneumonectomy) may, however, be mandatory in cases of large lesions, endobronchic involvement or resectable lymph-node metastases. In published series, wedge resections were performed in 50–68% of cases, lobectomies in 40–45% and pneumonectomies in 6–8%, and the total number of metastases resected in a single patient reached 12.[63,64,70–72]

Results

Postoperative mortality is low, ranging from 0% to 5%,[63,72] and postoperative morbidity varies from 2% to 12%, according to the preoperative status of the patient and the type of resection performed.[63,64,70]

Surgical resection of lung metastases significantly prolongs survival: 5-year survival rates observed in the principal reported series are given in Table 8.3.

Prognostic factors are similar to those associated with resection of liver metastases. Age, sex and type of resection have no impact on survival.[63,64,70–72] In the series of McAfee et al,[70] the outcome was related to the number of lesions, the 5-year survival rates being 36.5% for solitary nodules ($n = 98$), 19.3% for two deposits ($n = 28$) and 7.7% when three or more lesions

were resected ($n = 13$). Others reported 5-year survival rates ranging from 22% to 35% after resection of multiple metastases.[63,72] The delay between treatment of the primary tumor and the lung metastases had no prognostic value in most series.[63,64,70–72] The size of the largest metastasis had no impact on survival in some studies,[71,72] but lesions of more than 3 cm were associated with a worse outcome in others.[64] Patients who had previous resection of liver metastases before lung metastases had similar survival, with 5-year actuarial survival rates of 30.5–68%.[70,71] A preoperative plasma CEA level higher than 5 ng/ml was associated with a poor outcome, with a 5-year survival rate of 16% compared with 46.8% for those with normal CEA value. Complete removal of all metastatic disease appears to be the main prognostic factor in all series.

Following resection, the lung is the first site of recurrence in 50–70% of cases, followed by locoregional recurrences at the site of the primary, brain and liver metastases.[70,71] Repeat lung resections can be considered in some cases, since 5-year actuarial survival rates of 30% have been reported.[70]

Table 8.3 Five-year survival following pulmonary resection for lung metastases from colorectal cancer

Ref	Number of patients	5-year survival rate (%)
76	31	30
77	34	28
67	28	28
68	35	22
64	65	41
63	144	44
70	139	30.5

BRAIN METASTASES

These metastases of colorectal cancer are rare, and are associated with disseminated disease in most cases. The available data on the surgical management of brain metastases from colorectal cancer are scarce. Their prognosis is even worse than those of other metastases. The brain is rarely the sole site of disease, and only 10–30% of patients with brain metastases die from strictly neurological causes. Treatment of brain metastases is based on steroids, radiotherapy and surgery. In a controlled trial including patients with brain metastases of various origins, it has been shown that for solitary lesions, resection improved local control rates, overall survival and functional independence as compared with radiation. On the other hand, combined treatments increased survival and disease-free survival, and reduced the rate of recurrences at the original site.[78] In a series of 19 patients with brain metastases of colorectal origin, the mean survival was 4.9 months after resection (5 patients) and 2.6 months after radiation therapy (14 patients). The 6-month survival rates were 40% and 25% respectively, but there were no survivors at 1 year.[79] Others reported more encouraging results, with a mean survival of 8.3 months in a series of 73 patients who had a resection for brain metastases from colorectal cancer. One- and two-year survival rates were 31.5% and 5.5% respectively, and 5 patients were alive at 19, 39, 40, 60 and 126 months. Prognosis was better for supratentorial than for cerebellar localization. At the time of brain metastases, 36 patients had liver metastases (49%), 53 (73%) had lung metastases and 28 had metastases at both sites. Of the 36 patients who had recurrences, 15 were reoperated upon, and the mean survival time was 11.4 months.[80]

Surgical excision can be proposed for a very limited number of patients – especially in cases of solitary lesion and control of the metastatic disease at other sites.

REFERENCES

1. Stangl R, Altendorf-Hofmann A, Charnley RM, Scheele J, Factors influencing the natural history of colorectal liver metastases. *Lancet* 1994; **343:** 1405–10.
2. Iwatsuki S, Shaw BW, Starzl TE, Experience with 150 liver resections. *Ann Surg* 1983; **197:** 247.
3. Pugh RNH, Murray-Lyon IM, Danson JL et al, Transsection of esophagus for bleeding varices. *Br J Surg* 1973; **60:** 646.
4. Kawasaki S, Maakushi M, Kasaku T et al, Resection for multiple metastatic liver tumors after portal embolization. *Surgery* 1994; **115:** 674–7.
5. Elias D, Detroz B, Lasser P et al, Is simultaneous hepatectomy and intestinal anastomasis safe? *Am J Surg* 1995; **169:** 254–60.
6. Scheele J, Stangl R, Altendorf-Hofmann A, Gall FP, Indicators of prognosis after hepatic resection for colorectal secondaries. *Surgery* 1991; **110:** 13–29.
7. Nordlinger B, Jaeck D, Guiguet M et al, Surgical resection of hepatic metastases. Multicentric retrospective study by the French Association of Surgery. In: *Treatment of Hepatic Metastases of Colorectal Cancer* (Nordlinger B, Jaeck D, eds). Paris: Springer-Verlag, 1992; 129–46.
8. Wernecke K, Rummenny E, Bongartz G, Comparative sensitivities of sonography, CT, and MRI imaging. *AJR* 1991; **157:** 731–7
9. Ferrucci JT, Liver tumor imaging, current concepts. *AJR* 1990; **155:** 473–84.
10. Sitzmann JV, Coleman JA, Preoperative assessment of malignant hepatic tumors. *Am J Surg* 1991; **159:** 137–43.
11. Soyer P, Levesque M, Caudron C et al, MRI of liver metastases from colorectal cancer vs CT during arterial portography. *J Comput Assist Tomogr* 1993; **17:** 67–74.
12. Timothy GJ, Greig JD, Crosbie JL et al, Superior staging of liver tumors with laparoscopy and laparoscopic ultrasound. *Ann Surg* 1994; **6:** 711–19.
13. Castaing D, Emond J, Kunstlinger F, Bismuth H, Utility of operative ultrasound in the surgery of liver tumors. *Ann Surg* 1986; **204:** 600–5.
14. Castaing D, Kunstlinger F, Habib N, Bismuth H, Intraoperative ultrasonographic study of the liver. Methods and anatomic results. *Am J Surg* 1985; **149:** 676–82.
15. Pichlmayr R, Is there a place for liver grafting for malignancy? *Transpl Proc* 1988; **20:** 478–82.
16. Bismuth H, Houssin D, Castaing D, Major and minor segmentectomies 'réglées' in liver surgery. *World J Surg* 1982; **6:** 10–24.
17. Makuuchi M, Hasegawa H, Yamasaki S, Hasegawa H, Four new hepatectomy procedures for resection of the right hepatic vein and preservation of the inferior right hepatic vein. *Surg Gynecol Obstet* 1987; **164:** 69–73.
18. Starzl TE, Bell RH, Beart RW, Putnam CW, Hepatic trisegementectomy and other liver resections. *Surg Gynecol Obstet* 1975; **141:** 429–37.
19. Starzl TE, Iwatsuki S, Shaw B, left hepatic trisegmentectomy. *Surg Gynecol Obstet* 1982; **155:** 21–7.
20. Panis Y, Ribeiro J, Chretien Y et al, Métastases hépatiques dormantes; mise en évidence sur un modèle expérimental de métastases d'origine colorectale. *Ann Chir* 1989; **43:** 765–6.
21. Bismuth H, Castaing D, Garden OJ, Major hepatic resection under total vascular exclusion. *Ann Surg* 1989; **210:** 15–19.
22. Delva E, Camus Y, Nordlinger B et al, Vascular

occlusions for liver resections: operative management and tolerance to hepatic ischemia. *Ann Surg* 1989; **209:** 211–18.

23. Nagao T, Inove S, Mizuta T et al, One hundred hepatic resections. *Ann Surg* 1985; **202:** 42–9.

24. Takenaka K, Kanematsu T, Fukuzawa K, Sugimachi K, Can hepatic failure after surgery for hepatocellular carcinoma in cirrhotic patients be prevented? *World J Surg* 1990: **14:** 123–7.

25. Nagasue N, Yukaya H, Ogawa Y et al, Segmental and subsegmental resections of the cirrhotic liver under hepatic inflow and outflow occlusion. *Br J Surg* 1985; **72:** 565–8.

26. Smadja C, Kahwaji F, Berthoux L et al, Intérêt du clampage pédiculaire total dans les exérèses hépatiques pour carcinome hépatocellullaire chez le cirrhotique. *Ann Chir* 1987; **41:** 639–42.

27. Terblanche J, Krige JEJ, Bornman PC, Simplified hepatic resection with the use of prolonged vascular inflow occlusion. *Arch Surg* 1991; **126:** 298–301.

28. Huguet C, Nordlinger B, Bloch P, Conard J, Tolerance of the human liver to prolonged normothermic ischemia. *Arch Surg* 1978; **113:** 1448–51.

29. Pringle JH, Notes on the arrest of hepatic hemorrhage due to trauma. *Ann Surg* 1908; **48:** 541–9.

30. Elias D, Desruennes E, Lasser P, Prolonged intermittent clamping of the portal triad during hepatectomy. *Br J Surg* 1991; **78:** 42–4.

31. Delva E, Barberousse JP, Nordlinger B et al, Hemodynamic and biochemical monitoring during major liver resection with use of hepatic vascular exclusion. *Surgery* 1984; **95:** 309–17.

32. Huguet C, Nordlinger B, Galopin JJ et al, Normothermic hepatic vascular exclusion for extensive hepatectomy. *Surg Gynecol Obstet* 1978; **147:** 689–93.

33. Pichlmayr R, Grosse H, Haus J et al, Technique and preliminary results of extracorporeal liver surgery (bench procedure) and of surgery on the in situ perfused liver. *Br J Surg* 1988; **77:** 21–6.

34. Hannoun L, Panis Y, Balladur P et al, 'Ex situ–in vivo' liver surgery. *Lancet* 1991; **337:** 1616.

35. TonThat Tung, *Les résections majeures et mineures du foie*. Paris: Masson, 1979.

36. Andrus C, Kaminski DL, Segmental hepatic resection utilizing the ultrasonic dissector. *Arch Surg* 1986; **210:** 515–21.

37. Franco D, Smadja C, Kahwaji F et al, Segmentectomies in the management of liver tumors. *Arch Surg* 1988; **123:** 519–23.

38. Gennari L, Doci R, Bignami P, Bozetti F, Surgical treatment of hepatic metastasis from colorectal cancer. *Ann Surg* 1986; **203:** 49–54.

39. Holm A, Bradley E, Joaquim S, Aldrek S, Hepatic resection of metastasis from colorectal carcinoma. *Ann Surg* 1990; **209:** 428–33.

40. Hughes KS, Sugarbaker PH, Resection of the liver for metastatic solid tumors. In: *Surgical Treatment of Metastatic Cancer* (Rosenberg SA, ed). Philadelphia: JB Lippincott, 1984; 125–64.

41. Nordlinger B, Quilichini MA, Parc R et al, Hepatic resection for colorectal liver metastases. Influence on survival of preoperative factors and surgery for recurrence in 80 patients. *Ann Surg* 1987; **205:** 256–63.

42. Sesto ME, Vogt DP, Hermann RE, Hepatic resection in 128 patients: a 24 year experience. *Surgery* 1987; **102:** 846–51.

43. Bradpiece HA, Benjamin IS, Halevy A, Blumgart LH, Major hepatic resection for colorectal liver metastases. *Br J Surg* 1987; **74:** 324–6.

44. Butler J, Attiyeh FF, Daly JM, Hepatic resection for metastases of the colon and rectum. *Surg Gynecol Obstet* 1986; **162:** 109–13.

45. Cobourn CS, Makowka L, Langer B et al, Examination and patient selection and outcome for hepatic resection for metastatic disease. *Surg Gynecol Obstet* 1987; **165:** 239–46.

46. Ekberg H, Transberg KG, Andersson R et al, Determinants of survival in liver resection for colorectal secondaries. *Br J Surg* 1986; **73:** 727–31.

47. Wagner JS, Adson MA, Van Heerdeen JA et al, The natural history of hepatic metastases from colorectal cancer. A comparison with resective treatment. *Ann Surg* 1984; **199:** 502–8.

48. Hughes KS, Rosenbtein RB, Songhorabodi S et al, Resection of liver for colorectal carcinoma metastases. A multi-institutional study of long term survivors. *Dis Colon Rectum* 1988; **31:** 1–4.

49. Hughes KS, Simon R, Songhorabodi S et al, Resection of liver for colorectal liver metastases: a multi-institutional study of patterns of recurrence. *Surgery* 1986; **100:** 278–84.

50. Hughes KS and the Registry of Hepatic Metastases, Resection of the liver for colorectal carcinoma metastases: a multi-institutional study of indications for resection. *Surgery* 1988; **103:** 278–88.

51. Logan SE, Meier SJ, Ramming KP et al, Hepatic resection of metastatic colorectal carcinoma. A ten year experience. *Arch Surg* 1982; **117:** 25–8.

52. Foster JH, Berman MM, Solid liver tumors. *Major Probl Clin Surg* 1977; **22:** 242.

53. Iwatsuki S, Esquivel CO, Gordon RD, Starzl TE,

Liver resection for metastatic colorectal cancer. *Surgery* 1986; **100:** 804–10.

54. Younes RN, Rogakto A, Brenmam MF, The influence of intra-operative hypotension and perioperative blood transfusion on disease free survival in patients with complete resection of colorectal liver metastases. *Ann Surg* 1991; **214:** 107–13.

55. Hughes KS, Scheele J, Sugarbaker PH, Surgery for colorectal cancer metastatic to the liver: optimising the results of treatment. *Surg Clin North Am* 1989; **69:** 339–59.

56. Cady B, McDermott WV, Major hepatic resection for metachronous metastases from colon cancer. *Ann Surg* 1985; **201:** 204–9.

57. Dagradi AD, Mangiante GL, Marchiori LAM, Nicoli NM, Repeated hepatic resection. *Int Surg* 1987; **72:** 87–92.

58. Griffith KD, Sugarbaker PH, Chang A, Repeat hepatic resections for colorectal metastases. *Surgery* 1990; **107:** 101–4.

59. Huguet C, Bona S, Nordlinger B et al, Repeat hepatic resection for primary and metastatic carcinoma of the liver. *Surg Gynecol Obstet* 1990; **171:** 398–402.

60. Lange JF, Leese T, Castaing D, Bismuth H, Repeat hepatectomy for recurrent malignant tumors of the liver. *Surg Gynecol Obstet* 1989; **169:** 119–26.

61. Stone MD, Cady B, Jenkins RL et al, Surgical therapy for recurrent liver metastases from colorectal cancer. *Arch Surg* 1990; **125:** 718–22.

62. Nordlinger B, Vaillant JC, Guiguet M et al, Repeat liver resections for recurrent colorectal metastases: prolonged survivals. *J Clin Oncol* 1994; **12:** 1491–6.

63. McCormack PM, Burt ME, Bains MS et al, Lung resection for colorectal metastases. 10-year results. *Arch Surg* 1992; **127:** 1403–6.

64. Goya T, Miyazawa N, Kondo H et al, Surgical resection of pulmonary metastases from colorectal cancer. Ten-year follow-up. *Cancer* 1989; **64:** 1418–21.

65. Johnson MR, Median sternotomy for resection of pulmonary metastasis. *J Thorac Cardiovasc Surg* 1983; **85:** 516–21.

66. Regnard JF, Marzelle J, Cerrina J et al, Chirurgie des metastases pulmonaires. *Chirurgie* 1985; **111:** 512–22.

67. Mountain CF, McCurtrey MJ, Hermes KE, Surgery for pulmonary metastasis a twenty year experience. *Ann Thorac Surg* 1984; **38:** 323–30.

68. McCormack PM, Martini N, The changing role of surgery for pulmonary metastases. *Ann Thorac Surg* 1979; **28:** 139–45.

69. Takita H, Edgerton F, Karakousis C, Surgical management of metastases to the lung. *Surg Gynecol Obstet* 1981; **152:** 751–4.

70. McAfee MK, Allen MS, Trastek VF et al, Colorectal lung metastases: results of surgical excision. *Ann Thorac Surg* 1992; **53:** 780–6.

71. Yano T, Hara N, Ichonose Y et al, Results of pulmonary resection of metastatic colorectal cancer and its application. *J Thorac Cardiovasc Surg* 1993; **106:** 875–9.

72. Mori M, Tomoda H, Ishida T et al, Surgical resection of pulmonary metastases from colorectal adenocarcinoma. Special reference to repeated pulmonary resections. *Arch Surg* 1991; **126:** 1297–301.

73. Fortner JG, Silver JS, Golbey RB et al, Multivariate analysis of a personal series of 247 consecutive patients with liver metastasis from colorectal cancer. Treatment by hepatic resection. *Ann Surg* 1984; **199:** 306–16.

74. Adson MA, Van Heerden JA, Adson MH et al, Resection of hepatic metastases from colorectal cancer. *Arch Surg* 1984; **119:** 647–51.

75. Doci R, German L, Bigmani P et al, One hundred patients with hepatic metastases from colorectal cancer treated by resection: analysis of prognostic determinant. *Br J Surg* 1991; **78:** 797–801.

76. Cahan WG, Castro EB, Hajdu SI, The significance of a solitary lung shadow in patients with colon carcinoma. *Cancer* 1974; **33:** 414–21.

77. Wilkins EW Jr, Head JM, Burke JF, Pulmonary resection for metastatic neoplasms in the lung. *Am J Surg* 1978; **135:** 480–3.

78. Patchell RA, Tibbs PA, Walsh JW et al, A randomized trial of surgery in the treatment of single metastases to the brain. *N Engl J Med* 1990; **322:** 494–500.

79. Alden TD, Gianino JW, Saclarides TJ, Brain metastases from colorectal cancer. *Dis Colon Rectum* 1996; **39:** 541–5.

80. Wronski M, Arbit E, Bilsky M, Galicich JH, Resection of brain metastases from colorectal cancer. *Dis Colon Rectum* 1996; **39:** A33.

9

Postoperative histopathological evaluation: Implications for prognosis?

Fred T Bosman

CONTENTS • **Introduction** • **Pathological examination of a surgical resection specimen**
• **Prognostic significance of classical parameters** • **Prognostic significance of newer tumor parameters**
• **Conclusions**

INTRODUCTION

Histopathological examination of biopsy and surgical specimens plays an important role in the clinical management of patients with colorectal cancer. In order to establish a final diagnosis in endoscopically suspected cancer, histological examination of small biopsy specimens is indispensable. To verify the nature of a polyp, histological examination of the endoscopic resection specimen is important. This will also indicate whether or not additional treatment might be necessary. For verification of the diagnosis, and determination of stage and grade and the completeness of the resection, examination of surgical resection specimens of colorectal carcinoma is performed. It is the purpose of this chapter to briefly review the pathological procedures concerning the work-up of a resection specimen and to discuss in depth which pathological parameters play a role in clinical decision-making.

PATHOLOGICAL EXAMINATION OF A SURGICAL RESECTION SPECIMEN

Careful macroscopy is an essential first step in the work-up of a resection specimen. This will

differ slightly between colectomy and rectal resection specimens. For both, inspection of the lateral margins of resection is important. When the macroscopic tumor margin is less than 5 cm from the lateral resection margin, histological examination of this margin is essential. Serial sectioning of the tumor mass is important to judge the depth of infiltration into the bowel wall. Tissue samples will be taken of the area of deepest infiltration. The circumferential surface of rectal specimens will be inked, prior to serial sectioning perpendicular to the axis of the lumen. Detailed examination of the minimal distance between the circumferential (inked) margin and the point of deepest infiltration is important.[1] Pericolic/rectal fat will be carefully dissected in order to obtain a maximum number of lymph nodes for histological examination. To facilitate the detection of lymph nodes, clearance of the fat can be very helpful.[2] The site of lymph nodes will be carefully recorded:[3] adjacent to the tumor, proximal to the tumor, distal to the tumor and in the resection margin – along the larger vessels.

Microscopy will reveal the nature of the tumor (usually an adenocarcinoma), the subtype (mucinous or colloid carcinoma can be distinguished as subtypes), and the degree of differentiation, which is conventionally graded as well, moderately and poorly differentiated. Modern histochemical and molecular techniques allow a more detailed description of the characteristics of the tumor, as will be discussed later. The depth of invasion will be recorded for colonic carcinomas, and the minimal distance between the invasion front and the circumferential margin for rectal tumors.[1] Additional relevant parameters are angio-invasion, perineural invasion and lymphoid inflammatory response.[4-6] The resection margins will be histologically examined as well as the lymph nodes. The number of positive lymph nodes relative to the total number per level will be recorded. All of these parameters will be included in the final conclusion, which will end with a classification of the tumor according to stage. It is convenient to stage the tumors according to the Astler–Collins modification of the original Dukes classification, to the TNM classification and to the Jass classification. A comparison of these classifications is provided in Figure 9.1.

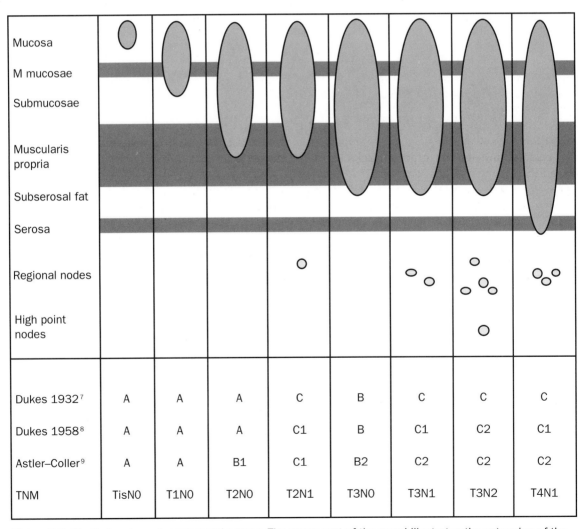

Figure 9.1 Staging systems for colorectal cancer. The upper part of the panel illustrates the extension of the primary tumor through the layers of the bowel wall.[7-9]

PROGNOSTIC SIGNIFICANCE OF CLASSICAL PARAMETERS

It is generally recognized that tumor stage, conventionally expressed in the Dukes classification, is the most powerful predictor of final outcome.[10] The five-year survival rate according to Dukes stage is presented in Table 9.1. The Dukes or TNM classifications do not take angio-invasion, perineural invasion and lymphoid inflammatory response into account. The TNM classification supplies a subdivision of the N status. Although there is a generally shared feeling that the prognosis deteriorates with more positive nodes and more widespread nodal involvement, this has not been adequately validated.[3] Angio-invasion is a repeatedly proven prognostically useful characteristic, and ought to be included in prognostic algorithms. This might also be true for perineural invasion, although this has not been adequately proved. Lymphocytic infiltrate, as proposed by Shepherd et al,[6] has also been used by others,[5,11] but has not been consistently validated as an important parameter. Its grading lacks reproducibility, which may be one of the reasons why it is a relatively weak prognostic indicator. In rectal cancer the minimal distance to the circumferential margin of resection is an important predictor for recurrent disease. This has led to the use of this parameter as a decisive element in determining whether or not post-operative adjuvant radiotherapy might be necessary.[12]

PROGNOSTIC SIGNIFICANCE OF NEWER TUMOR PARAMETERS

The introduction of methods developed in cell and molecular biology into diagnostic histopathology has enabled a much more detailed analysis of tumor cell characteristics. These developments include histochemical staining, which allows detailed characterization of differentiation at the level of proteins and mRNA, of proliferation and apoptotic activity, of invasive behavior and of metastatic spread, and also molecular genetic analysis, which allows detailed characterization of genetic aberrations in the tumor cells. In part, these new parameters have already been proved to be of prognostic relevance.

Parameters related to invasion and metastasis

The impact of lymph-node metastases on prognosis has been an important reason why several groups have studied the yield of lymph-node metastases by immunohistochemical staining for micrometastases, mostly using antibodies against cytokeratins. Several studies have

Table 9.1 Survival rates for colorectal cancer according to the Dukes and TNM classifications

Dukes stage	5-year survival rate (%)	TNM stage	5-year survival rate (%)
A	80	0	75
		I (A + B)	70
B	65	II	60
C	25	III	30
D	10	IV	5

indeed shown that this approach yields micrometastases in 25% of cases that could otherwise have been classified as node-negative.[13,14] The impact of this result on prognosis, however, is not yet resolved. Jeffers et al[13] did not find any relationship between lymph-node micrometastases and prognosis, whereas Greenson et al[14] found better prognosis in Dukes B patients without micrometastases than in those with them. Their case number, however, was rather limited, and additional studies are necessary to clarify this issue.

In line with the importance of metastases, the tumor or cellular characteristics indicative of invasive behavior have been studied in detail. An interesting approach was proposed by Hase et al,[15] who distinguished between two patterns of invasion: irregular tumor cell budding at the invasive front versus a straight 'pushing' tumor margin. Irregular invasion was associated with poorer survival, even after stratification for Dukes stage. The problem with these parameters is that they can only be assessed in a rather subjective way, and therefore often lack reproducibility. For this reason, such parameters will not solve problems of staging.

With rapidly advancing insights into mechanisms of tumor cell invasion, numerous attempts have already been made to develop new prognostic parameters based upon the molecular actors involved in this highly complex process. Invasion implies *proteolytic degradation of the extracellular matrix* surrounding the tumor cells, a *stromal response* to this aggressive tumor cell behavior, *dissolution of intercellular adhesion*, which is mediated by cell adhesion molecules, and *migration through the extracellular matrix*, which involves cell–matrix interaction and activation of the tumor cell cytoskeleton. All these processes have been studied in connection with prognosis.

Matrix proteases belonging to the plasminogen activator (PA)–plasmin system have been studied repeatedly as prognostic factors in colorectal cancer.[16–18] Urokinase (uPA) staining appeared to be predictive for the development of liver metastases.[16,17] Ganesh et al determined the components of the system, including uPA, (tissue) tPA and the inhibitors PAI-1 and -2 by immunoassay. A high ratio of uPA in cancer tissue to tPA in normal tissue and a high level of PAI-2 were predictive of poor outcome.[18] The prognostic value of expression of matrix metalloproteinase 1 (MMP-1), an interstitial collagenase, was studied by Murray et al.[19] High expression of MMP-1 was associated with poor prognosis.

Stromal response, in terms of basement membrane deposition in the tumor center, was studied by Havenith et al[20] and subsequently by Offerhaus et al.[21] Consistently, an extensive deposition of basement membrane material around tumor cell nests was indicative of a favorable prognosis. This phenomenon has been explained in terms of a positive host response towards the tumor. A somewhat contrasting observation is the association of a pronounced desmoplastic response at the tumor edge with unfavorable prognosis.[22]

Extensive attention has been paid to expression of cell adhesion molecules and prognosis, following the observation that loss of E-cadherin expression in carcinoma cells in model systems induced invasive behavior. More recently, it has become clear that not only E-cadherin but also the catenins are involved in maintaining cell adhesion in desmosomes, and reduced expression, due to mutations or due to downregulated transcription, might be involved in the invasive process. The gene responsible for adenomatous polyposis coli (APC) is also implicated in the interaction of the E-cadherin–catenin complex with the cytoskeleton.[23] The prognostic value of expression of members of this complex has recently been studied. It has become clear that cadherin and catenin mutations are rare, their apparent loss of expression during invasion being due to downregulated expression.[24] Expression levels were essentially parallel with differentiation level of the tumors. A prognostic value was reported for E-cadherin expression in colorectal cancer, but this was largely accounted for by tumor grade.[25,26] Interestingly, patterns of expression were almost identical in primary lesions and in corresponding metastases.[27,28] A practical limitation of E-cadherin expression is that loss of immunohistochemical staining is rather difficult to score. Cell adhesion therefore seems to be more of tumor-biological than of clinical interest.

The CD 44 family of hyaluronan receptors has attracted a lot of attention recently, following reports that expression of splice variants of CD 44 (most notably the v6 variant) was correlated with unfavorable prognosis.[29] Several papers confirm the value of CD 44 v6 expression as an independent prognostic variable,[30] but a recent report has contested this, leaving the importance of CD 44 v6 expression somewhat disputed.[31] Another group of genes with a disputed role in colorectal cancer prognosis are the nm23 genes. Loss of the expression of nm23 has been reported to correlate with the occurrence of distant metastases in colorectal cancer,[32] but others have been unable to confirm this finding.[33]

Parameters related to proliferation and apoptosis

Tumor behavior is determined to a significant extent by the capacity of the cancer cells to multiply and hence increase tumor volume. In recent years it has become clear that not only cell proliferation but also cell loss determines the rate of volume increase of a tumor. Cell loss is largely determined by apoptosis or programmed cell death.

Several possibilities are available for the determination of proliferative activity. The most conventional is a mitotic count, but this is not a very reliable parameter. Through cytometric analysis of cellular DNA content, the fraction of cancer cells in the S phase of the cell cycle can be determined. This technique has some limitations, however. Tumor cell populations tend to have multiple stem lines with variable DNA content, making the determination of an S-phase fraction unreliable. Also, when paraffin-embedded material is analyzed, which has become the most frequently applied method, determination of the S-phase fraction is unreliable.[34] Nonetheless, prognostic significance of a high S-phase fraction has been reported.[35]

Cell proliferation has become popular with the introduction of immunohistochemical methods to determine the growth fraction of a tumor cell population. The best available technique is labeling of the Ki-67 antigen, using the MIB-1 antibody in paraffin sections. An alternative possibility is staining for PCNA (a DNA polymerase-related protein). Using these techniques, multivariate analysis of patient populations has shown that cancer cell proliferative index is an independent predictor of tumor behavior – a high index indicating shorter survival.[36]

Techniques are now also available for the histochemical staining of apoptotic cells. These techniques rely on detection of the internucleosomal DNA fragmentation, which is an early phenomenon in apoptotic cells. This so-called in situ nick-end labeling (ISEL or TUNEL) has been used by several investigators. The findings are not yet conclusive, but tend to favor a positive correlation between higher apoptotic index and better prognosis.[37] Much has become known about the molecular events that precede apoptosis. The tumor suppressor gene TP53 and the oncogene bcl-2 are involved in the regulating pathways. TP53 blocks the cell cycle in a genetically damaged cell in order to allow DNA repair. When the damage is irreparable, TP53 induces apoptosis. In contrast, the upregulation of bcl-2 expression blocks apoptosis. Against this background, the prognostic value of TP53 and bcl-2 expression has been evaluated. High TP53 expression has been found to be correlated with poor prognosis,[38,39] and this correlation has also been found for bcl-2.[40] Both findings need to be confirmed in additional studies, however. Since it is likely that response to chemo- and radiotherapy involves the apoptotic pathway, it might be possible to use TP53 and bcl-2 expression to predict tumor response to these therapeutic modalities. A mutated TP53 and high bcl-2 expression would block the apoptotic pathway and render the tumor cell therapy-resistant. Indications that this approach might be clinically valid has been published, but this also needs to be confirmed in additional studies.[41]

Parameters related to tumor cell differentiation

Conventionally, in grading of carcinomas, cytonuclear features (nuclear pleomorphism and hyperchromasia and cytoplasmic characteristics) as well as architecture (formation of glands, cell stratification and polarity) are taken into account. This subjective appraisal usually leads to three grades: well, moderately and poorly differentiated. Grading has been reported to be prognostically significant. However, conventional grading is not very reproducible, and was of only borderline prognostic significance in a recent study of prognostic variables.[4] A plausible alternative to subjective grading would be the analysis of the expression of characteristic products of terminally differentiated cells. For goblet cells, a variety of antibodies allows the detection of mucin production. For columnar resorptive cells, staining for microvillus-associated proteins such as villin, or of membrane-associated disaccharidases such as sucrase-isomaltase, can be used. For Paneth cells, lysozyme is an adequate marker, and for endocrine cells, chromogranin A. A variety of studies have investigated the prognostic significance of these markers, either singly or in combination.[42] In general, tumors with highly differentiated cells tend to have a more favorable prognosis than those with predominantly undifferentiated cells. In contrast, several studies have indicated that tumors with endocrine cells tend to behave more aggressively.[43,44] The search for differentiation-related prognostic markers has clearly not yielded any markers whose impact comes close to that of tumor stage. From a conceptual point of view, this may be explained by the fact that differentiation takes only tumor cell characteristics into account, whereas stage- and growth-related parameters are a reflection of the interaction between cancer cells and the host.

Parameters related to oncogenes and tumor suppressor genes

Colorectal cancer is probably the most intensely studied tumor type as far as molecular genetic abnormalities are concerned. Pioneering work of Vogelstein's group led to the development of a model for the molecular events responsible for colorectal carcinogenesis.[45] This concept has led in turn to intensive searches for diagnostic and prognostic uses of these molecular parameters. The prognostic value of TP53 and bcl-2 and their potential use for the prediction of response to chemo- and radiotherapy have been briefly mentioned. Surprisingly, for general use in diagnosis and prognosis of colorectal cancer, molecular genetic parameters have as yet had very limited impact.

Gross genetic abnormalities, as reflected in cellular DNA content, have been studied repeatedly in the last decades. Ploidy analysis has become relatively simple, and this parameter could be useful – especially since it reflects an end stage in the development of the neoplasm and thus combines the effects of various individual genetic abnormalities. Most studies indicate that tumor ploidy is correlated with patient survival.[46,47] Tumor ploidy has, however, been found to be correlated with parameters including stage, grade and proliferative activity, and therefore its impact as an independent prognostic indicator has been limited.[48]

Of all specific genetic abnormalities, the Ki-ras mutations have probably received the most attention. Mutations in this gene have been found to be of prognostic significance: tumors with Ki-ras mutations (about 50%) were prognostically more unfavorable than those without[49] – even more so when combined with TP53. An interesting observation was made by Moerkerk et al[50] regarding Ki-ras mutations and Dukes stage. In Dukes B tumors predominantly G → A mutations were found in codon 12, whereas in Dukes C tumors predominantly G → C or G → T mutations occurred. This finding suggests that a Dukes C tumor might not be simply the sequel to a Dukes B tumor, but may be generated through a different molecular pathway. This finding, however, needs to be confirmed. Moreover, recent data indicate that considerable genetic heterogeneity exists in colorectal neoplasms, which calls for more extensive sampling of tumors for molecular genetic abnormalities.[51] Given the fact that Ki-ras mutations have been identified even in preneoplastic, non-dysplastic lesions, it is unlikely that as a single parameter they will have important prognostic significance.

For some of the other genes that figure in the Vogelstein model, APC, MCC and DCC,[45] a role in tumor behavior still needs to be established. These are large genes with a wide scattering of point mutations, which makes their analysis cumbersome and time-consuming. They have not as yet, been studied in a sufficient number of patients to allow any firm conclusions to be drawn regarding their prognostic role. The story will certainly not end with the genes discussed above. The discovery of the genes responsible for the Lynch syndrome – a family of genes playing a role in mismatch repair – has led to studies of the role of microsatellite instability, caused by mutations in these genes, in the diagnosis and prognosis of colorectal cancer. It has become clear that microsatellite instability occurs in a limited proportion of Lynch-syndrome-associated colorectal carcinomas, and in a limited proportion of sporadic colorectal cancers, but also in non-neoplastic (e.g. inflammatory) conditions.[52] The role of mismatch repair genes therefore needs to be further clarified before any general conclusions can be drawn. Other genes will follow. Jen et al[4] identified an important prognostic role for a gene on 18q, which might be the DCC at this locus. A new tumor suppressor gene might be located at a locus on 8p.[53] Worldwide, the search for new genetic defects in neoplastic disease, including colorectal cancer, is on, and this will undoubtedly lead to the discovery of new prognostic factors.

CONCLUSIONS

Where does this impressive collection of new tumor cell characteristics leave us with the management of today's colorectal cancer patients? For the Dukes A, C and D categories, the problem is less urgent. For Dukes B patients, however, the chance of progressive disease is far from remote, which calls for identification of high-risk groups to be included in adjuvant treatment protocols. The general risk profile is clear. A Dukes B tumor that has infiltrating borders, is angioinvasive, induces the expression of collagenase type IV, is mutated in TP53 and Ki-ras, has lost E-cadherin expression but gained expression of CD 44 v6, is bcl-2 positive, has a high proliferative index, is aneuploid and shows loss of heterozygosity of 18q runs a very high risk for recurrent disease. It is not yet clear which combination of these parameters is the most predictive. Nor do we know whether, when adjuvant therapy is administered based on the expression of a set of unfavorable markers, survival will improve in the long run. Additional clinical research will be necessary to bring clinical tumor-biological research into the realm of everyday clinical application.

REFERENCES

1. Adam IJ, Mohamdee MO, Martin IG et al, Role of circumferential margin involvement in the local recurrence of rectal cancer. *Lancet* 1994; **344:** 707–11.
2. Cawthorn SJ, Gibbs NM, Marks CG, Clearance technique for the detection of lymph nodes in colorectal cancer. *Br J Surg* 1986; **73:** 58–60.
3. Shida H, Ban K, Matsumoto M et al, Prognostic significance of location of lymph node metastases in colorectal cancer. *Dis Colon Rectum* 1992; **35:** 1046–50.
4. Jen J, Kim H, Piantadosi S et al, Allelic loss of chromosome 18q and prognosis in colorectal cancer. *N Engl J Med* 1994; **331:** 213–21.
5. Harrison JC, Dean PJ, el-Zeky F, Vander Zwaag R, Impact of the Crohn's-like lymphoid reaction on staging of right-sided colon cancer: results of multivariate analysis. *Hum Pathol* 1995; **26:** 31–8.
6. Shepherd NA, Saraga EP, Love SB, Jass JR, Prognostic factors in colonic cancer. *Histopathology* 1989; **14:** 613–20.
7. Dukes CE, The classification of cancer of the rectum. *J Pathol Bacteriol* 1932; **35:** 323–32.
8. Dukes CE, Bussey HJR, The spread of rectal

cancer and its effect on prognosis. *Br J Cancer* 1958; **12**: 309–20.

9. Astler VB, Coller FA, The prognostic significance of direct extension of carcinoma of the colon and rectum. *Ann Surg* 1954; **139**: 846–54.

10. Deans GT, Parks TG, Rowlands BJ, Spence RA, Prognostic factors in colorectal cancer. *Br J Surg* 1992; **79**: 608–13.

11. Di Giorgio A, Botti C, Tocchi A et al, The influence of tumor lymphocytic infiltration on long term survival of surgically treated colorectal cancer patients. *Int Surg* 1992; **77**: 256–60.

12. de Haas-Kock DF, Baeten CG, Jager JJ et al, Prgonostic significance of radial margins of clearance in rectal cancer. *Br J Surg* 1996; **83**: 781–5.

13. Jeffers MD, O'Dowd GM, Mulcahy H et al, The prognostic significance of immunohistochemically detected lymph node micrometastases in colorectal carcinoma. *J Pathol* 1994; **172**: 183–7.

14. Greenson JK, Isenhart CE, Rice R et al, Identification of occult micrometastases in pericolic lymph nodes of Duke's B colorectal cancer patients using monoclonal antibodies against cytokeratin and CC49. Correlation with long-term survival. *Cancer* 1994; **73**: 563–9.

15. Hase K, Shatney C, Johnson D et al, Prognostic value of tumor 'budding' in patients with colorectal cancer. *Dis Colon Rectum* 1993; **36**: 627–35.

16. Mulcahy HE, Duffy MJ, Gibbons D et al, Urokinase-type plasminogen activator and outcome in Dukes' B colorectal cancer. *Lancet* 1994; **344**: 583–4.

17. Sato T, Nishimura G, Yonemura Y et al, Association of immunohistochemical detection of urokinase-type plasminogen activator with metastasis and prognosis in colorectal cancer. *Oncology* 1995; **52**: 347–52.

18. Ganesh S, Sier CF, Griffioen G et al, Prognostic relevance of plasminogen activators and their inhibitors in colorectal cancer. *Cancer Res* 1994; **54**: 4065–71.

19. Murray GI, Duncan ME, O'Neil P et al, Matrix metalloproteinase-1 is associated with poor prognosis in colorectal cancer. *Nature Med* 1996; **2**: 461–2.

20. Havenith MG, Arends JW, Simon R et al, Type IV collagen immunoreactivity in colorectal cancer. Prognostic value of basement membrane deposition. *Cancer* 1988; **62**: 2207–11.

21. Offerhaus GJ, Giardiello FM, Bruijn JA et al, The value of immunohistochemistry for collagen IV expression in colorectal carcinomas. *Cancer* 1991; **67**: 99–105.

22. Halvorsen TB, Seim E, Association between invasiveness, inflammatory reaction, desmoplasia and survival in colorectal cancer. *J Clin Pathol* 1989; **42**: 162–6.

23. Su LK, Vogelstein B, Kinzler KW, Association of the APC tumor suppressor protein with catenins. *Science* 1993; **262**: 1734–7.

24. Streit M, Schmidt R, Hilgenfeld RU et al, Adhesion receptors in malignant transformation and dissemination of gastrointestinal tumors. *J Mol Med* 1996; **74**: 253–68.

25. Dorudi S, Sheffield JP, Poulsom R et al, E-cadherin expression in colorectal cancer. An immunocytochemical and in situ hybridization study. *Am J Pathol* 1993; **142**: 981–6.

26. Dorudi S, Hanby AM, Poulsom R et al, Level of expression of E-cadherin mRNA in colorectal cancer correlates with clinical outcome. *Br J Cancer* 1995; **71**: 614–16.

27. van der Wurff AA, Arends JW, van der Linden EP et al, L-CAM expression in lymph node and liver metastases of colorectal carcinomas. *J Pathol* 1994; **172**: 177–81.

28. van der Wurff AA, ten Kate J, van der Linden EP et al, L-CAM expression in normal, premalignant, and malignant colon mucosa. *J Pathol* 1992; **168**: 287–91.

29. Yamaguchi A, Urano T, Goi T et al, Expression of a CD44 variant containing exons 8 to 10 is a useful independent factor for the predicition of prognosis in colorectal cancer patients. *J Clin Oncol* 1996; **14**: 1122–7.

30. Mulder JW, Kruyt PM, Sewnath M et al, Colorectal cancer prognosis and expression of exon-v6-containing CD44 proteins. *Lancet* 1994; **344**: 1470–2.

31. Gotley D, Fawcet J, Walsh M et al, Expression of alternatively spliced variants of the cell adhesion molecule CD44 is not related to tumor progression in colorectal cancer. *Clin Exp Metastasis* 1996; **145**: 28.

32. Cohn KH, Wang FS, Desoto-LaPaix F et al, Association of nm23-H1 allelic deletions with distant metastases in colorectal carcinoma. *Lancet* 1991; **338**: 722–4.

33. Ichikawa W, Positive relationship between expression of CD44 and hepatic metastases in colorectal cancer. *Pathobiology* 1994; **62**: 172–9.

34. Yamazoe Y, Maetani S, Nishikawa T et al, The prognostic role of the DNA ploidy pattern in colorectal cancer analysis using paraffin-embedded

tissue by an improved method. *Surg Today* 1994; **24:** 30–6.

35. Schutte B, Reynders MM, Wiggers T et al, Retrospective analysis of the prognostic significance of DNA content and proliferative activity in large bowel carcinoma. *Cancer Res* 1987; **47:** 5494–6.

36. al-Sheneber IF, Shibata HR, Sampalis J, Jothy S, Prognostic significance of proliferating cell nuclear antigen expression in colorectal cancer. *Cancer* 1993; **71:** 1954–9.

37. Baretton GB, Diebold J, Christoforis G et al, Apoptosis and immunohistochemical bcl-2 expression in colorectal adenomas and carcinomas. Aspects of carcinogenesis and prognostic significance. *Cancer* 1996; **77:** 255–64.

38. Goh HS, Yao J, Smith DR, p53 point mutation and survival in colorectal cancer patients. *Cancer Res* 1995; **55:** 5217–21.

39. Hamelin R, Laurent-Puig P, Olschwang et al, Association of p53 mutations with short survival in colorectal cancer. *Gastroenterology* 1994; **106:** 42–8.

40. Ofner D, Riehemann K, Maier et al, Immunohistochemically detectable bcl-2 expression in colorectal carcinoma: correlation with tumor stage and patient survival. *Br J Cancer* 1995; **72:** 981–5.

41. Watson AJ, Merritt AJ, Jones LS et al, Evidence of reciprocity of bcl-2 and p53 expression in human colorectal adenomas and carcinomas. *Br J Cancer* 1996; **73:** 889–95.

42. Ho SB, Itzkowitz SH, Friera AM et al, Cell lineage markers in premalignant and malignant colonic mucosa. *Gastroenterology* 1989; **97:** 392–404.

43. Hamada Y, Oishi A, Shoji T et al, Endocrine cells and prognosis in patients with colorectal carcinoma. *Cancer* 1992; **69:** 2641–6.

44. de Bruine AP, Wiggers T, Beek C et al, Endocrine cells in colorectal adenocarcinomas: incidence, hormone profile and prognostic relevance. *Int J Cancer* 1993; **54:** 765–71.

45. Fearon ER, Vogelstein B, A genetic model for colorectal tumorigenesis. *Cell* 1990; **61:** 759–67.

46. Chapman MA, Hardcastle JD, Armitage NC, Five-year prospective study of DNA tumor ploidy and colorectal cancer survival. *Cancer* 1995; **76:** 383–7.

47. Baretton G, Gille J, Oevermann E, Lohrs U, Flow-cytometric analysis of the DNA-content in paraffin-embedded tissue from colorectal carcinomas and its prognostic significance. *Virchows Archiv B, Cell Pathol Mol Pathol* 1991; **60:** 123–31.

48. Sun XF, Carstensen JM, Stal O et al. Prognostic significance of p53 expression in relation to DNA ploidy in colorectal adenocarcinoma. *Virchows Archiv A, Pathol Anat Histopathol* 1993; **423:** 443–8.

49. Bell SM, Scott N, Cross D et al, Prognostic value of p53 overexpression and c-Ki-ras gene mutations in colorectal cancer. *Gastroenterology* 1993; **104:** 57–64.

50. Moerkerk P, Arends JW, van Driel et al, Type and number of Ki-ras point mutations relate to stage of human colorectal cancer. *Cancer Res* 1994; **54:** 3376–8.

51. Shibata D, Schaeffer J, Li ZH et al, Genetic heterogeneity of the c-K-ras locus in colorectal adenomas but not in adenocarcinomas. *J Natl Cancer Inst* 1993; **85:** 1058–63.

52. Bubb VJ, Curtis LJ, Cunningham C et al, Microsatellite instability and the role of hMSH2 in sporadic colorectalcancer. *Oncogene* 1996; **12:** 2641–9.

53. Farrington SM, Cunningham C, Boyle SM et al, Detailed physical and deletion mapping of 8p with isolation of YAC clones from tumour suppressor loci involved in colorectal cancer. *Oncogene* 1996; **12:** 1803–8.

10

Systemic adjuvant therapy of colon cancer

Rachel SJ Midgley, David J Kerr

CONTENTS • **Introduction** • **Early studies** • **5-Fluorouracil: alone and in combination** • **Current trials of adjuvant chemotherapy** • **The future of adjuvant therapy** • **Conclusions**

INTRODUCTION

With a predicted annual European incidence of approximately 150 000 and a mortality of around 95 000, colorectal-cancer chemotherapy is a focus of intensive research. Although public ignorance and perhaps embarrassment often delay the presentation of colonic malignancy, a macroscopically curative surgical resection is undertaken in 70–80% of cases. Unfortunately, experience dictates that in approximately half of these cases incurable tumour recurrence can be expected.[1] This failure of operative therapy to cure is a result of residual occult viable tumour cells whose bulk is below the threshold of detection of current radiological interventions, which have metastasized prior to primary tumour resection. They may be in the circulation (blood, lymph) or may indeed be aggregated microfoci of cells at either local or distant sites. Clearly the natural history of microscopic residual metastatic disease will not be affected by surgery, other than theoretical doubts that the growth fraction of these metastases may be increased following debulking of the primary cancer. This has led to the development of adjuvant cytotoxic therapy, administered with intent to target these low-burden, rapidly cycling foci of cancer cells and to eradicate them before they become established and therefore relatively refractory to intervention.

In any adjuvant therapy setting patients are expected to be free from symptoms directly related to the tumour. Therefore it is imperative that the risk-to-benefit ratio is considered carefully and that the suggested total doses of chemotherapy strike a balance between maximum chance of cure/prolonged survival and tolerance of side-effects. Thus in colorectal cancer, although any patient with Dukes stage A, B or C would theoretically be eligible for adjuvant therapy, the excellent 5-year survival rates of 80–90% for surgery alone in stage A patients have excluded this group from the majority of controlled trials.

The process of metastasis is stochastic, and two rather different models have been proposed. The first involves sequential or 'stepped' spread of local tumour to the liver via the portal vein and subsequent vascular dissemination to distant organ sites like the lung. The opposing theory suggests a more explosive, simultaneous dissemination via blood and lymph vessels to distant sites determined by the pattern of expression of cell surface recognition molecules such as the adherins. The relative importance of these two models may have bearing on the most appropriate route of administration of adjuvant chemotherapy. For example, if one is to believe the sequential model then it would appear logical to test the hypothesis that portal venous infusion of cytotoxic chemotherapy could increase colorectal cancer cure rates.

EARLY STUDIES

The first adjuvant chemotherapy trials on colorectal cancer began in the 1960s. These were often small, underpowered retrospective studies using a single agent, commonly 5-fluorouracil (5-FU), and they failed to demonstrate any therapeutic benefit with respect to either recurrence rate or survival.[2-4]

The late 1980s brought more promising evidence when the results of two large cooperative trials were published that suggested at least some statistically significant benefit for adjuvant chemotherapy.[5,6] Thus in 1988 the National Surgical Adjuvant Breast and Bowel Project (NSABP) reported the results of protocol C-01: comparing patients treated with surgery alone ($n = 394$) with those receiving post operative chemotherapy in the form of 5-fluorouracil, semustine and vincristine ($n = 379$), they found an overall improvement in disease-free survival (DFS) and overall survival (OS) in favour of the chemotherapy arm. At 5 years follow-up, patients treated with surgery alone were at 1.29 times the risk of developing treatment failure and 1.31 times the likelihood of dying as were patients treated with combination adjuvant chemotherapy ($p = 0.02$ and 0.05 respectively). A year later, the North Central Cancer Treatment Group and the Mayo Clinic reported similarly promising results with the use of levamisole and 5-fluorouracil.

However, the pivotal study that altered pessimistic attitudes towards adjuvant treatment and stimulated a flux of subsequent trials was the Intergroup trial reported by Moertel et al[7] in 1990. In this study, 318 patients with stage B colorectal malignancy were randomized for surgical treatment alone or surgery followed by 5-FU/levamisole. In addition, 929 stage C

patients received either surgery alone, surgery plus levamisole, or surgery plus 5-FU/levamisole. All chemotherapy was planned for an intended 12-month administration period. In the levamisole arm, 92% of patients continued treatment for at least 90% of the scheduled year or until death or disease progression. The corresponding figure for the levamisole/5-FU regime was 70%; the disparity is likely to be a consequence of increased toxicity of the combination. The authors demonstrated a 33% reduction in the odds of death and a 41% reduction of recurrence risk in patients who were treated with 5-FU/levamisole compared with surgery as a sole intervention. The overall survival percentage at $3\frac{1}{2}$ years were estimated at 77% and 55% in the treated and control arms respectively. Levamisole alone produced no additional benefit. Toxicity with levamisole alone was typically mild, and included arthralgia, myalgia and an abnormal metallic taste in the mouth. The predominant toxic effects of the combination were similar to those experienced previously with 5-FU alone, and comprised nausea, vomiting, diarrhoea, stomatitis, dermatitis and leukopenia, the latter being the commonest reason for dose limitation.

These striking results provoked the 1990 United States NIH Consensus Statement that 'all stage III patients who are unable to enter a clinical trial should be offered therapy with 5-fluorouracil and levamisole as administered in the Intergroup trial unless medical or psychosocial contraindications exist.'[8] This rapidly became an accepted regime in the USA. In the same year, the Seventh Kings Fund Forum was held in London with the formulation of a similar statement advising that any patient who could not be entered into the ongoing national AXIS trial of adjuvant therapy should be considered for systemic 5-FU/levamisole.[9]

The ramifications of this statement were twofold. Firstly, ethical considerations caused the premature closure of then-current trials that had a no-treatment arm. Secondly, it produced lively debate in Europe in the face of significant scepticism.

Not all of the suspicions were unjustified. There was no direct comparison with 5-FU as a single agent, and the post hoc rationale for an assumed synergism between 5-FU and levamisole was not convincing. Historically, levamisole has been used in veterinary medicine as an anti-helminthic drug, and its use in oncology was based on immunomodulatory effects observed in mice. Hypotheses now exist regarding a possible interaction of levamisole with histocompatibility antigens and subsequent induction of NK cell activity.[10] However, substantive proof of its immunomodulatory effect or of a synergism between it and 5-FU is still not forthcoming. More worryingly perhaps, further studies have associated levamisole both with a common reversible hepatotoxicity that may be confused with the onset of hepatic metastatic disease,[11] and with a rare devastating multifocal encephalopathy and an excess of non-cancer-related deaths.[12,13]

In addition, the survival benefit in the study was only seen on subgroup analysis of Dukes C and not B patients. Although there is a likely continuum of biological risk in colorectal cancer there were not enough stage B patients and subsequent events in this group to detect a significant survival effect. Advocates of meta-analysis have demonstrated that if the results of the Intergroup study are analysed in their entirety, the combination does not appear to be statistically better than single-agent 5-FU.[14]

5-FLUOROURACIL: ALONE AND IN COMBINATION

It is not difficult to appreciate that in the early 1990s the situation arose that although trials were closing on ethical grounds, no general consensus regarding the most appropriate therapy was adopted throughout Europe. Patients were being treated on an 'ad hoc' basis, and use of chemotherapy was largely restricted to those oncologists with a particular interest in colorectal cancer. Disappointingly, fewer than 1% of diagnosed cases were being randomized into clinical trials that may have shed further light on this situation.

Attention has already been drawn to the multiplicity of early studies of 5-FU-inclusive chemotherapy. Standing alone, most failed to demonstrate a statistically significant benefit in the treatment arm, although many suggested a trend in this direction. Gray et al[14] performed a meta-analysis on the collated data and concluded that adjuvant chemotherapy may reduce the odds of death in colorectal cancer by 10–15%. They stated that the confidence limits were large and that the results are of borderline statistical significance. However, it is readily apparent that even a small increase in 5-year survival in such a common disease would save thousands of lives per year throughout Europe. This encouraged oncologists to search for methods for maximizing the therapeutic benefits of 5-fluorouracil, including modulation by agents such as folinic acid.

5-Fluorouracil: modulation by folinic acid (leucovorin)

5-Fluorouracil is a thymidylate synthetase (TS) inhibitor that prevents formation of thymidine, and therefore impairs DNA synthesis. Addition of folinic acid stabilizes the 5-FU/TS complex, maximizing and prolonging the inhibition[15] (see Chapter 18). A meta-analysis of a large number of trials of the 5-FU/folinic acid (FA) combination in advanced colorectal cancer demonstrated useful activity, with an approximate doubling of response rate compared with 5-FU alone ($p < 10^{-7}$).[16–19]

Although results from these trials could not be translated directly into the adjuvant setting, they promoted renewed interest in the 5-FU/FA combination, and in 1993/1994 three large randomized adjuvant phase III trials produced confirmatory evidence of improved 3-year disease-free survival (DFS) and overall survival (OS) in 5-FU/FA treated patients compared with controls (see Table 10.1).

Thus a pooled analysis of three randomized studies from Italy, France and Canada reported that 5-FU/FA significantly reduced mortality by 22% (95% confidence interval (CI) 3–38; $p = 0.029$) and events by 35% (95% CI 22–46; $p < 0.0001$), increasing 3-year event-free

Table 10.1 Summary of three recent trials comparing 5-FU/FA against control in the adjuvant treatment of colon cancer

Trial (no. in study); randomized comparison; follow-up period	Survival			
	Disease-free survival		Overall survival	
	5-FU/FA	**Control**	**5-FU/FA**	**Control**
Overview of French, Italian and Canadian trials (n = 1493); 5-FU/HDFA vs observation;[20] 3 years	71%	62%	83%	78%
	($p < 0.0001$)		($p = 0.03$)	
Intergroup study (n = 309); 5-FU/LDFA vs observation,[21] 5 years	74%	58%	74%	63%
	($p = 0.004$)		($p = 0.02$)	
NSABP C-03 (n = 1080); 5-FU/HDFA vs MOF;[22] 3 years	73%	64%	84%	77%
	($p = 0.0004$)		($p = 0.003$)	

survival from 62% to 71% and overall survival from 78% to 83%.[20] Their cohorts consisted of 5-FU/high-dose FA (HDFA, 200 mg/m^2) versus observation alone. Compliance was good, and there was only one treatment-related death.

Furthermore, mature data from the American Intergroup study has confirmed that a 5-FU/low-dose FA regime decreased recurrence and conferred a survival advantage ($p = 0.02$).[21]

Finally, the National Surgical Adjuvant Breast and Bowel Project C-03 study compared 5-FU/high-dose FA (500 mg/m^2) against the regime MOF (methyl-CCNU/vincristine/5-FU) – a recognized schedule that they had carried over from previous trials. They demonstrated statistically significant benefits firstly with respect to 3-year disease-free survival (DFS): 73% (95% CI 69–77%) in the 5-FU/FA group compared with 64% (95% CI 60–80%) in the

MOF group ($p = 0.0004$). Secondly, overall mortality was decreased, with 84% of those randomized to receive 5-FU/FA surviving compared with 77% of those treated with MOF ($p = 0.003$). This represents a 32% reduction in mortality risk for patients randomized to receive 5-FU/FA compared with control. Perhaps more importantly, this improvement was established for Dukes B analysed as an individual subset: 3-year DFS 87% versus 82% and survival 95% versus 93%.[22]

The results in total suggested that 6 months treatment was probably adequate and that 5-FU/FA may be at least equivalent to 5-FU/levamisole when compared with the 1990 Intergroup study.[7]

In conclusion, evidence accrued that adjuvant chemotherapy using 5-FU/FA regimes can delay and reduce recurrence post-resection and have a modest impact on overall survival.

Table 10.2 Results of NSABP Protocol C-04

	5-year DFS	Cumulative odds	5-year survival	Cumulative odds
5-FU/LV	64%	–	74%	—
5-FU/LV/LEV	64%	0.98	72%	0.93
5-FU/LEV	60%	0.83 ($p < 0.05$)	69%	0.79 ($p < 0.05$)

CURRENT TRIALS OF ADJUVANT CHEMOTHERAPY

Having established the potential role of adjuvant therapy, particularly in stage C colon cancer patients, a number of questions remain incompletely answered.

What is the role of chemotherapy in lower-risk groups?

It is apparent that evidence to support a definite benefit from adjuvant chemotherapy in Dukes B patients has not been well described. Trials that include a surgery-alone arm such as the Nordic Study Group, the Dutch Study Group and the uncertain aim of QUASAR will help to clarify the role of adjuvant therapy in this subgroup.

What, if any, is the role of levamisole?

Two recent large US studies (Intergroup 0089 and NSABP C-04) have specifically addressed this question. In combination, they accrued over 5400 patients, and compared 5-FU/folinic acid (5-FU/LV) with 5-FU/levamisole (5-FU/LEV) and with a combination of all three drugs (5-FU/LV/LEV).

The NSABP results suggest an advantage for the 5-FU/LV (weekly or Roswell/GITSG schedule) over 5-FU/levamisole[23] (see Table 10.2). Between July 1989 and December 1990, 2151 patients with Dukes B and C colon cancer were randomized between the three arms. Global statistical analysis suggested no significant difference in disease-free survival (DFS) ($p = 0.12$) or survival (S) ($p = 0.14$) among the three arms. However, pairwise comparisons indicated DFS and S advantage for the 5-FU/LV over 5-FU/LEV. In the table, odds ratios of less than 1.0 indicate shorter DFS and S intervals than those observed in the control group (5-FU/LV). (Importantly, results form all four NSABP CRC trials indicate that benefit is maintained in stage B patients as a specific subset).[24] In contrast, preliminary results from the four-arm Intergroup trial have not yet demonstrated any significant differences between 5-FU/LEV and 5-FU/high-dose LV, either in terms of DFS (relative risk (RR) = 1.13, $p = 0.14$) or overall S (RR = 1.12, $p = 0.23$). However, the general trend favours the LV regime. The authors conclude that it would be premature to abandon the 5-FU/LEV as standard adjuvant treatment for stage III colon cancer.[25] This issue is clearly not resolved, and the 5-FU/LEV combination will therefore continue to feature in ongoing large randomized trials.

For what period should adjuvant therapy be given, and what is the most appropriate dosage regime for folinic acid?

With specific regard to the length of treatment, a recent joint trial of the North Central Cancer Treatment Group and the NCI Canada Clinical Trials Group was conducted to compare (a) 6 versus 12 months of continuous chemotherapy and (b) 5-FU/LEV versus 5-FU/LEV/LV as

Table 10.3 Results of NCI/NCCTG Trial (1996): adjuvant chemotherapy for colon cancer – regime and duration

Regime	Duration (months)	4-year DFS	p	4-year overall survival	p
5-FU/LV/LEV	6	70%		75%	
5-FU/LEV	12	69%	0.49	72%	0.03
5-FU/LV/LEV	12	66%		66%	
5-FU/LEV	6	64%		63%	

depicted in Table 10.3 ($n = 915$). With a follow-up of 4 years on multivariate global analysis, there was no significant change in DFS or overall S wrought by either drug regimen or duration, suggesting that 6 months of chemotherapy was sufficient, with no statistically significant additional benefit for longer regimes.[26] Interestingly, again with pairwise comparison, the 6-month 5-FU/LEV/LV regime was significantly superior to the 5-FU/LEV regime of the same duration.

Further evidence on the relevance of adjuvant chemotherapy and the optimal regime will be available with the maturity of the UK QUASAR study. This aims to randomize 7500 patients over a 3–4-year period to regimes shown in Figure 10.1. The projected accrual predicts a greater than 80% chance of detecting a true 5% difference in survival between chemotherapy and control (uncertain indication); between high-dose and low-dose FA

(HDFA versus LDFA) and between regimes including levamisole and those with placebo (clear indication).[27]

All patients treated with FA receive the pure *l* form rather than the racemic mixture, since it is the biologically active racemer and since the *d* form may in theory reduce the biomodulatory effect by competing with the *l* isomer for transport into the cell and subsequent polyglutamation.[28] However, a recent NCCTG trial has demonstrated no significant differences between the *l* racemer and the *d,l* mixture with respect to progression, toxicity or response in patients with advanced colorectal cancer.[29]

QUASAR has accrued 4000 patients in two years, mainly owing to adherence to its original principle of being Quick And Simple And Reliable, with minimal data collection and automated randomization and follow-up. Disappointingly, only 800 of these patients have been randomized in the uncertain indication,

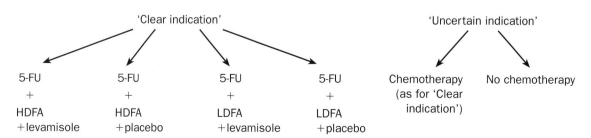

Figure 10.1 Treatment randomization in QUASAR.

probably because of the difficulties surrounding the process of informed consent and the prejudices of the randomizing clinicians.

Is infusional therapy superior to bolus in the adjuvant setting?

Studies in the USA on advanced colorectal cancer first suggested an improved response rate with continuous-infusion 5-FU compared with bolus injection. This was confirmed by Rougier et al[30] in France, with a response rate of 19% with infusional 5-FU therapy compared with 8% when a bolus regimen was utilized ($p < 0.02$, $n = 155$). However, no difference in survival was observed. Toxicity with continuous-infusion 5-FU appears to be mild, consisting mainly of reversible mucositis, and it appears to allow a greater dose intensity to be achieved before toxic side-effects become limiting. Modulation by FA of the continuous-infusion 5-FU was assessed in metastatic colon cancer in a French study, and a significantly higher response rate of 34% for the continuous-infusion versus 17% for bolus administration was observed.[31] Further studies in the USA have also indicated a trend in survival benefit and decreased toxicity for infusional schedules in advanced colorectal cancer.[32]

Ongoing studies that are addressing the role of systemic infusional treatment in the adjuvant setting include the US Mid Atlantic Oncology Program and the Intergroup 0153 trials. It will also be assessed in the EORTC Pan-European Phase III Intergroup trial, which is a collaborative effort involving the dominant adjuvant colorectal trials in the UK, Holland, Italy, France, Spain and Germany.

Is portal chemotherapy superior to the systemic approach?

Whereas *systemic* infusional 5-FU is relatively new in the adjuvant treatment of CRC, *portal* infusional therapy has been undergoing assessment for over a decade.[33] Theoretically, high first-pass metabolism should extract most of the drug locally in the liver, producing a high regional dose intensity but with little systemic escape and therefore reduced toxicity. In addition to the question of superiority of intraportal chemotherapy, there is the question of its efficacy as a complementary method used in parallel with systemic chemotherapy. This is the subject of the ongoing EORTC 40911 trial, which has already accrued 1580 patients. These issues are addressed in detail in Chapter 11.

Is intraperitoneal chemotherapy a viable option?

Relapsing colorectal disease is most commonly seen at the site of the anastomosis, as peritoneal seedlings or as metastatic liver disease. Phamacokinetic studies indicate that following intraperitoneal administration of 5-FU, high concentrations can be achieved and that 70% of the drug is cleared to the liver via the portal circulation.[34] It is thus commonsense to assume that the intraperitoneal route would be a useful therapeutic approach. However, in practice, such trials were hampered by the necessity for frequent diasylate changes complicated by the inherent risk of infective peritonitis.

However, subsequent to the development of a polymeric carrier solution with a potential intraperitoneal dwelling time of 24 hours, Kerr and co-workers undertook phase I toxicology and pharmacokinetic studies of prolonged i.p. infusion with 5-FU in cases of i.p. carcinomatosis from ovarian or GI malignancy who were refractory to standard therapy. It was possible to demonstrate that i.p. steady-state concentrations could be maintained at a level one thousand times that observed in the venous circulation.[35] It is envisaged that this finding could be utilized to maximize dose intensity whilst minimizing toxicity.

Indeed, a recently published study from Austria[36] gathered 236 patients with resected Dukes B and C cancer and randomized them to receive either control i.v. 5-FU/levamisole or investigational combined i.v. and i.p. 5-FU/FA. The results suggest a significant advantage in disease-free survival in favour of the experimental arm (17/94 versus 35/96 tumour recurrences, $p = 0.0015$). These findings bode well for the development of i.p. chemotherapy as an effective stratagem in the adjuvant setting. However, the unfortunate choice of 5-FU/levamisole as the control arm rather than 5-FU/FA limit the ability to assess the route of administration as a separate determining factor for outcome in this study.[36]

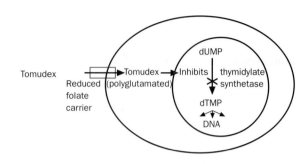

Figure 10.2 Mode of action of Tomudex.

THE FUTURE OF ADJUVANT THERAPY

The future in adjuvant therapy for colon cancer can be broadly split into four categories:

(1) novel cytotoxic drugs;
(2) immunotherapy;
(3) inhibitors of angiogenesis;
(4) gene therapy.

Novel cytotoxic drugs

5-Fluorouracil has been the chemotherapeutic mainstay of colorectal cancer treatment for 40 years, but the past 2 years have seen the introduction of a number of promising new agents.

Tomudex (ZD1694)
Tomudex is a direct and specific thymidylate synthetase (TS) inhibitor preventing the formation of thymidine triphosphate and curbing DNA synthesis.[37] It is a quinazoline folate analogue, which is transported by the reduced folate carrier. It undergoes polyglutamation by the intracellular enzyme folypolyglutamate synthetase to a more potent form, which provokes DNA fragmentation and cell death (Figure 10.2).[38]

Clarke et al[39] set a recommended dose of 3 mg/m^2 as a 15-minute infusion once every three weeks, and an objective response rate of 26% was obtained in a phase II trial involving 177 patients with advanced colorectal malignancy.[40]

Subsequently, the same dose regime was compared with 5-FU/FA administered for 5 days every four or five weeks, in an open randomized study of 439 patients with previously untreated advanced CRC. The response rate demonstrated that Tomudex was at least as effective as conventional chemotherapy (19.8% versus 12.7%; $p = 0.059$).[38]

Benefits noted in the Tomudex arm included significantly lower grade 3 and grade 4 toxicities such as leukopenia and mucositis, a decreased need for subsequent dose reduction, fewer days total treatment (9 versus 29) and fewer community visits (69 versus 230). The trial suggests a potential for improvement in quality of life and economic savings to both patients and health care providers – a point that needs to be addressed further in future studies.

Other trials are considering the further evaluation of Tomudex in the adjuvant setting, including the EORTC Pan European Trial.

Oxaliplatin
Oxaliplatin, a new third-generation platinum analogue, destabilizes nuclear structure by crosslinking DNA. In advanced colorectal cancer it has demonstrated a 10% response rate in patients with 5-FU-resistant tumours.[41] This is confirmed in studies by Levi et al[42] using a 5-day circadian regime. However, de Gramont et al[43] have demonstrated clinical synergism in combination with infusional 5-FU and folinic acid. Therefore it is likely that in the near future it will be randomized into prospective trials of adjuvant combination therapy.

Immunotherapy

Early attempts at controlling colonic cancer by immunological means traditionally utilized non-specific immunomodulators. Not surprisingly perhaps, none of these could be shown to significantly alter the course of the disease.

The NSABP C-01 trial reported a survival advantage in their cohort of patients treated with BCG compared with surgery-only controls (5-year survival 67% compared with 59%; $p = 0.03$).[5] They surmised that the BCG stimulated the host defences, provoking an antibody response against the tumour cells. Interestingly, however, further analysis revealed the survival advantage to be secondary to a decrease in non-cancer-related deaths, in particular cardio-vascular mortality!

A trial in 1993 treated patients in an adjuvant framework with autologous vaccines generated by incubation of the patients own tumour cells with BCG (active specific immunotherapy, ASI).[44] Ninety-eight patients were randomized to receive either surgery alone or surgery plus ASI. A statistically significant improvement in disease-free survival and overall survival was observed in colon patients only; an effect that was abolished by analysing colonic and rectal patients as a single population.

As hybridoma technology developed and the ability to produce monoclonal antibodies to a specific antigenic determinant was recognized, high expectations arose for their use in anti-cancer therapy. A major stumbling block has been the difficulty in defining tumour-specific antigens. However, in the early 1980s an anti-idiotypic anticolorectal cancer IgG2a antibody was developed. It induced cellular cytotoxicity with human effector cells, and prevented outgrowth of xenotransplanted human tumour cells in athymic mice.[45,46] Toxicity studies in advanced CRC patients in 1991 suggested it was well tolerated.[47]

This prompted Riethmuller to run a small randomized trial of the same antibody in adjuvant colorectal cancer treatment. 189 patients with Dukes C CRC were randomized to observation only versus four 100 mg infusions of the antibody. Median follow-up of 5 years revealed a 30% overall reduction in death rate and a 27% reduction in relapse rate in the treated group.[48] The effect of the antibody was most pronounced in patients who developed distant metastases as a first sign of relapse, and was not reproduced in patients with local relapse. The authors suggest that scar tissue and consequent poor blood supply may be responsible for the inefficacy of monoclonal antibody in reducing anastomotic recurrence rate.

Monoclonal antibody therapy is arguably particularly suitable for use in the adjuvant therapy of colorectal cancer for two reasons. Firstly, in the adjuvant setting, residual disease is assumed to be small-volume micrometastatic foci of cells. In mesenchymal tissues these will be surrounded by granulocytes, macrophages and killer cells, all effecting ready initiation of antibody-induced mechanisms of cytotoxicity and all potent inducers of apoptosis (cellular suicide). Secondly, CRC is characteristically a slowly growing tumour with only a minimal fraction of cells actively in the proliferating S phase of the cell cycle at any one time. This determines a certain resistance to antiproliferative agents such as 5-FU, and renders it most suitable for attack by cell-cycle-independent strategies, including immunotherapy.

It is therefore with interest and anticipation that the results of a current adjuvant trial combining the anti-CRC antibody with 5-FU/FA are awaited.

Inhibitors of angiogenesis

Recent advances in molecular biology have led to greater understanding of the mechanisms underlying the process of invasion and metastasis. Matrix metalloproteinases, an enzyme family including collagenase, elastase and gelatinase, are secreted by tumour cells, and degrade intercellular proteins and basement membrane, and therefore have an important role in tumour cell invasion. Marimastat, a potent and selective inhibitor of these enzymes, which is orally administered, appears to reduce the rate of carcino-embryonic antigen rise in advanced colorectal cancer,[49] and is likely to be a strong candidate for future adjuvant trials if its toxicity profile proves acceptable in this setting.

Gene therapy

Historically, the role of gene therapy has been against inherited disease, with the introduction of deficient genetic material into a cell to replace the machinery necessary for the production of a particular protein, the main candidate diseases being single-gene disorders. However, the concept of somatic gene therapy has now developed beyond this, and a wide variety of protocols for this form of treatment in cancer are under review.

Strategies include

(1) stimulation of cancer cells or host cells to produce cytokines or other molecules to alter the host response to malignancy;
(2) induction of expression of antigens (e.g. allogeneic HLA proteins) on tumour cells to promote the host response;
(3) introduction of tumour-suppressor genes to slow and abort cell growth;

(4) insertion of drug-resistance genes into normal cells to allow more aggressive chemotherapy;
(5) insertion of genes into cells that transcribe enzymes capable of metabolizing prodrugs.

The last method is probably the most exciting in colorectal cancer gene therapy, and is likely to be the most effectively applicable in the clinical setting. It is termed VDEPT – virus-directed enzyme prodrug therapy.

It is based on the recent formulation of retroviral vectors linking the carcino-embryonic antigen (CEA) promoter to the structural gene for the bacterial enzyme cytosine deaminase (which metabolizes the prodrug 5-fluorocytosine to 5-FU).[50] Viral transduction of this gene hybrid should occur only in CEA-expressing cells, i.e. CRC cells, conferring tumour selectivity for activation of the chemotherapeutic agent (see Figure 10.3). A 1000-fold higher concentration of 5-FU can be maintained in the tumour and in the immediately neighbouring bystander cells than in the systemic circulation.

Initially the method will be tested via hepatic artery infusion in hepatic metastatic colorectal malignancy. If significant benefit is observed,

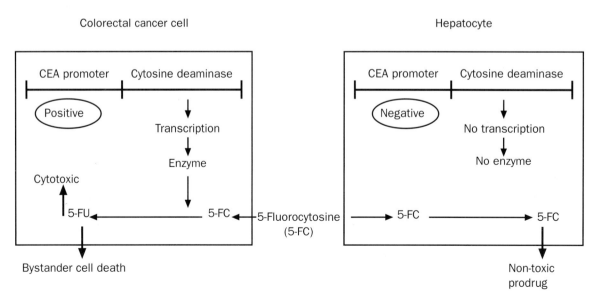

Figure 10.3 Gene therapy in colorectal cancer.

trials in the adjuvant setting via the portal vein are envisaged.

CONCLUSIONS

In summary, the last decade has demonstrated likely benefit for chemotherapy for colon cancer in the adjuvant setting.

The results of ongoing and planned large collaborative trials will determine the most effective routes, dosage regimes and combinations of the drugs presently in widespread use, in particular 5-FU, FA and levamisole.

New therapeutic agents are being considered that may prove superior with respect to response rates or side-effect profiles. Health economics and quality-of-life outcomes may be important factors when considering their implementation.

Finally, colorectal cancer will kill 19 000 people in the UK alone in the next 12 months. Therefore even apparently marginal improvements in survival through advances in adjuvant therapy will reap huge benefits in life years saved.

This should prove adequate stimulus to all clinicians to enter relevant patients into the current large controlled prospective trials in Europe.

REFERENCES

1. Abulafi AM, Williams NS, Local recurrence of colorectal cancer: the problems, the mechanisms, management and adjuvant treatment. *Br J Surg* 1994; **81:** 7–17.
2. Panettriere FJ, Goodman PJ, Conkinzi JJ et al, Adjuvant treatment in large bowel adenocarcinoma – long-term results of a Southwest Oncology Group Study. *J Clin Oncol* 1988; **6:** 947–55.
3. Higgins GA Jr, Amado JH, McElhinney J et al, Efficacy of prolonged intermittent treatment with combined 5FU and methyl CCNU following resection for carcinoma of the large bowel. *Cancer* 1984; **53:** 1–8.
4. Abdi EA, Harbora D, Hanson J et al, Adjuvant chemoimmuno and immunotherapy in stage B and C colorectal carcinoma. *Proc Am Soc Clin Oncol* 1987; **6:** 93.
5. Wolmark N, Fisher B, Rockette H et al, Post operative adjuvant chemotherapy or BCG for colon cancer: results from NSABP protocol C-01. *J Natl Cancer Inst* 1988; **80:** 30–6.
6. Laurie JA, Moertel CG, Fleming TR et al, Surgical adjuvant treatment of large bowel cancer; an evaluation of levamisole and the combination of levamisole and 5FU. A study of the North Central Cancer Treatment Group (NCCTG) and the Mayo Clinic. *J Clin Oncol* 1989; **7:** 1447–56.
7. Moertel CG, Fleming TH, MacDonald JS et al, Levamisole and fluorouracil for adjuvant treatment of resected colon cancer. *N Engl J Med* 1990; **322:** 352–8.
8. NIH Concensus Conference, Adjuvant therapy for patients with colon and rectal cancer. *J Am Med Assoc* 1990; **264:** 1444–50.
9. King's Fund Forum, Cancer of the colon and rectum. *Br J Surg* 1990; **77:** 1063–5.
10. Goodrich KH, Alvarez X, Holcombe RF et al, Effect of levamisole on MHC Class I expression in colorectal and breast cancer cell lines. *Cancer* 1993; **72:** 225–30.
11. Moertel CG, Fleming TR, MacDonald JS et al, Hepatic toxicity associated with 5FU plus levamisole adjuvant treatment. *J Clin Oncol* 1993; **11:** 2386–90.
12. Kimmel DW, Schutt AJ, Multifocal leukoencephalopathy; occurrence during 5FU and levamisole treatment and resolution after discontinuation of chemotherapy. *Mayo Clin Proc* 1993; **68:** 363–5.
13. Chlebowski RT, Lillington L, Nystrom JG, Sayre J, Late mortality and levamisole. Adjuvant treatment in colorectal cancer. *Br J Cancer* 1994; **69:** 1094–7.
14. Gray R, James R, Mossman J, Stenning S, AXIS: a suitable case for treatment. *Br J Cancer* 1991; **63:** 841–5.
15. Kerr DJ, 5-Fluouracil and folinic acid: interesting biochemistry or effective treatment? *Br J Cancer* 1989; **60:** 807–8.
16. Machover D, Goldschmidt E, Chollet P et al, Treatment of advanced colorectal and gastric adenocarcinomas with 5-fluorouracil combined with high dose folinic acid. *J Clin Oncol* 1986; **4:** 685–96.

17. Machover D, Schwartzenberg L, Goldshmidt E et al, Treatment of advanced colorectal and gastric adenocarcinomas with 5FU combined with high-dose folinic acid: a pilot study. *Cancer Treat Rep* 1982; **66:** 1803–7.

18. Madajewicz S, Petrelli N, Rustum Y et al, Phase I–II trial of high-dose calcium leucovorin and 5-fluorouracil in advanced colorectal cancer. *Cancer Res* 1984; **44:** 4667–9.

19. Buyse M, Piedbois P, Rustum Y – Advanced Colorectal Analysis Project, Modulation of 5-fluorouracil by leucovorin in patients with advanced colorectal cancer: evidence in terms of response rate. *J Clin Oncol* 1992; **10:** 896–903.

20. IMPACT trial, Efficacy of adjuvant fluorouracil and folinic acid in colon cancer. *Lancet* 1995; **345:** 939–44.

21. O'Connell M, Maillard J, MacDonald J et al, Controlled trial of fluorouracil and low-dose leucovorin given for six months as post-operative adjuvant therapy for colon cancer. *J Clin Oncol* 1997; **15:** 246–50.

22. Wolmark N, Rockette H, Fisher B et al, The benefit of leucovorin modulated 5-fluorouracil as post-operative adjuvant treatment for primary colon cancer: results from the Natl Surg Adjuv Breast and Bowel Project protocol C-03. *J Clin Oncol* 1993; **11:** 1879–88.

23. Wolmark N, Rockette H, Mamounas EP et al, The relative efficacy of 5-fluorouracil/leucovorin, 5-fluorouracil/levamisole and 5-fluorouracil/leucovorin/levamisole in patients with Dukes B and C carcinoma of the colon: first report of the NSABP protocol C-04. *Proc Am Soc Clin Oncol* 1996; **15:** 205 (abst).

24. Mamounas EP, Rockette H, Jones J et al, Comparative efficacy of adjuvant chemotherapy in patients with Dukes' B vs Dukes' C colon cancer: results from four NSABP adjuvant studies (C-01, C-02, C-03 and C-04). *Proc Am Soc Clin Oncol* 1996; **15:** 205 (abst).

25. Haller DG, Catalano PJ, MacDonald JS, Mayer RJ, Fluouracil, leucovorin and levamisole. Adjuvant treatment for colon cancer: preliminary results of INT 0089. *Proc Am Soc Clin Oncol* 1996; **15:** 211 (abst).

26. O'Connell MJ, Laurie JA, Shepherd L et al, a prospective evaluation of chemotherapy duration and regimen as surgical adjuvant treatment for high risk colon cancer; a collaborative trial of the North Central Cancer Treatment Group and the National Cancer Institute of Canada Clinical Trials Group. *Proc Am Soc Clin Oncol* 1996; **15:** 209 (abst).

27. *QUASAR – A UK CCR Study of Colorectal Cancer Treatment Protocol: UK Version*, December 1994.

28. Zittoun J, Marquet J, Pilkorger JJ et al, Comparative effect of 6S, 6R and 6RS on leucovorin on methotrexate rescue and modulation of 5-fluorouracil. *Br J Cancer* 1991; **63:** 885–8.

29. Goldberg RM, O'Connel MJ, Wieand HS et al, A prospective randomised trial of intensive course 5FU combined with a) the *l*-isomer of IV leucovorin, b) oral *d,l,* leucovorin or c) IV *d, l* leucovorin for the treatment of advanced colorectal cancer: a North Central Cancer Treatment Group trial. *Proc Am Soc Clin Oncol* 1996; **15:** 207 (abst).

30. Rougier Ph, Paillot B, Laplanche D et al, End results of a multicentric randomised trial comparing 5-fluorouracil in continuous systemic infusion (CI) to bolus administration (B) in measurable metastatic colorectal cancer (MCC). *Proc Am Soc Clin Oncol* 1992; **11:** 163 (abst).

31. De Grammont A, Bosset JF, Milan C et al, A prospectively randomised trial comparing 5-fluorouracil bolus with low-dose folinic acid and 5-fluorouracil bolus plus continuous infusion with high dose folinic acid for advanced colorectal cancer. *Proc Am Soc Clin Oncol* 1995; **14:** 194 (abst).

32. Leichman CG, Fleming TR, Muggia FM, A phase II study of 5-fluorouracil and its modulation in advanced colorectal cancer: a Southwest Oncology Group Study. *J Clin Oncol* 1995; **13:** 1303–11.

33. Taylor I, Machin D, Mullee M, A randomised controlled trial of adjuvant portal vein cytotoxic perfusion in colorectal cancer. *Br J Surg* 1985; **72:** 359.

34. Speyer JL, Sugarbaker PH, Collins JM et al, Portal levels and hepatic clearance of 5-fluorouracil after IP administration in tumours. *Cancer Res* 1981; **41:** 1916–22.

35. McArdle CS, Kerr DJ, O'Gorman P et al, Pharmacokinetic study of 5-fluorouracil in a novel dialysate solution; a long-term IP treatment approach for advanced colorectal cancer. *Br J Cancer* 1994; **70:** 762–6.

36. Scheithauer W, Marczell A, Depish D et al, Combined IV and IP chemotherapy with 5-fluorouracil and leucovorin vs 5-fluorouracil and levamisole for adjuvant treatment of resected colon carcinoma. *Proc Am Soc Clin Oncol* 1996; **15:** 216 (abst).

37. Jackman AL, Taylor GA, Gibson W et al, ICI D1964: a quinazoline antifolate thymidylate synthetase inhibitor that is a potent inhibitor of

L1210 tumour cell growth in vitro and in vivo; a new agent for clinical study. *Cancer Res* 1991; **51:** 5579–86.

38. Cunningham D, Zalcberg JR, Rath U et al, Tomudex ZD1694: results of a randomised trial in advanced colorectal cancer demonstrate efficacy and reduced mucositis and leukopenia. *Eur J Cancer* 1995; **31A:** 1945–54.

39. Clarke JS, Ward J, De Boer M et al, Phase I study of the new thymidylate synthetase inhibitor 'TOMUDEX' ZD1694 in advanced malignancy. *Ann Oncol* 5(Suppl 5): 132 (abst).

40. Zalcberg JR, Cunningham D, Van Cutsem E et al, ZD 1694: a novel thymidylate synthase inhibitor with substantial activity in the treatment of patients with advanced colorectal cancer. TOMUDEX colorectal cancer study group. *J Clin Oncol* 1996; **14:** 716–21.

41. Moreau S, Machover D, de Gramont A et al, A Phase II trial of oxaliplatin: l-OHP in patients with colorectal cancer previously resistant to 5-fluorouracil and folinic acid. *Proc Am Soc Clin Oncol* 1993; **12:** 645 (abst).

42. Levi F, Perpoint B, Garufi C et al, Oxaliplatin activity against metastatic colorectal cancer. A phase II study of 5 day continuous venous infusion at circadian rhythm modulated rate. *Eur J Cancer* 1993; **29A:** 1280–4.

43. De Gramont A, Vignoud J, Tournigand C et al, Oxaliplatin with high dose folinic acid and 5-fluorouracil 48 hr infusion in pre-treated metastatic colorectal cancer (CRC). *Eur J Cancer* 1995; **31A:** 716.

44. Hoover HC Jr, Brandhorst JS, Peters LC, Adjuvant ASI for human colorectal cancer: a 6.5 year median follow-up of a phase III prospective randomised trial. *J Clin Oncol* 1993; **11:** 390–9.

45. Herlyn M, Steplewski Z, Herlyn D, Koprowski H, Colorectal carcinoma-specific antigen: detection by means of monoclonal antibodies. *Proc Natl Acad Sci USA* 1979; **76:** 1438–42.

46. Herlyn M, Steplewski Z, Herlyn MF, Koprowski H, Inhibition of growth of colorectal carcinoma in nude mice by monoclonal antibody. *Cancer Res* 1980; **40:** 717–21.

47. Mellstedt H, Frodin JE, Masucci G et al, The therapeutic use of monoclonal antibodies in colorectal carcinoma. *Semin Oncol* 1991; **2:** 462–77.

48. Riethmuller G, Schneider-Gadicke E, Schlimok G, Randomised trial of monoclonal antibody for adjuvant treatment of resected Dukes C colorectal carcinoma. *Lancet* 1994; **343:** 1177–83.

49. Millar A, Brown P, 360 patient meta-analysis of studies of marimastat – a novel matrix metalloproteinase inhibitor. *Ann Oncol* 1996; **7**(Suppl 5): 123 (abst).

50. Huber BE, Austin EA, Good SS et al, In vivo anti-tumour activity of 5-fluorocytosine on human colorectal cancer cells genetically modified to express cytosine deaminase. *Cancer Res* 1993; **53:** 4619–26.

11

Adjuvant intraportal treatment

Urban Th Laffer, Urs Metzger

INTRODUCTION

Liver metastases are present on initial diagnosis of large-bowel cancer in 25–30% of patients.[1] After curative surgery of colorectal primary tumors, the liver again is the most frequent site of relapse.[2,3] Once liver metastases have developed, the prognosis is poor, with an expected median survival time of 6–9 months,[1,4] the extent of the tumor being the most important prognostic factor.[5] A great deal of work has been done to determine the factors that influence development of liver metastases. There is evidence that tumor cells embolize into the portal venous system via the mesenteric veins and enter the liver. In 1957, Dukes[6] found evidence of venous spread in 17% of operative rectal cancer specimens. Fisher and Turnbull[7] discovered tumor cells in the mesenteric venous blood of 32% of colorectal carcinoma patients at surgery. They suggested that manipulation of the tumor may force malignant cells into the circulation, and initiated the so-called no-touch isolation technique.[8,9] However, not all circulating cancer cells give rise to metastases. Several reports have shown that patients with malignant cells in the portal venous blood fare no worse than those without.[10,11]

Metachronous liver metastases may originate from microscopic deposits not visible at surgery for the primary tumor. These micrometastases are the most important target for adjuvant systemic therapy.[12,13] Since adjuvant systemic chemotherapy has mostly failed in several prospective randomized trials,[14,15] numerous studies have approached the issue of hepatic-artery or portal-vein infusion of fluorinated pyrimidines.

PATTERNS OF VASCULARITY OF LIVER TUMORS AND THEIR CONSEQUENCES FOR DIFFERENT THERAPEUTIC APPROACHES

In the therapeutic management of both primary and metastatic liver tumors, vascularity assumes major importance. The blood supply of these tumors constitutes a pathway for the delivery of antitumor agents. In addition, the possibility of diminishing or eliminating oxygen supply and blood flow to these tumors depends on knowledge of vascularity. The vascularity of liver tumors is more complicated than that of most other tumors because of the presence of both arterial and portal circulations. Both systems play a role in the perfusion of tumors, and arterioportal and arteriovenous shunting may further complicate the picture. Considerable work on the vascular patterns of experimental tumors has been carried out using pigmented silicone rubber (Microfil) injected into the arterial and portal circulations. The tumors investigated were Walker carcinosarcomas implanted in the livers of rats. In these studies by Ackerman,[16] tumors measuring less than 1 mm in diameter did not display any new vessel formation. Beyond this size, single, newly formed vessels began to encircle the tumors. The vessels were derived from either the arteriolar or the portal circulation in completely random fashion.

As tumors continued to grow, reaching diameters between 5 and 7 mm, the encircling plexus became more extensive and better developed. As this occurred, the arterial circulation became predominant, and in most specimens no portal circulation was seen. In general, portal vessels were compressed or displaced as the tumors grew. Similar results were obtained by Bassermann[17] and by Taylor et al,[18] who measured blood flow into colorectal liver metastases using ^{133}Xe clearance in patients undergoing surgery for colorectal cancer. Preoperative measurements made after direct parenchymal injection showed a mean flow of 41.5 ± 22.5 ml/min per 100 mg, which, after hepatic arterial occlusion, was reduced to a mean of 5% of the preocclusion value. Dynamic bloodflow studies using a gamma camera were performed in the postoperative period of administration of [131]Xe into both hepatic-artery and portal-vein catheters.

The initial distribution images indicated a predominantly arterial perfusion of the metastases, but, after hepatic-artery occlusion, portal-vein perfusion to the metastases was statistically significantly increased. Ridge et al[19] demonstrated a quantitative advantage of hepatic-artery infusion over portal-vein infusion of colorectal hepatic metastases using nitrogen-13 amino acids and ammonia with dynamic gamma-camera imaging. Data collected from the liver for 10 minutes after rapid bolus injection of nitrogen-13 L-glutamate, L-glutamine or ammonia were compared with ^{99m}Tc macroaggregated albumin (MAA) images produced after injection through the hepatic artery or portal vein in the same session. Tumor regions defined from the ^{99m}Tc sulfur colloid scans were compared with nearby liver areas of similar thickness. For the nitrogen-13 compounds, the area-normalized count rate at first-pass maximum (Q_{max}) and the tissue-extraction efficiency were computed. Results showed that more than twice as much of a nutrient substrate was delivered per volume of tumor relative to liver by the hepatic artery than by the portal vein. The delivery of substance in solution (such as nutrients or drugs) to tumor and liver tissue correlated with the distribution of colloids such as MAA after hepatic-artery and portal-vein injection.

It can be concluded from these studies that the arterial route is superior to the portal for established metastatic disease, whereas the portal route might be preferable for the adjuvant setting.

PHARMACOKINETICS OF INTRAPORTAL CHEMOTHERAPY

Almersjö et al[20] showed the safety of intraportal 5-fluorouracil (5-FU) continuous-infusion therapy. At the dose of 15 mg/kg body weight/24 hours, serum concentrations were generally below 100 ng/ml, whereas the same dose given intravenously resulted in serum levels of 100–300 ng/ml.

Increasing the dose to 30 mg/kg/24 hours resulted in serum concentrations less than 200 ng/ml using the portal-vein route, whereas intravenous systemic infusion was not feasible because of hematologic toxicity. Speyer et al[21] measured portal circulation levels and hepatic clearance of 5-FU in humans after intraperitoneal administration. They found high levels of 5-FU in the portal vein, comparable to concentrations after direct intraportal infusion, and calculated a hepatic extraction rate of 80–90%.

Berger et al[22] tested systemic and local toxicity in Sprague–Dawley rats after systemic or locoregional infusion or bolus injection over 5 days at equimolar doses (total dose 1220 µM/kg each). In this experimental model, continuous infusion resulted in lower systemic and local toxicities, and in general the locoregional administration was less toxic than administration via the vena cava.

INTRAPORTAL INFUSION AS AN ADJUVANT MODALITY FOR COLORECTAL CANCER

In 1957, Morales et al[23] advocated intraportal injection of cytotoxic agents at the time of surgery for colorectal cancer in an attempt to prevent liver metastases. It is generally accepted that adjuvant therapy should be started as soon as possible after surgery, when the tumor burden is minimal.[24,25] In addition, surgical stress, anesthetic and other drugs, hypercoagulability, blood transfusion, and impairment of immune function due to surgery possibly render the perioperative period a vulnerable phase for tumor promotion.

The renewed interest in portal adjuvant infusion is based on an early publication by Taylor et al,[26] who, in 1979, reported on a randomized study evaluating adjuvant cytotoxic liver infusion for colorectal cancer. After a mean follow-up of 26 months, 23 patients had died in the control group and 7 in the infusion group. The incidence of liver metastases in the two groups (13 control, 2 infusion) was statistically significantly different. Based on these results, several cooperative groups initiated prospective randomized trials comparing intraportal infusion of various regimens with surgery alone.

In a more recent analysis, Taylor et al[27] reported on 127 control patients and 117 patients who received adjuvant infusion. Thirteen patients were excluded following randomization: one had cirrhosis, three were found on laparotomy to have liver metastases, and in nine there were technical problems with catheter cannulation. After a median follow-up of 4 years, 53 patients had died with recurrent disease in the control group and 25 in the infusion group. The liver was the predominant site of recurrence: 22 patients in the control group and 5 in the infusion group developed haptic metastases. Overall survival appeared to be

improved in the infusion group; on closer examination, however, the only significant improvement in overall survival was among patients with Dukes B colon tumors.

In a three-arm study at St Mary's and surrounding hospitals in the UK, 398 patients have been randomized: 145 control patients, 123 heparin-treated patients (heparin 10 000 U/24 hours for 7 days), and 130 patients receiving heparin + 5-FU (1000 mg/24 hours for 7 days)[28,29]. In this study, 10.6% patients in the heparin-alone and 18.5% in the 5-FU plus heparin group failed to complete treatment, blockage or premature removal of the catheter being the principal reasons for these trial deviants. No patient had treatment stopped because of white-cell count. There were no statistically significant differences in the incidence of postoperative complications. However, there was a tendency for fewer postoperative complications in the control group. Four deaths were attributed to adjuvant therapy, one to 5-FU (septic complication) and three to the use of heparin (coagulopathy, presacral hematoma, retroperitoneal hemorrhage). All patients had at least five years of follow-up. Analysis of age-adjusted five-year survival data, based on intention to treat, revealed no statistically significant differences between groups (77.0% in the control, 72.7% in the heparin-alone, and 81.7% in the heparin plus 5-FU group). However, the survival data for patients with Dukes C disease showed a statistically significant survival advantage for the 5-FU plus heparin group of 16.3% as compared with the control group ($p < 0.03$), representing a 32.3% reduction in mortality associated with intraportal 5-FU and heparin adjuvant therapy. In the total trial group there were 49 liver metastases in the first five years of follow-up. There was the same evidence of fewer liver tumor recurrences in the 5-FU plus heparin group than the control group, but the numbers were too small to reach statistical significance.

In a Dutch trial, surgery alone, 5-FU (1000 mg/24 hours for 7 days) plus heparin (5000 U/24 hours for 7 days), and urokinase (10 000 U/hour for 24 hours only) have been compared in a randomized fashion. Portal adjuvant treatment was applied through a catheter placed in the dilated umbilical vein. A total of 304 patients were eligible: 102 in the control, 99 in the 5-FU plus heparin, and 103 patients in the urokinase group. The recently published results are based on a median follow-up of 44 months.[30] Development of septic complications was not related to treatment groups. Liver metastases developed in 23/102 patients (23%) in the control group, in 7/99 patients (7%) in the 5-FU/heparin group, and in 18/103 patients (18%) in the urokinase group ($p = 0.01$, 5-FU/heparin versus control). In a multivariate Cox regression analysis with the covariates tumor stage, tumor site, sex and age, the chance of developing liver metastases after portal infusion with 5-FU/heparin was one-third of the chance in the control group ($p < 0.001$). Infusion with urokinase had no significant effect on the development of liver metastases. However, the positive effect of reduction of the incidence of liver metastases was not reflected in a significant reduction of the death rate or an improvement in the overall or disease-free survival.

In the National Surgical Adjuvant Breast and Bowel Project (NSABP) Protocol C-02,[31] 1158 patients have been followed for an average time of 41.8 months. A comparison between the two groups of patients indicated both an improvement in disease-free survival (74% versus 64%, $p = 0.02$) and a survival advantage (81% versus 73%, $p = 0.07$) in favor of the chemotherapy-treated group. When compared with the treated group, patients who received no further treatment had 1.26 times the risk of developing a treatment failure and 1.25 times the likelihood of dying after four years. However, the trial failed to demonstrate an advantage from 5-FU in decreasing the incidence of hepatic metastases.

In 1981 the Swiss Group for Clinical Cancer Research (SAKK) started a randomized trial comparing adjuvant portal chemotherapy with 5-FU (500 mg/m²/24 hours for 7 days) and mitomycin C (10 mg/m²/2 hours in a single dose given at day one) with radical surgery alone. 533 patients with histologically proven adenocarcinoma of the colon or rectum who were candidates for a curative en-bloc resection

and were younger than 75 years were randomized. Randomization could be performed based upon absence of metastatic disease in the preoperative investigations, and 65 patients (12%) were diagnosed intraoperatively to have liver metastasis (29 patients) or incomplete resection (8 patients), or having different histology (26 patients). In two cases only, there was a protocol violation. The latter 28 patients were inevaluable for the time to and pattern of recurrence, but these remained in study according 'intent to treat' for survival analysis.

At a median follow-up of 8 years,[32] patients who were assigned to receive perioperative adjuvant portal chemotherapy had a significantly lower relapse rate than those who were not: the five-year disease-free survival percentages were $55 \pm 3\%$ among the patients who received perioperative chemotherapy and $45 \pm 3\%$ among the patients in the control group. The ratio of hazard functions for relapse of treated as compared with untreated patients based on a proportional hazards model stratified according to tumor site and with tumor stage and age as covariates was 0.78 (95% confidence interval, CI, 0.61–0.99, $p = 0.045$). 235 patients had died: 108 in the infusion group versus 127 in the control group. The five-year overall survival percentages favored the infusion group: $63 \pm 3\%$ versus $53 \pm 3\%$. The hazard ratio was 0.74 (95% CI 0.57–0.96, $p = 0.026$). Treatment benefits in terms of disease-free and overall survival were comparable in all subgroups, but suggested possibly larger differences for patients of positive nodal status and colon-cancer patients.

To the best of our knowledge, at least 12 prospective controlled studies have been done on adjuvant chemotherapy by portal infusion following radical surgery for colorectal cancer. Most of the trials were multicentric, and some did not include rectal cancer. The adjuvant treatment was given as continuous infusion for 5 to 7 days immediately after operation. According to three protocols, the effect of anticoagulants was tested, using heparin or urokinase alone. All but one[33] of these studies demonstrate an improvement of overall and disease-free survival and a reduction of the incidence of liver recurrences, particularly in the subgroups of colon-cancer patients and for patients with involvement of the regional lymph nodes (Dukes C). However, none of the randomized studies could demonstrate a statistically significant overall effect in the reduction of the incidence of liver metastases as Taylor did. Most of the authors argue that the effect of adjuvant portal chemotherapy on overall and disease-free survival may be attributed to a general reduction of tumor recurrences (i.e. local recurrences, liver metastases and other distant metastases), and it is speculated that these effects are a result of the systemic efficacy of portally applied 5-FU. This hypothesis has been evaluated in the second clinical trial of the Swiss Group for Clinical Cancer Research (SAKK) in a randomized three-arm study (control versus portal versus systemic adjuvant therapy) between 1987 and 1993. The median follow-up time is too short to draw any conclusions at present.

Toxic deaths have been recorded in at least three trials: one in Taylor's study, due to perirectal sepsis,[27] one in the St Mary's trial in a patient over 80 years old,[28,29] and one in the Swiss Group trial,[32] where an insulin-dependent male suffered Gram-negative septicemia and leukopenia during portal infusion. For further studies, it is recommended that

insulin-dependent diabetics, patients with a cumulative high risk for postoperative complications (i.e. obesity, cardiac and/or pulmonary disease), and patients with any evidence of intraabdominal sepsis at laparotomy or during the early postoperative period should be excluded. However, the overall operative mortality in all these trials was in the range of 3–4% or less, and is considerably lower than reported from previous multicenter trials. The reduced incidence of surgical complications indicates advances in surgical technique and in management before and after such elective cancer surgery. This allows adjuvant chemotherapy programs to be moved closer to the surgical interventions, and surgeons are becoming more familiar with the use of chemotherapy in the early postoperative phase in colorectal as well as in breast cancer and for tumors in other sites. If a short perioperative course of chemotherapy is as effective as a 6–12-month regimen, this will have significant impact on patients' quality of life and the costs of health care systems. For this reason, the Swiss Group for Clinical Cancer Research (SAKK) recently initiated a randomized multicenter trial comparing short-term adjuvant perioperative chemotherapy with long-term chemotherapy with 5-FU and levamisole, as recommended by the National Cancer Institute (NCI) in colon-cancer patients.

REFERENCES

1. Bengmark S, Hafström L, The natural history of primary and secondary malignant tumours of the liver. The prognosis for patients with hepatic metastases from colonic and rectal carcinoma by laparotomy. *Cancer* 1969; **23**: 198.
2. Cedermark BJ, Schultz SS, Bakshi S et al, Value of liver scan in the follow-up study of patients with adenocarcinoma of the colon and rectum. *Surg Gynecol Obstet* 1977; **144**: 745.
3. Weiss L. Grundmann E, Torhorst J et al, Haematogeneous metastatic patterns in colonic carcinoma: an analysis of 1541 necropsies. *J Pathol* 1986; **150**: 195.
4. Pestana C, Reitmeier RJ, Moertel CG et al, The natural history of carcinoma of the colon and rectum. *Am J Surg* 1964; **108**: 826.
5. Wanebo H, A staging system for liver metastases from colorectal cancer. *Proc Am Soc Clin Oncol* 1984; **3**: 143.
6. Dukes CE, Discussion on major surgery in carcinoma of the rectum, with or without colostomy, excluding the anal canal and including the rectosigmoid. *Proc R Soc Med* 1957; **50**: 1031.
7. Fisher ER, Turnbull RB, The cytological demonstration and significance of tumor cells in the mesenteric venous blood in patients with colorectal cancer. *Surg Gynecol Obstet* 1955; **100**: 102.
8. Turnbull RB, Kyhle K, Watson FR, Brett J, Cancer of the colon: the influence of the no-touch isolation technique on survival rates. *Ann Surg* 1967; **166**: 420.
9. Turnbull RB, Cancer of the colon: 5–10 years'

survival rates following resection utilizing the isolation technique. *Ann R Coll Surg Engl* 1970; **46**: 243.

10. Roberst S, Jonasson O, McGrath R et al, Clinical significance of cancer cells in the circulating blood: two- to five-year survivals. *Ann Surg* 1961; **154**: 362.

11. Sellwood RA, Kuper SW, Burn JI, Wallace EN, Circulating cancer cells: the influence of surgical operations. *Br J Surg* 1965; **52**: 69.

12. De Vita VT, The relationship between tumor mass and resistance to chemotherapy. Implications for surgical adjuvant treatment of cancer. The James Ewing Lecture. *Cancer* 1983; **51**: 1209.

13. Schabel FM, Concepts for systemic treatment of micrometastases. *Cancer* 1975; **35**: 15.

14. Metzger U, Schneider K, Largiader F, Adjuvante Therapie des Kolon- und Rektumkarzinoms. Übersicht über den heutigen Stand. *Onkologie* 1982; **5**: 228.

15. Holyoke ED, Moertel CG, O'Connell MJ, and the Gastrointestinal Tumor Study Group, Adjuvant therapy of colon cancer: results of a prospectively randomized trial. *N Engl J Med* 1984; **310**: 737.

16. Ackermann NB, The blood supply of experimental liver metastases. IV. Changes in vascularity with increasing tumor growth. *Surgery* 1974; **75**: 589.

17. Bassermann R, Changes of vascular pattern of tumors and surrounding tissue during different phases of metastatic growth. *Cancer Res* 1986; **100**: 256.

18. Taylor I, Bennett R, Sherriff S, The blood supply of colorectal liver metastases. *Br J Cancer* 1974; **39**: 749.

19. Ridge JA, Bading JR, Gelbard AS et al, Perfusion of colorectal hepatic metastases. *Cancer* 1987; **59**: 1547.

20. Almersjö O, Brandberg A, Gustavsson B, Concentration of biological active 5-fluorouracil in general circulation during continuous portal infusion in man. *Cancer Lett* 1975; **1**: 113.

21. Speyer JL, Sugarbaker PH, Collins JM et al, Portal levels and hepatic clearance of 5-fluorouracil after intraperitoneal administration in humans. *Cancer Res* 1981; **41**: 1916.

22. Berger MR, Henne TH, Aguiar JLA et al, Experiments on the toxicity of locoregional liver chemotherapy with 5-fluoro-2'-deoxyuridine and 5-fluorouracil in an animal model. *Rec Results Cancer Res* 1986; **100**: 148.

23. Morales F, Bell M, McDonald GD, Cole WH, The prophylactic treatment of cancer at time of operation. *Ann Surg* 1957; **146**: 588.

24. Burchenal JH, Adjuvant therapy – theory, practice, and potential. The James Ewing Lecture. *Cancer* 1976; **37**: 46.

25. Fisher B, Gunduz N, Saffer EA, Influence of the interval between primary tumor removal and chemotherapy on kinetics and growth of metastases. *Cancer Res* 1983; **43**: 1488.

26. Taylor I, Rowling JT, West C, Adjuvant cytotoxic liver perfusion for colorectal cancer. *Br J Surg* 1979; **66**: 833.

27. Taylor I, Machin D, Mullee M et al, A randomized controlled trial of adjuvant portal vein cytotoxic XX perfusion in colorectal cancer. *Br J Surg* 1985; **72**: 359.

28. Fielding LP, Hittinger R, Grace RH, Fry JS, Randomised controlled trial of adjuvant chemotherapy by portal-vein perfusion after curative resection for colorectal adenocarcinoma. *Lancet* 1992; **340**: 502.

29. Kingston RD, Fielding JW, Palmer MK, Perioperative heparin: a possible adjuvant to surgery in colo-rectal cancer? *Int J Colorectal Dis* 1993; **8**: 111.

30. Wereldsma JC, Bruggink ED, Meijer WS et al, Adjuvant portal liver infusion in colorectal cancer with 5-fluorouracil/heparin versus urokinase versus control. Results of a prospective randomized clinical trial (colorectal adenocarcinoma trial I). *Cancer* 1990; **65**: 425.

31. Wolmark N, Rockette H, Wickerham DL et al, Adjuvant therapy of Dukes' A, B, and C adenocarcinoma of the colon with portal-vein fluorouracil hepatic infusion: preliminary results of National Surgical Adjuvant Breast and Bowel Project Protocol C-02. *J Clin Oncol* 1990; **8**: 1466.

32. The Swiss Group for Clinical Cancer Research (SAKK), Laffer U, Metzger U, Aeberhard P et al, A single course of adjuvant intraportal chemotherapy for colorectal cancer: long-term results. *Lancet* 1995; **345**: 345

33. Beart RWJ, Moertel CG, Wieand HS et al, Adjuvant therapy for resectable colorectal carcinoma with fluorouracil administered by portal vein infusion. A study of the Mayo Clinic and the North Central Cancer Treatment Group. *Arch Surg* 1990; **125**: 897.

12

Guidelines for the safe administration of perioperative intraperitoneal chemotherapy

Arvil D Stephens, Susan K White, Paul H Sugarbaker

CONTENTS • Introduction • Methods and materials • Results • Conclusions

INTRODUCTION

Health care providers are subjected daily to occupational health risks such as exposure to hepatitis, HIV and tuberculosis, any infectious process, inadvertent inhalation of anesthetics, exposure to residual ethylene oxide, and exposure to radiation. Another current concern is exposure to cytotoxic agents. Because adjuvant chemotherapy for colon and rectal cancers has been accepted by the medical community, cytotoxic drugs are administered in a wide variety of medical settings. The infusion center is no longer the only site for administering chemotherapeutic drugs. Adjuvant chemotherapy has found its way into the operating room, the postanesthesia care unit, the surgical intensive care unit, the postsurgical ward and the private physician's office.

Questions have been raised regarding the long-term, low-dose exposure to cytotoxic agents and their cumulative effects on health care providers. Clinical research protocols are based on the understanding of the known toxicities of these drugs at therapeutic levels.[1,2] Conservative policies regarding occupational exposure have been implemented at the Washington Hospital Center, based on the possibility that some of

these toxic manifestations may present themselves with the low-dose chronic exposure. The paramount considerations of institutional policies should include protection of both the patient and health care providers.

Malignancies that present within the abdomino-pelvic cavity often cause their greatest morbidity and mortality through progressive involvement of the peritoneal surfaces.[3] Examples of this can be seen in patients with appendiceal cancer, ovarian cancer, colorectal cancer, gastric cancer, mesothelioma, and both retroperitoneal and visceral sarcoma. The most common sites for gastrointestinal cancer recurrence are the resection site and peritoneal surfaces.[3] These sites are involved not only by preoperative tumor dissemination, but also by intraoperative and perioperative dissemination of tumor. Treatments that maintain these patients disease-free at the resection site, and on peritoneal surfaces, should contribute to improvements in survival.

METHODS AND MATERIALS

The clinical pathway for treatment of peritoneal carcinomatosis from colorectal cancer at

Washington Hospital Center is presented in Figure 12.1. These treatments include adjuvant intraoperative, early postoperative and delayed postoperative chemotherapy. Chemotherapeutic drugs used in the operating room should be non-cell-cycle-dependent and possess a pharmacokinetic advantage when administered intraperitoneally, and their cytotoxicity should be enhanced when heated.[4] Mitomycin C is a chemotherapeutic drug that is commonly prescribed for colorectal malignancies. It inhibits DNA synthesis by alkylation of DNA strands, generation of free radicals and cross-linking of DNA strands, and by causing single-strand breaks in DNA.[1] The rationale for combining cytoreductive surgery and hyperthermic intraperitoneal chemotherapy are as follows:[4]

(1) to destroy residual cancer cells in the tumor bed or free cancer cells before postoperative changes in tumor cell kinetics occur and while tumor burden is minimal;

(2) to ensure favorable drug access to all surfaces at risk for recurrence before cancer cells are entrapped by wound healing or covered by surgical reconstructions;

(3) to provide dose-intensive, timely regional chemotherapy with a concentration of cytotoxic drug not achievable by intravenous administration;

(4) to minimize the possibility of toxicity by close monitoring of physiologic parameters;

(5) to administer a reasonable adjuvant treatment at minimal extra cost and without additional hospitalization.

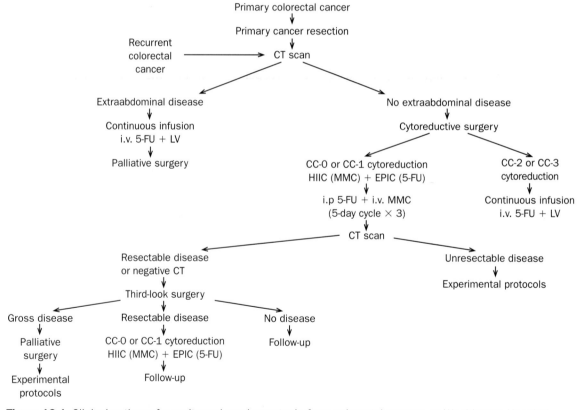

Figure 12.1 Clinical pathway for peritoneal carcinomatosis from colorectal cancers at Washington Hospital Center. *Abbreviations:* CT, computed tomography; i.v., intravenous; i.p., intraperitoneal; HIIC, hyperthermic intraoperative intraperitoneal chemotherapy; 5-FU, 5-fluorouracil; MMC, mitomycin C; LV, leucovorin; CC-0, completeness of cytoreduction – no macroscopic residual disease; CC-1, completeness of cytoreduction – residual disease < 2.5 mm in greatest diameter; CC-2, completeness of cytoreduction – residual disease 2.5–25 mm; CC-3, completeness of reduction – residual disease > 25 mm.

Cytoreductive surgery

Cytoreductive surgery is a combination of peri-toneal stripping procedures and resections that remove all macroscopic tumor from the abdom-inal cavity of patients with peritoneal carcino-matosis.[5,6] The intent is local control of disease in the peritoneal cavity. Cytoreductive surgery is composed of six different procedures:[5,6]

- omentectomy–splenectomy;
- left subdiaphragmatic peritonectomy;
- right subdiaphragmatic peritonectomy;
- pelvic peritonectomy–sigmoidectomy;
- cholecystectomy–lesser omentectomy;
- antrectomy.

Each has a definite en bloc resection that requires an orderly sequence of surgical maneuvers in order to create an optimum cytoreduction. The techniques have been described by Sugarbaker,[6] and have been applied to peritoneal carcinomatosis from lesions of low-grade malignancy, such as grade I mucinous adenocarcinoma or malignant pseudomyxoma peritonei. Cytoreductive surgery with hyperthermic intraoperative intraperitoneal chemotherapy (HIIC) may require as long as 10–14 hours in the operating room; therefore it is imperative for the peri-operative staff to be well trained and informed. At the Washington Hospital Center, a chemotherapy course is offered annually for in-house certification. The course is required for all nurses who work with cytotoxic agents.

The perioperative care of patients under-going cytoreductive surgery and early post-operative intraperitoneal chemotherapy has been described previously.[7] The potential chronic toxicities of mitomycin C include microangio-pathic hemolytic anemia, hemolytic–uremic syndrome and cumulative bone marrow sup-pression. The most important acute toxicity is renal toxicity. Adequate hydration is critical for patient safety. Large intravenous fluid chal-lenge, renal-dose dopamine or furosemide may be used to maintain urine output of at least 100 ml every 15 minutes during the intraopera-tive heated chemotherapy administration and for at least one hour thereafter.

Technique for intraoperative chemotherapy

Cytoreductive surgery is attempted to make each patient macroscopically disease-free.[6] At the end of the procedure, closed suction catheters are placed through the abdominal wall, using stab incisions, to lie beneath the right and left hemidiaphragms and within the pelvis (Figure 12.2). A curled intraperitoneal catheter is similarly placed in the abdominal cavity. The curled catheter is placed in the area at greatest risk for recurrence, and functions as an inflow line. The closed suction catheters are used as drainage lines. Two temperature probes are then placed over the edge of the abdominal incision. One temperature probe is secured to the inflow catheter. The other temperature probe is tied to a closed suction drain at a distant location from the inflow catheter. All transabdominal tubes are secured to the skin and to the peritoneum with purse string sutures to prevent fluid leakage. The abdomen is not closed; the skin edges are suspended from the Thompson retractor (Thompson Surgical Instruments, Traverse City, MI) with a number 2 running nylon suture. To prevent spillage of the chemotherapy and to con-trol potential chemotherapy vapors, a plastic sheet is sutured to the wound edges (Figure 12.3). A slit incision is then made in the center of the plastic sheet to allow the surgeon access to all intraabdominal surfaces and to manually con-trol the fluid distribution (Figure 12.4). The use of the Thompson retractor and a sterile plastic sheet is unique to our institution, and provides better drug distribution than closed abdominal techniques. After the hyperthermic perfusion is complete, any necessary reconstructive proce-dures are performed.

Early postoperative intraperitoneal chemotherapy

In addition to intraoperative hyperthermic per-fusion, all patients who have colorectal adeno-carcinoma or who have an incomplete cytoreduction receive five days of early postop-erative intraperitoneal chemotherapy with 5-fluorouracil.[4,5] These five days of chemotherapy

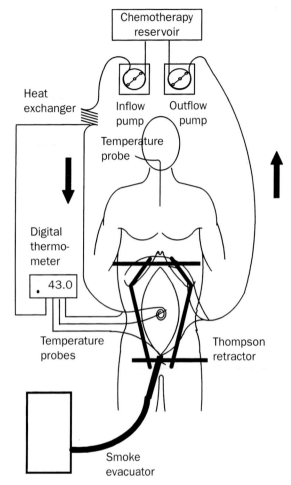

Figure 12.2 Hyperthermic intraoperative intraperitoneal chemotherapy administration. The equipment required for the intraoperative administration of hyperthermic chemotherapy includes three closed suction drains, a Tenckhoff catheter and two esophageal temperature probes. The abdominal wall is suspended from the Thompson retractor and covered with a sterile plastic sheet. The smoke evacuator is placed beneath one edge of the plastic sheet and run at a low rate during the perfusion. (Adapted, with permission, from Sugarbaker PH, Averbach AM, Jacquet P et al, A simplified approach to hyperthermic intraoperative intraperitoneal chemotherapy (HIIC) using a self-retaining retractor. In: *Peritoneal Carcinomatosis: Principles of Management* (Sugarbaker PH, ed). Boston: Kluwer, 1996; 415–21.)

are given on postoperative days 1–5. Each dose is prepared in 1000–2000 cm^3 of 1.5% dextrose peritoneal dialysis solution, depending on body surface area. Each dose is infused as quickly as possible (approximately 15–45 minutes) and allowed to dwell for 23 hours, then drained for 1 hour prior to the next infusion.

RESULTS

Safety considerations for chemotherapy administration

Blood and body fluids from patients receiving chemotherapy are considered contaminated for 48 hours after the last dose is administered.[8] The precautions described below should be applied to any patient who has received chemotherapy within 48 hours. Routes of exposure for health care providers include inhalation, contact, ingestion and injection. It is essential that certain equipment be available and appropriately utilized by personnel who come in contact with cytotoxic agents. This equipment includes impervious sterile gowns, protective eye wear, respirator mask (if a spill occurs), a spill kit, impenetrable hazardous waste containers, specially marked linen bags and appropriate cytotoxic agent labels. Unpowdered latex gloves should be worn when chemotherapy is administered. The powder used in the latex curing process tends to make the gloves more porous.

Three major advisory groups in the USA provide guidelines for the use of cytotoxic agents. Each institution in the USA that uses cytotoxic agents is expected to develop individual policies and procedures based on the principles of these guidelines. The major regulatory groups are the National Cancer Institute (NCI),[9] the Occupational Safety and Health Administration (OSHA)[8] and the Joint Commission on Accreditation of Health Care Organizations (JCAHO).[10] A summary of each group's guidelines is presented in Table 12.1; however, the complete references should be considered required reading for all personnel involved with cytotoxic agents.

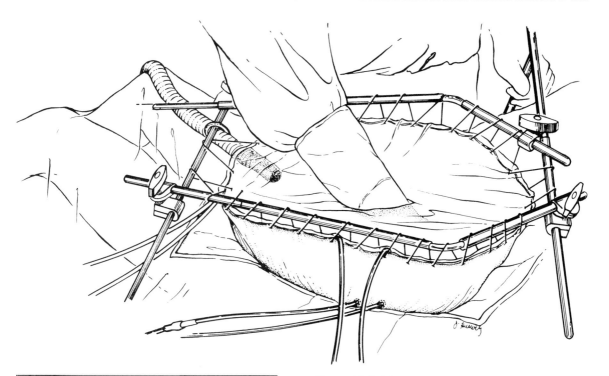

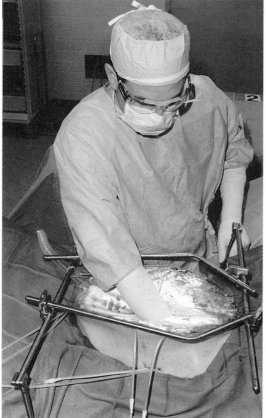

Figure 12.3 Midline abdominal incision suspended from Thompson retractor during HIIC. The abdominal incision is covered with a sterile plastic sheet during the HIIC administration. The edges of the incision are suspended from the Thompson retractor with a running number 2 nylon suture. The smoke evacuator is running continuously on a low setting.

Figure 12.4 Manipulation of the viscera during hyperthermic intraoperative intraperitoneal chemotherapy. Manipulation of the viscera during heated chemotherapy administration ensures adequate exposure of drug to all peritoneal surfaces, and distributes heat more homogeneously throughout the abdominal cavity. (From Sugarbaker PH, Ronnett BM, Archer A et al, Pseudomyxoma peritonei syndrome. *Adv Surg* 1996; **30**: 233–80, with permission.)

Table 12.1 Safety regulations pertaining to cytotoxic agents

National Cancer Institute (NCI)

1. Disposable surgical latex gloves are recommended for all procedures involving cytotoxic drugs. Polyvinyl chloride gloves should not be worn while handling cytotoxic agents.
2. Gloves should be routinely changed approximately every 30 minutes when working steadily with cytotoxic agents. Gloves should be changed immediately after overt contamination.
3. Double gloving is recommended for cleaning up of spills.
4. Protective barrier garments should be worn for all procedures involving the preparation, use and disposal of cytotoxic agents.
5. All potentially contaminated garments must not be worn outside the work area.

Occupational Safety and Health Administration (OSHA)

1. All personnel involved in handling cytotoxic drugs must receive orientation regarding techniques, procedures and policies.
2. The main routes of exposure are through inhalation of drug dust or droplets, absorption through the skin, and ingestion through contact with contaminated food and cigarettes.
3. Powderless surgical latex gloves should always be used. Double-gloving is recommended if it does not interfere with technique.
4. A protective disposable gown made of lint-free, low-permeability fabric with closed front, long sleeves and closed cuffs must be worn, with the cuffs tucked under gloves.
5. Surgical masks do not protect against breathing aerosols.

Joint Commission for the Accreditation of Health Care Organizations (JCAHO)

1. Nursing department personnel are prepared through appropriate education and training programs for their responsibilities in the provision of nursing care.
2. Written policies and procedures that reflect optimal standards of nursing care guide the provision of nursing care.
3. As part of the hospital's quality assurance program, the quality and appropriateness of the patient care provided by the nursing department are monitored and evaluated, and identified problems are resolved.

Routine clean-up of the patient care area is safe and effective if strict adherence to universal precautions is maintained. Any material in contact with chemotherapy should be separated from the standard trash or linen and placed in appropriate receptacles. At our institution, chemotherapy waste is stored on-site for 48 hours, then disposed by a licensed hazardous waste facility. All instruments that have come in contact with a patient's blood or body fluids should be labeled by the nursing staff with 'Cytotoxic Agent' prior to leaving the patient care area. All blood and pathology specimens obtained after the start of chemotherapy perfusion should also be labeled with 'Cytotoxic Agent'. Bactericidal solutions should not be used to clean contaminated items, because they may cause chemical reactions with the chemotherapy agent and they do not inactivate the chemotherapy.[8] OSHA recommends 70% isopropyl alcohol for clean-up. Seventy percent isopropyl alcohol is an effective solvent for chemotherapy agents, and does not contain additives that may interact with the chemotherapy.

Clean-up of chemotherapy spills should be directed by specific hospital policies and procedures that are based upon OSHA, JCAHO and NCI guidelines. All spills should be contained and cleaned up immediately by trained personnel. The procedures will be dictated by the size of the spill. If any personnel make direct contact with cytotoxic agents, they should immediately remove the contaminated apparel and discard in a hazardous waste container. The affected skin should be immediately washed with pure soap. Pure soap is recommended because it does not contain additives that may interact with the chemotherapy, i.e. dyes, perfumes, antibacterial agents, etc. If the eyes are affected, they should be immediately flooded with water or isotonic saline for five minutes. The personnel should then report to occupational health or to the emergency room. If only the clothing is contaminated, the article should be removed as soon as possible and placed in a cytotoxic linen bag.

Chemotherapy spill kits are commercially available, and should be readily available. A spill kit should include a respirator mask, goggles, powderless latex surgical gloves, an impervious gown, impervious shoe covers, at least two sheets of absorbent material, a small scoop and brush, 70% isopropyl alcohol and/or pure soap, 'Cytotoxic Agent' labels, a 'Caution' sign and large waste-disposal bags.

OSHA defines a small chemotherapy spill as less than 5 g or 5 ml of undiluted drug.[8] Personnel should wear impervious gowns, double powderless surgical latex gloves and eye protection when cleaning any chemotherapy spill. Liquids should be blotted dry with absorbent pads, and solid spills should be wiped with wet absorbent pads. The spill area will then be washed three times with 70% isopropyl alcohol or pure soap followed by clean water. After decontamination of the spill area, routine cleaning procedures may be used.

A large spill mandates the use of a spill kit, which should be readily available wherever chemotherapy is handled. Large spills should be immediately contained with absorbent pads, towels, etc. to prevent spreading. A respirator mask should be worn in addition to the standard protective clothing. Care must be taken to prevent the formation of aerosols. Access to the spill area should be restricted.

CONCLUSIONS

With the treatment regimen described in this clinical pathway, it is possible to administer a reasonable adjuvant treatment at minimal extra cost and without additional hospitalization days. The risks to personnel handling cytotoxic agents as part of this clinical pathway are a combined result of the amount of drugs used, the unique toxicity of each drug, and the extent to which personnel are directly exposed to the cytotoxic agents. The main routes of exposure are absorption through the skin, ingestion through contact with contaminated food or cigarettes, and the inhalation of drug dusts or droplets.

A renewed emphasis should be placed on the education and instruction of health care staff in the use and hazards of cytotoxic drugs. Formal courses for certification are recommended to ensure that all staff working with cytotoxic agents are adequately prepared. Specific detailed policies and procedures regarding the safe handling of these agents are an absolute must, and should be required reading by all staff on an annual basis. A starting point for each institution's policies and procedures should be the guidelines set forth by OSHA, JCAHO and the NCI.

Because the toxicities of low-level cumulative exposure are not well defined,[1] personnel who have specific medical concerns should be excluded from the chemotherapy environment. These include pregnant or breast-feeding women, men *or* women who are planning a family in the near future, personnel with known blood dyscrasias or who are immunocompromised, and personnel taking hematologically toxic medications. The NCI recommends that personnel involved with cytotoxic agents on a full-time basis be given periodic health examinations in accordance with institutional policy.[9]

REFERENCES

1. Harrison BR, Safe handling of cytotoxic drugs: a review. In: *The Chemotherapy Book* (Perry C, ed). Baltimore: Williams and Wilkins, 1992.
2. DeVita VT, Hellman S, Rosenberg SA (eds), *Principles and Practice of Oncology*, 3rd edn. Philadelphia: JB Lippincott, 1989.
3. Sugarbaker PH, Observations concerning cancer spread within the peritoneal cavity and concepts supporting an ordered pathophysiology. In: *Peritoneal Carcinomatosis: Diagnosis and Management* (Sugarbaker PH, ed). Boston: Kluwer, 1995.
4. Stephens AD, White SK, Brewer A et al, *Hyperthermic Intraoperative Intraperitoneal Chemotherapy: A Multidisciplinary Manual for Operating Room Staff*. Washington, DC: Washington Hospital Center Press, 1995.
5. Sugarbaker PH, *Intraperitoneal Chemotherapy and Cytoreductive Surgery: A Manual for Physicians and Nurses*. Grand Rapids, MI: The Ludann Company, 1993.
6. Sugarbaker PH, Peritonectomy procedures. *Ann Surg* 1995; **221:** 29–42.
7. Hallenbeck P, Sanniez CK, Ryan AB et al, Cytoreductive surgery and intraperitoneal chemotherapy. *AORN J* 1992; **56:** 50–72.
8. OSHA Work-practice guidelines for personnel dealing with cytotoxic (antineoplastic) drugs. *Am J Hosp Pharm* 1986; **43:** 1193–204.
9. National Study Commission on Cytotoxic Exposure, *Recommendations for Handling Cytotoxic Agents*, 1984.
10. Joint Commission on Accreditation of Health Care Organizations, *Accreditation Manual for Hospitals*, 1989.

13

Preoperative treatment of rectal cancer

Lars Påhlman

INTRODUCTION

The rationale for using preoperative radiotherapy, sometimes in combination with chemotherapy, in the management of primary rectal cancer is twofold. In patients with a mobile (resectable) rectal cancer, the objective is to eradicate micrometastases outside the surgical plane of dissection. With such an approach, the local recurrence rates will decrease, and this reduction would have an impact on overall survival. However, if the tumour is fixed (non-resectable), the rationale for preoperative treatment is to convert the tumour to a resectable one.

This chapter discusses the role of combining preoperative radiotherapy, chemotherapy and surgery in the treatment of rectal cancer. The two main treatment modalities, namely the supportive treatment in non-resectable rectal cancer and the role of adjuvant treatment in resectable tumours, will be discussed.

WHY RADIOTHERAPY IN THE MANAGEMENT OF RECTAL CANCER?

Surgery is the mainstay in the treatment of rectal cancer. However, after surgical resection of a rectal cancer, local failure is common. The exact proportion of patients who develop a clinically relevant local recurrence has varied considerably. Figures from less than 5% to more than 50% has been reported.[1-10] Definition of radicality, follow-up routines, definition of local failure, the skill of the surgeons and the selection of patients are probably important factors that might explain these discrepancies. The local recurrence rate has always exceeded 20% in the surgery-alone group in all reported controlled randomized trials during the last two decades in which radiotherapy (pre- or postoperative) has been compared with surgery alone (see Table 13.3 below). The recurrence rate most often exceeds 30%, a figure that probably represents the results in standard surgery for rectal cancer worldwide. The low figures reported from institutional series are most likely due to devoted and well-trained surgeons.[9,11,12] Sometimes more radical procedures have been used, with a clear risk of increased morbidity regarding sexual and bladder function.[12,13]

Since radiotherapy rarely fails at the periphery of the tumour, where the number of tumour cells is limited and the area is well vascularized and well-oxygenated cells are present, and surgery is often restricted to preserve normal tissues adjacent to the tumour, it is obvious to combine the two modalities. The radiation doses that can safely be given to the extrarectal areas at risk of containing tumour deposits not easily removed by surgery are sufficient to kill microscopic foci of tumour cells, at most a few millimetres in size, with high probability. Since the mechanism of failure is different for the two techniques, a combination of surgery and radiotherapy would seem highly rational. Whether or not chemotherapy should be added is not clear, and the scientific basis for such a regimen is not obvious.

A local recurrence has to be prevented, since the possibility of having a second curative procedure for local recurrence is less than 5% in unselected patient material.[14,15] The unacceptably high local failure rate after standardized surgery for rectal cancer, together with the high morbidity associated with most local failures, indicates that there is a need for improvements in surgery, additional treatment, or both.

PATIENT SELECTION

It is important to evaluate resectability preoperatively on clinical grounds, which can sometimes be difficult. If questions arise regarding resectability, an examination under anaesthetic will often facilitate this assessment regarding fixity. Other staging procedures, such as endorectal ultrasonography, computed tomography and magnetic resonance imaging, may also facilitate this assessment. Despite these modern technical staging procedures, the most important part is clinical judgement, including digital rectal examination.[16]

In patients with a resectable tumour, radiotherapy is aimed at eradicating suspicious microscopic populations of tumour cells that cannot be excised without a major risk of postoperative complications. If the tumour is considered non-resectable, for example a fixed tumour where it is likely that the tumour cannot be resected radically because of tumour overgrowth to adjacent non-resectable organs, the rationale for giving the patient radiotherapy is to achieve shrinkage of the tumour and consequent downstaging.

TARGET VOLUME

The lateral lymph nodes close to the pelvic wall, which are not always excised during surgery, and the lymph nodes along the internal iliac artery are common areas of recurrences, as are the areas of the posterior parts of the bladder, prostate or vagina.[3,15] That is why the entire dorsal part of the pelvic cavity should be included in the target volume, indicating that the posterior region of the prostrate or the posterior of the vaginal wall and the posterior part of the urinary bladder must constitute the anterior delineation of the target. Laterally the margins have to extend to the bony pelvis, and dorsally the target must reach the anterior part of the sacrum. A more difficult question is the extent of the target caudally and cranially.

Caudally, the question may be raised as to whether or not the anal region including the sphincter should be in the target. In very low-growing tumours close to the anal canal, the sphincter must be included. However, if an anterior resection is planned, it might be advisable not to include the sphincter in the irradiation target, since there are some reports indicating that bowel function might be impaired after adjuvant radiotherapy. Theoretically, irradiation might damage the sphincter.[17,18] Moreover, rectal cancer rarely has an intramural distal growth of more than a few millimetres.[19,20] Distally located lymph node metastases in the mesorectum can, however, be located more than 2 cm distal to the lower tumour margin, indicating that the lower border of the target should not be higher than the mesorectum or about 4 cm from the anal verge.[21,22]

Cranially, it can be questioned whether to enlarge the target to the lymph nodes along the proximal part of the inferior mesenteric artery. In most patients, tumour cells within these nodes indicate disseminated disease, and even if these cells are eradicated, the chance of cure is almost nil or less than 2%.[23,24] In several trials these lymph nodes have been included (see below), to prevent local failure and improve survival, but we have learned from these studies that much of the morbidity associated with adjuvant radiotherapy can be ascribed to irradiation of tissues above the pelvic cavity.[25,26]

DOSE LEVEL

The radiation effect within the irradiated volume is mainly dependent upon the number of tumour cells to be killed and the sensitivity of the surrounding tissues. To be able to eradicate macroscopic deposits, i.e. deposits more than 1 cm in diameter or about 10^9 cells, a dose of at least 60–70 gray (Gy) given in 6–7 weeks is necessary. Such a dose will also damage the surrounding normal tissue. On the other hand, the minimum dose required to kill micrometastases (less than a few millimetres in diameter, at most 10^8 cells) with a high probability is about 50 Gy given in 5 weeks.[27,28] There is also evidence to indicate that a higher dose (60–70 Gy) is required postoperatively to achieve similar effects on micrometastases due to repopulation of tumour cells in the time interval between surgery and the start of radiotherapy,[27,28] or due to the hypoxic state of tumour cells in the surgical bed.[29]

In this chapter a comparison is made of different regimens in a number of trials. Since the radiation effect depends not only on the total dose but also on the dose at each fraction and the overall treatment time, the biological effect of the irradiation has been estimated using the linear–quadratic (LQ) formula with a time correction factor for immediate effects,[30] and the cumulative irradiation effect (CRE),[31] with corrections for late effects.[32] In the LQ-time estimations, the common linear–quadratic quotient α/β was chosen as 10 Gy for tumour and immediate effects and 3 Gy for late effects, the repair ratio α/γ as 0.6 Gy/day and the initial delay time T_K as 7 days.[30]

To achieve a dose of 50 Gy with conventional fractionation (1.8–2 Gy daily), i.e. the minimum dose required to kill micrometastases with high probability, patients have to be treated for 5 weeks. This treatment time can be reduced if the dose at each fraction is increased to 5 Gy. According to both the CRE concept and the LQ formula, 5×5 Gy during one week, i.e. a total dose of 25 Gy, corresponds approximately to the effect attained when conventional irradiation to 40–50 Gy is given.

NON-RESECTABLE RECTAL CANCER

In most unselected patient material, 10–15% of all rectal carcinomas are fixed to the surrounding tissues. This fixity often makes the tumour locally non-resectable, owing to extensive infiltration of organs that cannot be removed surgically without severely disabling the patient. Moreover, only 50% in this group of patients have distant metastases at the time of diagnosis.[33–35] Untreated, this subgroup of patients has a median survival time of 6–8 months, often with severe symptoms such as pain, haemorrhage, faecal incontinence, and urinary or vaginal problems.

With preoperative radiotherapy, a locally extensive tumour considered to be inoperable at presentation can be converted to an operable one. Conversion rates to resectability have been achieved in 35% to over 75% of cases,[36–41] but the local treatment failure rate despite optimal preoperative radiotherapy is often high (about 50%) among resected patients, indicating the enormous challenge with this patient category. However, a proportion of patients have been cured.

Fixity to another organ has almost always been evaluated by palpation or during sigmoidoscopy. This assessment is uncertain even in experienced hands, since it is difficult to decide whether there actually is tumour overgrowth or only extensive fibrosis adjacent to the tumour.[16,34] The most appropriate way to evaluate non-resectability is of course to verify this by a laparotomy before radiotherapy, as has been done in some of the above-mentioned studies, which might be one explanation for the wide range of resectability reported. In cases where the fixation ultimately turns out to be the result of tumour infiltration, radiotherapy is essential. It has been shown by magnetic resonance imaging – at least in a high proportion of cases – that it can be seen whether fixation is a result of tumour infiltration or of fibrosis.[42]

External irradiation

High-dose, short-term irradiation (dose fractions >2 Gy) used in many adjuvant settings has no place in the group of patients with non-resectable tumours, since down-staging is essential and never occurs rapidly. Therefore conventional irradiation with 1.8–2 Gy fractions is ideal. Such a prolonged course of preoperative radiotherapy to a dose of 45–50 Gy can be delivered without any substantial risk to the patient. The results from major reported trials are given in Table 13.1. The great discrepancies in resectability rates are probably due to differences in surgical aggressiveness in combination with the criteria for non-resectability and different radiotherapy doses and techniques.[33,36,38,40,41,43,44] The most commonly used dose has been between 40 and 50 Gy. To allow further tumour regression, surgery has usually been performed 3–4 weeks later. The optimal irradiation dose has not, however, been estab-

lished. In a small non-randomized study the local control rate was 67% after 40 Gy and 91% after 50 Gy, giving some indications – but no firm conclusions can be drawn, because of the small number of patients.[35] According to the above discussion, a dose to 60–70 Gy is needed to have an impact on macroscopic disease, but with such a high dose the risk of damaging normal tissue within the target is substantial.

Combinations of radiotherapy and chemotherapy should theoretically give improvement, since the cell-killing mechanisms differ between the two techniques and synergistic effects may occur. The rationale for combining these two treatments is the different mechanism of effect: chemotherapy on systemic disease, and radiotherapy on local disease. However, it could be that the combined treatment will have an improved effect on local disease, by achieving a therapeutic gain with an increased effect on tumours without simultaneously enhancing important normal tissue reactions.[45,46] The exact knowledge of how to combine these two regimens and whether or not this is necessary in a preoperative setting is limited at present owing to a lack of randomized trials, since the simultaneous use can lead to a potential risk of more severe adverse effects. This was also found in a

Table 13.1 Resectability rates after preoperative radiotherapy in patients with locally non-resectable rectal cancer

Study	Dose (Gy)	CRE value	LQ time (Gy)	Additional chemotherapy	Number of patients	Resectable after irradiation	
						Number	%
Rotterdam[44]	34.5	13.0	35.2	Yes	25	40	40
Uppsala[38]	40	14.0	36.0	Yes	21	16	76
Bergen[33]	45	14.5	36.9	No	37	16	43
Mayo[36]	40–45	14.0–14.5	36.0–39.8	No	25	18	72
Odense[43]	23–73	11.0–17.8	24–50	Yes	18	3	17
Uppsala[41]	46–60	14.8–17.6	40.8–47.4	No	44	17	39
New York[40]	50.4	15.7	43.8	Yes	20	17	85

Dutch trial using preoperative chemo-radio-therapy, where more adverse effects occurred in the postoperative phase after combined treatment.[44] A Danish trial had to be halted because of adverse effects in the combined arm.[43] It has still not been determined whether the use of different cytostatic regimens, particularly those based on 5-FU, concomitantly with irradiation will produce greater tumour shrinkage than irradiation alone, as has been claimed.[45,46] In several non-randomized comparisons with radiotherapy alone versus chemo-radiotherapy, the initial results indicate a better effect on the local tumour burden if the combined treatment is used,[40,42] but with a substantially increased morbidity with combined treatment.[42,44] The concept has been studied in two randomized trials, but the combined treatment was not superior when compared with radiotherapy alone.[43,47] Thus today it may be said that scientific evidence for superiority of the combined approach is virtually lacking. Nevertheless, combined therapy is considered to be the standard at several centres, particularly in the USA.[40,47]

Intraoperative irradiation

To improve treatment results even further in patients with non-respectable tumours, the use of intraoperative irradiation with electrons alone or – more often – in combination with external irradiation has been suggested. The rationale for using intraoperative radiotherapy is the possibility of delivering a high dose to a small tumour-containing volume without damaging surrounding tissues. It is a tempting alternative, but experience is still very limited, although it has been available at several centres for more than a decade. However, no firm conclusions can yet be drawn owing to a lack of properly performed randomized trials. Since facilities for intraoperative treatment are expensive and the treatment is time-consuming and still only available in a few centres in each country, there is an urgent need for randomized trials to compare preoperative external beam therapy with intraoperative radiotherapy

in addition to preoperative external radiotherapy.

Summary: radiotherapy in non-resectable rectal cancer

With the assumption that a fixed tumour must be at least at a locally advanced stage, i.e. a Dukes stage B or C cancer, patients with such cancer will run a high risk of local failure even if the tumour can be resected for cure. These patients will therefore probably benefit from preoperative irradiation – and this is definitely true in cases where the fixation proves to be the result of tumour infiltration. A prolonged course of preoperative radiotherapy with the aim of producing tumour shrinkage should be used in this group of patients to doses of 45–50 Gy or even higher without any substantial risk to the patient. Still the question of whether or not irradiation should be combined with chemotherapy has to be answered with properly designed randomized trials. Also, the use intraoperative radiotherapy must be questioned, in view of the lack of results from randomized clinical trials.

RESECTABLE RECTAL CANCER

Radiotherapy is an attractive alternative in patients with resectable rectal cancer, since it can easily be delivered to a defined tissue volume with negligible damage to both non-irradiated and irradiated tissues. The timing of treatment, i.e. pre- or postoperative, has been discussed extensively, and both pros and cons are more or less obvious, as given in Table 13.2. As will be illustrated in this chapter, most data from the literature support the idea that preoperative treatment is more dose-efficient than postoperative irradiation.

Local recurrence rates

To kill micrometastases, a dose corresponding to a CRE value of about 14.5 (LQ time$_{acute}$ about

Table 13.2 Advantages and disadvantages of pre- and postoperative irradiation

	Preoperative irradiation	Postoperative irradiation
Dukes A lesions excluded	No	Yes
Patients with distant metastases can be excluded	No	Yes
Influence on wound healing	Yes	No
Delay in administering irradiation due to wound healing	No	Yes
Surgery delayed	Yes	No
Hypoxic cells in the periphery of the tumours at irradiation – reducing radiosensitivity	No	Yes
Tumour cell repopulation	No	Yes
Reduced circulating viable tumour cells at surgery	Yes	No
Reduction of local tumour, increasing resectability	Yes	No
With postoperative adhesions, small bowel may be at greater risk	No	Yes

40 Gy) is required to have an effect with a high probability of killing micrometastases. Subsequently no effects on local recurrence rates have been demonstrated in trials where considerably lower doses (CRE <11, LQ time <25 Gy) have been used, and only marginally (10%) effects on local recurrence rates have been found when the dose has been slightly higher.

Table 13.3 summarizes all controlled trials reported so far using pre- or postoperative radiotherapy, and the trials are compiled with regard to the LQ formula. The reduction in local recurrence rate at a given dose was lower in the trials where postoperative irradiation was given, but, despite a lower dose, a better reduction in the local failure rates has been demonstrated with preoperative irradiation. Moreover, a clear dose–response relationship concerning reduction in local recurrence rates is obvious.

With conventional fractionation using pre-operative irradiation to a moderate dose (CRE 11.1–13.0, LQ time 26–8.35.2 Gy), a reduction in the local recurrence rate has been demonstra-ted.[52,55] In the four trials where 5-Gy fractions were given 3–5 times a week,[50,54,56,57] a clear

Table 13.3 Pelvic recurrence after a combination of surgery and radiotherapy in rectal carcinoma (controlled trials with a surgery-alone group)

Study	Irradiation Dose (Gy)/ number of fractions	CRE value	LQ time (Gy)	Surgery alone: number of local recurrences/total (%)		Surgery + radiotherapy: number of local recurrences/total (%)		p value[a]	Percentage reduction in local failure rates
Preoperative									
Toronto[48]	5/1	5.0	7.5	b					
MRC 1[49]	5/1	5.0	7.5	c					
	20/10	8.7	20.4	c					
St Mark's[50]	15/3	9.7	22.5	51/210	(24)	31/185	(17)	NS	29
VASOG II[51]	31.5/18	11.1	26.8	b					
Bergen[52]	31.5/18	11.1	26.8	31/131	(24)	24/138	(17)	NS	29
VASOG I[53]	25/10	10.8	27.5	32/87	(37)	27/93	(22)	NS	22
North-West[54]	20/4	12.3	30.0	58/141	(41)	26/143	(18)	**	63
EORTC[55]	34.5/15	13.0	35.2	49/175	(28)	24/166	(14)	**	50
MRC2[d,e]	40/20	13.6	36.0	50/132	(38)	41/129	(32)	NS	16
SRCSG[56]	25/5	13.9	37.5	120/485	(28)	61/424	(14)	**	50
SRCT[57]	25/5	13.9	37.5	131/557	(24)	51/553	(9)	***	63
Postoperative									
Odense[58]	50/25	14.9	35.4	57/250	(23)	46/244	(19)	NS	17
MRC3[d]	40/20	13.6	36.0	69/235	(29)	46/234	(20)	**	31
GITSG[59]	40–48/22	13.6	36.0	27/106	(25)	15/96	(16)	NS	36
NSABP[60]	46.5/26	14.9	39.3	45/184	(24)	30/184	(16)	NS	33
EORTC[f]	46/23	14.9	40.8	30/88	(34)	25/84	(30)	NS	13
Rotterdam[61]	50/25	15.7	43.8	28/84	(33)	21/88	(24)	NS	41

[a] NS, $p > 0.05$; **, $p < 0.01$; ***, $p < 0.001$.
[b] Not reported.
[c] Only actuarial data reported, with no difference between groups.
[d] Only tethered rumours.
[e] MRC Trial Office, personal communication.
[f] EORTC Trial Office, personal communication.

dose–response relationship is observed. According to the effect on the local recurrence rates, the dose must at least exceed 4×5 Gy[54] or preferably 5×5 Gy.[56,57] In the largest trial (the Swedish Rectal Cancer Trial) a relative reduction in the local recurrence rate of 61% was present.[57]

As illustrated in Table 13.3, postoperative radiotherapy has less good effect on local recurrence rates than preoperative irradiation, despite the dose being 15–20 Gy higher when given postoperatively. Even if the postoperative dose was 50 Gy (CRE 14.9, LQ time 35.4 Gy) as in the Danish trial, no significant reduction in the local recurrence rate was found.[58] This was also true for the two American trials,[59,60] but if postoperative radiotherapy was combined with chemotherapy (see below), a more pronounced effect was noticed on the local failure rates. Only one trial using postoperative radiotherapy has shown a significant reduction in the local recurrence rates – the MRC3 trial, in which 40 Gy was given in 4 weeks (MRC Trial Office, British Medical Research Council, personal communication). In a Dutch trial from Rotterdam (50 Gy in 25 fractions), a tendency towards a reduced local recurrence rate was found in the irradiated group.[45]

The question whether or not preoperative radiotherapy is superior to postoperative has been addressed in only one trial – the Uppsala trial in Sweden, where patients were randomly allocated to preoperative or to postoperative radiotherapy.[62,63] In the preoperative group a total of 25.5 Gy was given during five fractions of 5.1 Gy daily over a 5–7-day period (CRE 14.0, LQ time 38.0 Gy). Surgery was performed early in the following week. Only patients with a tumour in Dukes stage B or C and allocated to the postoperative irradiation group received the radiotherapy. The postoperative treatment was planned to start within 6 weeks. Irradiation was given with 2 Gy fractions daily, 5 days a week in 4–5 weeks. After 40 Gy, a split of 10–14 days was planned; further irradiation was given for a period of 2 weeks, up to a total dose of 60 Gy (CRE 16.9, LQ time 46.9 Gy). This is the highest dose ever used as an adjuvant postoperative treatment, but, despite this, a statistically significantly reduced local recurrence rate after a minimum of 5 years' follow-up was found in the preoperatively irradiated group (12%) compared with the postoperative group (21%) ($p < 0.02$).[62]

To summarize, preoperative irradiation is more dose-effective than postoperative. Two possible explanations for the higher efficacy of preoperative radiotherapy are the repopulation of cells after surgery (the cells to be killed are simply more numerous after than before surgery), and/or that the cells to be killed in the infiltrating zones may be better oxygenated before surgery.

Influence on survival

Radiotherapy alone

Obviously, radiotherapy to the primary tumour cannot affect occult distant metastases in the liver and lung, which are the most commonly sites for recurrent disease. However, local recurrences can be reduced, and since such a failure is the only sign of a residual tumour in at least 20% of all patients resected for cure, the radiotherapy will have an impact on survival after prolonged follow-up. In a meta-analysis including all controlled trials published up to 1984, a slight improvement of survival by 4.3% was noted in the irradiated group of patients.[64] However, the more recently published trials using moderate to high doses were not included, namely the North-West trial in England,[54] the trial from the Imperial Cancer Research Fund in England,[50] and the Swedish Rectal Cancer Trial.[57] The latter trial was designed large enough to detect a survival benefit of 10%. After a minimum of 5 years follow-up, a statistically significantly overall survival benefit (48% versus 58%) was found if one-week preoperative radiotherapy (5×5 Gy) was used (Swedish Rectal Cancer Trial office, personal communication). In the trials where postoperative radiotherapy alone has been used, no effect on survival has been demonstrated.[58,61] In the only trial where preoperative radiotherapy has been tested against postoperative – the Uppsala trial – no survival difference between the two treatment groups was found.[62]

Combination with chemotherapy

As discussed above for non-resectable rectal cancer, a chemo-radiotherapy approach might have a better effect. Since the effects on local recurrence rates appear to be slightly improved when chemotherapy is combined with postoperative radiotherapy, survival will, theoretically, be improved. This modality has been used extensively in the USA, and in the GITSG trial survival was improved in the group of patients who received both radiotherapy and chemotherapy.[59] In a second American trial (NSABP) postoperative radiotherapy combined with chemotherapy was found to improve survival when compared with surgery alone.[60] The chemotherapeutic drugs used in these two trials were 5-FU and methyl-CCNU. In a third American randomized trial, the North Central Cancer Treatment Group (NCCTG), postoperative radiotherapy alone was compared with postoperative radiotherapy plus chemotherapy. As in the other two trials from the USA, 5-FU and methyl-CCNU were used. Improved survival was noted among the patients receiving radio-chemotherapy.[65] On the basis of the results in these three American trials, the consensus conference sponsored by the National Institute of Health in the USA recommended that standard treatment for patients with a tumour in Dukes stage B and C should be postoperative adjuvant radiotherapy (45–50 Gy in 4–6 weeks) together with chemotherapy.[66] In two subsequent trials performed by GITSG and NCCTG, it has been shown that the addition of methyl-CCNU to 5-FU is not required.[67,68] Moreover, in a not yet published Norwegian controlled randomized trial in which 46 Gy (CRE 14.9, LQ time 39.3 Gy) combined with 5-FU reduced the local recurrence rates by 50%, and this reduction had an impact on overall survival (Tveit et al, personal communication).

This survival benefit with the combined approach is not obvious. It is possible that the survival benefit can be ascribed more or less solely to a chemotherapy effect, since patients allocated to the radio-chemotherapy arm continued chemotherapy for one year in some trials. However, the survival improvements observed in the Swedish Rectal Cancer Trial are of the same magnitude as those reported from the American postoperative combined radio-chemotherapy trials. Since preoperative radiotherapy is more dose-effective than postoperative, it seems logical to give patients preoperative radiotherapy and to add chemotherapy postoperatively in those with more advanced cancer, i.e. tumours in Dukes stages B and C.

Is adjuvant radiotherapy safe?

The main concern when preoperative irradiation is used is the risk of overtreatment. This is the case for patients with a tumour in Dukes stage A, and patients with disseminated disease found at surgery. Although it is possible to identify Dukes A lesions with preoperative endoluminal ultrasound of the rectum, it is important to reduce morbidity as much as possible.

Postoperative mortality

Preoperative, but not postoperative, radiotherapy may have an impact on postoperative recovery. In two trials increased postoperative mortality has been noticed after preoperative irradiation.[50,56] In the Stockholm–Malmö trial the mortality was 8% in the irradiated group and 2% in the surgery-alone group.[56] In the other trial, from St Mark's Hospital, a similar finding was noted, namely an increased postoperative mortality among elderly patients (>75 years of age) and in those with generalized disease discovered at surgery.[50]

In the two trials reporting increased postoperative mortality, the irradiation was given with one dorsal and one frontal field. Large volumes of the abdomen were then unnecessarily irradiated. In the Uppsala trial, where the same dose was used as in the Stockholm–Malmö trial, the irradiation technique was designed to avoid irradiation of those parts of the pelvis and abdomen that were not included in the target volume. No increased postoperative mortality was noted, even though no upper age limit was used, thus establishing that preoperative radiotherapy with a high dose (25.5 Gy in one week, giving a CRE of 14.5 and an LQ time of 38 Gy) can be delivered without affecting postoperative mortality.[62] It may be speculated that the differences in techniques between the two Swedish trials are responsible for the differences in postoperative mortality.[26] This difference between the two Swedish trials was one reason why the Swedish Rectal Cancer Trial (5 × 5 Gy in one week) was undertaken, and postoperative mortality was one of the end points. According to the protocol, the use of three or four portals was mandatory, but in four hospitals the two-portal technique was used. In that group of patients the mortality was significantly increased compared with that in patients treated according to the protocol with a three- or four-portal technique,[69] but the most important finding was that the mortality in the surgery-alone arm and among the patients irradiated with a three- or four-portal technique was exactly the same (2.6% versus 2.6%). These data indicate that it is possible to give preoperative high-dose, short-course radiotherapy without increasing postoperative mortality.

Postoperative morbidity

A common complication of rectal cancer surgery is wound infection. In most trials in which preoperative radiotherapy is used, the risk of having a perineal wound infection after an abdominoperineal excision is increased from 10% to 20%.[62,69,70] This is still a relative low incidence in the light of the fact that all patients had a perineal sinus earlier due to surgical considerations. Twenty years ago, the perineal wound was left open for secondary healing, and a perineal wound will heal within one or two months in most patients.[62] A rare but very uncommon complication, a perineal sinus, is not more common if radiotherapy has been given.[63] No increase in other infectious complications of, for example, the abdominal wound, pulmonary tract or urinary tract has been seen in controlled trials after preoperative irradiation.

Preoperative radiotherapy might have an impact on anastomotic healing, but experimental data has not shown this,[71] and subsequently no increase in anastomotic dehiscence has been found after preoperative radiotherapy in all controlled randomized trials.[50,55,62,69,70]

The experience with conventional fractionation is well known. However, the short-course, high-dose radiotherapy used preferentially in the Swedish trials should be considered further, mainly because of unexpected complications. One such complication is that found in the Uppsala trial, where preoperative irradiation of 25.5 Gy (5×5.1 Gy) was used. Acute neurogenic pain in the lower lumbar region has been reported a few hours after irradiation.[62] This pain was usually of short duration, but could persist in some patients for several months, and in some of the affected patients these acute neurogenic symptoms have led to an inability to walk. The exact magnitude of this rather unexpected finding has been reviewed in Uppsala. Out of a total of 550 patients treated with 5×5 Gy within prospective protocols from 1980 to 1994, 19 (3%), reported pain, and in 6 patients (1%) the pain lasted for more than a few days. Four of the six patients with prolonged postoperative pain developed subacute neurogenic symptoms. No technical or human error in the treatment employed could be found, but it is more common in women than in men and appeared to be more common in obese patients and in patients with diabetes or previous neurological disorders.[26]

Tolerance to treatment

The most important issue to discuss is compliance. Depending upon this factor, the tolerance can be evaluated. Preoperative treatment has, by definition, more or less 100% compliance, whereas postoperative irradiation has less, mainly because of the prolonged postoperative course but also because of radiotherapy complications. In the Uppsala trial, where the acute adverse effects of pre- and postoperative radiotherapy were studied prospectively, it was found that preoperative treatment was well tolerated and that the compliance was 99.6% (only one of the patients who were allocated to preoperative irradiation did not receive the treatment). In contrast, postoperative irradiation was completed without any complications in only 9% of the patients. Similar data have recently been reported from the AXIS trial in the UK, where the compliance in the preoperative arm was 96% compared with 58% in the postoperatively treated group of patients (AXIS trial centre, personal communication). Difficulties of the same magnitude were reported from the Danish trial using postoperative radiotherapy, where only 85% of the patients who started postoperative irradiation completed the treatment.[42]

If postoperative chemo-radiotherapy is used, acute toxicity is even more pronounced. Most trials report an increased risk of dermatitis in the irradiated area, and several patients have had diarrhoea. Chemotherapy-dependent side-effects such as leucopenia occur in approximately 10% of patients.[59,60]

Late adverse effects

The most commonly studied late morbidity is intestinal obstruction and changed bowel habits like chronic diarrhoea. Available data from the literature indicate that such complications are not more common after preoperative radiotherapy than after surgery alone,[63,72] whereas after postoperative radiotherapy they are significantly more common, mainly owing to irradiation of fixed small-bowel loops in the pelvis.[58,62] When postoperative radiotherapy has been given, several techniques have been used to prevent the small bowel from falling down into the lesser pelvis.

Other complications one might expect after pelvic irradiation should come from areas within the target. In the Uppsala trial all patients have been followed up extensively and re-examined with respect to late adverse effects of irradiation, but no other possible late adverse effects compared with those having surgery alone was found.[63] A similar follow-up has been carried out in the Stockholm trial.[72] In that trial a slightly increased risk of venous thromboembolism, femoral neck or pelvis fractures, and fistulas was found. The risk of late small-bowel obstruction was clearly correlated with the size of the target. Another concern after adjuvant radiotherapy is sphincter function. After postoperative radiotherapy, this might be impaired,[17] and preliminary data from Uppsala indicate that preoperative radiotherapy also alters sphincter function,[18] which has recently been confirmed in a questionnaire study from the Swedish Rectal Cancer Trial (manuscript in preparation).

Summary: adjuvant radiotherapy in resectable cancer

All data from the collected international experience indicate that if radiotherapy is to be used, preoperative treatment is to be preferred, since it is more dose-effective. With the use of this preoperative approach, there are some concerns about irradiating patients with Dukes A lesions and patients with metastatic disease. However, with modern imaging techniques, these two patient categories can easily be identified by endoluminal ultrasonography, and/or computed tomography of the liver and lung, or ultrasonography of the liver combined with pulmonary X-ray examination.

In conclusion, preoperative radiotherapy has been convincingly shown to reduce local failure rates by more than 50%. This statement is true for 'standard' surgery. Since more 'optimized' surgery, as compared with so-called standard surgery, might decrease local failure rates,[9,11,12] it can be argued whether or not adjuvant radiotherapy is superfluous. This question is specifically addressed in a recently started Dutch trial, where 'optimized' surgery is mandatory, but the patients are randomly allocated to preoperative (5×5 Gy) radiotherapy or not.

CONCLUSIONS AND FUTURE PROSPECTS

In an adjuvant setting, i.e. in patients with primarily resectable rectal cancer, preoperative radiotherapy is more dose-effective than postoperative irradiation. Moreover, the latter is more resource-demanding than preoperative schedules have been, and therefore preoperative radiotherapy should be recommended. An important question to solve is which type of fractionation schedule should be used – short-term, high-dose preoperative irradiation ($4–5 \times 5$ Gy) or a more conventional fractionation. Another question is whether or not it is necessary to integrate chemotherapy in order to improve the surgical results further. With good surgery and preoperative radiotherapy, it is likely that local rectal cancer failure could more or less be eradicated. Other important aspects of adjuvant radiotherapy are compliance and economic considerations. Again, data from the literature support the use of preoperative radiotherapy. In particular, short preoperative schedules have proved effective and safe provided that the techniques are appropriate, and must therefore be more cost-effective than postoperative courses.

In patients with fixed tumours and where resectability can be discussed, preoperative prolonged radiotherapy is mandatory. The use of chemotherapy in combination with radiotherapy has not yet been settled, and results from ongoing randomized trials are awaited.

REFERENCES

1. Morson BC, Bussey HJR, Surgical pathology of rectal cancer in relation to adjuvant radiotherapy. *Br J Radiol* 1967; **40**: 161–5.

2. Berge T, Ekelund G, Mellner C et al, Carcinoma of the colon and rectum in a defined population. *Acta Chir Scand* 1973; (Suppl 438): 174.

3. Gunderson LL, Sosin H, Areas of failure found at reoperation (second or symptomatic look) following 'curative surgery' for adenocarcinoma of the rectum. *Cancer* 1974; **34**: 1278–92.

4. Pheils MT, Chapuis PH, Newland RC, Colquhoun M, Local recurrence following curative resection for carcinoma of the rectum. *Dis Colon Rectum* 1983; **26**: 98–102.

5. Påhlman L, Glimelius B, Local recurrences after surgical treatment for rectal carcinoma. *Acta Chir Scand* 1984; **150**: 331–5.

6. Phillips RKS, Hittinger R, Blesovsky L et al, Local recurrence following 'curative' surgery for large bowel cancer. I. The overall picture. *Br J Surg* 1984; **71**: 12–16.

7. Williams NS, Johnston D, Survival and recurrence after sphincter saving resection and abdominoperineal resection for carcinoma of the middle third of the rectum. *Br J Surg* 1984; **71**: 460–2.

8. McDermott FT, Hughes ESR, Pihl EA, Milne BJ, Local recurrence after potentially curative resection for rectal cancer in a series of 1008 patients. *Br J Surg* 1985; **72**: 34–6.

9. MacFarlane JK, Ryall RD, Heald RJ, Mesorectal excision for rectal cancer. *Lancet* 1993; **341**: 457–60.

10. McCall JJ, Cox MR, Wattchow DA, Analysis of local recurrence rates after surgery alone for rectal cancer. *Int J Colorect Dis* 1995; **10**: 126–32.

11. Enker WE, Laffer UT, Block GE, Enhanced survival of patients with colon and rectal cancer is based upon wide anatomic resection. *Ann Surg* 1979; **190**: 350–60.

12. Moriya Y, Hojo K, Sawada T, Koyama Y, Significance of lateral node dissection for advanced rectal carcinoma at or below the peritoneal reflection. *Dis Colon Rectum* 1989; **32**: 307–15.

13. Hojo K, Sawada T, Moroija Y, An analysis of survival and voiding, sexual function after wide iliopelvic lymph-adenectomy in patients with carcinoma of the rectum, compared with conventional lymphadenectomy. *Dis Colon Rectum* 1989; **32**: 128–33.

14. Holm T, Cedermark B, Rutqvist L-E, Local recurrence of rectal adenocarcimona after 'curative' surgery with and without preoperative radiotherapy. *Br J Surg* 1994; **81**: 452–5.

15. Jansson-Frykholm G, Påhlman L, Glimelius B, Treatment of local recurrences of rectal carcinoma. *Radiother Oncol* 1995; **34**: 185–94.

16. Nicholls RJ, York Mason A, Morson BC et al, The clinical staging of rectal cancer. *Br J Surg* 1982; **69**: 404–9.

17. Lewis WG, Williamson MER, Kuzu A et al, Potential disadvantages of postoperative adjuvant radiotherapy after anterior resection for rectal cancer: a pilot study of sphincter function, rectal capacity and clinical outcome. *Int J Colorect Dis* 1995; **10**: 133–7.

18. Graf W, Ekström K, Glimelius B, Påhlman L, Factors influencing bowel function after colorectal anastomosis. *Dis Colon Rectum* 1996; **39**: 593–600.

19. Grinell RS, Distal intramural spread of carcinoma of the rectum and rectosigmoid. *Surg Gynecol Obstet* 1954; **99**: 421–39.

20. Sondenaa K, Kjellevold KH, A prospective study of the length of the distal margin after low anterior resection for rectal cancer. *Int J Colorect Dis* 1990; **5**: 103–5.

21. Heald RJ, Husband EM, Ryall RDH, The mesorectum in rectal cancer surgery – the clue to pelvic recurrence? *Br J Surg* 1982; **69**: 613–16.

22. Scott N, Jackson P, Al-Jaberi T et al, Total mesorectal excision and local recurrence: a study of tumour spread in the mesorectum distal to rectal cancer. *Br J Surg* 1995; **82**: 1031–3.

23. Grinell RS, Results of ligation of inferior mesenteric artery at the aorta in resections of carcinoma of the descending and sigmoid colon and rectum. *Surg Gynecol Obstet* 1965; **120**: 1031–6.

24. Pezim ME, Nicholls RJ, Survival after high or low ligation of the inferior mesenteric artery during curative surgery for rectal cancer. *Ann Surg* 1984; **200**: 729–33.

25. Letchert JGJ; Lebesdue JV, de Boer RW et al, Dose-volume correlation in radiation-induced late small-bowel complications: a clinical study. *Radiother Oncol* 1990; **18**: 307–20.

26. Jansson-Frykholm G, Sintorn K, Montelius A et al, Preoperative radiotherapy in rectal carcinoma – aspects of acute adverse effects and radiation technique. *Int J Radiat Oncol Biol Phys* 1996; **35**: 1039–48.

27. Fletcher GH, Subclinical disease. *Cancer* 1984; **53:** 1274–84.

28. Withers HR, Peter LJ, Taylor JMG, Dose–response relationship for radiation therapy of subclinical diseases. *Int J Radiat Oncol Biol Phys* 1995; **31:** 353–9.

29. Trotti A, Klotch D, Endicott J et al, A prospective trial of accelerated radiotherapy in the postoperative treatment of high risk squamous cell carcinoma of the head and neck. In: *Head and Neck Cancer*, Vol 26 (Johnson JJ, Didoklar MS, eds). Amsterdam: Elsevier, 1993; 13–21.

30. Fowler JF, The linear–quadratic formula and progress in fractionated radiotherapy. *Br J Radiol* 1989; **62:** 679–94.

31. Kirk J, Gray WM, Watson ER, Cumulative radiation effect. Part I. Fractionated treatment regimes. *Clin Radiol* 1971; **22:** 145–55.

32. Turesson I, Fractionation and dose rate in radiotherapy. An experimental and clinical study of cumulative radiation effect. Thesis, Göteborg, 1978.

33. Bjerkeset T, Dahl O, Irradiation and surgery for primarily inoperable rectal adenocarcinoma. *Dis Colon Rectum* 1980; **23:** 298–303.

34. Durdey P, Williams NS, The effect of malignant and inflammatory fixation of rectal carcinoma on prognosis after rectal excision. *Br J Surg* 1984; **71:** 787–90.

35. Fortier GA, Krochak RJ, Kim JA, Constable WC, Dose response to preoperative irradiation in rectal cancer: implications for local control and complications associated with sphincter sparing surgery and abdominoperineal resection. *Int J Radiat Oncol Biol Phys* 1989; **12:** 1559–63.

36. Dosoretz DE, Gunderson LL, Hedberg S et al, Preoperative irradiation for unresectable rectal and rectosigmoid carcinomas. *Cancer* 1989; **52:** 814–18.

37. Emami B, Pilepich M, Willet C et al, Effect of preoperative irradiation on resectability of colorectal carcinomas. *Int J Radiat Oncol Biol Phys* 1982; **8:** 1295–9.

38. Frykholm G, Påhlman L, Glimelius B, Preoperative irradiation with and without chemotherapy (MFL) in the treatment of primarily nonresectable adenocarcinoma of the rectum. Results from two consecutive studies. *Eur J Clin Oncol* 1989; **25:** 1535–41.

39. James RD, Schofield PF, Resection of 'inoperable' rectal cancer following radiotherapy. *Br J Surg* 1985; **70:** 469–72.

40. Minsky BD, Cohen AM, Kemeny N et al, Preoperative 5-FU, and low dose leucovorin and sequential radiation therapy for unresectable rectal cancer. *Int J Radiat Oncol Biol Phys* 1993; **25:** 821–7.

41. Påhlman L, Glimelius B, Ginman C et al, Preoperative irradiation of primary non-resectable adenocarcinoma of the rectum and rectosigmoid. *Acta Radiol Oncol* 1985; **24:** 35–9.

42. Frykholm G, Hemmingsson A, Nyman R et al, Non-resectable adenocarcinoma of the rectum assessed by MR imaging before and after chemotherapy and irradiation. *Acta Radiol* 1992; **33:** 447–52.

43. Overgaard M, Overgaard J, Sell A, Dose–response relationship for radiation therapy of recurrent, residual, and primarily inoperable colorectal cancer. *Radiat Oncol* 1984; **1:** 217–22.

44. Wassif-Boulis S, The role of preoperative adjuvant therapy in management of borderline operability of rectal cancer. *Clin Radiol* 1982; **33:** 353–8.

45. Byfield J, Calabro-Jones P, Klisak I, Kulhanian F, Pharmacologic requirements for obtaining sensitization of human tumor cells in vitro to combined 5-fluorouracil or Ftorafur and X-rays. *Int J Radiat Oncol Biol Phys* 1982; **8:** 1923–33.

46. von der Maase H, Experimental studies on interactions of radiation and cancer chemotherapeutic drugs in normal tissues and a solid tumour. *Radiat Oncol* 1986; **7:** 47–68.

47. Rominger CJ, Gelber RD, Gunderson LL, Conner N, Radiation therapy alone or in combination with chemotherapy in the treatment of residual or inoperable carcinoma of the rectum an rectosigmoid or pelvic recurrence following colorectal surgery. *Am J Clin Oncol* 1985; **8:** 118–27.

48. Rider WD, Palmer JA, Mahoney LJ, Robertson CT, Preoperative irradiation in operable cancer of the rectum. *Can J Surg* 1977; **20:** 335–8.

49. Duncan W, Smith AN, Freedman LS et al, The evaluation of low dose preoperative X-ray therapy in the management of operable rectal cancer; results of a randomly controlled trial. *Br J Surg* 1984; **71:** 21–5.

50. Goldberg PA, Nicholls RJ, Porter NH et al, Long-term results of a randomised trial of short-course low-dose adjuvant pre-operative radiotherapy for rectal cancer. Reduction in local treatment failure. *Eur J Cancer* 1994; **30A:** 1602–6.

51. Higgins G, Humphrey E, Dwight R et al, Preoperative radiation and surgery for cancer of the rectum. VASOG trial II. *Cancer* 1986; **58:** 352–9.

52. Horn A, Halvorsen JF, Dahl O, Preoperative

radiotherapy in operable rectal cancer. *Dis Colon Rectum* 1990; **33:** 823–8.

53. Roswit B, Higgins G, Keehn R, Preoperative irradiation for carcinoma of the rectum and rectosigmoid colon: Report of a National Veterans Administration randomized study. *Cancer* 1975; **35:** 1597–602.

54. James RD, Haboubi N, Schofield PF et al, Prognostic factors in colorectal carcinoma treated by preoperative radiotherapy and immediate surgery. *Dis Colon Rectum* 1991; **34:** 546–51.

55. Gérard A, Buyse M, Nordlinger B et al, Preoperative radiotherapy as adjuvant treatment in rectal cancer. *Ann Surg* 1988; **208:** 606–14.

56. SRCSG (Stockholm Rectal Cancer Study Group), Preoperative short-term radiation therapy in operable rectal carcinoma. *Cancer* 1990; **66:** 49–53.

57. SRCT (Swedish Rectal Cancer Trial), Local recurrence rate in a randomized multicentre trial of preoperative radiotherapy compared to surgery alone in resectable rectal carcinoma. *Eur J Surg* 1996; **162:** 397–402.

58. Balslev I, Pedersen M, Teglbjaerg PS et al, Postoperative radiotherapy in Dukes' B and C carcinoma of the rectum and rectosigmoid. A randomized multicenter study. *Cancer* 1986; **58:** 22–8.

59. GITSG (Gastro Intestinal Tumour Study Group), Prolongation of the disease-free interval in surgically treated rectal carcinoma. *N Engl J Med* 1985; **312:** 1464–72.

60. Fisher B, Wolmark N, Rockette H et al, Postoperative adjuvant chemotherapy or radiation therapy for rectal cancer: results from NSABP Protocol R-01. *J Natl Cancer Inst* 1988; **80:** 21–9.

61. Treuniet-Donker AD, van Putten WLJ, Postoperative radiation therapy for rectal cancer. *Cancer* 1991; **67:** 2042–8.

62. Påhlman L, Glimelius B, Pre- and postoperative radiotherapy in rectal carcinoma: report from a randomized multicenter trial. *Ann Surg* 1990; **211:** 187–95.

63. Jansson-Frykholm G, Glimelius B, Påhlman L, Preoperative or postoperative irradiation in adenocarcinoma of the rectum: final treatment results of a randomized trial and an evaluation of late secondary effects. *Dis Colon Rectum* 1993; **36:** 564–72.

64. Buyse M, Zeleniuch-Jacquotte A, Chalmers TC, Adjuvant therapy of colorectal cancer. Why we still don't know. *J Am Med Assoc* 1988; **259:** 3571–8.

65. Krook JE, Moertel CG, Gunderson LL et al, Effective surgical adjuvant therapy for high-risk rectal carcinoma. *N Engl J Med* 1991; **324:** 709–15.

66. NCI, Clinical announcement: Adjuvant therapy for rectal cancer, 14 March 1991.

67. GITSG (Gastro Intestinal Tumour Study Group), Radiation therapy and fluorouracil with or without semustine for the treatment of patients with surgical adjuvant adenocarcinoma of the rectum. *J Clin Oncol* 1992; **10:** 549–57.

68. O'Connell MJ, Martenson JA, Wieand HS et al, Improving adjuvant therapy for rectal cancer by combining protracted infusion fluorouracil with radiation therapy after curative surgery. *N Engl J Med* 1994; **331:** 502–7.

69. SRCT (Swedish Rectal Cancer Trial), Preoperative irradiation followed by surgery vs surgery alone in resectable rectal carcinoma – postoperative morbidity and mortality in a Swedish multicenter trial. *Br J Surg* 1993; **80:** 1333–6.

70. Bubrik MP, Rolfmeyers ES, Schauer RM et al, Effects of high-dose and low-dose preoperative irradiation on low anterior anastomosis in dogs. *Dis Colon Rectum* 1982; **25:** 406–15.

71. Bubrik MP, Rolfmeyers ES, Schauer RM et al, Effects of high-dose and low-dose preoperative irradiation on low anterior anastomosis in dogs. *Dis Colon Rectum* 1982; **25:** 406–15.

72. Holm T, Singnomklao T, Rutqvist L-E, Cedermark B, Adjuvant preoperative radiotherapy in patients with rectal carcinoma. Adverse effects during long term follow-up of two randomized trials. *Cancer* 1996; **78:** 968–76.

14

Adjuvant systemic treatment of colorectal cancer: Duration of therapy

Gernot Hartung, Wolfgang Queißer

CONTENTS • **Introduction** • **Rationale for adjuvant treatment: duration of therapy with 5-FU in early trials** • **Effective adjuvant therapy: treatment duration in first studies** • **Development of adjuvant treatment up to 1996: currently available data on treatment duration and effect of different regimens** • **Ongoing studies** • **Monoclonal antibody 17-1A: a perspective for shorter and less intense adjuvant treatment** • **Conclusions and outlook**

INTRODUCTION

Until 1990, it was a controversial issue whether or not high-risk stages of colorectal cancer should be treated with adjuvant chemotherapy. The Intergroup-0035 study published by Moertel et al[1] gave a major impulse for the wide acceptance of adjuvant treatment in patients with high-risk colon cancer (TNM stage III, Dukes C).[2] Since then, the positive effect of adjuvant treatment has been confirmed in several studies, and new modified treatment regimens have been introduced (for reviews see references 3 and 4). There are still major controversies regarding which drugs should be applied and for what time period treatment should be given. Recent data from several multicenter trials allow a preliminary answer to this latter question.

RATIONALE FOR ADJUVANT TREATMENT: DURATION OF THERAPY WITH 5-FU IN EARLY TRIALS

The rationale for adjuvant therapy in colorectal cancer was based on the presumption that undetectable microscopic residual disease at the primary tumor site would cause local relapse, whereas disseminated tumor cells might develop into distant metastases. As the most active and tolerable single drug in palliative treatment with response rates from 5% to 15%,[5,6] 5-fluorouracil (5-FU) alone was administered in the early adjuvant trials of the 1970s and 1980s. Treatment duration in these studies was chosen from 12 up to 18 months, and a low dose of the drug was administered. However, a meta-analysis performed by Buyse et al[7] in 1988 revealed a disappointing result. A marginal benefit of 3.4% for the cumulative survival advantage in treated patients was found. The need for new and more efficient drug combinations and schedules was evident.

EFFECTIVE ADJUVANT THERAPY: TREATMENT DURATION IN FIRST STUDIES

In the first studies to show significant positive results for adjuvant treatment, 5-FU-based therapy was given for periods from 12 to 18 months. In 1988 the National Surgical Adjuvant Breast and Bowel Project (NSABP) published a first report on significant benefit from adjuvant chemotherapy.[8] Treatment for 18 months with

Table 14.1 Adjuvant therapy in colorectal cancer: major studies published until 1995 – outcome of recurrence and mortality

Study	Tumour stage (Dukes)	Treatment group	Duration of therapy	Control group	Duration of therapy	Reduction in recurrence (%)	Reduction in mortality (%)
Colon cancer							
NSABP C 01[8]	B + C	MOF (n = 358)	18 months	Follow-up only (n = 383)		17 (p = 0.02)	24 (p = 0.05)
Intergroup 0035[1,9]	C	5-FU + Lev (n = 304)	12 months	Follow-up only (n = 315)		40 (p = 0.0001)	33 (p = 0.0007)
	B2	(n = 159)		(n = 159)		No effect	No effect
NSABP C 03[10]	B + C	5-FU + FA (n = 521)	12 months	MOF (n = 524)	12 months	30 (p = 0.0004)	32 (p = 0.003)
Italian[11]	C	5-FU + FA (n = 57)	12 months	Follow-up only (n = 58)		44 (p = 0.0016)	39 (p = 0.0025)
	B2	(n = 59)		(n = 60)		No effect	No effect
IMPACT[12]	C	5-FU + FA (n = 318)	6 months	Follow-up only (n = 334)		35 (p = 0.0001)	22 (p = 0.029)
	B	(n = 418)		(n = 423)		No effect	No effect
Rectal cancer							
NCCTG 794751[13]	B2 + C	Radiation + 5-FU + Me-CCNU (n = 104)	12 months	Radiation only (n = 100)	12 months	34 (p = 0.0016)	29 (p = 0.025)
GITSG 7180[14]	B2 + C	Radiation + 5-FU (n = 109)	6 months	Radiation + 5-FU + ME-CCNU, (n = 101)	12 months	11 (not significant)	14 (not significant)
NCCTG[15]	B2 + C	Radiation + 5-FU *protracted infusion,* (n = 328)[a]	6 months	Radiation + 5-FU *bolus injection,* (n = 332)[b]	6 months	27 (p = 0.01)	31 (p = 0.005)

Abbreviations: NSABP = National Surgical Adjuvant Breast and Bowel Project; IMPACT = International Multicenter Pooled Analysis of Colon Cancer Trials; GITSG = Gastrointestinal Tumour Study Group; NCCTG = North Central Cancer Treatment Group; 5-FU = 5-fluorouracil; FA = folinic acid; MOF = Me-CCNU, vincristine, 5-FU; Lev = levamisole.

[a] The first 114 patients received Me-CCNU in addition.
[b] The first 112 patients received Me-CCNU in addition.

methyl-CNNU, oncovin (vincristine) and 5-FU (MOF) slightly improved recurrence rate and survival compared with surgery alone.

Further trials using 5-FU in combination with either levamisole or folinic acid (FA) confirmed the patient's benefit from adjuvant chemotherapy.[9–15] In addition, in rectal cancer the combination of chemotherapy and radiation showed promising results (for an overview see Table 14.1).

Treatment with 5-FU + levamisole was recommended as standard in the USA and Europe for Dukes C colon cancer after publication of the 3.5-year median follow-up data of the Intergroup 0035 study by Moertel et al.[1] In this study three groups were randomized to receive either no further treatment postoperatively, levamisole alone for 12 months or 5-FU + levamisole for 12 months. Dukes B patients were not randomized for the single-agent levamisole arm. 929 patients with Dukes' C tumors were analysed. In the 5-FU + levamisole group 63% of the patients had a 5-year disease-free survival compared with 47% for surgery alone. The difference was highly significant ($p = 0.0001$). For overall survival after 3.5 years (71% versus 55%, $p = 0.0064$), the results were impressive. The decrease in the risk of tumor relapse was calculated at 41%, and that in the risk of death at 33%. However, for Dukes B patients, no significant results could be found. The data were confirmed at a 7-year follow-up.[9]

The combination of 5-FU and FA was introduced into adjuvant therapy because of the high effectiveness and tolerability it had shown in palliative treatment.[5,6] Two studies by the NSABP (protocol C-03)[10] and an Italian group[11] indicated high effectivity of 12-month regimens with 5-FU and FA, which were comparable, if not superior, to that known from 5-FU and levamisole. A further trial by the IMPACT group[12] showed similar results in Dukes C patients, even if treatment with 5-FU and FA was applied for 6 months only.

Based on available data up to 1995, the following questions (among others) on adjuvant treatment in colorectal cancer were of major interest: Would it be possible to shorten treatment duration in the different regimens from 12 down to 6 months? If so, which drug combination should be applied?

DEVELOPMENT OF ADJUVANT TREATMENT UP TO 1996: CURRENTLY AVAILABLE DATA ON TREATMENT DURATION AND EFFECT OF DIFFERENT REGIMENS

During the late 1980s, several studies were initiated in the USA, which are now mature enough to give first answers to the above questions. They were presented for the first time at the ASCO Meeting in 1996.

The issue of optimal duration of 5-FU-based adjuvant chemotherapy of colon cancer was investigated in a study by the NCCTG initiated in 1989 (see Table 14.2).[16] In this study 915 patients at high risk of relapse were randomized to four arms of therapy:

(1) 5-FU + levamisole for 6 months;
(2) 5-FU + low-dose FA + levamisole for 6 months;
(3) 5-FU + levamisole for 12 months;
(4) 5-FU + low-dose FA + levamisole for 12 months.

Of these patients, 17% had TNM stage II (Dukes B2), while 83% had TNM stage III (Dukes C) disease. 890 patients (97%) were eligible for analysis at time of presentation, with a median follow up of 4.2 years; 163 (99%) of the protocol-targeted 165 recurrences were then observed.

Overall, there were no differences in disease-free survival (DFS) among the four treatment arms ($p = 0.49$). However, the examination of overall survival (OS) for every individual treatment arm revealed that mortality was highest in patients treated with 5-FU + levamisole for only 6 months (37%) and lowest in patients treated with 5-FU + low-dose FA + levamisole for 6 months (25%, $p = 0.005$). This was the only significant difference in pairwise comparison. Treatment with either regimen for up to 12 months did not show any benefit. However, patients receiving the triple-drug regimens suffered a greater incidence of grade 3–4 diarrhea (20–25%) and stomatitis (9.5–11%).[17]

Table 14.2 North Central Cancer Treatment Group (NCCTG) trial:[16] duration of adjuvant fluorouracil-based therapy in TNM stage II or III (Dukes B2 or C) colon cancer, evaluation of four combinations with 5-FU, FA or levamisole in 915 patients

	Treatment regimen	Duration (months)	DFS (%)	OS (%)
Group 1	5-FU 450 mg/m^2 daily i.v. $\times$ 5 days; then 450 mg/m^2 weekly from day 29, + levamisole 3 $\times$ 50 mg orally $\times$ 3 days every 2 weeks	6	64	63
Group 2	5-FU 370 mg/m^2 + FA 20 mg/m^2 daily i.v. $\times$ 5 days, repeated at 4 and 8 weeks and every 5 weeks thereafter, + levamisole 3 $\times$ 50 mg orally $\times$ 3 days every 2 weeks	6	70	75 ($p < 0.005$) with group 1
Group 3	5-FU 450 mg/m^2 daily i.v. $\times$ 5 days; then 450 mg/m^2 weekly from day 29, + levamisole 3 $\times$ 50 mg orally $\times$ 3 days every 2 weeks	12	69	72
Group 4	5-FU 370 mg/m^2 + FA 20 mg/m^2 daily i.v. $\times$ 5 days, repeated at 4 and 8 weeks and every 5 weeks thereafter, + levamisole 3 $\times$ 50 mg orally $\times$ 3 days every 2 weeks	12	66	66

Abbreviations: 5-FU = 5-fluorouracil; FA = folinic acid; DFS = disease-free survival; OS = overall survival.

Table 14.3 National Surgical Adjuvant Breast and Bowel Project (NSABP) C-04 trial:[18] comparison of adjuvant fluorouracil-based therapy with FA or levamisole in TNM stage II or III (Dukes B2 or C) colon cancer, evaluation of three combinations in 2151 patients

	Treatment regimen	Duration (months)	DFS (%)	Cumulative odds	OS (%)	Cumulative odds
Group 1	5-FU 500/mg/m^2 bolus i.v. + FA 500 mg/m^2 over 2 hours each week for 6 weeks, repeated for 6 cycles	12	64	—	74	—
Group 2	5-FU 450 mg/m^2 daily i.v. × 5 days; then 450 mg/m^2 weekly from day 29, + levamisole 3 × 50 mg orally × 3 days every 2 weeks	12	60	0.83 ($p < 0.05$)	69	0.79 ($p < 0.05$)
Group 3	5-FU 500/mg/m^2 bolus i.v. + FA 500 mg/m^2 over 2 hours each week for 6 weeks, repeated for 6 cycles, + levamisole 3 × 50 mg orally × 3 days every 2 weeks	12	64	0.98	72	0.93

Abbreviations: 5-FU = 5-fluorouracil; FA = folinic acid; DFS = disease-free survival; OS = overall survival.

The investigators concluded that

- 12 months of adjuvant chemotherapy does not provide a significant benefit over 6 months treatment;
- 5-FU + low-dose FA + levamisole for 6 months is more effective than 5-FU + levamisole for 6 months, though more toxic.

The question that remains unanswered by the NCCTG trial is whether the combination of 5-FU + FA might be equally effective as treatment with 5-FU and levamisole for 12 months or the triple-drug regimen. This matter was investigated in two studies by the NSABP (protocol C-04)[18,19] and by the Intergroup (protocol 0089).[20,21]

The NSABP C-04 study (see Table 14.3) was initiated in 1989. In this study 2151 patients with TNM stage II (40%) or III (60%) were randomized to one of three treatment arms:

(1) 5-FU + high-dose FA up to 12 months;
(2) 5-FU + levamisole for 12 months;
(3) 5-FU + high-dose FA + levamisole up to 12 months.

No significant differences in 5-year DFS or mortality were found after a median follow-up of 70 months. However, in pairwise comparison, group 1 was superior to group 2, with a slight increase of DFS ($p = 0.05$) and reduced mortality (183 deaths versus 213 in group 2, $p < 0.05$). Toxicity was similar in all three groups, with grade 3–4 toxicity in 28–38% of patients. Grade 3–4 diarrhea was more prevalent in group 1 than in group 2 (27% versus 9%); stomatitis and hematological toxicities were more frequent in group 2. Global analysis showed that the magnitude of response was similar in stage II and III patients.

The investigators concluded that

- 5-FU + FA for 12 months, though more toxic with respect to grade 3–4 diarrhea, might be superior to 5-FU + levamisole in terms of outcome, and should therefore be preferred as control in future studies;
- there was no benefit from a triple-drug regimen;
- the study indicated that Dukes B2 patients might profit from adjuvant chemotherapy as well.

The Intergroup 0089 trial addressed the question of which dose of FA should be applied and how long therapy should be given compared with standard 5-FU + levamisole (see Table 14.4). The study was initiated in 1988: 3759 patients have been recruited (20% TNM stage II, Dukes B2; 80% TNM stage III, Dukes C) and randomized to one of four groups:

(1) 5-FU + low-dose FA up to 6 months;
(2) 5-FU + high-dose FA up to 12 months;
(3) 5-FU + levamisole for 12 months;
(4) 5-FU + low-dose FA + levamisole up to 6 months.

After 83% of predicted recurrences and 72% of expected deaths had been observed, an interim analysis was performed. Three comparisons were unblinded. There were no significant differences in DFS and OS between the following groups: 1 versus 2, 3 versus 2, and 1 versus 4.

However, grade 3–4 diarrhea was significantly more pronounced in the FA-containing regimens compared with 5-FU + levamisole. Stomatitis occurred more often in the 5-day than with the weekly 5-FU regimens. If toxicity was analysed for age groups, myelosuppression resulted in a higher risk of infection in patients aged >70 years.[21]

The investigators concluded from this interim analysis that

- 5-FU + low-dose FA up to 6 months and 5-FU + high-dose FA up to 12 months are equally effective;
- 5-FU + high-dose FA up to 12 months and 5-FU + levamisole for 12 months are equivalent in terms of outcome;
- there was no benefit from a triple-drug regimen;
- patient characteristics and toxicity profiles should be considered for choosing an optimal adjuvant therapy for the individual patient.

ONGOING STUDIES

Some ongoing studies are expected to provide additional information in the near future for the

Table 14.4 Intergroup 0089 trial:[20] comparison of adjuvant fluorouracil-based therapy with high- or low-dose FA or levamisole in TNM stage II or III (Dukes B2 or C) colon cancer, evaluation of four combinations in 3759 patients

	Treatment regimen	Duration (months)
Group 1 (5-FU + LD FA)	5-FU 425 mg/m^2 + FA 20 mg/m^2 daily i.v. × 5 days, repeated every month	6
Group 2 (5-FU + HD FA)	5-FU 500 mg/m^2 bolus i.v. at 1 hour during FA 500 mg/m^2 over 2 hours every week for 6 weeks, then every 2 months	12
Group 3 (5-FU + Lev)	5-FU 450 mg/m^2 daily i.v. × 5 days; then 450 mg/m^2 weekly from day 29, + levamisole 3 × 50 mg orally × 3 days every 2 weeks	12
Group 4 (5-FU + LD FA + Lev)	5-FU 425 mg/m^2 + FA 20 mg/m^2 daily i.v. × 5 days, repeated every month, + levamisole 3 × 50 mg orally × 3 days every 2 weeks	6

Comparison (trends were in favor of second regimen in each comparison)	DFS	OS
5-FU + HD FA vs 5-FU + LD FA	nsd	nsd
5-FU + Lev vs 5-FU + HD FA	nsd	nsd
5-FU + LD FA vs 5-FU + LD FA + Lev	nsd	nsd

Abbreviations: 5-FU = 5-fluorouracil; FA = folinic acid; Lev = levamisole; DFS = disease-free survival; OS = overall survival; nsd = no significant difference.

question of treatment duration (see Table 14.5 for study designs). The AIO (Arbeitsgemein-schaft Internistische Onkologie) in Germany initiated two multicenter studies in 1993 to address the question of treatment duration with identical 5-FU + FA regimens. Colon cancer patients (Dukes C) are randomized to receive 5-FU + levamisole for 12 months, or 5-FU and medium-dose FA for 6 months or 12 months. Rectal cancer patients (Dukes B2 and C) receive postoperative chemotherapy with 5-FU and medium-dose FA for either 6 months or 12 months.[22] The Gastrointestinal Tumour Study Group of the EORTC is currently investigating postoperative chemotherapy with 5-FU + lev-amisole for 6 months and with 5-FU + FA (L-isomer) for 6 months in Dukes B2 and C colon cancer; rectal cancer patients receive post-operative radiation in addition. Several groups are comparing different 12 months drug regi-mens in colon and rectal cancer patients (for an overview of selected studies see Table 14.6).

MONOCLONAL ANTIBODY 17-1A: A PERSPECTIVE FOR SHORTER AND LESS INTENSE ADJUVANT TREATMENT

A new principle for adjuvant treatment of col-orectal cancer has been established with the

Table 14.5 Ongoing studies to compare duration of adjuvant therapy in colon and rectal cancer

AIO Study, Germany: Studiengruppe Mannheim

Colon cancer Dukes C	Treatment regimen	Duration (months)
Group 1 5-FU + Lev	5-FU + levamisole (standard)	12
Group 2 5-FU + FA	5-FU 450 mg/m^2 + FA 100 mg/m^2 daily i.v. × 5 days, repeated every month (12 cycles)	12
Group 3 5-FU + FA	5-FU 450 mg/m^2 + FA 100 mg/m^2 daily i.v. × 5 days, repeated every month (6 cycles)	6

Rectal cancer Dukes B2 + C	Treatment regimen	Duration (months)
Group 1 5-FU + FA	5-FU 450 mg/m^2 + FA 100 mg/m^2 daily i.v. × 5 days, repeated every month (12 cycles)	12
Group 2 5-FU + FA	5-FU 450 mg/m^2 + FA 100 mg/m^2 daily i.v. × 5 days, repeated every month (6 cycles)	6

Radiation (50.4 Gy) and weekly chemotherapy 5-FU 350 mg/m^2 + FA 100 mg/m^2 during 2nd cycle

EORTC Study (40911)

Colon and rectal cancer Dukes B2 and C	Treatment regimen	Duration (months)
Group 1[a]	5-FU + levamisole (standard)	6
Group 2[a]	5-FU 375 mg/m^2 + FA (L-isomer) 100 mg/m^2 daily i.v. × 5 days, repeated every month (6 cycles)	6

For rectal cancer patients: additional 50 Gy radiotherapy.

Abbreviations: 5-FU = 5-fluorouracil; FA = folinic acid.
[a] With or without local postoperative chemotherapy (intraportal or intraperitoneal) according to a second randomization (factorial design).

monoclonal antibody (mAb) 17-1A.[23] In one randomized study with 155 evaluable patients with Dukes C colorectal carcinoma, postoperative application of 17-1A (1 × 500 mg, 4 × 100 mg every 4 weeks, total treatment duration 4–5 months) reduced the mortality rate by 32% ($p < 0.01$) and the recurrence rate by 23% ($p < 0.014$) after 7 years median follow-up.[24] The mAb appears to be more active in preventing disseminating disease than local recurrence. The toxicity is low; only mild adverse events have been reported. Therapy is short (and potentially more economical), and patients can be treated on an outpatient basis, with only 5

Table 14.6 Ongoing studies to compare different 12-month regimens of adjuvant therapy in colon and rectal cancer

Intergroup Study 0114, USA

Rectal cancer Dukes B2 and C	Treatment regimen	Duration (months)
Group 1	5-FU	12
Group 2	5-FU + levamisole (standard)	12
Group 3	5-FU + low-dose FA	12
Group 2	5-FU + FA + levamisole	12

Additional 50 Gy radiotherapy.

Tumorzentrum Ulm Study, Germany

Colon (Dukes C) and rectal (Dukes B2 and C) cancer	Treatment regimen	Duration (months)
Group 1	5-FU + levamisole (standard)	12
Group 2	5-FU + levamisole (standard) + FA	12
Group 3	5-FU + levamisole (standard) + interferon alpha	12

For rectal cancer patients: additional 50 Gy radiotherapy.

AGEO-NRW, Germany

Colon cancer (Dukes C)	Treatment regimen	Duration (months)
Group	15-FU + levamisole (standard)	12
Group 2	5-FU + FA	12

Abbreviations: 5-FU = 5-fluorouracil; FA = folinic acid.

visits necessary for the application of the complete treatment regimen. Overall, the improvements in DFS and mortality observed with 17-1A as monotherapy are similar to those achieved with 5-FU + levamisole or 5-FU + FA. Therefore, for Dukes C patients, mAb17-1A may be considered as an alternative to adjuvant chemotherapy, if chemotherapy does not seem appropriate for the patient. Theoretically, 17-1A may possess activity against tumor cells that are either dormant or chemotherapy-resistant. Currently, the combination of the antibody + 5-FU based chemotherapy is being investigated (see Table 14.7).

Table 14.7 Ongoing studies with mAb 17-1A in colon cancer

Protocol 157-002, Europe and other countries (except USA)

Colon cancer Dukes C	Treatment regimen	Duration (months)
Group 1	5-FU + FA	6
Group 2	5-FU + FA + mAb 17-1A	7
Group 3	mAb 17-1A	5

Protocol 157-003, USA

Colon cancer Dukes C	Treatment regimen	Duration (months)
Group 1	5-FU + (Lev *or* FA)	6
Group 2	5-FU + (Lev *or* FA) + mAb 17-1A	7

Studiengruppe Mannheim, Germany

Colon cancer Dukes B2–B3	Treatment regimen	Duration (months)
Group 1	mAb 17-1A	5
Group 2	No treatment	—

Abbreviations: 5-FU = 5-fluorouracil; FA = folinic acid; Lev = levamisole; mAb 17-1A = monoclonal antibody 17-1A (Panorex).

CONCLUSIONS AND OUTLOOK

In summary, no definite recommendation on adjuvant chemotherapy of Dukes C colon carcinoma can be given at this time. The combination of 5-FU with high-dose FA (weekly schedule) does not seem to be superior to 5-FU + levamisole, if therapy is continued for 12 months. However, a 6-month therapy with 5-FU + low-dose FA (5-day regimen) is probably equivalent to either 12-month regimens with 5-FU + levamisole or 5-FU + high-dose FA or the combination of all three drugs. Therefore 5-FU + low-dose FA for 6 months may be considered as a promising alternative to the standard 12-month treatment with 5-FU + levamisole. The choice of treatment should depend on toxicity and quality-of-life considerations. While a shorter treatment duration for the 5-FU + FA regimen would enable patients to be reintegrated faster into normal and professional life, higher rates of gastrointestinal toxicity may be expected. The question whether 12 months of 5-FU + low-dose or intermediate-dose FA is superior to 6 months remains unanswered, and is being investigated in ongoing studies.[22]

The issue of duration of chemotherapy in rectal cancer is also still unanswered. At present, treatment with 5-FU for 6 months and postoperative local radiation is recommended according to the NCI statement and European groups[2,25] for Dukes B2 and C patients. Data from randomized studies comparing the durations of identical postoperative chemotherapy schedules are presently not available, but may be expected within the next few years.[22] It may be assumed that optimal treatment durations in colon and rectal cancer would be similar. Therefore the positive data for 6-month treatment schedules in colon cancer support the current recommendations for adjuvant treatment in rectal cancer as well.

In colon cancer, mAb 17-1A might be a good and less toxic alternative to conventional chemotherapy. This would allow a less time-consuming and possibly more economical treatment strategy, if the currently available positive data can be confirmed on ongoing studies. Since the data presently available rely on only one trial with a rather small patient number,

final conclusions concerning the true value of mAb 17-1A are not possible yet. It will be of interest whether combined treatment with the antibody and chemotherapy in 6-month regimens may optimize treatment outcome.

Further new agents active in metastatic disease have recently been identified, including thymidilate synthase inhibitors, camptothecin derivatives, oxaliplatin, and fluorouracil prodrugs.[26] Also, the continuous application of high-dose 5-FU in combination with FA according to the Ardalan regimen has shown to be more effective than the current 5-FU-based regimens.[27] These new treatment options may become candidates for future adjuvant trials with the perspective that more active drugs and regimens allow shorter adjuvant therapy.

REFERENCES

1. Moertel CG, Fleming TR, MacDonald JS et al, Levamisole and fluorouracil for adjuvant treatment of resected colon carcinoma. *N Engl J Med* 1990; **322**: 352–8.
2. NIH Consensus Conference, Adjuvant therapy for patients with colon and rectal cancer. *J Am Med Assoc* 1990; **264**: 1444–50.
3. Hartung G, Diezler P, Hagmüller E, Queißer W, New approaches to adjuvant therapy of colorectal carcinoma including current German activities. *Onkologie* 1993; **16**: 416–24.
4. Köhne-Wömpner CH, Schöffski P, Schmoll HJ, Adjuvant therapy of colon adenocarcinoma: current status of clinical investigation. *Ann Oncol* 1994; **5**(Suppl 3): 97–104.
5. Moertel CG, Chemotherapy for colorectal cancer. *N Engl J Med* 1994; **330**: 1136–42.
6. Cohen AM, Minsky BS, Schilsky RL, Colorectal cancer. In: *Cancer, Principles and Practice of Oncology*, 4th edn (de Vita V, ed). 1993; 929–77.
7. Buyse M, Zeleniuch-Jaquotte A, Chalmers TC, Adjuvant therapy of colorectal cancer. Why we still don't know. *J Am Med Assoc* 1988; **259**: 3571–8.
8. Wolmark N, Fisher B, Rockette H et al, Postoperative adjuvant chemotherapy or BCG for colon cancer: results from NSABP protocol C-01. *J Natl Cancer Inst* 1988; **80**: 30–6.
9. Moertel CG, Fleming TR, MacDonald JS et al, Fluorouracil and levamisole as effective adjuvant therapy after resection of stage III colon carci-

noma: a final report. *Ann Intern Med* 1995; **122**: 321–6.
10. Wolmark N, Rockette H, Fisher B et al, The benefit of leucovorin-modulated fluorouracil as postoperative adjuvant therapy for primary colon cancer: results from National Surgical Adjuvant Breast and bowel project protocol C-03. *J Clin Oncol* 1993; **11**: 1879–87.
11. Francini G, Petrioli R, Lorenzini L et al, Folinic acid and 5-fluorouracil as adjuvant chemotherapy in colon cancer. *Gastroenterology* 1994; **106**: 899–906.
12. International Multicentre Pooled Analysis of Colon Cancer Trials (IMPACT) Investigators, Efficacy of adjuvant fluorouracil and folinic acid in colon cancer. *Lancet* 1995; **354**: 939–4.
13. Krook JE, Moertel CG, Gunderson LL et al, Effective surgical adjuvant therapy for high risk rectal carcinoma. *N Engl J Med* 1991; **324**: 709–15.
14. Gastrointestinal Tumor Study Group, Radiation therapy and fluorouracil with or without semustine for treatment of patients with surgical adjuvant adenocarcinoma of the rectum. *J Clin Oncol* 1992; **10**: 549–57.
15. O'Connell MJ, Martenson JA, Wieand HS et al, Improving adjuvant therapy for rectal cancer by combining protracted infusion fluorouracil with radiation therapy after curative surgery. *N Engl J Med* 1994; **331**: 502–7.
16. O'Connell MJ, Laurie JA, Shepherd L et al, A prospective evaluation of chemotherapy

duration and regimen as surgical adjuvant treatment for high-risk colon cancer: a collaborative trial of the North Central Cancer Treatment Group and the National Cancer Institute of Canada clinical trials. *Proc Am Soc Clin Oncol* 1996; **15**: 478.

17. Erlichmann C, Optimal duration of fluorouracil based adjuvant chemotherapy. *Inpharma* 1996; Suppl 4: 8.

18. Wolmark N, Rockette H, Mamounas EP et al, The relative efficacy of 5-fluorouracil and leucovorin and levamisole (FU-LV-LEV) in patients with Dukes B and C carcinoma of the colon: first report of NSABP C-04. *Proc Am Soc Clin Oncol* 1996; **15**: 460.

19. Wolmark N, Efficacy of fluorouracil combined with levamisole and/or calcium folinate. *Inpharma* 1996; Suppl 4: 7.

20. Haller DG, Catalano PJ, Macdonald JS, Mayer RJ, Eastern cooperative oncology group (ECOG); Southwest oncology group (SWOG); Cancer and acute leukemia group b (CALGB), fluorouracil (FU), leucovorin (LV) and levamisole (LEV) adjuvant therapy for colon cancer: preliminary results of Int-0089. *Proc Am Soc Clin Oncol* 1996; **15**: 486.

21. Haller D, Calcium folinate: low dose or high dose? *Inpharma* 1996; Suppl 4: 7–8.

22. Hartung G, Queißer W, Diezler P et al, Adjuvant chemotherapy with 5-fluorouracil and folinic acid in colorectal cancer: evaluation of toxicity. *Onkologie* 1996; **19**: 62–7.

23. Riethmüller G, Schneider-Gädicke E, Schlimok G et al, Randomised trial of monoclonal antibody for adjuvant therapy of resected Dukes C colorectal carcinoma. *Lancet* 1994; **343**: 1177–83.

24. Riethmüller G, Holz E, Schlimok G et al, Monoclonal antibody (MAB) adjuvant therapy of Dukes C colorectal carcinoma: 7-year update of a prospective randomized trial. *Proc Am Soc Clin Oncol* 1996; **15**: 1385.

25. CAO, AIO, ARO, Konsensus CAO/AIO/ARO zur adjuvanten Therapie bei Colon- und Rektumkarzinom vom 11.01.1994. *Onkologie* 1994; **17**: 291–3.

26. Schmoll HJ, Colorectal carcinoma: current problems and future perspectives. *Ann Oncol* 1994; **5**(Suppl 3): 115–21.

27. Köhne CH, Wilke HH, Hecker P et al, Interferon-alpha does not improve the antineoplastic efficacy of high dose infusional 5-fluorouracil plus folinic acid in advanced colorectal cancer. First results of a randomized multicenter study by the Association of Medical Oncology of the German Cancer Society (AIO). *Ann Oncol* 1995; **6**: 461–6.

15

The future of radiotherapy in rectal carcinoma

Jean Bourhis, Antoine Lusinchi, François Eschwège

CONTENTS • **Introduction** • **Ballistics improvements** • **Biological modifiers** • **Modified fractionation** • **Combination radio-chemotherapy** • **Gene transfer** • **Conclusions**

INTRODUCTION

Radiotherapy has been used for several decades in the management of patients with rectal adenocarcinoma. Randomized trials have shown a benefit in favor of radiotherapy at doses higher than 20 Gy prior to surgery. One of these trials was conducted by the EORTC (40761) Gastro Intestinal Group, and showed that 34.5 Gy given in 3.5 weeks significantly reduced the rate of locoregional relapse.[1] Other randomized trials have been performed,[2–5] using either lower or higher total doses (40–45 Gy) as preoperative or as postoperative treatment. An overview of these randomized trials has been conducted by the Oxford and Institut Gustave Roussy meta-analysis group, showing a significant (20%) reduction in the rate of locoregional relapse, which was more pronounced for pre- than for postoperative radiotherapy.[6] A small but statistically significant difference in survival (5%) was also observed in favor of the use of radiotherapy compared with no treatment adjuvant to surgery (Pignon, personal communication). A direct comparison of preoperative versus postoperative radiotherapy has been performed by a Swedish group,[7] showing, in a series of 236 patients, that preoperative irradiation was more efficient in reducing local relapse. It was also better tolerated.

In summary, adjuvant radiotherapy has been shown to be effective in reducing the probability of locoregional relapse in rectal carcinoma, and this may ultimately lead to a survival benefit. Radiotherapy also plays an essential role in the management of fixed (T4), inoperable rectal carcinomas, as well as in recurrent ones.[8,9]

The future of radiotherapy in rectal carcinoma depends upon the possibilities of improving the therapeutic index of radiotherapy and of better integrating radiotherapy in combination with other cytotoxic agents. Several directions should be tested (and are briefly presented in this chapter), with the aim of increasing the biological effect of radiotherapy on tumor cells, while minimizing the toxicity to normal tissues surrounding the tumor. Thus new protocols should take advantage of advances in radiation research in general, including new techniques to improve ballistics, the addition of biological modifiers, modified fractionation, etc.

BALLISTICS IMPROVEMENTS

The response of adenocarcinoma of the rectum to radiation probably depends on the ability to apply a sufficiently high dose of radiation to the tumor without exceeding the tolerance limits of the normal pelvic tissues.[10] The concept of increased probability of tumor control as the total dose of radiation increases has been illustrated by studies using contact therapy alone or combined with external radiation in a highly selected group of patients with inoperable rectal carcinoma. In this series the use of very high-dose radiation (>70 Gy) resulted in high local control rates.[11,12]

On the basis of these data, it is conceivable that a dose–effect relationship could also exist for larger tumors: increasing the dose of radiation to the tumor while sparing normal tissues might be useful to improve the resectability of fixed (T4) or recurrent rectal carcinomas, and to increase the rate of sphincter preservation[10] in operable carcinoma of the distal part of the rectum. Several approaches can be proposed to increase the radiation dose selectively delivered to the tumor, including three-dimensional conformal radiotherapy, which has recently been developed, and allows the delivery of high doses of radiation in volumes more accurately determined compared with conventional radiotherapy. A second approach has been used, consisting of intraoperative radiotherapy.[13] The principle is to give 45–50 Gy/5 weeks of external radiation therapy followed by a 10–15 Gy boost in the posterior pelvis or in the tumor bed during the surgical procedure. Promising results have been reported in pilot studies including mainly tumors fixed to the pelvic wall, and tumor recurrences in the pelvis. The value of this method is currently being evaluated in a multicenter randomized trial in patients with locally advanced tumors.

Keeping the tolerance of pelvic normal tissues as high as possible is critical when treating rectal carcinoma with radiotherapy. With that aim, an optimal radiation technique should be used, with linear accelerators, multiple beams, and computerized dose distribution. In addition, whenever possible, irradiation of the small bowel should be avoided, for example by implanting in the pelvis during the surgical procedure a mammary prosthesis, which allows the small bowel to be spared during the postoperative irradiation.[5]

BIOLOGICAL MODIFIERS

Recently, new biological parameters have been investigated that could contribute to better predictions of the outcome of radiotherapy. Indeed, it has been suggested that the results of radiotherapy might be improved if the treatment could be modified according to biological features known to be correlated with radiation resistance in experimental tumors. Among these biological parameters, tumor hypoxia,[14,15] intrinsic radiosensitivity[16] and tumor cell kinetics[17] have been proposed to predict response to radiation. The identification of such parameters for each patient could be used to modulate radiotherapy individually, according to these biological findings. Indeed, accelerated radiotherapy[18,19] could be used in cases of rapid tumor cell kinetics. Out of these biological parameters, hypoxia is also likely to be important in influencing tumor response to radiotherapy.[14,15] Changes in tumor oxygenation can be obtained by several means: oxygen partial pressure increases dramatically with carbogen breathing (95% O_2, 5% CO_2), with an increase in mean and median pO_2 for most tumors tested.[20] The potential benefit associated with carbogen breathing is currently under investigation in patients with different tumor types, and should be tested in rectal carcinoma if the results of these studies are promising. New approaches also have to be evaluated with compounds cytotoxic under hypoxic conditions, such as tirapazamine (SR4233).

MODIFIED FRACTIONATION

Considerable interest has arisen recently in unconventional fractionation schemes in radiation therapy. Although most studies have been performed on carcinomas of the upper digestive tract, this approach should be evaluated in other tumor types, such as rectal carcinoma, given the promising results that have been obtained in some recently completed randomized trials. Hyperfractionation consists in decreasing the dose per fraction to minimize late radiation toxicity, and by this means it is possible to increase the total dose to the tumor. This hypothesis was confirmed for head and neck cancer in the EORTC 22791 randomized trial,[21] in which the dose per fraction was decreased (1.15 Gy twice daily), and consequently the total dose could be raised to 80.5 Gy without increasing the probability of late toxicity. A statistically significant 20% improvement in local control was seen in favor of the hyperfractionated arm. In addition to such pure hyperfractionated trials, accelerated radiotherapy has been investigated in several studies showing that high total doses of radiation can be delivered in overall treatment times much shorter compared with conventional radiation therapy. The rationale for accelerating radiotherapy is to minimize the repopulation of surviving tumor cells during the course of treatment. The benefit of accelerated radiation therapy has been shown in head and neck carcinoma in a recently completed EORTC randomized trial (22851), suggesting that rapid repopulation of surviving tumor cells during radiation therapy might be critical for obtaining a cure in this type of tumor. Whether this approach is feasible and of benefit in rectal carcinoma needs further investigation. An analysis of tumor cell kinetics has been performed for rectal carcinoma, showing that the potential doubling time could be predictive of tumor response after preoperative radio-chemotherapy, and suggesting that rapidly proliferating rectal tumors might benefit from acceleration of radiotherapy.[9,22,23]

COMBINATION RADIO-CHEMOTHERAPY

The combination of postoperative radiotherapy plus chemotherapy has been shown to be effective in improving disease-free survival for surgically treated rectal carcinoma. In addition, the GITSG randomized trial[24] showed, in a series of 202 patients with B2-C tumors, that the combination of postoperative pelvic irradiation with 5-FU and methyl-CCNU was superior to postoperative radiotherapy alone in terms of local control and distant metastases. The EORTC is currently conducting a randomized trial

(EORTC 22921) to determine whether the addition of 5-FU and low-dose leucovorin to preoperative pelvic irradiation (45 Gy/4.5 weeks) in resectable T3–4 tumors is superior to the same radiotherapy alone.

The type of drug and its route of delivery could also be of particular importance in the design of optimal radio-chemotherapy combinations, as suggested by the randomized trial conducted by O'Connell et al (NCCTG),[8,25] showing that continuous infusion of 5-FU during the course of radiation treatment led to a significant improvement in patient outcome. New effective drugs for colorectal carcinoma have recently been reported, such as CPT 11, gemcitabin and oxaliplatin. The combination of these drugs with radiation has to be tested, at least in locally advanced rectal carcinoma.

GENE TRANSFER

New strategies to improve the efficacy of radiation therapy might include gene transfer of genes known to have an impact on cellular response to radiation, such as the p53 tumor suppressor gene. Alteration of the p53 gene is a common genetic feature in colorectal carcinoma. The wild-type p53 gene is required for apoptotic death after irradiation in many experimental models.[26,27] In addition, several investigations have shown that the wild-type p53 gene is able to increase the effect of radiation in human cancer cell lines.[28,29] Recently, a synergy between the transfer of wild-type p53 and radiation has been shown in a xenograft model of a human colorectal carcinoma. The combination of a small dose of radiation (5 Gy) with intratumoral injection of wild-type p53 via a recombinant adenovirus defective for replication (Ad5CMVp53) induced a tumor regrowth delay that is significantly higher than for AD5CMVp53 injection alone or for radiation alone.[29] This study strongly suggests that there is a potentiation between ionizing radiation and Ad5CMVp53 in this type of cancer.

CONCLUSIONS

Several approaches are currently being tested to evaluate whether the effectiveness of radiotherapy for rectal tumors can be improved without increasing toxicity to pelvic normal tissues. Many of them take advantage of progress in radiation research in general. Ongoing and future clinical trials will determine the efficacy and the usefulness of these new methods.

REFERENCES

1. Gerard JP, Buyse M, Nordlinger B, Pre-operative radiotherapy as adjuvant treatment in rectal cancer. Final results of a randomized study of the EORTC. *Ann Surg* 1988; **208:** 606–14.
2. Bosset JF, Horiot JC, Adjuvant treatment in the curative management of rectal cancer: a critical review of the results of clinical randomized trials. *Eur J Cancer* 1993; **29:** 770–4.
3. Higgins GA, Huumprey EW, Dwight RW, Pre-operative radiation and surgery for cancer of the rectum. Veterans Administration Surgical Oncology Group Trial II. *Cancer* 1986; **58:** 352–9.
4. Stockholm Rectal Cancer Study Group, Pre-operative short term radiation therapy in operable rectal carcinoma. A prospective randomized trial. *Cancer* 1990; **66:** 49–55.
5. Treurniet Donner A, Van Putten W, Wereldsma J, Postoperative radiation therapy for rectal cancer: an interim analysis of a prospective randomized multicentre trial in the Netherlands. *Cancer* 1991; **67:** 2042–8.
6. Minski BD, Cohen AM, Keeny N, Combined modality therapy of rectal cancer: decreased acute toxicity with the pre-operative approach. *J Clin Oncol* 1992; **10:** 1218–24.
7. Frikholm GJ, Glimelius B, Pahlman L, Pre-operative or post-operative irradiation in adenocarcinoma of the rectum: final treatment results of a randomized trial and an evaluation of late secondary effects. *Dis Colon Rectum* 1993; **36:** 564–82.
8. Marsh R, Chu NC, Vauthey JN et al, Preoperative treatment of patients with locally advanced unresectable rectal adenocarcinoma utilizing continuous chronobiologically shaped 5-FU infusion and radiation therapy. *Cancer* 1996; **78:** 217–25.
9. Rich T, Seubber J, Meistrich M, Pre-operative chemoradiation for T3 rectal cancers produces high rate of pathological downstaging. *Proc Euro Soc Therapeut Radiol Oncol (ESTRO)* 1994; Abst 629.
10. Marks C, Mohiuddin M, Gludstein S, Sphincter preservation for cancer of the distal rectum using high dose pre-operative radiation. *Int J Radiat Oncol Biol Phys* 1988; **15:** 1065–8.
11. Papillon J, *Rectal and Anal Cancers. Conservative Treatment by Irradiation. An Alternative to Radical Surgery.* Berlin: Springer-Verlag, 1982.
12. Sischy B, Hildebrandt V, Dhom G, Definitive radiation therapy for selected cancers of the rectum. *Br J Surg* 1988; **75:** 901–3.
13. Willet CG, Shellito PC, Eliseo R, Intra-operative electron beam therapy for primary locally advanced rectal or rectosigmoid carcinoma. *J Clin Oncol* 1991; **9:** 843–9.
14. Lartigau E, Vitu L, Haie-Meder C, Measurements of oxygen tension in uterine cervix carcinoma: a feasibility study. *Eur J Cancer* 1992; **28:** 1354–7.
15. Lartigau E, Le Ridant AM, Lambin P, Oxygenation of head and neck tumors. *Cancer* 1993; **71:** 2319–25.
16. West C, Davidson S, Roberts S, Hunter R, Intrinsic radiosensitivity and prediction of patients response to radiotherapy for carcinoma of the cervix. *Br J Cancer* 1993; **68:** 819–23.
17. Fowler JF, Rapid repopulation in radiotherapy: debate on mechanism. The phantom of tumor treatment continually rapid repopulation unmasked. *Radiother Oncol* 1991; **22:** 156–8.
18. Bourhis J, Fortin A, Dupuis O et al, Very accelerated radiotherapy: preliminary results in locally unresectable head and neck squamous cell carcinoma. *Int J Radiat Oncol Biol Phys* 1995; **32:** 747–52.
19. Dische S, Saunders M, The rationale for continuous hyperfractionated accelerated radiotherapy (CHART). *Int J Radiat Oncol Biol Phys* 1990; **19:** 1317–20.
20. Martin L, Lartigau E, Weeger P, Changes in the oxygenation of head and neck tumors during carbogen breathing. *Radiother Oncol* 1993; **27:** 123–30.
21. Horiot, JC, LeFur P, N'Guyen T et al, Hyperfractionated compared with conventional radiotherapy in oropharyngeal carcinoma: an

EORTC randomized trial. *Eur J Cancer* 1990; **26:** 779–80.

22. Rew D, Wilson GD, Taylor I, Weaver PC, Proliferation characteristics of human colorectal carcinomas measured in vivo. *Br J Surg* 1991; **78:** 60–6.

23. Willet CG, Warland G, Coen J et al, Rectal cancer: the influence of tumor proliferation on response to pre-operative irradiation. *Int J Radiat Oncol Biol Phys* 1995; **32:** 57–61.

24. GITSG, Prolongation of the disease-free interval in surgically treated rectal carcinoma. *N Engl J Med* 1985; **312:** 1465–70.

25. O'Connell MJ, Martenson J, Wieland HS, Improving adjuvant therapy for rectal cancer by combining protracted-infusion 5FU with radiation therapy after curative surgery. *N Engl J Med* 1994; **331:** 502–7.

26. Clarke A, Gledhill S, Hooper M et al, p53 dependence of early apoptotic and proliferative response within the mouse intestinal epithelium following γ-irradiation. *Oncogene* 1994; **9:** 1767–73.

27. Lee JM, Bernstein A, p53 mutations increase resistance to ionizing radiation. *Proc Natl Acad Sci USA* 1993; **90:** 5742–6.

28. Gallardo D, Drazan K, McBride W, Adenovirus-based transfer of wild p53 gne increases ovarian tumor radiosensitivity. *Cancer Res* 1996; **56:** 4891–93.

29. Spitz FR, Nguyen D, Skibber J et al, Adenoviral mediated p53 gene therapy enhances radiation sensitivity of colorectal cancer cell lines. *Proc Am Assoc Cancer Res* 1996; **37:** 347.

16

Adjuvant treatment following curative resection of liver metastases from colorectal carcinoma

Donato Nitti, Alberto Marchet, Pierpaolo Da Pian, Pier Luigi Pilati, Mario Lise

CONTENTS • **Introduction** • **Intra-arterial chemotherapy** • **Intraportal and intraperitoneal chemotherapy** • **Systemic chemotherapy** • **Conclusions**

INTRODUCTION

The liver is the main site for metastases from colorectal carcinoma. Of patients who undergo radical surgery for primary colorectal carcinoma, 14–25% have synchronous metastases,[1] and 8–25% will develop hepatic recurrences.[1,2] For untreated patients, the median survival time ranges from 3 to 19 months after diagnosis,[3–5] although long-term survivals have occasionally been reported. Liver resection can be performed in only 14–30% of cases,[6–8] but it is still the most effective treatment available for metastases from colorectal carcinoma, 5-year survivals of 25–35% being reported in the larger series.[9–15] No prospective randomized trials have been conducted to establish the real efficacy of liver resection for metastases. Different retrospective studies with historical control groups have, however, shown a benefit in the survival and disease-free interval of patients who undergo 'radical' hepatic resection.

Although the reported findings are not in complete agreement, factors that seem associated with a better prognosis following resection are disease-free interval after primary tumor resection and hepatic resection margins.[13,16,17]

Other more controversial factors include primary tumor stage, preoperative CEA values, number of metastases, and type of liver resection performed.[6,13,17,18] In a recent study,[19] patients with metastases from colorectal carcinoma were, on the basis of the more important prognostic factors, subdivided into three risk groups with different 2-year survival rates, and a simple prognostic scoring system was proposed to evaluate the chances of cure following hepatic resection.

Whether or not the above prognostic factors are present, resection should be attempted in all patients with resectable hepatic metastases, the main criterion for selection of patients being the possibility of performing 'radical' resection.

However, by the third year following potentially curative hepatic resection, most patients relapse. Reported recurrence rates vary considerably, partly because some series include resection with a non-curative aim. The residual liver is the most frequent site of metastatic recurrences (18–69%), followed by the lung (28–31%).[20–24] Recurrence in the liver depends mainly on the presence of microscopic neoplastic residue in the hepatic parenchyma before or during surgery. It therefore appears justified to associate liver resection for metastases with adjuvant chemotherapy, in an attempt to improve surgical results and to reduce the risk of relapse.

Although systemic chemotherapy is the most widely used type of treatment, locoregional therapy (intra-arterial, intraportal or intraperitoneal) has also been proposed. However, since few of the studies done to investigate the efficacy of adjuvant chemotherapy have a control group, it is difficult to make a reliable comparison between the results of surgery alone and those of surgery plus chemotherapy.

INTRA-ARTERIAL CHEMOTHERAPY

Experimental and clinical data have demonstrated that liver metastases larger than 1 cm derive most of their blood supply from the hepatic artery.[25] Infusional therapy through the hepatic artery is likely to be more toxic to the metastases than to the normal liver, which is mainly supplied by the portal vein.[26] With hepatic arterial chemotherapy infusion (HAI), drug concentrations delivered into the liver are higher, and by using drugs with a high hepatic extraction, such as fluoropyrimidines, systemic side-effects are minimized.[26–28]

HAI has been widely used in patients with unresectable liver metastases from colorectal carcinoma using different drugs and times of administration (i.e. bolus versus continuous infusion).[29–32]

In a recent meta-analysis made on 654 patients with unresectable liver metastases, the Meta-Analysis Group in Cancer[33] reported a 41% tumor response rate for patients who received HAI compared with 14% for patients who received intravenous chemotherapy (IVC) (response odds ratio 0.25%, 95% CI 0.16–0.40, $p < 10^{-10}$). Survival analyses showed a statistically significant advantage for HAI with floxuridine (FUDR) compared with the control group when all trials were taken into account ($p = 0.0009$), but not when the survival analysis was restricted to trials comparing HAI with FUDR and IVC with FUDR or 5-fluorouracil (5-FU) ($p = 0.14$).

In view of the positive effect of local control, adjuvant HAI has also been given following radical resection of liver metastases. In a series of 35 patients with resectable liver metastases, Wagman and Kemeny[34] found in a subgroup of 11 patients with single metastases that postoperative intra-arterial FUDR treatment reduced the time to failure (TTF) to the liver with respect to the control arm (30.7 versus 8.7 months, $p = 0.03$), but had no significant influence on survival (37.3 versus 28.3 months, $p = 0.66$). In a subgroup of 24 patients with multiple liver metastases, no significant differences were found between the TTF and the median survival of those who underwent liver resection and intra-arterial FUDR with respect to patients treated with only intra-arterial FUDR (TTF = 15.6 versus 9.4 months, $p = 0.18$; median survival = 19.8 versus 22.4 months, $p = 0.42$).

The results of adjuvant HAI reported in three other clinical trials[35–37] are contradictory, and the conclusions drawn are difficult to evaluate. In a study by Moriya and colleagues,[35] 16 patients who underwent radical resection of liver metastases were given HAI with 5-FU plus mitomycin C (MMC) and oral 5-FU. At a 21-month mean follow-up, 6 patients (38%) had recurrences (4 in the residual liver only, 1 in the liver and the lung, and 1 in the lung only), with a recurrence rate of 31% in the residual liver. The overall 2-year survival rate was 74%. In a study by Lorenz and colleagues,[36] HAI with FUDR (with or without folinic acid) was given to 51/90 patients who had undergone radical liver resection for metastases from colorectal cancer. The hepatic recurrence was delayed in the HAI group with respect to the group treated with surgery alone (52 versus 14 months, $p = 0.036$) and disease-free survival was also longer in the treated group (19 versus 12 months, $p = 0.08$). Overall survival showed a trend in favor of the HAI group ($p = 0.07$). In a study by Curley and colleagues,[37] 18 evaluable patients underwent adjuvant HAI with bolus injection of 5-FU following liver resection. After a median follow-up of 33 months, 9/18 patients (50%) developed recurrences, and in only 3 of the 9 cases was the recurrence confined to the liver. The median survival of patients without disease was 39 months, compared with 27 months for those with recurrences, the difference between the two groups being statistically significant ($p < 0.01$). The authors conclude that the rate of recurrence in patients treated with HAI is significantly lower than that in historical controls treated with surgery alone.[37]

In 15–20% of patients receiving HAI, severe toxicity due to gastrointestinal ulceration, chemical hepatitis and sclerosing cholangitis (only partially prevented by dexamethasone infusion) has been reported[29,30,34] when an Infusaid pump with FUDR continuous infusion is used, but not with other techniques or protocols.[38] In some cases these complications have been fatal. The frequency of technical complications related to the placement of hepatic artery catheters varies in the different studies, depending on the surgeons' experience and the arterial anatomy of the patients.[39]

At present, HAI may be considered the best available way of delivering regional chemotherapy, but the real benefit from this treatment modality following liver resection must be investigated in multicenter controlled randomized clinical trials. At the Memorial Sloan-Kettering Cancer Center, New York, randomized randomized studies are underway to evaluate the effect of adjuvant HAI and systemic chemotherapy versus adjuvant systemic chemotherapy alone after hepatic resection of metastases from colorectal cancer.[30]

INTRAPORTAL AND INTRAPERITONEAL CHEMOTHERAPY

Tumor invasion into the mesenteric vein causes the spread of malignant cells to the portal vein, and may result in microscopic metastases to the liver. Moreover, it has been suggested that during the early phase of metastatic growth, the tumoral blood supply originates in the portal vein, whereas well-established liver metastases are supplied by the hepatic artery.[40] It is reasonable to assume that, in patients with subclinical disease, infusion of chemotherapy via the portal vein might more closely simulate the route of

tumor emboli, thus reaching the small deposits.

Intraportal chemotherapy (IPC), using 5-FU with heparin, has been widely used as adjuvant treatment following resection of colorectal cancer. A meta-analysis based on individual data was conducted in nine randomized trials on a total of 3824 patients.[41] The mortality rate was significantly lower in the group of patients who received postoperative IPC than in the group submitted to surgery alone (risk reduction $13 \pm 6\%$, $p = 0.02$). The benefit from IPC was more evident in terms of disease-free survival (risk reduction $14 \pm 5\%$, $p = 0.007$) and time to metastases (risk reduction 27%, $p = 0.0008$).

IPC has also been proposed following liver resection of metastases from colorectal cancer. In a study by Fortner and colleagues,[17] no significant difference was found between the survival of patients treated with locoregional chemotherapy and that of patients treated with systemic chemotherapy after liver resection. No reduction in the incidence of liver recurrence was observed in the group treated with IPC. However, these authors stopped using IPC after a death, which occurred following portal-vein thrombosis. In a study by Elias and colleagues,[42] 12 consecutive patients received IPC with 5-FU after liver surgery of colorectal cancer, but technical failures, including infection and venous thrombosis, occurred in 50% of the cases. Only 40% of the patients received a full course of chemotherapy, and no useful tumor-response data were obtained. In the study by Tsujitani and colleagues,[43] five patients underwent adjuvant IPC with 5-FU and MMC and 17 received systemic chemotherapy mainly using MMC. Neither technical failures nor operative deaths occurred in the IPC group, and the morbidity rate in these patients was similar to that in patients treated with i.v. chemotherapy. In this study, IPC did not lead to a reduction in recurrences to the liver when compared with systemic chemotherapy, probably because of the low 5-FU dosage.

Intraperitoneal chemotherapy using a Tenckhoff catheter would both allow the delivery of high drug concentrations to the portal vein and result in a systemic effect during prolonged treatment, while obviating technical difficulties associated with intraportal or intra-arterial catheterization.[6,21,30] In August's study on 33 patients with resectable liver metastases,[6] post-resection intraperitoneal 5-FU (21 patients) appeared to improve survival in the subgroup of 17 patients with one to five metastases when compared with 12 patients not receiving adjuvant therapy, but the follow-up was inadequate and no statistically significant difference was found between the survivals $(p > 0.05)$. Moreover, when the 33 operated patients were considered overall, there was no difference between the survival of patients who received intraperitoneal 5-FU and that of patients who had surgery alone.

SYSTEMIC CHEMOTHERAPY

The combination most widely used for hepatic metastases from colorectal carcinoma is 5-FU and leucovorin (5-FU/LV). Numerous randomized trials on 5-FU/LV versus 5-FU alone have appeared in the literature.[44] A meta-analysis performed on nine randomized clinical trials[44]

showed a significant benefit for the 5-FU/LV arm (administered either as weekly or monthly regimens) with respect to the 5-FU arm in terms of tumor response rate (23% versus 11%, OR 0.45, $p < 10^{-7}$). However, any advantage in response did not lead to improvement in overall survival (OR 0.97, $p = 0.57$).

It therefore appears justified to use the 5-FU/LV regimen as systemic adjuvant chemotherapy after resection of hepatic metastases. Until now, most studies have been conducted on small series, often with different drugs in different dosages.[7,18,45–51] Finally, the i.v. 5-FU/LV regimen, which is considered one of the more effective combinations, has been used only in a small number of patients.

Of the studies published so far (Table 16.1), only two[49,50] have found that patients treated with surgery plus chemotherapy have a slight advantage over those who undergo surgery alone. In the study by Iwatsuki and colleagues,[49] 22/60 patients were given systemic chemotherapy after liver resection, most receiving 5-FU for 6–18 months. The 5-year survival rate of 22 treated patients was significantly

Table 16.1 Colorectal liver metastases: adjuvant systemic chemotherapy (C) following hepatic resection (HR)

Ref	Treatment	Number of patients		Survival
		HR + C	HR	HR + C versus HR
18	ne	18	21[a]	ne
47	Various regimens	13	17[a]	ns
48	5-FU	5	4[a]	ne
46	5-FU + semustine	26	141[b]	ns
49	5-FU	22	38[a]	$p < 0.05$
45	5-FU	11	51[a]	ns
7	Various regimens	24	25[a]	ns
50	Various regimens	155	367[a]	$p < 0.05$
51	5-FU ± folinic acid	14	62[a]	ns

[a] Retrospective. [b] Prospective not random. ne, not evaluable; ns, not significant.

higher than that of 38 patients treated with surgery alone ($p < 0.05$). In a multicenter report from 24 institutions, Hughes and colleagues[50] found that patients who received postoperative adjuvant chemotherapy had a better overall survival than those who underwent surgery alone.

Three Italian institutions made a retrospective study on 102 patients to evaluate the role of adjuvant chemotherapy following liver resection for metastases from colorectal carcinoma.[51] Out of 102 patients who underwent liver resection, 40 received postoperative chemotherapy, with 5-FU alone or in association with folinic acid or with other drugs. When results were adjusted for the prognostic factors that were unbalanced in this series, the 3-year disease-free survival was 39% for patients who received chemotherapy after liver resection and 36% for those who underwent surgery alone, while the 3-year survivals were 46% versus 42% for the

two groups respectively. On multivariate survival analysis, the relative risk of death associated with treatment was 0.53 (95% CI = 0.27–1.05, $p = 0.06$).

In 1994, the GI Cancer Cooperative Group of the EORTC, the National Cancer Institute of Canada and the GIVIO group from Italy proposed a phase III clinical trial of chemotherapy with 5-FU plus leucovorin following potentially curative resection of liver metastases from colorectal carcinoma. After surgery, the patients will be randomized in two arms (Figure 16.1):

(1) adjuvant systemic chemotherapy with 5-FU ($370 \, \text{mg/m}^2$ for 5 days) plus l-leucovorin ($100 \, \text{mg/m}^2$ i.v. for 5 days) repeated for six cycles at 28 day intervals; or
(2) delayed chemotherapy (at the time of documented unresectable recurrent disease).

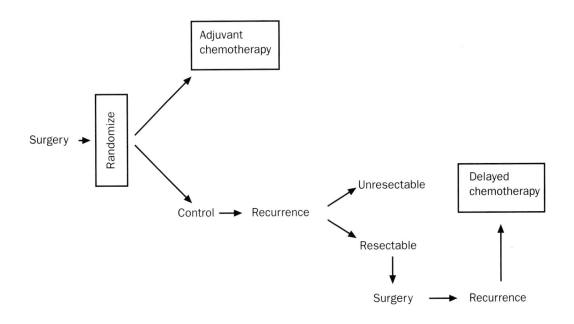

Figure 16.1 Chemotherapy following resection of metastases from colorectal carcinoma: ENG (EORTC, NCIC, GIVIO) trial.

The objectives of the study are as follows:
(i) to evaluate the efficacy of adjuvant chemotherapy by comparing the overall survival of treated patients with that of controls who undergo surgery alone;
(ii) to compare disease-free survivals of treated and control patients;
(iii) to compare the effects of these treatment modalities on quality of life.

Accrual of patients was started in March 1994, and is still ongoing.

CONCLUSIONS

In conclusion, in spite of all the caveats intrinsic to the retrospective nature of the studies that have appeared in the literature, it is suggested that chemotherapy following liver resection of metastases from colorectal carcinoma can be effective – but any efficacy has yet to be proven. Therefore, since hepatic resection for colorectal metastases is not performed that often, the only way to definitely establish whether systemic or locoregional chemotherapy really improves surgical results, and, if so, to what extent, would be to participate in the ongoing multi-center controlled randomized studies.

ACKNOWLEDGEMENTS

We are grateful to Ms Sara Pearcey for her editorial assistance.

This work was supported in part by Grant 011709 from the ACRO Project of the Consiglio Nazionalle delle Ricerche (CNR), Rome.

REFERENCES

1. Finlay IG, Meek DR, Gray HW et al, Incidence and detection of occult hepatic metastases in colorectal carcinoma. *Br Med J* 1982; **284:** 803–5.
2. Bengtsson G, Carlsson G, Fafstrom L et al, Natural history of patients with untreated liver metastases from colorectal cancer. *Am J Surg* 1981; **141:** 586–9.
3. Bengmark S, Halfstrom L, The natural history of primary and secondary malignant tumors of the liver. The prognosis of patients with hepatic metastases from colon and rectal carcinoma verified by laparotomy. *Cancer* 1969; **23:** 198–202.
4. Nielsen J, Balslev I, Jensen HE, Carcinoma of the colon with liver metastases. *Acta Chir Scand* 1971; **137:** 463–5.
5. Cady B, McDermott WV, Major hepatic resection for metachronous metastases from colon cancer. *Ann Surg* 1985; **201:** 204–9.
6. August D, Sugarbaker P, Ottow R et al, Hepatic resection of colorectal metastases. Influence of clinical factors and adjuvant intraperitoneal 5-fluorouracil via Tenckoff catheter on survival. *Ann Surg* 1985; **201:** 210–18.
7. Fortner JG, Recurrence of colorectal cancer after hepatic resection. *Am J Surg* 1988; **155:** 378–82.
8. Wagner JS, Adson MA, van Heerden JA et al, The natural history of hepatic metastases from colorectal cancer. *Ann Surg* 1984; **199:** 502–8.
9. Scheele J, Stangl R, Altendorf-Hofmann A, Gall F, Indicators of prognosis after hepatic resection for colorectal secondaries. *Surgery* 1991; **110:** 13–19.
10. Sardi A, Multiple operations for recurrent colorectal cancer. *Semin Surg Oncol* 1991; **7:** 146–56.
11. Austgen T, Souba W, Bland K, Reoperation for colorectal carcinoma. *Surg Clin N Am* 1991; **71:** 175–92.
12. Saenz N, Cady B, McDermott W, Steele G, Experience with colorectal cancer metastatic to the liver. *Surg Clin N Am* 1989; **69:** 361–70.
13. Hughes K, Scheele J, Sugarbaker P, Surgery for colorectal cancer metastatic to the liver. Optimizing the results of treatment. *Surg Clin N Am* 1989; **69:** 339–59.
14. Cady B, Stone M, The role of surgical resection of liver metastases in colorectal carcinoma. *Semin Oncol* 1991; **18:** 399–406.
15. Lise M, Da Pian PP, Nitti D et al, Colorectal metastases to the liver: present status of management. *Dis Col Rectum* 1990; **8:** 688–94.
16. Registry of Hepatic Metastases, Resection of the liver for colorectal carcinoma metastases: a

multi-institutional study of indications for resection. *Surgery* 1988; **103**: 270–88.

17. Fortner J, Silva J, Golbey R et al, Multivariate analysis of a personal series of 247 consecutive patients with liver metastases from colorectal cancer. *Ann Surg* 1984; **199**: 306–16.

18. Bengmark S, Hafstrom L, Jeppsson B et al, Metastatic disease in the liver from colorectal cancer: an appraisal of liver surgery. *World J Surg* 1982; **6**: 61–5.

19. Nordlinger B, Guiguet M, Vaillant J-C et al, Surgical resection of colorectal carcinoma metastases to the liver. A prognostic scoring system to improve case selection, based on 1568 patients. *Cancer* 1996; **77**: 1254–62.

20. Hughes KS, Simon R, Songlorabadi S, Resection of the liver for colorectal carcinoma metastases. A multi-institutional study of patterns of recurrence. *Surgery* 1986; **100**: 278–84.

21. Lise M, Da Pian PP, Nitti D, Pilati PL, Colorectal metastases to the liver: present status and future strategies. *J Surg Oncol* 1991; **2**: 69–73.

22. Ekberg H, Tranberg KG, Andersson R et al, Pattern of recurrence in liver resection for colorectal secondaries. *World J Surg* 1987; **11**: 541–7.

23. Bozzetti F, Bignami P, Morabito A et al, Patterns of failure following surgical resection of colorectal cancer liver metastases. *Ann Surg* 1987; **205**: 264–70.

24. Hohenberger P, Schlag P, Schwartz V, Herfarth C, Tumor recurrence and options for further treatment after resection of liver metastases in patients with colorectal cancer. *J Surg Oncol* 1990; **44**: 245–51.

25. Breedis C, Young C, The blood supply of neoplasms in the liver. *Am J Pathol* 1954; **30**: 969.

26. Chen HSG, Gross JF, Intra-arterial infusion of anticancer drugs: theoretic aspects of drug delivery and review of responses. *Cancer Treat Rep* 1980; **64**: 31–40.

27. Ensminger WD, Rosowsky A, Raso V, A clinical pharmacological evaluation of hepatic arterial infusion of 5-fluoro-2-deoxy-uridine and 5-fluorouracil. *Cancer Res* 1978; **38**: 3784–92.

28. Sigurdson ER, Ridge JA, Kemeny N, Tumor and liver drug uptake following hepatic artery and portal vein infusion. *J Clin Oncol* 1987; **5**: 1836–40.

29. Patt Y, Regional hepatic arterial chemotherapy for colorectal cancer metastatic to the liver: the controversy continues. *J Clin Oncol* 1993; **11**: 815–19.

30. Blumgart L, Fong Y, Surgical options in the treatment of hepatic metastasis from colorectal cancer. *Curr Probl Surg* 1995; **32**: 333–428.

31. Kemeny N, Lokich J, Anderson N, Ahlgren J, Recent advances in the treatment of advanced colorectal cancer. *Cancer* 1993; **71**: 9–18.

32. Rougier Ph, Laplanche A, Huguier M et al, Hepatic arterial infusion of floxuridine in patients with liver metastases from colorectal carcinoma: long-term results of a prospective randomized trial. *J Clin Oncol* 1992; **10**: 1112–18.

33. Meta-Analysis Group in Cancer, Reappraisal of hepatic arterial infusion in the treatment of non-resectable liver metastases from colorectal cancer. *J Natl Cancer Inst* 1996; **88**: 252–8.

34. Wagman L, Kemeny M, Leong L et al, A prospective, randomized evaluation of the treatment of colorectal cancer metastatic to the liver. *J Clin Oncol* 1990; **8**: 1885–93.

35. Moriya Y, Sugihara K, Hojo K, Makuuchi M, Adjuvant hepatic intra-arterial chemotherapy after potentially curative hepatectomy for liver metastases from colorectal cancer: a pilot study. *Eur J Surg Oncol* 1991; **17**: 519–25.

36. Lorenz M, Hottenrott Ch, Enke A, Adjuvante, regionale chemotherapie nach resektion von lebermetastasen kolorektaler primartumoren. *Zentralbl Chir* 1993; **118**: 279–89.

37. Curley S, Roh M, Chase J, Hohn D, Adjuvant hepatic arterial infusion chemotherapy after curative resection of colorectal liver metastases. *Am J Surg* 1993; **166**: 743–8.

38. Safi F, Hepp G, Beger HG, Simultaneous adjuvant regional and systemic chemotherapy after resection of liver metastases of colorectal cancer. *Proc Am Soc Clin Oncol* 1996; **15**: 226.

39. Campbell K, Burns C, Sitzmann J et al, Regional chemotherapy devices: effect of experience and anatomy on complications. *J Clin Oncol* 1993; **11**: 822–6.

40. Storer EH, Akin TJ, Chemotherapy of hepatic neoplasm on the umbelical portal vein. *Am J Surg* 1966; **11**: 56–8.

41. Piedbois P, Buyse M, Gray R et al, Portal vein infusion is an effective adjuvant treatment for patients with colorectal cancer. *Proc Am Soc Clin Oncol* 1995; **14**: 192.

42. Elias D, Lasser Ph, Rougier Ph et al, Early adjuvant intraportal chemotherapy after curative hepatectomy for colorectal liver metastases – a pilot study. *Eur J Surg Oncol* 1987; **13**: 247–50.

43. Tsujitani S, Watanbe A, Kakeji Y et al, Hepatic recurrence not prevented with low-dosage long-term intraportal 5-FU infusion after resection of

colorectal liver metastasis. *Eur J Surg Oncol* 1991; **17:** 526–9.

44. Advanced Colorectal Cancer Meta-Analysis Project, Modulation of fluorouracil by leucovorin in patients with advanced colorectal cancer: evidence in terms of response rate. *J Clin Oncol* 1992; **10:** 896–903.

45. Butler J, Attiyeh FF, Daly JM et al, Hepatic resection for metastases of the colon and rectum. *Surg Gynec Obstet* 1986; **162:** 109–13.

46. O'Connel MJ, Adson MA, Schutt AJ et al, Clinical trial of adjuvant chemotherapy after surgical resection of colorectal cancer metastatic to the liver. *Mayo Clin Proc* 1985; **60:** 517–20.

47. Rajapal S, Dasmahapatra KS, Ledesma EJ et al, Extensive resections of isolated metastases from

carcinoma of the colon and rectum. *Surg Gynec Obstet* 1982; **115:** 813–16.

48. Nims TA, Resection of the liver for metastatic cancer. *Surg Gynec Obstet* 1984; **159:** 46–8.

49. Iwatsuki S, Esquivel CO, Gordon RD et al, Liver resection for metastatic colorectal cancer. *Surgery* 1986; **100:** 804–10

50. Hughes K, Fortner J, The role of adjuvant chemotherapy following curative hepatic resection of colorectal metastases. *Proc Am Soc Clin Oncol* 1991; **10:** 145.

51. Nitti D, Civalleri D, Samori G et al, Retrospective study on adjuvant chemotherapy after surgical resection of colorectal cancer metastatic to the liver. *Eur J Surg Oncol* 1994; **20:** 454–60.

17

How much are we convinced that adjuvant treatment is effective?

Anders Jakobsen

INTRODUCTION

Adjuvant treatment is usually a treatment given to patients already undergoing another treatment modality with curative intent – this implies that the adjuvant treatment is inevitably given to some patients who are already cured. Let us consider a malignant disease with a cure rate of 50% by surgery. If an adjuvant treatment is 100% effective then the cure rate will increase to 100%, but half of the patients are treated in vain because they were cured by operation. Adjuvant therapy is rarely if ever 100% effective, and a more realistic figure is 20%, which means, in this example, that the cure rate increases to 60%, but 90% of the patients will not benefit from the treatment, if we neglect a possible delay of recurrence. This implies that adjuvant treatment should be considered carefully before it is established as standard, especially if it is toxic. The scientific evidence of effect must be convincing, as proved by a substantial improvement in survival that clearly outweighs the treatment side-effects. Adjuvant therapy has a limited effect in most malignant diseases. Therefore large clinical trials are required. Based on the log rank test, an

improvement in survival rate by 10% (e.g. from 35% to 45%) necessitates approximately 570 events, meaning a sample size of approximately 1000 patients (significance level 5%, power 90%).

Colorectal cancer is a major health problem in the Western world, and adjuvant treatment of all patients would require considerable resources. On the other hand, an increased cure rate of, for example, 10% would save many lives because of the high incidence of the disease.

ADJUVANT CHEMOTHERAPY IN COLON CANCER

Radiotherapy cannot be used in the adjuvant setting of colon cancer except for the sigmoid colon, since radiation in a sufficient dose to the upper abdomen involves a high risk of serious side-effects. The discussion can therefore be limited to adjuvant chemotherapy. Until the late 1980s, there was no definitive proof that adjuvant chemotherapy was effective in colon cancer.[1] The situation changed with two large randomized trials from the USA in 1989 and

1990.[2,3] Both trials showed a significant improvement in survival for Dukes C patients receiving 5-fluorouracil (5-FU) and levamisole. These results led to a very rapid acceptance of this treatment as standard adjuvant therapy in the USA,[4] and further studies with a control group were abandoned.

A more sceptical attitude has prevailed in Europe, and there are still a number of ongoing studies with a control group treated by surgery only. This scepticism is based on several reservations concerning the US trials. First, it is well known that these trials only included a minor fraction of all potential candidates. Many trials in the USA usually include on the order of 1% of the potential candidates, and selection influencing the outcome cannot be ruled out. Therefore such trials do not prove that the results apply to a general population of cancer patients. It should also be mentioned that one of the trials[3] was closed on the basis of an interim analysis, and the statistics should therefore be interpreted with caution. Furthermore, it is difficult to explain the effect of levamisole. So far, we do not know how it works, and it may have an adverse effect, as suggested by a small trial comparing levamisole with placebo. For patients surviving 5 years from randomization, the mortality was significantly higher in the levamisole group.[5]

It is also remarkable that the treatment did not improve the survival of Dukes B patients. This also applies to the long-term follow-up.[6] One explanation may be that the number of events was too small to detect a minor difference in this group.

A recent retrospective analysis of four NSABP trials with different regimens indicates that adjuvant chemotherapy also has an effect on Dukes B tumours.[7]

Despite these reservations, the two trials are strongly suggestive as to the effect of 5-FU and levamisole in Dukes C colon cancer. This is further underlined by the publication of long-term results from the Moertel study.[8] The improvement in survival was highly significant in the treated Dukes C group.

The IMPACT study,[9] which is a combination of three trials, also speaks strongly in favour of adjuvant treatment of patients with Dukes C colon cancer. The patients were randomized to treatment with 5-FU and leucovorin for 6 months versus control. The results of this large study (1493 patients) showed an improvement in survival comparable to that of 5-FU and levamisole. Also in this study, the improvement was clear in Dukes C only. The pooling of data implies a risk of errors, and the results should be interpreted with caution. On the other hand, the authors describe their methods carefully, and the results clearly support their conclusion that 5-FU plus leucovorin is an effective adjuvant regimen. This statement is also underlined by the fact that 5-FU and leucovorin provided a better effect than a regimen combining 5-FU, vincristine and lomustine (MOF) in the NSABP trial.[10] Furthermore, a recent trial[11] with 317 patients, stage II and stage III colon cancer, added further evidence to the effect of adjuvant treatment with 5-FU and leucovorin.

Preliminary results from several other trials are now emerging mainly from the USA. They all compare different adjuvant chemotherapy regimens, especially 5-FU, levamisole and leucovorin in different combinations. So far, 5-FU and leucovorin for 6 months seems to be at least as effective as 5-FU and levamisole for 12 months,[12,13] but a final conclusion must await a longer follow-up.

Adjuvant portal-vein infusion therapy has been applied in nine randomized trials with more than 4000 patients. The results from a meta-analysis[14] confirm a significantly lower mortality in patients treated this way ($p = 0.02$), but the trials present different results with respect to the reduction in liver metastases. It has not been proven that the effect is primarily on liver micrometastases. It may well be due to the systemic effect of the perioperative chemotherapy. Adjuvant intraperitoneal chemotherapy with 5-FU and leucovorin is used in a number of ongoing studies, but the results must await further follow-up.

An interesting approach to adjuvant immunotherapy was published in 1994.[15] Patients with Dukes C colorectal cancer were randomly assigned to treatment with a monoclonal murine antibody (17-1A) or control. The 5-year survival rate was significantly higher in the treatment group, and the reduction in mortality was comparable to that of adjuvant cytotoxic treatment. This is the first randomized trial that states a clear effect of adjuvant passive immunotherapy, and the area needs further exploration. The role of this modality alone or in combination with cytostatic drugs should be elucidated in large-scale trials before a conclusion can be drawn.

Taken together, several trials now show, beyond reasonable doubt, that adjuvant chemotherapy has an effect in Dukes C colon cancer, but a possible effect in Dukes B has not been clearly proven. The improvement in 5-year survival rate is probably on the order of 10%, and serious side-effects occur only in a small percentage of patients. Treatment-related deaths are very rare (<0.1%), but very little is known about the effect on daily life. New protocols should include quality-of-life studies according to standardized methods. Such information is lacking in the papers published so far. Most 5-FU-based regimens are expected to have minor or moderate influence on daily activity, but objective information is certainly needed. The same applies to analyses of the cost–effectiveness of the treatment.

Do the benefits outweigh the side-effects. Or, in other words, should adjuvant chemotherapy be used as standard treatment? Compared with other progresses in oncology, the answer must be 'yes'. A reasonable standard would be 5-FU and leucovorin for 6 months, but there is still a long way to go before we have the optimal treatment. This problem should be faced in large, well-designed, randomized trials.

ADJUVANT CHEMOTHERAPY IN RECTAL CANCER

There is less clear evidence that adjuvant chemotherapy alone has a substantial effect in rectal cancer. One explanation is that chemotherapy has been combined with radiotherapy in many trials, and this set-up may of course have confused the results. The exact contribution of each modality is difficult to estimate. The combined treatment is well established in the USA, and in 1991 it was approved by the NCI as standard treatment in Dukes B and C rectal cancer. The theoretical advantage of the combined treatment is that systemic therapy preferentially reduces the risk of distant metastases, whereas locoregional failures are probably less affected, as suggested by observations from adjuvant colon cancer trials. Adjuvant radiotherapy, on the other hand, has of course only a local effect.

The independent effect of adjuvant chemotherapy was investigated in the NSABP R-01 protocol[16] with three arms, comparing surgery with surgery plus chemotherapy or radiotherapy. The results showed a significant improvement in survival in the patients treated with adjuvant chemotherapy. A similar approach was used in the GITSG study,[17] except that it also included an arm with combined treatment. The results, favouring combined treatment, should, however, be taken with caution because of the small sample size ($n = 202$). The Intergroup study[18] with postoperative radiotherapy in both arms and randomization to 5-FU bolus injection versus protracted infusion during pelvic radiation also provided indirect evidence on the effect of chemotherapy.

The contribution of postoperative pelvic irradiation to systemic chemotherapy is not convincing. The problem was addressed in the NSABP R-02 protocol[19] with randomization to adjuvant chemotherapy versus postoperative combined treatment. The preliminary data indicated no significant difference in disease-free or overall survival.

Our present knowledge does not allow any firm conclusions to be drawn regarding the adjuvant chemotherapy of rectal cancer. The current literature provides evidence of at least a marginal effect on survival, but further proof is needed before adjuvant chemotherapy should be used as a general standard. It is to be hoped that a number of ongoing studies, especially two large British trials (Quasar and Axis), will provide a definitive conclusion.

ADJUVANT RADIOTHERAPY IN RECTAL CANCER

Adjuvant radiotherapy to the primary tumour area does not affect distant metastases, and therefore it can improve the cure rate only if a reduced frequency of local recurrence also leads to improved survival. There is indirect evidence that this may be the case. In approximately 20% of cases the local recurrence is the only manifestation of the disease, and thus – at least on a theoretical basis – a reduction in local recurrence rate should increase survival.

The interpretation of current results is difficult because of variations in treatment technique, dose and interval between operation and start of radiation treatment.

Preoperative adjuvant radiotherapy appears to have some potential advantages. It reduces the number of viable malignant cells, which may reduce the risk of both local and distant relapse. There is a higher probability of achieving curative resection. The treatment may lead to 'downstaging' of the resected tumour.

However, some disadvantages should also be considered. Preoperative radiation may delay curative surgery. It may also increase the risk of postoperative morbidity and mortality. The treatment is inevitably given to some patients who are unlikely to have any benefit. Patients with Dukes A tumours have a low risk of local recurrence, and preoperative radiation for this category seems dubious. The same holds true for patients with metastases at operation.

Despite these objections, preoperative radiotherapy may have an important role in the treatment of rectal cancer. There are now 11 randomized trials, of which two used one fraction (5 Gy) only and one did not report the frequency of local recurrence. Six of the eight remaining trials showed a significant reduction in local recurrence in the group receiving preoperative radiation. The Stockholm trial[20] furthermore indicated an improved survival of the patients randomized to radiation. This only applied to the subgroup undergoing radical operation, and may be due to selection; however, the latest Swedish trial suggests a survival benefit of preoperative radiation for the whole

group treated with this modality,[21] but scepticism still prevails.[22]

Postoperative radiotherapy alternatively can be reserved for patients with a high risk of local recurrence, and it does not interfere with surgery. The disadvantage is a substantial risk of radiation side-effects. Postoperative adjuvant radiation alone has been evaluated in six randomized trials, of which only one showed a significant decrease in local recurrence, and none of the trials indicated any impact on survival.

The important issue now is whether the benefit of radiation outweighs the side-effects. Preoperative radiation leads to a substantial reduction in local recurrence, and there is suggestive evidence of improved survival. The short course, as used in Sweden, does not delay the operation. Furthermore, the complication rate appears small if the treatment is given only to the pelvis, with a three- or four-field technique. However, the benefit needs to be further evaluated in randomized trials, especially in combination with a more radical operation (TME). There is also an obvious need to evaluate preoperative radiation in combination with postoperative chemotherapy.

Postoperative radiation has a certain risk of serious side-effects, and it has only a minor influence on the frequency of local recurrence. Survival is not improved. Therefore postoperative radiation alone can only be justified in clinical trials in combination with other adjuvant modalities.

CONCLUSIONS

In 1988 Marc Buyse raised a question in the heading of his paper on adjuvant therapy of colorectal cancer:[1] 'Why we still don't know'. In the meantime, several randomized trials have addressed the issue, and today we do know at least part of the answer. We have proof that adjuvant chemotherapy improves the survival of Dukes C colon cancer, and this fact can no longer be ignored. New trials with a control group are not justified, and the time has come to use adjuvant chemotherapy as standard treatment. This is not a 'breakthrough', but it does represent a major step forward in the treatment of a serious disease. Compared with other progresses in oncology seen over the last decade, it certainly ranks high – but new approaches are needed for a radical improvement of prognosis, which is not likely to be obtained even with new more effective cytostatic regimens or immunotherapy.

The situation concerning Dukes B needs further clarification, and large randomized trials with a control group should be launched.

So far, neither pre- nor postoperative radiation can be considered as standard treatment in rectal cancer, but there is an urgent need to investigate preoperative radiation in combination with a new surgical strategy (TME). It may be hoped that the combination reduces the frequency of local recurrence to a few percent. There is no logical reason why adjuvant chemotherapy should not have an effect in rectal cancer, since it is effective in colon cancer, but definitive proof is still lacking. This issue should be faced in large randomized trials.

REFERENCES

1. Buyse M, Zeleniuch-Jacquotte A, Chalmers TC, Adjuvant therapy of colorectal cancer. *J Am Med Assoc* 1988; **259:** 3571–8.
2. Laurie JA, Moertel CG, Fleming TR et al, Surgical adjuvant therapy of large-bowel carcinoma: an evaluation of levamisole and the combination of levamisole and fluorouracil. *J Clin Oncol* 1989; **7:** 1447–56.
3. Moertel CG, Fleming TR, Macdonald JS et al, Levamisole and fluorouracil for adjuvant therapy of resected colon carcinoma. *N Engl J Med* 1990; **322:** 352–8.
4. Consensus Statements: Adjuvant therapy for patients with colon and rectum cancer. NCI, 1990.
5. Chlebowski RT, Lillington L, Nystrom JS, Sayre J, Late mortality and levamisole adjuvant therapy in colorectal cancer. *Br J Cancer* 1994; **69:** 1094–7.
6. Moertel CG, Fleming TR, Macdonald JS et al, Intergroup study of fluorouracil plus levamisole as adjuvant therapy for stage II/Dukes' B2 colon cancer. *J Clin Oncol* 1995; **13:** 2936.
7. Mamounas EP, Rockette H, Jones J et al, Comparative efficacy of adjuvant chemotherapy in patients with Dukes' B vs Dukes' C colon cancer: results from four NSABP adjuvant studies. *Proc Am Soc Clin Oncol* 1996; **15:** 205.
8. Moertel CG, Fleming TR, Macdonald JS et al, Fluorouracil plus levamisole after resection of stage III colon carcinoma: a final report. *Ann Intern Med* 1995; **122:** 321–6.
9. IMPACT Investigation, Efficacy of fluorouracil and folinic acid in colon cancer. *Lancet* 1995; **345:** 939–44.
10. Wolmark N, Rockette H, Fisher B et al, The benefit of leucovorin-modulated fluorouracil as postoperative adjuvant therapy for primary colon cancer: results from national surgical adjuvant breast and bowel project protocol C-03. *J Clin Oncol* 1993; **11:** 1879–87.
11. O'Connell MJ, Mailliord JA et al, Controlled trial of fluorouralcil and low-dose leucovorin given for 6 months as postoperative adjuvant therapy for colon cancer. *J Clin Oncol* 1997; **1:** 246–50.
12. O'Connell MJ, Laurie JA, Shepherd L et al, A prospective evaluation of chemotherapy duration and regimen as surgical adjuvant treatment for high-risk colon cancer: a collaborative trial of the North Central Cancer Treatment Group and the National Cancer Institute of Canada Clinical Trials Group. *Proc Am Soc Clin Oncol* 1996; **15:** 209.
13. Haller DG, Catalano PJ, Macdonald JS et al, Fluorouracil (FU) leucovorin (LV) and levamisole (LEV) adjuvant therapy for colon cancer; four-year results of INT-0089. *Proc Am Soc Clin Oncol* 1997; **16:** 265a.
14. Piedbois P, Buyse M, Gray R et al, Portal vein infusion as an effective adjuvant treatment for patients with colorectal cancer. *Proc Am Soc Clin Oncol* 1995; **14:** 192.
15. Riethmüller G, Schneider-Gädicke E, Schlimok G et al, Randomised trial of monoclonal antibody for adjuvant therapy of resected Dukes' C colorectal carcinoma. *Lancet* 1994; **343:** 1177–83.
16. Fisher B, Wolmark N, Rockette H et al, Postoperative adjuvant chemotherapy of radiation therapy for rectal cancer: Results from NSABP protocol R-01. *J Natl Cancer Inst* 1988; **80:** 21–9.
17. Gastrointestinal Tumor Study Group,

Prolongation of the disease-free interval in surgically treated rectal carcinoma. *N Engl J Med* 1985; **312:** 1464–72.

18. Gastrointestinal Tumor Study Group, Radiation therapy and fluorouracil with or without semustine for the treatment of patients with surgical adjuvant adenocarcinoma of the rectum. *J Clin Oncol* 1992; **10:** 549–57.

19. Rockette H, Deutsch M, Petrelli N, Effect of postoperative radiation therapy (RTX) when used with adjuvant chemotherapy in Dukes' B and C rectal cancer: results from NSABP R-02. *Proc Am Soc Clin Oncol* 1994; **13:** 193.

20. Cedermark B, The Stockholm II trial on preoperative short term radiotherapy in operable rectal carcinoma. A prospective randomized trial. *Proc Am Soc Clin Oncol* 1994; **13:** 577.

21. Swedish Rectal Cancer Trial, Improved survival with preoperative radiotherapy in resectable rectal cancer. *N Engl J Med* 1997; **336:** 980–7.

22. Minsky BD, Adjuvant therapy for rectal cancer – a good first step. *N Engl J Med* 1997; **336:** 1016–17.

18

Mechanism of drug action in colorectal cancer treatment

Alberto F Sobrero

CONTENTS • Introduction • 5-Fluorouracil • Biochemical modulation of 5-FU • Other fluoropyrimidines • Agents interfering with 5-FU catabolism • New, pure TS inhibitors • Irinotecan • Oxaliplatin

INTRODUCTION

Every chemotherapeutic agent available on the market today has been tested against advanced colorectal cancer. Hormonal agents and biological response modifiers have also been investigated in this disease. However, this chapter is restricted to two main classes of compounds:

(a) those agents that are most often employed in the clinical treatment of advanced colorectal cancer;
(b) those agents that appear most promising in this field.

Thus alkylating and intercalating agents, vinca alkaloids, topoisomerase II inhibitors and taxanes will not be considered here. Cisplatin has also been excluded. Despite the bulky literature on the use of this drug in combination with 5-fluorouracil (5-FU), the clinical evidence suggesting inactivity (or activity at the cost of prohibitive toxicity) is overwhelming.[1] It is therefore fair to say that 5-FU + cisplatin combinations are as little to be recommended as the MOF or MOF–STREP combinations (methyl-CCNU, vincristine, 5-FU and streptozotocin) that were so popular in the early 1980s.

Table 18.1 reports the classification of agents

Table 18.1 Potentially active agents against advanced colorectal cancer

- 5-Fluorouracil (5-FU)
- Other fluoropyrimidines
  - 5-Fluorouridine
  - 5-Fluoro-2'-deoxyuridine, floxuridine
  - 5'-Deoxy-5-fluorouridine, doxifluridine,
  - Furtulon
  - Ftorafur, Tegafur, Futraful
  - Capecitabine
- Agents interfering with 5-FU catabolism
  - UFT
  - Ethynyluracil
  - S1
- Selective thymidylate synthase inhibitors
  - ZD 1694, raltitrexed, Tomudex
  - ZD 9331
  - GW1843 U89
  - AG 331
  - AG 337, Thymitaq
  - LY 231514
- Topoisomerase I inhibitors
  - Irinotecan, CPT-11, Campto
- Oxaliplatin

with intrinsic activity against colorectal cancer. This list has expanded substantially in the last five years, with irinotecan, new thymidylate synthase inhibitors, agents that interfere with 5-FU catabolism and oxaliplatin representing very promising new drugs for this disease.

5-FLUOROURACIL

Development

5-Fluorouracil represents one of the few examples of 'rational drug design': it was developed after the observation that cancer cells utilize uracil more avidly than normal cells.[2] Uracil metabolism was thus perceived as a possible target for selective antineoplastic drug development. The hydrogen atom in position 5 was substituted with a fluorine atom. This halogen was chosen for two reasons: its size similarity with hydrogen and its profound effects on the properties of the resulting compounds. To better understand this point, it helps to compare acetic acid, which is a normal component of our metabolism, with fluoroacetic acid, which is a potent poison. Similarly, the fluorine atom was expected to convert uracil into a poison for those cells that preferentially utilize uracil. This was indeed found to be the case, and 5-FU has a wide spectrum of antineoplastic activity.

Mechanism of action

5-FU by itself is inactive. It needs metabolic activation.[3] The similarity between the fluorine atom and the hydrogen is such that 5-FU utilizes the same transport system and activation pathways as uracil, but, once activated, it may alter cellular function, resulting in cell death. Figure 18.1 illustrates the metabolic pathways of fluoropyrimidine activation and degradation. There are three key active metabolites

- *5-fluorodeoxyuridylate* (5-FdUMP) inhibits the enzyme in the rate-limiting step in DNA synthesis, thymidylate synthase (TS);
- *5-fluorouridine triphosphate* (5-FUTP) is

incorporated into RNA, causing crucial alterations in its processing and function;
- *5-fluorodeoxyuridine triphosphate* (5-FdUTP) (or deoxyuridine triphosphate, dUTP) may be incorporated into DNA instead of deoxythymidine triphosphate (dTTP), the normal substrate for DNA polymerase.

The first two mechanisms predominate in the great majority of experimental tumor systems, while the third seems to operate only in a few others. In addition, it has long been postulated, and demonstrated in animal tumor models, that the antitumor activity of 5-FU depends upon its 'anti-DNA effect', while its toxicity is caused by the anti-RNA mechanism. However, the relative contribution to cytotoxicity of three mechanisms of action is not so well understood. Table 18.2 gives a good idea of the complexity of this system. It summarizes the determinants of sensitivity and resistance to fluoropyrimidines:[3] the complexity is such that one can easily understand why it is so difficult to predict the sensitivity and the toxicity of this drug in an individual patient's tumor. The determinants are subdivided into those contributing to the anti-DNA effects of 5-FU (TS inhibition), those contributing to the anti-RNA effects, and those responsible for the incorporation of fraudulent nucleotides (5-FdUTP or dUTP) into DNA. Another factor may be relevant in this respect, namely 5-FU scheduling.

Importance of 5-FU scheduling

The existence of a relationship between the schedule of 5-FU administration and a specific mechanism of action is suggested by several observations.

1. Plasma levels above the threshold for cytotoxic effects (1 μM) following conventional i.v. bolus doses are maintained for only a few hours.[4] TS inhibition is strictly S-phase-dependent. It is thus unlikely that this enzyme represents a major site of action under conditions of short-term, high-dose exposure. Rather, continuous exposure is likely to affect this mechanism. Conversely,

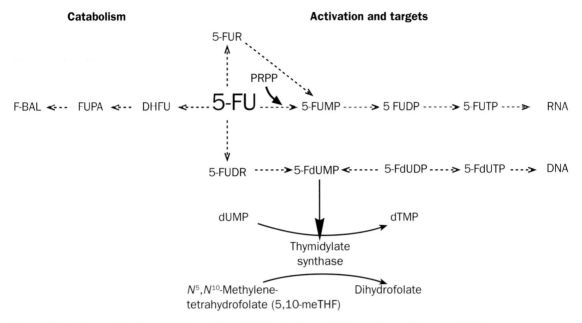

Figure 18.1 The mechanism of action of 5-FU. *Abbreviations*: 5-FUR, 5-fluorouridine; 5-FUDR, 5-fluorodeoxyuridine; DHFU, dihydrofluorouracil; FUPA, β-ureido-α-fluoropropionate; F-BAL, α-fluoro-β-alanine.

the relative independence of 5-FU incorporation into RNA from a specific cell-cycle phase is compatible with significant cytotoxicity, even under conditions of short-term administration. 5-FU peak concentration, rather than duration of exposure, may be the key factor for incorporation into RNA.[5]

2. Prolonged low-dose 5-FU produces cytotoxicity that is prevented by thymidine, whereas, in general, short-term, high-dose 5-FU administration results in growth inhibition refractory to thymidine protection.[6]

3. Finally, long-term, low-dose repeated exposure to 5-FU results in resistance due to impaired stability of TS inhibition, while short-term, high-dose exposure is associated with resistance due to decreased incorporation into RNA.[7] And cells resistant to pulse 5-FU still retain sensitivity to a prolonged exposure to the fluoropyrimidine.[8]

These observations support the contention that 5-FU may be considered as two different drugs, depending on the dose and schedule of administration.[1]

BIOCHEMICAL MODULATION OF 5-FU

General rationale

The mechanism of action of 5-FU is very complex, and the number of biochemical determinants of cytotoxicity are very high. It is therefore reasonable to look for strategies that may favor the activation of the fluoropyrimidine towards this or that active metabolite in order to increase the activity or decrease the toxicity of this drug. For example, if it is true that TS inhibition accounts for the antitumor effect, while the anti-RNA effect is only responsible for toxicity, then optimizing the conditions

Table 18.2 Determinants of sensitivity to fluoropyrimidines

(1) TS-related mechanism
    (A) Enzyme-related
        (a) Baseline activity of enzyme
        (b) Affinity of TS for 5-FdUMP
        (c) Upregulation of TS expression following 5-FU exposure
    (B) Substrate-related
        (a) Baseline dUMP concentration
        (b) dUMP expansion following 5-FU exposure
    (C) Cofactor-related
        (a) Concentration of N^5,N^{10}-methylenetetrahydrofolate (5,10-meTHF)
        (b) Polyglutamylation of 5,10-meTHF
    (D) Inhibitor-related (5-FdUMP)
        (a) Concentration of FdUMP following 5-FU exposure
          • Cellular entry
          • Activity of anabolic and catabolic enzymes
          • Availability of substrates and cofactors
        (b) Duration of 5-FdUMP levels above cytotoxic concentration
    (E) Product-related (dTTP)
    Capacity to salvage endogenous thymidine
(2) RNA-incorporation-related mechanism
    (A) 5-FUPT-related
        (a) Concentration of 5-FUTP following 5-FU exposure
          • Cellular entry
          • Activity of anabolic and catabolic enzymes
          • Availability of substrates and cofactors
        (b) Extent of 5-FUTP incorporation into RNA
    (B) UTP-related
        (a) Concentration of uridine triphosphate (UTP) and cytidine triphosphate (CTP)
        (b) Capacity to salvage endogenous uridine
(3) DNA-damage-related mechanism
    (A) Fraudulent nucleotide
        (a) Extent of 5-FdUTP incorporation into DNA
        (b) Extent of dUTP incorporation into DNA
    (B) DNA repair
        (a) dUTP hydrolase activity
        (b) Uracil DNA glycosylase activity

for prolonged and complete TS inhibition should enhance the efficacy of 5-FU. This could be obtained by exogenous leucovorin (5-formyl-tetrahydrofolate, LV) or by decreasing the rise in dUMP that follows 5-FU exposure. However, we still do not know if the rationale behind this example holds for every case; it is very likely that some colorectal cancers are more sensitive to TS inhibition, while others may be more sensitive to the consequences of 5-FUTP incorporation into RNA. What may be an effective strategy against one patient's cancer may be deleterious for the next patient. Predictive tests would be essential for biochemical modulation, but the number of determinants, the complexity of the assays and the ethical problems connected with sampling limit the results of these studies. Finally, if it is true that the mechanism of action of 5-FU depends upon the schedule of administration, biochemical modulation of the fluoropyrimidine should be schedule-oriented.[9–11] In particular, enhancement of 5-FU cytotoxicity with LV might be greater when the fluoropyrimidine is administered as a continuous infusion while channeling 5-FUra into RNA using methotrexate (MTX), trimetrexate or N-phosphonoacetyl-L-aspartate (PALA) might improve results when high-dose, short-term administration is used. These factors have not been taken into account in most clinical trials.

Enhanced cytotoxicity versus reduced host toxicity

In general, biochemical modulation can be divided into strategies to enhance antitumor cytotoxicity and those to decrease toxicity. An example of the latter approach is delayed uridine rescue from RNA-directed toxicity of 5-FU.[12] But the intrinsic toxicity of the rescue nucleoside and the risk of interfering with the antitumor activity of 5-FU has limited its use. Similarly, allopurinol may antagonize 5-FU by inhibiting its activation to 5-fluorouridylate (5-FUMP).[13] Therefore in general attempts to reduce toxicity are not so popular.

Another important consideration in this respect is the low clinical activity of unmodulated 5-FU (a response rate of only 10–20%): it makes little sense to reduce the toxicity of an agent that is so little active. Most of the time, it would not be used anyway. Thus a higher antitumor activity at the cost of the same toxicity must be reached first. Then pursuing strategies to reduce toxicity will make much more sense.

5-FU plus LV

This is the most popular of all modulations. Inhibition of TS is considered the most important mechanism of cytotoxicity of 5-FU. This enzyme catalyzes the last step in the de novo synthesis of thymidylate (dTMP), and it is the rate-limiting step for DNA synthesis.

In the absence of inhibitors, this enzyme binds the substrate, deoxyuridylate (dUMP), and adds a methyl group to it, producing dTMP. This is phosphorylated to deoxythymidine triphosphate (dTTP) and incorporated into DNA. In this reaction, the source of the methyl group is the reduced folate cofactor N^5,N^{10}-methylenetetrahydrofolate (5,10-meTHF). After binding dUMP, TS binds 5,10-meTHF and transfers the methyl group to dUMP. This is made possible by the elimination of the hydrogen attached to the C-5 position of uracil.[3]

Following 5-FU exposure and adequate 5-FdUMP formation, the methyl transfer does not take place, because the fluorine atom in the C-5 position of 5-FdUMP is much more tightly bound than hydrogen. The enzyme is then trapped in a slowly reversible ternary complex. The presence of 5,10-meTHF (or its polyglutamates) is essential for tight binding of 5-FdUMP to TS. The longer excess 5,10-meTHF is around, the longer TS is blocked, and the more likely the cells will die. Conversely, if insufficient 5,10-meTHF is present, the extent and particularly the duration of TS inhibition will be limited, and the cell may survive. Since endogenous reduced folate levels are suboptimal, supplementation with exogenous folates should enhance TS inhibition.

Besides the biochemical determinants listed in Table 18.2, there are three pharmacologic variables affecting the outcome of this combination:

- the schedule of 5-FU employed;
- the dose of reduced folates;
- the length of exposure to excess exogenous reduced folates.

The importance of the schedule of 5-FU has already been addressed, and specifically investigated in experimental[14] and clinical studies.[9,15]

The dose of reduced folate is important in that concentrations of LV below 1 μM are insufficient to expand intracellular folate pools, and 10 μM is usually considered the target concentration. But the duration of exposure to LV is also crucial. In fact, prolonged exposure to the reduced folates allows extensive polyglutamylation of 5,10-meTHF, which promotes ternary-complex formation much more efficiently than 5,10-meTHF.[16]

5-FU plus inhibitors of de novo pyrimidine synthesis

The dUMP accumulation that occurs following 5-FU exposure may reverse the cytotoxic effects of the fluoropyrimidine via competition with 5-FdUMP binding to TS. In addition, uridine triphosphate (UTP) may compete with 5-FUTP for binding to RNA polymerase, thereby limiting the anti-RNA effects of 5-FU. Inhibitors of pyrimidine biosynthesis might be used to enhance 5-FU activity by depleting the natural uridine nucleotide pools (dUMP and UTP) and promoting the utilization of fraudulent pyrimidine nucleotides, such as 5-FdUMP and 5-FUTP.

The de novo synthesis of pyrimidines begins from simple components and proceeds to uridylate through six reactions. A number of compounds are available to inhibit each of these reactions. The most interesting are PALA and Brequinar.

PALA, N-phosphonoacetyl-L-aspartate, is an inhibitor of aspartate transcarbamoylase, the second step in de novo pyrimidine synthesis, producing substantial decreases in UTP and CTP pools. Two features are particularly appealing in the biochemical modulation of 5-FU with this drug. First, non-cytotoxic doses of PALA are sufficient to lower ribonucleotide pools, and, second, these changes appear to spare normal tissues. Therefore low, non-toxic doses of PALA might successfully modulate 5-FU activity, allowing the use of maximally tolerated doses of 5-FU.[17]

Brequinar sodium potently inhibits dihydroorotate dehydrogenase, the fourth enzyme of the de novo pyrimidine biosynthetic pathway that may be rate-limiting for UMP synthesis. Brequinar increases the cytotoxicity of 5-FU by the general mechanism explained for all these inhibitors.[18]

5-FU plus inhibitors of de novo purine synthesis

The conversion of 5-FU to 5-FUMP by orotate phosphoribosyl transferase (OPRTase) requires 5-phosphoribosyl 1-pyrophosphate (PRPP) as a cofactor. Its level is an important determinant of 5-FU cytotoxicity, and depends on the activity of the enzyme PRPP synthetase as well as on its rate of utilization in reactions of nucleotide biosynthesis. 6-Methylmercaptopurine ribonucleoside (MMPR) is an inhibitor of the first enzyme of the de novo pathway of purine biosynthesis,[19] producing increased availability of PRPP. The same occurs when other inhibitors of de novo purine biosynthesis, such as azaserine (O-diazoacetyl-L-serine) and DON (6-diazo-5-oxo-L-norleucine) are used.

5-FU plus antifolates

All three major mechanisms of 5-FU cytotoxicity may be implicated in this complex schedule-dependent synergistic interaction.

1. When TS is not blocked, it consumes 5,10-meTHF; inhibition of dihydrofolate reductase (DHFR) by antifolates therefore results in progressive depletion of 5,10-meTHF. The whole reduced folate pool decreases, including 10-formyltetrahydrofolate, a required substrate for purine synthesis (Figure 18.2). In addition, dihydrofolate increases, and this cofactor inhibits purine biosynthesis by itself. Because of this antipurine effect, the PRPP pool expands, thereby enhancing 5-FU anabolism to 5-FUMP and its RNA-directed cytotoxicity.[20] This occurs only if antifolates are given before fluoropyrimidines. Conversely, antagonism occurs[21] when antifolates are given after fluoropyrimidines, because the inhibition of TS by 5-FdUMP prevents the

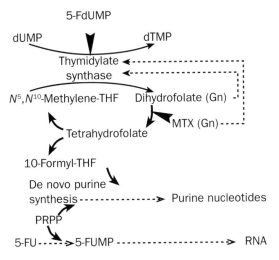

Figure 18.2 The interactions between MTX and 5-FU.

3. Finally, the reduced dTTP levels, as a consequence of TS inhibition by MTX,[26] may promote 5-FdUTP or dUTP incorporation into DNA and contribute to the synergism.

5-FU plus interferon

A host of biochemical, molecular, pharmacologic and immunomodulatory effects have been described[3] as the basis for the reported synergy between the cytokine and 5-FU. However, since several recent large randomized studies[27] have failed to confirm any clinical usefulness of this combination in advanced colorectal cancer, 5-FU–interferon should be regarded like the 5-FU–cisplatin and the MOF combinations.

OTHER FLUOROPYRIMIDINES

5-Fluorouridine and 5-fluoro-2'-deoxyuridine are the ribonucleoside and deoxyribonucleoside derivatives of 5-FU respectively. The rationale for their development may be found in their different metabolic activation pathways. Following phosphorylation, 5-fluorouridine is incorporated into RNA, while 5-fluoro-2'-deoxyuridine inhibits TS. Phosphorylases, however, may convert these nucleosides back to 5-FU, therefore limiting the approach to selectively target one or the other major mechanism of fluoropyrimidine action.

5-Fluorouridine has long been dropped from clinical use owing to its toxicity. 5-Fluoro-2'-deoxyuridine is much more efficiently metabolized by the liver than 5-FU. This is why its major clinical use is in hepatic arterial administration for colorectal cancer with metastases limited to the liver.[28]

Ftorafur is a prodrug of 5-FU. It is a highly lipophilic molecule (a furan nucleoside), and this property accounts for its nearly complete oral bioavailability.[29] In addition, conversion to 5-FU is slow (via a two-step enzymic reaction that takes place mainly in the liver), and the plasma half-life is very long (around 10 hours). As a consequence of these properties, repeated oral administrations of ftorafur should simulate

consumption of 5,10-meTHF, preserving the tetrahydrofolate pool for purine and protein synthesis, thereby antagonizing the effects of MTX on both of these pathways. The sequence of administration of the two agents is thus critical.

2. Enhanced TS inhibition has also been implicated in the synergism: this may be a consequence of a marked increase in the activity of ribonucleotide reductase[22] (triggered by MTX-induced lower dTTP pools), an enzyme that converts 5-FUDP into 5-FdUDP; alternatively,[23] dihydrofolate polyglutamates, accumulating as a consequence of MTX inhibition of DHFR, may tighten the binding of 5-FdUMP to TS, enhancing ternary complex stability. MTX and, in particular, its polyglutamate derivatives may also enhance the binding of 5-FdUMP to TS, by substituting for 5,10-meTHF.[24] However, the fact that trimetrexate[25] (an antifolate with the same mechanism of action as MTX, but incapable of polyglutamylation) still synergizes with fluoropyrimidines in the same sequence-dependent manner makes this last mechanism unlikely.

continuous infusion of 5-FU, without the inconvenience of catheter implantation and the cost of infusion pumps.

Doxifluridine (5'-deoxy-5-fluorouridine) cannot be converted as such into fluorinated nucleotides, because it has the deoxy structure in position 5', which is where phosphorylation occurs.[30] In order to become active, this compound must be converted into 5-FU by the enzyme pyrimidine nucleoside phosphorylase. The rationale for its development is the postulate that the activating enzyme is principally located in tumor tissues and in the intestinal tract, whereas normal proliferating tissues have only low activity.[31] The oral administration of doxifluridine results in 5-FU within the intestinal tract. This is why the major dose-limiting toxicity of this agent is diarrhea. In an attempt to overcome this limitation, capecitabine[32] was developed: this orally active compound is designed to pass the intestinal barrier as the intact molecule. Much less diarrhea occurs. Once in the liver, it is converted to doxifluridine by two enzymes, and hence into 5-FU.

AGENTS INTERFERING WITH 5-FU CATABOLISM

Deficiency in enzymes responsible for 5-FU catabolism, mainly dihydropyrimidine dehydrogenase (DPD), is the cause of the rare but very severe toxicity following conventional doses of the fluoropyrimidine. Interference with 5-FU catabolism (Figure 18.1) is therefore being pursued. Ethinyluracil[33] and S1[34] are examples of agents in phase I clinical studies that are based upon this approach. Inhibition of 5-FU breakdown causes a dramatic reduction in the maximum tolerated dose of 5-FU that can be administered. The key to the success of this strategy lies in its potential selectivity of action.

NEW, PURE TS INHIBITORS

Like 5-FU, these drugs are antimetabolites. Like 5-FU, they inhibit the enzyme TS. But, unlike 5-FU, these compounds are pure inhibitors of TS. In general, they have no other relevant mechanism of action. Most of these compounds are analogues of folic acid, but some (331, 337) are structurally unrelated.

Two key features distinguish all these compounds from each other:[35] the way in which they enter cells (whether or not they utilize the reduced folate carrier) and whether or not they are polyglutamylated. The reason for seeking analogues that differ in terms of these properties is that altered transport and polyglutamylation are known potential mechanisms of resistance. Table 18.3 compares these properties among TS inhibitors that have proven or potential activity against colorectal cancer.

The best known of these compounds is ZD 1694, raltitrexed (Tomudex),[36] which is currently in phase III clinical trials. Once inside the cell, Tomudex is polyglutamylated, and this has two main consequences: it enhances the affinity for binding to TS (up to 100-fold) and it prolongs the intracellular retention time – the large, polyglutamylated molecules do not efflux from the cells as easily as the parent compound.

Following exposure to a therapeutic dose of Tomudex, TS is completely inhibited, and remains so long after drug removal. No new thymidylate is synthesized, and its level falls, resulting ultimately in DNA single- and double-strand breaks and cell deaths.[37]

The theoretical advantages of all these compounds over 5-FU are twofold:

(1) there are no problems associated with the incorporation into nucleic acids;
(2) the increase in deoxyuridylate level, which follows TS inhibition and might compromise further binding of 5-FdUMP to TS, could only be beneficial to ternary complex formation with a folate-based TS inhibitor.

IRINOTECAN (CPT-11)

Irinotecan is an analogue of camptothecin, a natural alkaloid that inhibits the DNA-unwinding enzyme topoisomerase I.[38] This drug is much larger than the parent compound, and it is almost inactive on its own. It needs activation

Table 18.3 TS inhibitors with proven or potential activity against colorectal cancer

Compound	Manufacturer	Clinical development	Toxicity	Use of RFC[a]	Polyglutamylated
ZD 1694, raltitrexed, Tomudex	Zeneca	Phase III	Asthenia, diarrhea, nausea/vomiting, ↑ transaminases	Yes	Yes
ZD 9331	Zeneca	Phase I	To be defined	Yes	No
AG 331	Agouron	Phase I	Nausea/vomiting, flushing	No	No
AG 337, Thymitaq	Agouron	Phase II	Myelotoxicity, mucositis	No	No
GW 1843U89	Glaxo–Wellcome	Phase I	Diarrhea	Yes	Yes, up to diglutamate
LY 231514	Eli–Lilly	Phase II	Neutropenia	Yes	Yes

[a] RFC = reduced folate carrier.

by a carboxylesterase converting enzyme that generates SN38, a compound that is a 1000-fold more potent inhibitor of topoisomerase I than irinotecan. Both the prodrug and SN38 are in two forms: the active, lactone, form and the inactive, carboxylate form. The mechanism of action of SN38 is not completely elucidated, but cytotoxicity appears to be mainly mediated by the interference with topoisomerase I (Figure 18.3). This enzyme allows relaxation of torsional strain in DNA. It binds to supercoiled double-stranded DNA, and produces a nick in one of the DNA chains, allowing free rotation of the DNA molecule on the axis of the intact DNA chain. When SN38 or camptothecin are present, they bind to the complex topisomerase I DNA, and inhibit the so-called re-ligation step of the reaction, i.e. the detachment of the enzyme from the relaxed DNA and the reconstitution of the continuity of the DNA strand that was initially opened. These alterations can be rapidly repaired; the real damage occurs only when a DNA replication fork encounters these complexes (camptothecin–SN38–DNA), resulting in double-strand DNA breaks.

Its partial activity against 5-FU-resistant tumors makes this agent extremely promising, despite the high incidence of severe diarrhea that almost always complicates its administration.[39]

OXALIPLATIN

This is the only platinum analogue with demonstrated single-agent activity against colorectal cancer.[40] Its mechanism of action is the same as that of cisplatin, with DNA as the major target. Intrastrand DNA adducts and interstrand crosslinks are the most relevant type of DNA damage. This agent has no renal toxicity, but substantial neurotoxicity. It synergizes with 5-FU,[41] and is being used in combination with fluoropyrimidines.

ACKNOWLEDGEMENT

This work was supported in part by a grant of the AIRC 1996.

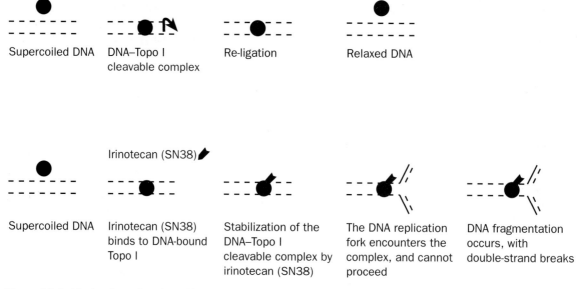

Figure 18.3 Mechanism of action of irinotecan. The upper lines show the role of topoisomerase (Topo) I; the black dot represents Topo I. The lower panels show the effects of the interaction with irinotecan.

REFERENCES

1. Sobrero AF, Aschele C, Bertino JR, Five fluorouracil bolus and continuous infusion: a tale of two drugs. Implications for biochemical modulation in colorectal cancer. *J Clin Oncol* 1997; **15:** 368–81.

2. Heidelberger C, Chauduari NK, Danenberg P et al, Fluorinated pyrimidines. A new class of tumor inhibitory compounds. *Nature* 1957; **179:** 663–4.

3. Grem J, 5-Fluoropyrimidines. In: *Cancer Chemotherapy and Biotherapy Principles and Practice* (Chabner BA, Longo D, eds). Philadelphia: Lippincott Raven, 1996; 149–211.

4. Fraile RJ, Baker LH, Buroker TR et al, Pharmacokinetics of 5-fluorouracil administered orally, by rapid intravenous and by slow infusion. *Cancer Res* 1980; **40:** 2223–8.

5. Nord LD, Stolfi RL, Martin DS, Biochemical modulation of 5-fluorouracil with leucovorin or delayed uridine rescue: correlation of antitumor activity with dosage and FUra incorporation into RNA. *Biochem Pharmacol* 1992; **43:** 2543–9.

6. Evans RM, Laskin JD, Hakala MT, Assessment of growth-limiting events caused by 5-fluorouracil in mouse cells and in human cells. *Cancer Res* 1980; **40:** 4113–22.

7. Aschele C, Sobrero A, Faderan MA et al, Novel mechanism(s) of resistance to 5-fluorouracil in human colon cancer (HCT-8) sublines following exposure to two different clinically relevant dose schedules. *Cancer Res* 1992; **52:** 1855–64.

8. Sobrero A, Aschele C, Guglielmi A et al, Synergism and lack of cross-resistance between short-term and continuous exposure to fluorouracil in human colon adenocarcinoma cells. *J Natl Cancer Inst* 1993; **85:** 1937–44.

9. Sobrero AF, Aschele C, Guglielmi A et al, Schedule-selective biochemical modulation of 5-fluorouracil: a phase II study in advanced colorectal cancer. *Clin Cancer Res* 1995; **1:** 955–60.

10. Santelli G, Valeriote F, Schedule-dependent cytotoxicity of 5-fluorouracil in mice. *J Natl Cancer Inst* 1986; **76:** 159–64.

11. Calabro-Jones PM, Byfield JE, Ward JF et al, Time–dose relationships for 5-fluorouracil cytotoxicity against human epithelial cancer cells in vitro. *Cancer Res* 1982; **42:** 4413–20.

12. Leyva A, Van Groeningen CJ, Kraal I, Phase I

and pharmacokinetic studies of high dose uridine intended for rescue from 5-FU toxicity. *Cancer Res* 1984; **44:** 5928–33.

13. Wooley P, Ayoob M, Smith FP, A controlled trial of the effect of 4-hydroxypyrazolopyrimidine (allopurinol) on the toxicity of a single bolus dose of 5-fluorouracil. *J Clin Oncol* 1985; **3:** 103–9.

14. Moran RG, Scanlon KL, Schedule-dependent enhancement of the cytotoxicity of fluoropyrimidines to human carcinoma cells in the presence of folinic acid. *Cancer Res* 1991; **51:** 4618–23.

15. Leichman CG, Leichman L, Spears CP et al, Prolonged infusion of fluorouracil with weekly bolus leucovorin: a phase II study in patients with disseminated colorectal cancer. *J Natl Cancer Inst* 1993; **85:** 41–4.

16. Nadal JC, Van Groeningen CJ, Pinedo HM et al, In vivo potentiation of 5-fluorouracil by leucovorin in murine colon carcinoma. *Biomed Pharmacother* 1988; **42:** 387–93.

17. Martin DS, Stolfi LR, Sawyer RC et al, Therapeutic utility of utilizing low doses of N-(phosphonacetyl)-L-aspartic acid in combination with 5-fluorouracil: a murine study with clinical relevance. *Cancer Res* 1983; **43:** 2317–21.

18. Pizzorno G, Wiegand RA, Lentz SK, Hanschumacher RE, Brequinar potentiates 5-fluorouracil antitumor activity in a murine model colon 38 tumor by tissue-specific modulation of uridine nucleotide pools. *Cancer Res* 1992; **52:** 1660–5.

19. Paterson ARP, Wang MC, Mechanism of the growth inhibition potentiation arising from combination of 6-mercaptopurine with 6-(methylmercapto)purine ribonucleoside. *Cancer Res* 1970; **30:** 2379–87.

20. Cadman E, Heimer R, Davis L, Enhanced 5-fluorouracil nucleotide formation after methotrexate administration: explanation for drug synergism. *Science* 1979; **205:** 1135–7.

21. Bowen D, Folsch E, Guernsey LA, Fluoropyrimidine-induced antagonism to free and tightly bound methotrexate: suppression of 14C formate incorporation into RNA and protein. *Eur J Cancer* 1980; **16:** 893–9.

22. Elford HC, Bonner EL, Kerr BH et al, Effect of methotrexate and 5-fluorodeoxyuridine and ribonucleotide reductase activity in mammalian cells. *Cancer Res* 1977; **37:** 4389–94.

23. Fernandes DJ, Bertino JR, 5-Fluorouracil–methotrexate synergy. Enhancement of 5-fluorodeoxyuridine binding to thymidylate synthetasa by dihydropteroylpolyglutamates. *Proc Natl Acad Sci USA* 1980; **77:** 5663–7.

24. Santi DV, McHenry CS, Sommer H, Mechanism of interaction of thymidylate synthetase with 5-fluorodeoxyuridylate. *Biochemistry* 1974; **13:** 471–81.

25. Romanini A, Li WW, Colofiore JR, Bertino JR, Leucovorin enhances cytotoxicity of trimetrexate/fluorouracil, but not methotrexate/fluorouracil, in CCRF-CEM cells. *J Natl Cancer Inst* 1992; **84:** 1033–8.

26. Goulian M, Bleile B, Tseng BY, The effects of methotrexate on levels of dUTP in animal cells. *J Biol Chem* 1980; **225:** 10 630–7.

27. Raderer M, Scheithauer W, Treatment of advanced colorectal cancer with 5-fluorouracil and interferon alpha: an overview of clinical trials. *Eur J Cancer* 1995; **31:** 1002–8.

28. Kemeny N, Daly J, Reichman B et al, Intrahepatic or systemic infusion of fluorodeoxyuridine in patients with liver metastases from colorectal carcinoma. *Ann Internal Med* 1987; **107:** 459–65.

29. Au J, Wu AT, Friedman MA, Sadee W, Pharmacokinetics and metabolism of ftorafur in man. *Cancer Treat Rep* 1979; **63:** 343–50.

30. Geng YM, Gheuens E, De Bruijn EA, Activation and cytotoxicity of 5′-deoxy-5-fluorouridine in c-Ha-ras transfected NIH 3T3 cells. *Biochem Pharmacol* 1991; **41:** 301–7.

31. Suzuky S, Hongu Y, Fukazawa H et al, Tissue distribution of 5′-deoxy-5-fluorouridine and derived 5-fluorouracil in tumor bearing mice and rats. *Gann* 1980; **71:** 238–45.

32. Twelwes C, Budman DR, Creaven PJ et al, Pharmacokinetics and pharmacodynamics of capecitabine in two phase I studies. *Proc Am Soc Clin Oncol* 1996; **15:** 1509.

33. Shilsky RL, Burris H, Ratain M et al, Phase I clinical and pharmacologic study of 776C85 plus 5-fluorouracil in patients with advanced cancer. *Proc Am Soc Clin Oncol* 1996; **15:** 1544.

34. Horikoshy N, Mitachi Y, Sugimaky K, Taguchi T, S1, new oral fluoropyrimidine is very active in patients with advanced gastric cancer. *Proc Am Soc Clin Oncol* 1996; **15:** 466.

35. Tuoroutoglu N, Pazdur R, Thymidylate synthase inhibitors. *Clin Cancer Res* 1996; **2:** 227–43.

36. Jackman AL, Farrugia DC, Gibson W et al, ZD 1694 (Tomudex): a new thymidylate synthase inhibitor with activity in colorectal cancer. *Eur J Cancer* 1995; **31A:** 1277–82.

37. Jackman AL, Taylor GA, Gibson W et al, ICI DI

1694, a quinazoline antifolate thymidylate synthase inhibitor that is a potent inhibitor of L1210 tumor growth in vitro and in vivo: a new agent for clinical study. *Cancer Res* 1991; **51:** 5579–86.

38. Takimoto C, Arbuck S, The camptothecins. In: *Cancer Chemotherapy and Biotherapy Principles and Practice* (Chabner BA, Longo D, eds). Philadelphia: Lippincott Raven, 1996; 463–84.

39. Armand JP, Ducreux M, Mahjoubyi M et al, CPT-11 (irinotecan) in the treatment of colorectal cancer. *Eur J Cancer* 1995; **31A:** 1283–7.

40. Diaz Rubio E, Zaniboni A, Gastiaburu J et al, Phase II multicentric trial of oxaliplatin as first line chemotherapy in metastatic colorectal cancer. *Proc Am Soc Clin Oncol* 1996; **15:** 468.

41. Louvet C, Bleiberg H, Gamelin E, Oxaliplatin synergistic clinical activity with 5 fluorouracil in FU resistant colorectal cancer patients is independent of FU plus folinic acid schedule. *Proc Am Soc Clin Oncol* 1996; **15:** 467.

19

Single-agent chemotherapy of colorectal cancer

Thierry Conroy

CONTENTS • **Introduction** • **5-Fluorouracil alone** • **Other fluoropyrimidines** • **Traditional drugs** • **Other agents** • **New drugs**

INTRODUCTION

For nearly 30 years, 5-fluorouracil (5-FU) has remained the only cytotoxic drug available for the treatment of metastatic colorectal cancer (MCC). Recent important developments such as the coadministration of biochemical modulators and the efficacy of adjuvant treatment are described in other chapters. This chapter will focus on several drugs with proven activity against MCC, mainly fluorinated pyrimidines, and some promising drugs: raltitrexed, irinotecan and oxaliplatin.

5-FLUOROURACIL ALONE

5-FU is still the most widely used agent in the treatment of unresectable MCC. However, the drug's real efficiency and the optimal schedule are still being discussed. The range of response rates to 5-FU reported in the literature is wide (3–45%), and depends mostly on dose, schedule and type of study. Monocentric phase II studies with 5-FU (±a modulator) sometimes report high response rates of up to 63% in small groups of patients. Most multicentric phase III studies administering the same schedules to larger patient groups do not reach a 25% response rate.[1–3] This is why our review will focus on the results of randomized studies.

These discrepancies are explained by recruitment bias and methodological differences. Criteria of response are sometimes different. Many studies published in the 1980s considered a 30% decrease in measurements of malignant hepatomegaly below costal margin as a partial response. European trials use WHO criteria, but in nearly all American studies, confirmation of a response is not requested by a second assessment 4 weeks later. In a recent SWOG study,[1] 31% of the responses were unconfirmed, and the response rate increased from 16.7% to 24.2% with the inclusion of responders who had no second confirmatory tests. Quality control is also a recent requirement, and an external review of responses by an independent panel of radiologists improves reliability of data quality.

The response rate to intravenous (i.v.) bolus 5-FU, whatever the dose and schedule used, was evaluated in two meta-analyses. The first included 10 trials comparing bolus 5-FU with 5-FU modulated by leucovorin.[4] The response rate was 11% for bolus 5-FU, including 3% of complete responses. In the subsequent meta-analysis of 8 trials comparing 5-FU versus 5-FU modulated by methotrexate, the response rate of 5-FU alone was 10%, with 2% of complete responses. On excluding data with infusional 5-FU, the results remain the same. The median survival time was 9.1 months. The performance status was the only clinical significant predictor of response and survival,[5] and was identified as the most important factor for survival in many other studies.[2,6–12]

Toxicities of bolus 5-FU are dose-dependent and usually mild. Dose-limiting toxicities are leukopenia and mucositis. Oral cryotherapy decreases the incidence and severity of stomatitis due to bolus 5-FU. Other frequent toxicities are diarrhoea, phlebitis and minor conjunctivitis. The risk of toxic death (around 1%) increases in the rare patients with dihydropyrimidine dehydrogenase deficiency. Women present a higher risk of severe toxicity, including leukopenia, infection, diarrhoea and vomiting. An age of 70 years or more is also a risk factor for severe toxicity, and requires close monitoring of chemotherapy.[13]

Dose response for bolus 5-FU?

Using retrospective data (1967–1986) from phase II and phase III studies on weekly bolus 5-FU, Hryniuk et al[14] suggested a dose-intensity effect for 5-FU. Unfortunately, until now, no randomized studies testing different 5-FU dose intensities have been available to support this hypothesis. However, three randomized trials used bolus 5-FU as control arm, with dose escalation until dose-limiting toxicity. The dose intensity ranged from 472 to 546 mg/m^2/week, and 37–56% of the patients had grade 3 or 4 toxicity. In two trials, confirmation of the response with a second assessment four weeks later was not required. In two of these trials regression of hepatomegaly was accepted as a response criterion, and, in the third study, responses were not externally reviewed. Using these methods, response rates were 12.1%, 17.3% and 23%. The median duration of response was 6 months,[15] and the median time to treatment failure was 3.7 to 4.5 weeks.[16,17] The median survival time ranged from 10.6 to 12.5 months. These results do not appear better than those obtained with standard bolus 5-FU without dose escalation.

Two- or five-day loading bolus 5-FU schedule

5-FU administered as a daily i.v. bolus for five consecutive days every 3–5 weeks was the standard treatment at the beginning of the 1980s. At least eight randomized studies used this schedule as control arm. Results are summarized in Table 19.1. As Hryniuk et al[14] pointed out after analysis of previous trials, a trend towards higher responses rates and longer survival is observed for patients included in trials with the highest projected dose intensity, but patients' characteristics and methods differ from one study to another. Toxicity of this schedule may be severe,[20] and leukopenia is the dose-limiting toxicity.[15] Using a two-day course, with a 600 mg/m^2/week dose intensity of 5-FU, Glimelius et al[8] obtained poor results. Response rate (confirmed by external review) was 3% (95% confidence interval 0–7%) in 91 evaluable patients. The time to treatment failure was 2 months and the median survival time was 6 months.

Three- or five-day loading-dose bolus 5-FU then weekly bolus 5-FU

Three randomized studies had a control arm consisting of an initial loading dose of 5-FU for 3–5 days, followed in 2 weeks by weekly bolus injection (Table 19.2). The major toxicity is leukopenia, following the loading course. In the ECOG study,[12] grade 3 and 4 haematological toxicity was observed in 45% of the patients, with two sepsis-related deaths. In these intensive schedules, response rates ranged from 17.3% to 23%, with median survival time from 10.4 to 12.5 months. Weekly bolus schedules without loading course appear to have the same range of activity (Table 19.2), with very low haematological toxicity.[7,22,23]

High-dose weekly infusional 5-FU

In a phase I/II trial, Ardalan et al[24] identified a 2.6 g/m^2 dose of 5-FU as the maximum tolerated dose administered as a 24-hour infusion on

Table 19.1 Randomized trials with loading i.v. bolus 5-FU schedule

Ref	Projected dose intensity (mg/m²/ week)	Dose escala- tion	Number included	Number evaluable	External review of responses	Response rate (%)	95% CI (%)	CR (%)	Median duration of response (months)	TTF (months)	Median survival (months)
6	750	No	172	74	No	17.6	9.7–28.2	2.7	7.8	ns	14.1
18	687.5	No	90	78	Yes	18	9–27	7.7	13	4.6	14.3
15	625	Yes	113	107	Yes	12.1	ns	ns	6	ns	10.6
19	625	No	78	78	ns	9	ns	ns	ns	5	8
20	500	No	91	87	Yes	7	3–14	0	ns	ns	11
9	500	No	70	39	No	10	ns	ns	ns	3.5	7.7
10	500	No	90	90	No	10	4–16	3.3	ns	6	11
21	462.5	Yes	61	61	No	7	0–13	ns	2.7	2.9	9.6

ns, not stated; TTF, time to treatment failure.

Table 19.2 Randomized trials with weekly i.v. bolus 5-FU

Ref	Loading dose	Weekly dose	Dose escala- tion	Number included	Number evaluable	External review of responses	Response rate (%)	95% CI (%)	Median duration of response (months)	TTF (months)	Median survival (months)
12	500 mg/m²/d × 5	600 mg/m²	No	153	153	No	18	ns	ns	5.1	10.4
16	12 mg/kg/d × 5 d	15 mg/kg	Yes	55	52	Yes	17.3	16–18	ns	4.5	11.3
17	375 mg/m²/d × 3 d	400 mg/m²	Yes	112	102	No	23	ns	ns	3.7	12.5
22	No	15 mg/kg (18 wk)	No	71	68	No	19	10–30.5	9	ns	9.2
23	No	600 mg/m²	No	73	72	No	8.3	2–14.6	ns	3	11
7	No	600 mg/m²	No	69	64	No	16	ns	ns	ns	10.3
11	No	600 mg/m²	Yes	116	ns	ns	6	2–12	ns	3.1	10

ns, not stated; TTF, time to treatment failure.

a weekly basis. This schedule appeared promising, and was tested in an SWOG randomized study.[1] In 63 patients with measurable disease, the response rate was 15%, the median progression-free survival time was 6 months and the median survival time was 15 months.

The EORTC also tested the high-dose infusional 5-FU regimen.[2] The treatment consisted of 60 mg/kg of 5-FU over 48 hours given weekly for 4 weeks and thereafter every 2–3 weeks. Responses were extramurally reviewed. Twelve out of 110 patients (11%) achieved a response. The median survival time was 9.3 months, and myelosuppression was negligible.

Five-day continuous infusion

Five-day 5-FU infusion demonstrated superior efficacy with lower myelotoxicity versus bolus 5-FU in the historic trial by Seifert et al.[25] Two studies confirmed the low toxicity of this regimen. Response rates were 3% and 23% in 55 and 74 patients respectively. The median time to progression was 3.4 months,[27] and the median duration of response was 4.7 months.[25] The median survival times were 12 and 13.8 months respectively. An infusion extended to 14 days at a 5-FU dose of 350 mg/m^2 with a 2-week rest period did not increase 5-FU efficiency.[28] In 88 patients, the response rate was 12.5%, the time to treatment failure was 3.8 months and the median survival time was 10 months.

Long-term continuous infusion

Initiated by Jacob Lokich, protracted 5-FU infusion is a safe and efficient way to administer 5-FU. This treatment modality is discussed in detail in Chapter 23. Briefly, long-term infusional 5-FU was evaluated in 7 randomized studies including 726 patients with measurable disease. The mean response rate was 27% (range 18–45.8%). The median duration of response was 5.5 months,[29] and the median time to disease progression was from 6 to 8 months. In the ECOG study,[12] the median time

to treatment failure was 6.2 months for patients treated with the infusional schedule compared with 5.1 months for bolus 5-FU ($p = 0.007$). Toxicity profiles also favoured infusional 5-FU, which induced no haematological toxicity. However, no statistically significant survival differences were observed in the three trials comparing bolus and infusional 5-FU.[1,12,20] When used as second-line treatment in patients with MCC resistant to bolus 5-FU, the response rate averages 10%.

OTHER FLUOROPYRIMIDINES

Floxuridine (5-fluoro-2'-deoxyxuridine, 5-FUdR)

Floxuridine as a systemic agent showed no advantage over 5-FU in two randomized studies performed in the 1960s. More recently, three randomized trials compared continuous i.v. versus hepatic intraarterial floxuridine in patients with colorectal cancer metastatic to the liver.[30] Systemic floxuridine was given at a dose of 0.075 mg/kg/day (with 0.25/mg/kg/day steps escalation) to 0.125 mg/kg/day for 14 days every 28 days. Dose-limiting toxicity was diarrhoea. The mean response rate was 12.1% (range 7.9–16.3%). Intrahepatic infusion of floxuridine is discussed in detail in Chapter 29.

Doxifluridine (5'-deoxy-5-fluorouridine, 5'-dFUrd)

Doxifluridine is a synthetic 5-FU derivative, which is converted into 5-FU inside the cells by a pyrimidine phosphorylase. In animal models, this enzyme shows especially high activity in tumoral tissues. The drug should therefore have a better therapeutic index than 5-FU. However, the results of a recent randomized phase III study comparing i.v. doxifluridine and 5-FU show a high rate of neurotoxicity (22.3%, including 6% grade 3–4). A daily dose of 4 g/m^2 for 5 days yielded a response rate of 5% (95% confidence interval 2–11%) in 112 patients, and the median survival was 11 months.[31] The oral route is an attractive way to administer doxifluridine. A response rate of 14% (95% confidence interval 5–29%) was reported in a series of 36 elderly patients. The most common side-effect was diarrhoea.[32] Doxifluridine was also evaluated with leucovorin.[33] Both drugs were administered orally. Of 62 patients, 20 (32%; 95% confidence interval 21–45%) achieved a response with a median duration of 4 months. The treatment was well tolerated, but the incidence of diarrhoea was high (29% grade 3 or 4).

Tegafur (Ftorafur, 1-(2-tetrahydrofuranyl)-5-fluorouracil)

Tegafur, a fluoropyrimidine synthesized in 1967, is converted to 5-FU in vivo. Initial studies with i.v. regimens concluded that there was unacceptable CNS toxicity. Daily oral treatment is better tolerated and clinically active, but tegafur has failed to achieve wide acceptance outside Japan and Russia. New interest has arisen in the combination with low-dose oral leucovorin, which has proved to be effective for MCC.[34]

UFT, commercially available in Japan, is composed of tegafur and uracil in a molar ratio of 1:4. Uracil prevents 5-FU degradation, and allows the delivery of a lower total dose of tegafur, thus reducing its neurological toxicity. Phase II studies performed in Japan showed a partial response rate of 25% in 56 patients. Promising results were reported with oral UFT and leucovorin:[35] in a phase II study, the response was 39% (95% confidence interval 28–50%) in 75 evaluable patients. A randomized study versus conventional i.v. 5-FU and leucovorin is warranted.

S-1, a new oral fluorinated pyrimidine, is a combination of tegafur with two modulators, 5-chloro-2,4-dihydroxypyridine (CDHP) and potassium oxonate (oxo). CDHP inhibits 5-FU degradation in the liver to enhance its antitumour effect, and oxo inhibits phosphorylation in the digestive tract to reduce side-effects. Phase II trials are ongoing.

Capecitabine

Capecitabine is a 5-FU prodrug administered orally and absorbed as an intact molecule. It is subsequently activated by a cascade of enzymes, resulting in the preferential release of 5-FU at the tumour site. A partial response in MCC was observed in a phase I study in combination with oral leucovorin.

TRADITIONAL DRUGS

Mitomycin C

Mitomycin C has been used in the treatment of MCC since 1959. Several studies performed before 1977 in previously treated and untreated patients reported a response rate ranging from 12% to 33%, and it was considered at least equal to 5-FU,[36] but myelosuppression was dose-limiting. Recently, a randomized study was performed to assess the protective effect of amifostine on mitomycin haematological toxicity. Ninety-seven patients with MCC resistant to 5-FU received mitomycin 20 mg/m^2 (with or without amifostine) every 6 weeks. Using the WHO criteria, the response rate was 0% and the time to progression was 2.5 months.[37]

Nitrosoureas

Nitrosoureas have long been considered as active drugs in MCC. A response rate of 10–15% for lomustine, carmustine, semustine and streptozocin was described in previously untreated patients.[36] No recent trial has evaluated these drugs with standard criteria of response.

Despite initial reports claiming the benefit of combining 5-FU with semustine and vincristine (MOF), ± streptozocin (MOF-S), subsequent studies failed to confirm any advantage for MOF or any nitrosourea-containing combination therapy, when compared with 5-FU alone.[7] Recent studies have also shown that new nitrosoureas have at best very limited activity (6–7% response rate). This is the case for

ACNU, PCNU and fotemustine. Cystemustine is ineffective. Tauromustine (TCNU) showed promising results in a phase II study including 57 patients, with a response rate of 14%. Two parallel phase III trials were performed, comparing TCNU with best supportive care or with bolus 5-FU. A total of 434 patients were randomized. The response rates were only 1% and 6% for TCNU. The median survival times were 5 or 6 months for TCNU, 6 months for best supportive care, and 10 months for 5-FU ($p = 0.03$ versus TCNU). The median time between progression and death was shorter for patients who received TCNU in both trials, indicating a detrimental effect of the drug.[11]

OTHER AGENTS

Other chemotherapeutic agents, such as alkylating agents, anthracyclines, vinca alkaloids, etoposide, teniposide, cisplatin, carboplatin and taxoids, as well as biological response modifiers such as interferons, tumor necrosis factor and interleukin-2, were found to be ineffective. Octreotide, a somatostatin analogue, was also shown to be ineffective in asymptomatic patients with MCC.

NEW DRUGS

Raltitrexed (Tomudex, ZD1694)

This is an antifolate, and is the first available specific thymidylate synthase inhibitor. Its main advantages are the absence of cardiac toxicity and the convenience of the dosing schedule ($3\,mg/m^2$ i.v. once every 3 weeks). The main toxicities (grade 3–4) are diarrhoea (13%), leukopenia (10%), increase in transaminases (10%) and fatigue (5%). Dose modifications are warranted in patients with renal insufficiency or in the case of hepatic or haematological toxicities. Special attention must be given to vigorous in-hospital management of diarrhoea, especially if associated with neutropenia. In the case of severe toxicity, i.v. folinic acid rescue may reduce toxicity, but can abrogate the antitumour effect.

Raltitrexed has shown interesting activity in MCC: in a large phase II study including 177 patients untreated for advanced disease, the response rate was encouraging (26%; 95% confidence interval 19–33%). The median duration of response was 5.6 months and the median survival time was 9.6 months.[38]

A subsequent randomized study compared raltitrexed versus 5-FU and low-dose leucovorin. Toxicities were statistically different. Patients who received raltitrexed had more anaemia and increased transaminases, but a lower incidence of severe mucositis and leukopenia. There were no differences in response rate (19.8% versus 12.7%), median time to progression, survival or quality of life using the EORTC core questionnaire.[39] Results from the other two randomized studies are needed before considering raltitrexed as an option for first-line treatment of metastatic disease.

Numerous other thymidylate synthase inhibitors are at various phases of clinical development.

Irinotecan (CPT 11)

This is a camptothecin analogue, and has a unique mechanism of action, inhibiting DNA topoisomerase I. The main function of this enzyme is to relax DNA torsional tension as it arises during replication. Irinotecan stabilizes the interaction between the enzyme and DNA, leading to the arrest of replication and to irreversible DNA strand breaks, and eventually to cell death. Irinotecan is an S-phase-specific agent, unaffected by the P-glycoprotein-mediated multidrug-resistant phenotype.

In European clinical studies, irinotecan was administered at a dosage of $350\,mg/m^2$ i.v. every 3 weeks (as a 30–120 minute infusion). Limiting toxicities were diarrhoea and neutropenia. Severe diarrhoea (grade 3 or 4) developed in 13–37% of patients and 8–13.5% of cycles. The risk of diarrhoea increases in patients with performance status >1, age over 65 and previous abdominal radiotherapy. Analysis of four completed phase II studies in patients with MCC that has progressed during 5-FU-based therapy indicates that irinotecan is active in this situation. The overall response rate is 363 evaluable patients is 11.6%, with a median duration of response of 6.7 months. Of the patients previously progressing while on 5-FU, 30% are alive without progression at 6 months, and 14% experienced minor responses or unconfirmed PR. Only half of the responses were observed after 3 cycles, so that, if toxicity is acceptable, treatment should not be interrupted in cases of no change after the first assessment.[40] Results of phase II trials are reported in Table 19.3. The effect of irinotecan on survival has not yet been determined in randomized clinical trials.

Two trials with 49 and 41 patients respectively included exclusively chemotherapy-naive patients.[44,45] Toxicities have been similar and response rates have varied from 25% to 32%. Interestingly, the median response duration was 8.1–8.5 months. Phase II trials with irinotecan combined with 5-FU-containing regimens are ongoing.

Other camptothecin analogues

These have demonstrated activity in preclinical studies. GC 211 and 9-aminocamptothecin were tested in phase II studies in patients with MCC. At the doses and schedules used, these drugs showed no activity. Another topoisomerase I inhibitor, topotecan, has yielded disappointing results, using a daily-times-five i.v. drug administration. The response rate was 0–7% in a total of 76 patients. Administered as a 21-day continuous infusion, topotecan exerted minor activity in untreated patients with MCC. The response rate was 10% of 41 evaluable patients, and the median response duration was 7 months.[46]

Oxaliplatin

This is a platinum complex (*trans-l*-1,2-diaminocyclohexane oxalatoplatinum, L-OHP) with no nephrotoxicity. The main side-effects are cold-induced paresthesias, vomiting and

Table 19.3 Phase II studies of irinotecan in 5-FU-resistant patients

Ref	Irinotecan dose	Number included	Number evaluable	Number of CR + PR (%)	95% CI (%)	Median duration of response (months)
41	100 mg/m^2/wk or 150 mg/m^2/2 wk	51[a]	46	10 (22)	ns	ns
42	125 mg/m^2/wk × 4 −2 wk rest	41[a]	21	5 (24)	ns	ns
43	125–150 mg/m^2/wk × 4 −2 wk rest	48	43	9 (23)	10–36	6
40	350 mg/m^2 q 3 wk	455	363	42 (11.6)	8.5–15.3	6.4

[a] Patients with prior 5-FU-containing regimen, not necessarily resistant to 5-FU.

Table 19.4 Phase II studies of oxaliplatin in fluoropyrimidine-resistant patients

Ref	Oxaliplatin dose (q 21 d)	Number included	Number evaluable	Number of PR (%)	95% CI (%)	Median duration of response (months)
47	30 mg/m²/d × 5 d	30	29	3 (10)	2–27	6
48	130 mg/m²	58	55	6 (11)	3–19	6
48	130 mg/m²	51	51	5 (10)	1.7–18	4.5+

diarrhoea. Three phase II studies have been performed in 135 patients with evaluable MCC resistant to fluoropyrimidines. The overall response rate was 10.4% (Table 19.4). Three partial responses have also been reported out of 14 evaluable patients treated as first-line chemotherapy.[49] Several phase II studies have documented the synergistic effect of oxaliplatin plus 5-FU in 5-FU-resistant MCC patients, with response rates above 25%.[50] Oxaliplatin appears to be a very promising drug, at least in combination with 5-FU second-line treatment, and warrants further evaluation in randomized trials.

REFERENCES

1. Leichman CG, Fleming TR, Muggia FM et al, Phase II study of fluorouracil and its modulation in advanced colorectal cancer: a Southwest Oncology Group Study. *J Clin Oncol* 1995; **13:** 1303–11.
2. Blijham G, Wagener T, Wils J et al, Modulation of high-dose infusional fluorouracil by low-dose methotrexate in patients with advanced or metastatic colorectal cancer: final results of a randomized European Organisation for Research and Treatment of Cancer study. *J Clin Oncol* 1996; **14:** 2266–73.
3. Dufour P, Husseni F, Dreyfus B et al, 5-Fluorouracil versus 5-fluorouracil plus α-interferon as treatment of metastatic colorectal carcinoma. A randomized study. *Ann Oncol* 1996; **7:** 575–9.
4. The Advanced Colorectal Cancer Meta-Analysis Project, Modulation of fluorouracil by leucovorin in patients with advanced colorectal cancer: evidence in terms of response rate. *J Clin Oncol* 1992; **10:** 896–903.
5. The Advanced Colorectal Cancer Meta-Analysis Project, Meta-analysis of randomized trials testing the biochemical modulation of fluorouracil by methotrexate in metastatic colorectal cancer. *J Clin Oncol* 1994; **12:** 960–9.
6. Herrmann R, Knuth A, Kleeberg U et al, Sequential methotrexate and 5-fluorouracil (FU) vs FU alone in metastatic colorectal cancer. Results of a randomized multicenter trial. *Ann Oncol* 1992; **3:** 539–43.
7. Richards F, Case LD, White DR et al, Combination chemotherapy (5-fluorouracil, methyl-CCNU, mitomycine C) versus 5-fluorouracil alone for advanced previously untreated colorectal carcinoma. A phase III trial of the Piedmont Oncology Association. *J Clin Oncol* 1986; **4:** 565–70.
8. Nordic Gastrointestinal Tumor Adjuvant Therapy Group, Superiority of sequential methotrexate, fluorouracil, and leucovorin to fluorouracil alone in advanced symptomatic colorectal carcinoma: a randomized trial. *J Clin Oncol* 1989; **7:** 1437–46.
9. Poon MA, O'Connell MJ, Moertel CG et al,

Biochemical modulation of fluorouracil: evidence of significant improvement of survival and quality of life in patients with advanced colorectal carcinoma. *J Clin Oncol* 1989; **7**: 1407–18.

10. Labianca R, Pancera G, Aitini E et al, Folinic-acid + 5-fluorouracil (5-FU) versus equidose 5-FU in advanced colorectal cancer. Phase III study of GISCAD (Italian Group for the Study of Digestive Tract Cancer). *Ann Oncol* 1991; **2**: 673–9.

11. Smyth JF, Hardcastle JD, Denton G et al, Two phase III trials of tauromustine (TNCU) in advanced colorectal cancer. *Ann Oncol* 1995; **6**: 948–9.

12. Hansen RM, Ryan L, Anderson T et al, Phase III study of bolus versus infusion fluorouracil with or without cisplatin in advanced colorectal cancer. *J Natl Cancer Inst* 1996; **88**: 668–74.

13. Stein BN, Petrelli NJ, Douglass HO et al, Age and sex are independent predictors of 5-fluorouracil toxicity. Analysis of a large phase III trial. *Cancer* 1995; **75**: 11–17.

14. Hryniuk WM, Figueredo A, Goodyear M, Applications of dose intensity to problems in chemotherapy of breast and colorectal cancer. *Semin Oncol* 1987; **14**: 3–11.

15. Petrelli N, Douglas HO, Herrera L et al, The modulation of fluorouracil with leucovorin in metastatic colorectal carcinoma: a prospective randomized phase III trial. *J Clin Oncol* 1989; **7**: 1419–26.

16. Valone FH, Friedman MA, Wittlinger PS et al, Treatment of patients with advanced colorectal carcinomas with fluorouracil alone, high-dose leucovorin plus fluorouracil, or sequential methotrexate, fluorouracil, and leucovorin: a randomized trial of the Northern California Oncology Group. *J Clin Oncol* 1989; **7**: 1427–36.

17. Laufman LR, Bukowski RM, Collier MA et al, A randomized, double-blind trial of fluorouracil plus placebo versus fluorouracil plus oral leucovorin in patients with metastatic colorectal cancer. *J Clin Oncol* 1993; **11**: 1888–93.

18. Di Costanzo F, Bartolucci R, Calabresi F et al, Fluorouracil alone versus high-dose folinic acid and fluorouracil in advanced colorectal cancer: a randomized trial of the Italian Oncology Group for Clinical Research (GOIRC). *Ann Oncol* 1992; **3**: 371–6.

19. Rougier P, Paillot B, Laplanche A et al, End results of a multicentric randomized trial comparing 5-FU continuous systemic infusion (CI) to bolus administration chemotherapy (B) in mea-

surable metastatic colorectal cancer (MCC). *Proc Am Soc Clin Oncol* 1992; **11**: 163 (abst).

20. Lokich JL, Ahlgren JD, Gullo JJ et al, A prospective randomized comparison of continuous infusion fluorouracil with a conventional bolus schedule in metastatic colorectal carcinoma: a Mid-Atlantic Oncology Program study. *J Clin Oncol* 1989; **7**: 425–32.

21. Erlichman C, Fine S, Wong A, Elhakim T, A randomized trial of fluorouracil and folinic acid in patients with metastatic colorectal carcinoma. *J Clin Oncol* 1988; **6**: 469–75.

22. Loehrer PJ, Turner S, Kubilis P et al, A prospective randomized trial of fluorouracil versus fluorouracil plus cisplatin in the treatment of metastatic colorectal cancer: a Hoosier Oncology Group trial. *J Clin Oncol* 1988; **6**: 642–8.

23. Nobile MT, Rosso R, Sertoli MR et al, Randomized comparison of weekly bolus 5-fluorouracil with or without leucovorin in metastatic colorectal carcinoma. *Eur J Cancer* 1992; **28A**: 1823–7.

24. Ardalan B, Singh G, Silberman H, A randomized phase I and II study of short-term infusion of high-dose fluorouracil with or without *N*-(phosphonacetyl)-L-aspartic acid in patients with advanced pancreatic and colorectal cancers. *J Clin Oncol* 1988; **6**: 1053–8.

25. Seifert P, Baker LH, Reed ML, Vaitkevicius VK, Comparison of continuous 5-fluorouracil with bolus injection in treatment of patients with colorectal adenocarcinoma. *Cancer* 1975; **36**: 123–8.

26. Kemeny N, Israel K, Niedzwiecki D et al, Randomized study of continuous infusion fluorouracil versus fluorouracil plus cisplatin in patients with metastatic colorectal cancer. *J Clin Oncol* 1990; **8**: 313–18.

27. Diaz-Rubio E, Jimeno J, Anton A et al, A prospective randomized trial of continuous infusion fluorouracil (5-FU) versus 5-FU plus cisplatin in patients with advanced colorectal cancer. *Am J Clin Oncol* 1992; **15**: 56–60.

28. Weinerman B, Shah A, Fields A et al, Systemic infusion versus bolus chemotherapy with 5-fluorouracil in measurable metastatic colorectal cancer. *Am J Clin Oncol* 1992; **15**: 518–23.

29. Lokich JJ, Ahlgren JD, Cantrell J et al, A prospective randomized comparison of protracted infusional 5-fluorouracil with or without weekly bolus cisplatin in metastatic colorectal carcinoma. A Mid-Atlantic Oncology Program study. *Cancer* 1991; **67**: 14–19.

30. Meta-Analysis Group in Cancer, Reappraisal of

hepatic arterial infusion in the treatment of nonresectable liver metastases from colorectal cancer. *J Natl Cancer Inst* 1996; **88**: 252–8.

31. Bajetta E, Colleoni M, Rosso R et al, Prospective randomized trial comparing fluorouracil versus doxifluridine for the treatment of advanced colorectal cancer. *Eur J Cancer* 1993; **29A**: 1658–63.

32. Falcone A, Pfanner E, Ricci S et al, Oral doxifluridine in elderly patients with metastatic colorectal cancer. A multicenter phase-II study. *Ann Oncol* 1994; **5**: 760–2.

33. Bajetta E, Colleoni M, Di Bartolomeo M et al, Doxifluridine and leucovorin: an oral treatment combination in advanced colorectal cancer. *J Clin Oncol* 1995; **13**: 2613–19.

34. Nogue M, Segui MA, Batiste E et al, Phase II study of oral tegafur (TF) and low-dose oral leucovorin (LV) in advanced colorectal cancer (ACC). *Proc Am Soc Clin Oncol* 1996; **15** 201 (abst).

35. Gonzalez-Baron M, Feliu J, De la Gandara I et al, Efficacy of oral tegafur modulation by uracil and leucovorin in advanced colorectal cancer. A phase II study. *Eur J Cancer* 1995; **31A**: 2215–19.

36. Petrelli NJ, Mittelman A, An analysis of chemotherapy for colorectal carcinoma. *J Surg Oncol* 1984; **25**: 201–6.

37. Poplin EA, Lorusso P, Lokich JJ et al, Randomized clinical trial of mitomycin-C with or without pretreatment with WR-2721 in patients with advanced colorectal cancer. *Cancer Chemother Pharmacol* 1994; **33**: 415–19.

38. Zalcberg JR, Cunningham D, Van Cutsem E et al, A novel thymidylate synthase inhibitor with substantial activity in the treatment of patients with colorectal cancer. *J Clin Oncol* 1996; **14**: 716–21.

39. Cunningham D, Zalcberg JR, Rath U et al, Tomudex (ZD1694): results of a randomized trial in advanced colorectal cancer demonstrate efficacy and reduced mucositis and leucopenia. *Eur J Cancer* 1995; **31A**: 1945–54.

40. Rougier P, Bugat R, Marty M et al, Efficacy of CPT-11 in CRC patients progressive on 5-FU-based chemotherapy. In: *Proceedings of VIth EORTC GITCCG Symposium: An Update after 25 Years of Experience, Nijmegen*, 1996; 97 (abst).

41. Shimada Y, Yoshino M, Wakui A et al, A phase II study of CPT-11, a new camptothecin derivative, in metastatic colorectal cancer. *J Clin Oncol* 1993; **11**: 909–13.

42. Pitot HC, Wender D, O'Connell MJ et al, Phase II trial of CPT-11 (Irinotecan) in patients with metastatic colorectal cancer: a North Central Cancer Treatment Group (NCCTG) study. *Proc Am Soc Clin Oncol* 1994; **13**: 197 (abst).

43. Rothenberg ML, Eckardt JR, Kuhn JG et al, Phase II trial of irinotecan in patients with progressive or rapidly recurrent colorectal cancer. *J Clin Oncol* 1996; **14**: 1128–35.

44. Rougier P, Culine S, Bugat R et al, Multicentric phase II study of first line CPT-11 (irinotecan) in advanced colorectal cancer (CRC): preliminary results. *Proc Am Soc Clin Oncol* 1994; **13**: 200 (abst).

45. Conti JA, Kemeny NE, Saltz LB et al, Irinotecan is an active agent in untreated patients with metastatic colorectal cancer. *J Clin Oncol* 1996; **14**: 709–15.

46. Creemers GJ, Gerrits CJH, Schellens JHM et al, A phase II and pharmacologic study of Topotecan administered as a 21-day continuous infusion to patients with colorectal cancer. *J Clin Oncol* 1996; **14**: 2540–5.

47. Levi F, Perpoint B, Garufi B et al, Oxaliplatin activity against metastatic colorectal cancer. A phase II study of 5-day continuous venous infusion at circadian rhythm modulated rate. *Eur J Cancer* 1993; **29A**: 1280–4.

48. Machover D, Diaz-Rubio E, De Gramont A et al, Two consecutive phase II studies of oxaliplatin (L-OHP) for treatment of patients with advanced colorectal carcinoma who were resistant to previous treatment with fluoropyrimidines. *Ann Oncol* 1996; **7**: 95–8.

49. Diaz-Rubio E, Zaniboni A, Gastiaburu J et al, Phase II multicentric trial of oxaliplatin (L-OHP) as first line chemotherapy in metastatic colorectal carcinoma (MCRC). *Proc Am Soc Clin Oncol* 1996; **15**: 207 (abst).

50. Louvet C, Bleiberg H, Gamelin E et al, Oxaliplatin (L-OHP) synergistic clinical activity with 5-fluorouracil (FU) in FU resistant colorectal cancer (CRC) patients (pts) is independent of FU ± folinic acid (FA) schedule. *Proc Am Soc Clin Oncol* 1996; **15**: 206 (abst).

20

Past combination chemotherapy of colorectal cancer

Werner Scheithauer

INTRODUCTION

The cure of childhood leukemias and Hodgkin's disease with combination chemotherapy in the 1960s proved that human cancers, even in their advanced stages, could be cured by drugs. The application of chemotherapy to solid tumours then began.

Based on animal studies published by Goldin and Mantel[1] in 1957, and 'with the hope that a larger proportion of cancer cells can be killed by the simultaneous administration of several antitumour agents without increasing their harmful effects on normal tissues', in 1965 Horton and co-workers[2] investigated a combination of 5-fluorouracil (5-FU), mitomycin C, vincristine and thiotepa in advanced malignancies, including 12 patients with colorectal cancer. They observed 'a sufficient number of regressions to indicate that the combination of drugs had a definite antitumour effect', i.e. four of the 37 evaluated patients had a tumour regression greater than 50%, and 7 other patients, including 2 with colon cancer, had a regression of 25–49%. The authors noted that the duration of remission was generally short (4–11 weeks) and that the use of a high dose of the four drugs resulted in a 'quite pronounced toxicity', including 4 (9%) treatment-related deaths due to severe leukopenia. The authors commented that '... The clinical status of some patients whose tumours regressed was improved by the combination treatment and the toxic effects were undoubtedly worthwhile. Others derived no clinical benefit from the temporary shrinkage of their tumours and were in fact probably made more ill by treatment.' Continuation of the study of combinations of drugs in advanced cancer was planned with the intent to use lower doses and to perform a comparison with control patients treated by a single drug from the combination.

EMPIRICAL COMBINATION REGIMENS

In the following three decades, numerous other cytotoxic drug combinations were investigated in the search for more effective treatments of colorectal cancer. Because of the limited number of chemotherapeutic options, most attempts to improve systemic treatment have consisted in empirically adding other drugs to 5-fluorouracil. Early studies of such combination chemotherapy regimens, including MIFUC (mitomycin C, cytosine arabinoside and

5-FU),[3-5] 5-FU + Cytoxan, CYFUCA (Cytoxan, 5-FU and cytosine arabinoside), 5-FU + BCNU or BCNU + mitomycin C[6,7] were very unsuccessful – no therapeutic advantage over 5-FU was noted. In 1975, however, Moertel and co-workers[8] at the Mayo Clinic recorded a 43.5% objective response rate with a combination of 5-FU, methyl-CCNU and vincristine. This was significantly superior in a randomized comparison to the usual 19% with 5-FU alone. Subsequently, similar advantages over 5-FU

alone were demonstrated in controlled studies with 5-FU, methyl-CCNU and vincristine by Falkson[9] and with 5-FU and methyl-CCNU by the Southwest Oncology Group.[10] In the latter randomized trial, 271 patients were included and treated with intravenous 5-FU (400 mg/m²/week), either alone or combined with oral methyl-CCNU (175 mg/m²/week). The response to 5-FU alone was 14%, whereas 38 of 128 patients (30%) responded to the combination regimen. Unfortunately, apart from an

Table 20.1 Studies of MOF ± streptozotocin combination regimens in advanced colorectal cancer

Reference	Regimen	No. of patients	Response rate (%)
Baker et al[10]	5-FU + methyl-CCNU[a]	128	30
Moertel[11]	5-FU + methyl-CCNU	62	16
Posey et al[12]	5-FU + methyl-CCNU	37	37
Lavin et al[13]	5-FU + methyl-CCNU[a]	88	10
Buroker et al[14]	5-FU + methyl-CCNU[a]	111	17
Lokich et al[15]	5-FU + methyl-CCNU	52	3
Engstrom et al[16]	5-FU + methyl-CCNU[a]	103	9
Moertel et al[8]	Methyl-CCNU + vincristine + 5-FU[a]	39	43.5
Moertel[11]	Methyl-CCNU + vincristine + 5-FU	137	27
Falkson and Falkson[9]	Methyl-CCNU + vincristine + 5-FU[a]	46	37
Lavin et al[13]	Methyl-CCNU + vincristine + 5-FU[a]	81	12
Engstrom et al[16]	Methyl-CCNU + vincristine + 5-FU[a]	92	11
Macdonald et al[17]	Methyl-CCNU + vincristine + 5-FU	25	40
Kemeny et al[18]	Methyl-CCNU + vincristine + 5-FU	69	10
Kemeny et al[20]	MOF + streptozotocin[a]	77	32
Weltz et al[21]	MOF + streptozotocin	40	25
GITSG[22]	MOF + streptozotocin	40	10
Buroker et al[23]	MOF + streptozotocin[a]	38	34

[a]Part of a randomized trial.

increase in toxicity with the combined treatment, in none of these studies was a significant survival advantage observed. Further attempts to confirm the superiority of MOF- or MF-type regimens have not been uniformly successful (Table 20.1). Even the Mayo Clinic group, analyzing an expanded population of 137 patients, showed their response rates to have fallen from 43.5% to 27%.[11] Overall, response rates for MOF- or MF-type regimens have ranged from 4% to 40%,[8–18] a heterogeneity that does not seem surprising in view of the reported response rates of 5-FU alone, which vary tenfold.

Simple attempts to substitute or add another alkylating-type agent, such as mitomycin C, for the nitrosourea have not resulted in reproducible and clinically meaningful differences.[14,19] There have been attempts to combine multiple alkylating-type agents such as 5-FU, methyl-CCNU, mitomycin or MOF and streptozotocin[20–23] (Table 20.1). Randomized trials with appropriate control groups have again failed to duplicate these results and to demonstrate a significant survival superiority for any such combination.[20,24] In 1978, Moertel[25] wrote that '... it must be concluded that there is no chemotherapy approach to gastrointestinal carcinoma valuable enough to justify application of standard clinical treatment.' And in subsequent correspondence: 'I cannot accept the contention that gastrointestinal cancer patients' most ideal and frequently only opportunity to receive beneficial chemotherapy should be wasted by exposure to routine 5-FU at either toxic or non-toxic doses. On the other hand, I do think that pessimism about treatment for these patients can be dispelled by thoughtfully designed clinical research programmes which offer the hope of realistic gain.'

PRECLINICALLY DESIGNED COMBINATION REGIMENS

Despite subsequent improvements in anticancer drug screening models,[27–31] and continuing extensive preclinical as well as clinical research efforts, regrettably, until today no major advances have been achieved, at least concerning the effectiveness of conventional combination chemotherapy in advanced colorectal cancer.

Other cytotoxic agents that have been added to fluorouracil regimens, and that were evaluated clinically on the basis of promising in vitro response activity of the combination in human tumour cell lines and/or nude mouse transplant tumours, include triazinate, a potent dihydrofolate reductase inhibitor,[32,33] razoxane (ICRF-159), an orally administered piperazine derivative,[33] melphalan,[34–36] doxorubicin and other anthracyclines,[37–39] mitoxantrone,[40] vindesine[41] and spirogermanium, an azaspiran–germanium compound.[42,43] Therapeutic results in humans have not only remained disappointing, but since these additional agents contribute their own toxicity profiles, adverse reactions associated with these combination regimens have been necessarily greater than with 5-FU alone.

More recently, cisplatin/5-fluorouracil regimens have been tried against colon cancer by many investigators, largely because of the activity of this heavy-metal complex against other solid tumours and its putative synergy with 5-FU.[44] Experimental data accumulated by Schabel and associates[44] suggested that the most synergistically active combination of drugs in L1210 leukemia murine models was cisplatin plus 5-FU, which produced a 60% cure rate. In 1987 Cantrell et al[45] reported a substantially improved response rate in patients with colorectal cancer when they were treated with a combination of 5-FU infusion and weekly low-dose cisplatin. In that study, 20 of 32 evaluable patients achieved either complete or partial response. Enhanced effectiveness with this combination was consistent in a number of phase II studies in advanced colon cancer,[46] and improved benefit was seen in head and neck and esophageal cancers at that time.[47,48] Toxicity, however, was severe. It was subsequently demonstrated that the dose-limiting myelosuppression of the combination was much more manageable when 5-FU was given by infusion rather than bolus administration. Similarly, the objective response rates seemed

Table 20.2 Randomized studies of 5-fluorouracil + cisplatin compared with 5-fluorouracil alone in patients with advanced colorectal cancer

Reference	5-FU dose	Cisplatin dose	No. of patients	Response rate (%)	and survival (wk)
Labianca et al[49]	600 mg/m²/wk		28	15	56
	600 mg/m²/wk	60 mg/m² q 3 wk	26	20	43
Loehrer et al[50]	15 mg/kg/wk		68	19	39
	15 mg/kg/wk	60 mg/m² q 3 wk	64	22	40
Poon et al[51]	500 mg/m²/d × 5 d		28	10	31
	325 mg/m²/d × 5 d	20 mg/m²/d × 5 d	26	15	30
Díaz-Rubio[52]	1000 mg/m²/d CI × 5 d		18	23	39
	1000 mg/m²/d CI × 5 d	100 mg/m² q 4 wk	21	21	51
Lokich et al[53]	300 mg/m²/d CI × 10 wk		54	33	42
	300 mg/m²/d CI × 10 wk	20 mg/m²/wk	54	31	48
Kemeny et al[54]	1000 mg/m²/d × 5 CI q 4 wk		59	3	52
	1000 mg/m²/d × 5 CI q 4 wk	20 mg/m²/d × 5 q 4 wk	16	25	43
Hansen et al[55]	500 mg/m²/d × 5 d >×1/wk		153	18	42
	500 mg/m²/d × 5 d >×1/wk	20 mg/m²/wk[a]	12	—	—
	300 mg/m²/d CI		159	28	52
	300 mg/m²/d CI	20 mg/m²/wk	153	31	52[a]

[a]Discontinued because of excessive toxicity after only 12 patients had begun treatment.

higher when 5-FU was coadministered as a continuous infusion.[46] Randomized trials comparing intravenous push,[49,50] prolonged i.v. infusion[51–54] and both administration schedules of 5-FU,[55] however, confirmed neither higher response rates nor prolongation of survival time for the combination treatment. The only exception is a study by Kemeny et al.[54] This trial revealed a higher response rate for 5-FU/cisplatin – but again no impact on survival. The combined data of the phase III trials shown in Table 20.2 thus do not support the use of cisplatin/5-FU combinations for the treatment of colorectal cancer outside clinical trials. Concomitant treatment with cisplatin seems to cause added toxicity and complexity of treatment without providing a major clinical benefit.

For the first time, new agents, including Tomudex, CPT-11 and oxaliplatin, have been shown to be active in colorectal cancer. It is hoped that their combinations with 5-FU will ultimately improve the clinical outcome of patients with advanced disease.

REFERENCES

1. Goldin A, Mantel N, The employment of combinations of drugs in the chemotherapy of neoplasia: a review. *Cancer Res* 1957; **17**: 635–54.
2. Horton J, Olson KB, Gehrt P, Spear M, Combination therapy with 5-fluorouracil (NSC-19893), mitomycin C (NSC-26980), vincristine (NSC-67574), and thiotepa (NSC-6396) for advanced cancer. *Cancer Chemother Rep* 1965; **49**: 59–61.
3. Ota K, Kurita S, Nishimura M et al, Combination therapy with mitomycin C (NSC-26980), 5-fluorouracil (NSC-19893), and cytosine arabinoside (NSC-63878) for advanced cancer in man. *Cancer Chemother Rep* 1972; **56**: 373–85.
4. Yagoda A, Lippman A, Winn R et al, Mitomycin C, 5-FU, and cytosine arabinoside (MiFuCa) in adenocarcinomas. *Proc Am Assoc Cancer Res and Am Soc Clin Oncol* 1974; **15**: 190 (abst).
5. DeJager RL, Magill GB, Golbey RB, Combination chemotherapy with mitomycin C, 5-fluorouracil, and cytosine arabinoside in gastrointestinal cancer. *Cancer Treat Rep* 1976; **60**: 1373–5.
6. Carter SK, Large bowel cancer – the current status of treatment. *J Natl Cancer Inst* 1974; **56**: 3–10.
7. Carter SK, Friedman M, Integration of chemotherapy into combined modality treatment of solid tumors. *Cancer Treat Rev* 1974; **1**: 111–29.
8. Moertel CG, Schutt AJ, Hahn RG, Reitemeier RJ, Therapy of advanced colorectal cancer with a combination of 5-fluorouracil, methyl-1,3-*cis*-(chloroethyl)-1-nitrosurea + vincristine. *J Natl Cancer Inst* 1975; **65**: 69–71.
9. Falkson G, Falkson HC, Fluorouracil, methyl-CCNU + vincristine in cancer of the colon. *Cancer* 1976; **38**: 1468–70.
10. Baker LH, Vaitkevicius VK, Gehan E, and the Gastrointestinal Committee of the Southwest Oncology Group, Randomized prospective trial comparing 5-fluorouracil (NSC 19893) to 5-fluorouracil and methyl CCNU (NSC 95441) in advanced gastrointestinal cancer. *Cancer Treat Rep* 1976; **60**: 733–7.
11. Moertel CG, Chemotherapy of gastrointestinal cancer. *N Engl J Med* 1978; **299**: 1049–52.
12. Posey L, Morgan LR, Methyl CCNU versus methyl CCNU and 5-fluorouracil in carcinoma of the large bowel. *Cancer Treat Rep* 1977; **61**: 1453–8.
13. Lavin P, Mittleman A, Douglass H et al, Survival and response to chemotherapy for advanced colorectal adenocarcinoma. An Eastern Cooperative Oncology Group report. *Cancer* 1980; **46**: 1536–43.
14. Buroker T, Kim PN, Groppe C et al, 5-FU infusion with mitomycin C vs. 5-FU infusion with methyl CCNU in the treatment of advanced colon cancer. *Cancer* 1978; **42**: 1228–33.
15. Lokich JJ, Skarin AT, Mayer RJ, Frei E, Lack of effectiveness of combined 5-FU and methyl-CCNU therapy in advanced colorectal cancer. *Cancer* 1977; **40**: 2792–6.
16. Engstrom P, MacIntyre JM, Douglass HO Jr et al, Combination chemotherapy of advanced colorectal cancer utilizing 5-fluorouracil, semustine, dacarbazine, vincristine, and hydroxurea: a phase III trial by the Eastern Cooperative Oncology Group (EST 4275). *Cancer* 1982; **49**: 1555–60.
17. Macdonald JS, Kisner DF, Smythe T, 5-Fluorouracil (5-FU), methyl CCNU and vincristine in the treatment of advanced colorectal cancer: phase II study utilizing weekly 5-FU. *Cancer Treat Rep* 1976; **60**: 1597–600.
18. Kemeny N, Yagoda A, Braun D Jr, Golbey R, A randomized study of two different schedules of methyl CCNU, 5-FU, and vincristine for metastatic colorectal adenocarcinoma. *Cancer* 1980; **46**: 1536–43.
19. Ramming KP, Tesler AS, Haskell CM, Gastrointestinal tract neoplasms. In: *Cancer Treatment* (Haskel CM, ed). Philadelphia: WB Saunders, 1980: 300–72.
20. Kemeny N, Yagoda A, Braun J, Metastatic colorectal carcinoma: a prospective trial of methyl CCNU, 5-fluorouracil (5-FU) and vincristine (MOF) versus MOF plus streptozotocin (MOF-Strep). *Cancer* 1983; **51**: 20–5.
21. Weltz MD, Perry DJ, Blom J, Methyl CCNU, 5-fluorouracil, vincristine, and streptozotocin (MOF-Strep) in metastatic colorectal carcinoma. *J Clin Oncol* 1983; **1**: 135–7.
22. Gastrointestinal Tumor Study Group, Phase II study of MOF-Strep (methyl CCNU, vincristine, 5-fluorouracil, streptozotocin) in advanced measurable colorectal carcinoma. *J Clin Oncol* 1984; **2**: 770–2.
23. Buroker TR, Moertel CG, Fleming TR et al, A control evaluation of recent approaches to biochemical modulation or enhancement of 5-fluorouracil in colorectal carcinoma. *J Clin Oncol* 1985; **3**: 1624–31.

24. Richards FD, Case LD, White DR et al, Combination chemotherapy (5-fluorouracil, methyl-CCNU, mitomycin C) versus 5-fluoro-uracil alone for advanced previously untreated colorectal cancer: a phase III study of the Piedmont Oncology Association. *J Clin Oncol* 1986; **4**: 565–70.

25. Moertel CG, Current concepts in cancer: chemotherapy of gastrointestinal cancer. *N Engl J Med* 1978; **299**: 1049–52.

26. Moertel CG, Letter. *N Engl J Med* 1979; **301**: 329.

27. Shoemaker RH, Wolpert-DeFilippes MK, Kern DH et al, Application of a human tumor colony-forming assay to new drug screening. *Cancer Res* 1985; **45**: 2145–53.

28. Peckham MJ, Courtenay VD, Steel GG, Experimental chemotherapy of gastrointestinal carcinoma xenografts. *Cancer Treat Rev* 1979; **6**(Suppl): 43–50.

29. Finlay GJ, Baguley BC, The use of human cancer cell lines as a primary screening system for anti-neoplastic compounds. *Eur J Cancer Clin Oncol* 1984; **20**: 947–54.

30. Edelstein MB, Smink T, Ruiter DJ et al, Improvements and limitations of the subrenale capsule assay for determining tumor sensitivity to cytostatic drugs. *Eur J Cancer Clin Oncol* 1984; **20**: 1549–56.

31. Scheithauer W, Clark GM, Moyer MP, Von Hoff DD, New screening system for selection of anti-cancer drugs for treatment of human colorectal cancer. *Cancer Res* 1986; **46**: 2703–8.

32. Shaw MT, Bonnet JD, Wilson H, Heilbrun LK, Bakers' antifol in combination with 5-fluorouracil and methyl CCNU in the treatment of metastatic colorectal cancer: a Southwest Oncology Group study (protocol 7764). *Cancer Treat Rep* 1980; **64**: 247.

33. Windschitl H, Scott M, Schutt A et al, Randomized phase II studies in advanced colorectal carcinoma: a North Central Cancer Treatment Group study. *Cancer Treat Rep* 1983; **67**: 1001–8.

34. Gough IR, Furnival CM, Burnett W, Melphalan and 5-fluorouracil in advanced gastrointestinal carcinoma: a preliminary report. *Cancer Treat Rev* 1979; **6**(Suppl): 127–9.

35. Gough IR, Furnival CM, Thynne GSJ, Phase II trial of 5-FU plus melphalan in advanced colorectal carcinoma. *Cancer Treat Rep* 1981; **65**: 735–6.

36. Gough IR, Furnival CM, High-dose intermittent iv 5-FU and melphalan in advanced colorectal carcinoma. *Cancer Treat Rep* 1983; **67**: 595–6.

37. O'Connell MJ, Moertel CG, Rubin J et al, Lack of clinical therapeutic synergism between cyclophosphamide, adriamycin, and *cis*-dichlorodiammine-platinum(II) in metastatic human colorectal carcinoma. *Cancer Treat Rep* 1980; **64**: 311–12.

38. Haller DG, Woolley PV, Macdonald JS et al, Phase II trial of 5-fluorouracil, adriamycin, and mitomycin C in advanced colorectal cancer. *Cancer Treat Rep* 1978; **62**: 563–655.

39. White LA Jr, Perry MC, Kardinal CG et al, Phase II study of 5-fluorouracil, methyl-CCNU, and daunorubicin in colorectal cancer: a Cancer and Leukemia Group B study. *Cancer Treat Rep* 1979; **63**: 154–6.

40. Schroeder M, Donhuijsen-Ant R, Westerhausen M, 5-Fluorouracil plus mitoxantrone in the treatment of advanced colorectal cancer: initial experiences. *Blut* 1986; **53**: 211 (abst).

41. Planting A, Hillen H, Dejong M, Phase II study: vindesine + 5-fluorouracil combination chemotherapy in advanced colorectal cancer. *Eur J Cancer Clin Oncol* 1986; **22**: 533.

42. McMaster ML, Greco FA, Johnson DH, Hainsworth JD, An evaluation of combination 5-fluorouracil and spirogermanium in the treatment of advanced colorectal carcinoma. *Invest New Drugs* 1990; **8**: 87–92.

43. Williamson SK, Slavik M, Phase I evaluation of spirogermanium and 5-fluorouracil in colorectal carcinoma. *Invest New Drugs* 1991; **9**: 49–52.

44. Schabel FM, Trade MW, Laster WR et al, *Cis*-dichlorodiammine-platinum(II): combination chemotherapy and cross resistance studies with tumors in mice. *Cancer Treat Rep* 1979; **63**: 1459–73.

45. Cantrell JE Jr, Hart RD, Raylor RF, Harvey JH Jr, Pilot trial of prolonged continuous-infusion 5-fluorouracil and weekly cisplatin in advanced colorectal cancer. *Cancer Treat Rep* 1987; **71**: 615–18.

46. Köhne-Wömper CH, Schmoll JH, Harstrick A, Rustum YM. Chemotherapeutic strategies in metastatic colorectal cancer: an overview of current clinical trials. *J Clin Oncol* 1992; **19**(Suppl 3): 105–25.

47. Weaver A, Fleming S, Vandenberg H, Cisplatinum and 5-fluorouracil as initial therapy in advanced epidermoid cancers of the head and neck. *Head Neck Surg* 1982; **4**: 370–3.

48. Leichmann L, Seydel HG, Steiger Z, Preoperative adjuvant therapy for squamous cell cancer of the esophagus: SWOG and RTOG trials. *Proc Am Soc Clin Oncol* 1984; **3**: 147 (abst).

49. Labianca R, Pancera G, Cesana B et al, Cisplatin + 5-fluorouracil versus 5-fluorouracil alone in advanced colorectal cancer: a randomized study. *Eur J Cancer* 1988; **24:** 1579–81.

50. Loehrer PJS, Turner S, Kubilis P et al, A prospective randomized trial of fluorouracil versus flourouracil plus cisplatin in the treatment of metastatic colorectal cancer: a Hoosier Oncology Group trial. *J Clin Oncol* 1988; **6:** 642–8.

51. Poon MA, O'Connell MJ, Moertel CG et al, Biochemical modulation of fluorouracil: evidence of a significant improvement of survival and quality of life in patients with advanced colorectal carcinoma. *J Clin Oncol* 1989; **7:** 1407–18.

52. Díaz-Rubio E, Milla A, Jimero J, Belon J, Aranda E, Díaz Faes J et al, Lack of clinical synergism between cisplatin (CDDP) and 5-fluorouracil (5-FU) in advanced colorectal cancer (CRC). Results of a randomized study. *Proc Am Soc Clin Oncol* 1988; **7:** 110 (abst).

53. Lokich JJ, Cantrell JE, Ahlgren JD, Phillips J, A phase III trial of protracted infusional 5-FU (PIF) vs. PIF plus weekly bolus cisplatin (CDDP) in advanced measurable colon cancer (MAOP protocol 5286). *Proc Am Soc Clin Oncol* 1989; **8:** 104 (abst).

54. Kemeny N, Israel K, Niedzwiecki D et al, Randomized study of continuous infusion fluorouracil versus fluorouracil plus cisplatin in patients with metastatic colorectal cancer. *J Clin Oncol* 1990; **8:** 313–18.

55. Hansen RM, Ryan L, Anderson T et al, Phase III study of bolus versus infusion fluorouracil with or without cisplatin in advanced colorectal cancer. *J Natl Cancer Inst* 1996; **88:** 668–73.

21

Metabolic modulation of 5-fluorouracil by high-dose leucovorin: Preclinical rationale and clinical efficacy

Youcef M Rustum, Shousong Cao

INTRODUCTION

5-Fluorouracil (5-FU) is known to exert its antiproliferative effects following its metabolic activation. 5-FU can be preferentially metabolized via either the deoxyribonucleotide pathway or the ribonucleotide pathway, depending on the relative activity of the enzymes involved and the relative availability of deoxyribose-1-P or ribose-1-P (Figure 21.1). Along the ribonucleotide pathway, 5-FU is anabolized to 5-fluorouridine triphosphate (5-FUTP), which is incorporated into RNA;[1-3] the consequence of this incorporation is the production of fraudulent RNA, which can ultimately cause cell death. Along the deoxyribonucleotide pathway, 5-FU is anabolized to 5-fluorodeoxyuridine monophosphate (5-FdUMP), which is a potent inhibitor of the enzyme thymidylate synthase (TS);[4-11] this enzyme inhibition leads to decreased thymidine triphosphate pools and to inhibition of DNA synthesis. These two mechanisms of action cooperate to determine 5-FU cytotoxicity, but their relative importance to 5-FU therapeutic selectivity may depend on the tumor type and on the schedule of drug administration. The pools of 5-FdUMP are also derived from the conversion of 5-FUDP to 5-FdUDP via the ribonucleotide reductase. It is known that in some cell lines, 5-FdUTP is incorporated into cellular DNA, and it has been proposed that this incorporation is the determinant of 5-FU action in vitro.

In addition to being anabolized, 5-FU is degraded to the level of carbon dioxide (CO_2) by dihydrouracil dehydrogenase. In fact, this degradation is rapid, and over 90% of the injected dose ends up as CO_2 within a few minutes. Of the approximately 10% or so of the drug available for anabolism, 80–90% is present intracellularly as acid-soluble (5-FUTP) and acid-insoluble (F-RNA). Thus, only a small fraction of the injected dose is in the form of 5-FdUMP, the potent inhibitor of TS.

In the reaction catalyzed by TS, the normal substrate 2′-deoxyuridine 5′-monophosphate (dUMP) is converted to 2′-deoxythymidine 5′-monophosphate (dTMP), which is required for DNA synthesis (Figure 22.1). In this reaction, the reduced folate N^5,N^{10}-methylene-tetrahydrofolate (N^5,N^{10}-CH_2FH_4) serves as the required cofactor, since the methylene group of

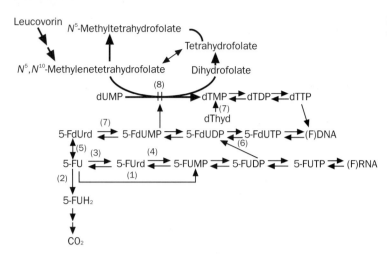

Figure 21.1 Metabolic pathway of fluoropyrimidines and leucovorin.

(1) phosphoribosyltransferase; (2) uracil dehydrogenase; (3) uracil phosphorylase;
(4) uridine kinase; (5) thymidine phosphorylase; (6) ribonucleotide reductase;
(7) thymidine kinase; (8) thymidylate synthase

the folate is added to the 5 position of the heterocyclic ring, and is subsequently reduced to the CH_3 state to form dTMP. The active metabolite of 5-FU, 5-FdUMP, inhibits this reaction in a competitive manner with respect to the normal substrate dUMP. In the absence of the reduced folate cofactor, the 5-FdUMP forms a bivalent complex with the enzyme ($K_d = 10^5$ M), whereas in the presence of N^5,N^{10}-CH_2FH_4 a covalent ternary complex is formed between the enzyme, the folate cofactor and 5-FdUMP, in which 5-FdUMP is bound more tightly, with a $K_d \approx 10^{-12}$ M. This observation has led numerous investigators to suggest that the therapeutic efficacy of 5-FU may be critically dependent on the intracellular levels of the reduced folate cofactor, namely of N^5,N^{10}-CH_2FH_4.

Metabolic modulation involves a demonstrated change in the metabolism of the target cell of a cytotoxic anticancer drug by normal metabolites (modulators) such that the activity of the anticancer drug is augmented in the target cell; the modulators by themselves need not be cytotoxic. This approach is distinctly different from drug combination treatments, which are based on cooperative interactions among cytotoxic agents in target cell populations comprising cell subsets of different sensitivities to the individual drug used in that combination; in this case, no interaction in the same cell is required. A classical metabolic modulation treatment would be represented by the use of leucovorin, uridine, deoxyinosine or thymidine as a modulator of an agent such as 5-FU. These normal metabolites by themselves have no toxic manifestations at doses that produce modulation.

During the past 10 years or so, several approaches have been pursued in an attempt to modulate the cellular effects of 5-FU towards augmented therapeutic efficacy. These investigations were initially carried out in in vitro and in vivo model systems, and clinical trials were designed on the basis of the available laboratory knowledge.

The observed increase in therapeutic efficacy of 5-FU by leucovorin (LV) in several preclinical model systems was confirmed clinically in patients with advanced colorectal cancers and in an adjuvant setting. Although the dose of LV per se does not appear to play a major role in the modulation of the response to 5-FU, the schedule of 5-FU/LV appears to be critical in terms of toxicity and perhaps efficacy. Factors critical to an effective modulation of 5-FU by LV are listed in Table 21.1.

The key determinant is a stabilization of the ternary complex, resulting in pronounced and prolonged inhibition of the target enzyme TS and inhibition of DNA synthesis – factors strongly influenced by the dose and schedule of LV. The duration of TS inhibition in the presence of leucovorin is also influenced by the extent of the polyglutamation of N^5,N^{10}-CH_2FH_4, which is a function of LV schedule of administration.

METABOLISM OF LEUCOVORIN

Leucovorin exists commercially as a diastereomer: 6-d- or (6R)-LV is the presumed biologically inactive isomer and 6-l- or (6S)-LV is the biologically active isomer. These two isomers are prepared in equal amounts for clinical use. As shown in Figure 21.1, LV is extensively metabolized to various folate cofactors. In blood, however, the three major metabolites present following an i.v. dose of (6R, S)-LV are (6S)-LV, (6R)-LV and N^5-methyltetrahydrofolate (N^5-CH_3FH_4). The concentration of the biologically active cofactor, N^5,N^{10}-CH_2FH_4, in tissues is a function of the dose, schedule and route of administration of (6R,S)-LV. This cofactor is present as monoglutamate and as polyg-lutamate (up to 6 glutamic acid residues). The polyglutamate of N^5,N^{10}-CH_2FH_4 yields greater potentiation of 5-FU action than the monoglutamate, as demonstrated by a higher rate constant (Table 21.2).

PHARMACOKINETIC PARAMETERS

The pharmacokinetic parameters of high-dose (6R,S)-LV (500 mg/m^2) have been investigated.[12] The concentrations of (6R,S)-LV, (6S)-LV and N^5-CH_3FH_4 at different time points during and following the 2-hour i.v. infusion of (6R,S)-LV have been investigated. The (6R,S)-LV concentrations peaked at the end of the 2-hour infusion, while the N^5-CH_3FH_4 peak concentration was observed from 1–3 hours after the end of treatment. (6S)-LV concentrations above 10 μM were reached 1 hour after the start of the 2-hour infusion, and maintained for about 2 hours. The plasma concentration of N^5-CH_3FH_4 exceeded 10 μM for a period of about 6 hours. Mean $t_{1/2}$ and plasma clearance of (6S)-LV were respectively 10- and 18-fold faster than those of (6R,S)-LV. Under these conditions, the percentage of (6S) isomer in the HPLC-detected (6R,S)-LV dropped from 50% at the beginning of drug administration to less than 10% 2 hours after the termination of drug infusion. The contribution of the (6S) isomer to

Table 21.1 Critical factors for the potentiation of the therapeutic efficacy of 5-fluorouracil by leucovorin

- Stabilization of the ternary complex: 5-FdUMP–dTMP-synthase–N^5,N^{10}-CH_2FH_4
- Level of thymidylate synthase
- Intracellular concentration of reduced folates
- Circulating level of thymidine
- Intracellular concentration of 5-deoxyuridine monophosphate

Table 21.2 Rate constant of ternary complex formation of N^5,N^{10}-CH_2FH_4 as a function of polyglutamate chain length

Polyglutamate chain length n	Rate constant (min^{-1})
1	0.05
2	0.15
3	0.22
4	0.23
5	0.24
6	0.35

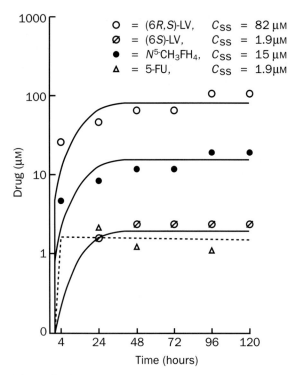

Figure 21.2 Pharmacokinetic properties of leucovorin and its metabolites in patients treated with (6R,S)-LV.

major role in the intracellular accumulation of N^5, N^{10}-CH$_2$FH$_4$.

PRECLINICAL ANTITUMOR ACTIVITY AND TOXICITY OF 5-FU MODULATED BY LV: ROLE OF DOSE AND SCHEDULE

Three schedules were used at the maximum tolerated doses (MTDs) of 5-FU:

(I) continuous infusion of 5-FU for 4 days, with or without daily 2-hour intravenous infusion of LV (20 or 200 mg/kg body weight);
(II) intravenous push of 5-FU alone or after 1 hour of LV infusion, followed by a 1-hour intravenous infusion of LV (20 or 200 mg/kg) daily for 4 days;
(III) intravenous push of 5-FU alone or after 1 hour of LV infusion, followed by a 1-hour intravenous infusion of LV (20 or 200 mg/kg), weekly for 3 weeks.

Figure 21.3 shows the proportions of rats bearing advanced Ward colorectal carcinoma that achieved CR 28 days after treatment with

the (6R,S)-LV AUC was less than 4%.

A five-day continuous i.v. infusion of (6R,S)-LV (500 mg/m^2/d $\times$ 5) yielded a steady-state concentration of 82 μM, 1.9 μM and 15 μM for (6R,S)-LV, (6S)-LV and N^5-CH$_3$FH$_4$ respectively (Figure 21.2). Pharmacokinetic studies of oral (6R,S)-LV (125 mg/m^2 q 4 h $\times$ 4 h) were carried out in patients with advanced colorectal carcinoma, and the results indicate that the plasma concentrations of (6S)-LV seen in these patients receiving oral (6R,S)-LV were below 0.5 μM.

In brief, LV is rapidly metabolized to various cofactors, with (6R)-LV, N^5-CH$_3$FH$_4$ and (6S)-LV being the dominant plasma cofactors. Significant differences in elimination plasma half-life do exist among these metabolites. Since it has been demonstrated that both (6S)-LV and N^5-CH$_3$FH$_4$ can modulate the cytotoxicity of 5-FU, it is not known whether each alone or both together of these active metabolites play a

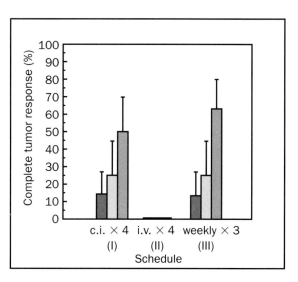

Figure 21.3 Complete response (CR) of 5-FU ± LV at the MTD in rats bearing Ward colorectal carcinoma. ■, 5-FU alone; □, 5-FU + LV 20 mg/kg/d; ▨, 5-FU + LV 200 mg/kg/d.

5-FU, plus or minus LV, according to the three schedules.[13] The data indicate that, except for schedule II (where only PRs were achieved), LV potentiated 5-FU antitumor activity in a dose-dependent manner. The role of LV dose in achieving higher CR proportions was clearly evident when FU was administered by the weekly schedule (schedule III). With schedule I, but not with schedule II, LV modulation of 5-FU antitumor activity was observed; but the greatest effect was seen with schedule III, where the difference in CR frequency between the low dose and the high dose of LV was statistically significant ($p < 0.005$).

The toxicity of 5-FU/LV was a function of the schedule of 5-FU/LV, but independent of the dose of LV: there was diarrhea with the weekly schedule and stomatitis/diarrhea with the daily $\times$ 5 schedule. The antitumor activity and toxicity profile of 5-FU/LV observed in the rat model were similar to those observed clinically. Furthermore, the results obtained in rats with 5-FU/LV indicated that, independently of the dose of LV used (low versus high), the dose of 5-FU had to be reduced by 25%. These results are similar to those obtained clinically.

CLINICAL RESPONSE

Madjaewicz et al[14] utilized a high-dose LV protocol in a phase I trial in which patients received 500 mg/m² LV as a 2-hour infusion with escalating doses of 5-FU administered midway into infusion. This therapy was repeated once a week for 6 weeks, with a 2-week rest between the courses of treatment. This dose of LV was chosen in an attempt to achieve a plasma concentration of (6S)-LV that would exceed 10 µM. In this regimen, the recommended dose of 5-FU was 600 mg/m² (i.v. push). This treatment modality produced 9 partial responses (PR) among 23 patients with advanced colorectal cancer. The median duration of response was 10 months (6–18 months).

Petrelli et al[15–17] completed a three-arm phase III trial evaluating 5-FU/LV (LV 500 mg/m², 2-h infusion/wk $\times$ 6 + 5-FU 600 mg/m² i.v. push mid-infusion/wk $\times$ 6) versus sequential MTX before 5-FU (MTX: 50 mg/m², 4 h before 5-FU: 600 mg/m², i.v. push weekly) versus 5-FU alone (5-FU 450 mg/m² i.v. push $\times$ 5 days then 200 mg/m² i.v. push, q other day $\times$ 6 doses) in previously untreated patients with colon carcinoma (Table 21.3). The response rate of patients treated with LV plus 5-FU (CR + PR = 48%) was significantly greater than that of patients treated with other regimens (11% PR for 5-FU alone and 5% PR for MTX before 5-FU). Similar results were reported by Hines et al,[18] who achieved a 45% response rate in patients with colon carcinoma who were treated with the 5-FU/LV regimen. In all of these investigations, diarrhea was the dose-limiting toxicity, with no significant stomatitis or hematological toxicity.

Although the clinical results with 5-FU + (6R, S)-LV demonstrated a significantly better response rate than treatment with 5-FU alone, the impact of this treatment on survival

Table 21.3 Response to therapy				
Regimen (No. of patients)	Partial response (%)	Complete response (%)	Stable (%)	Progression (%)
5-FU (19)	2 (11)	0	1 (5)	16 (84)
5-FU + MTX (21)	1 (5)	0	2 (9)	18 (86)
5-FU + LV (25)	11 (44)	1 (4)	4 (16)	9 (36)

was not documented.[19] Because of the unacceptable toxicity with the 600 mg/m^2 5-FU weekly schedule, the dose of 5-FU was reduced to 500 mg/m^2 for any further clinical trials. Doroshow and colleagues[20] demonstrated that the response rate for 5-FU plus high-dose LV was superior to 5-FU alone ($p = 0.0019$). Complete responses were observed in 7.2% and 2.8% of patients receiving high-dose LV plus 5-FU and 5-FU respectively.[21] Partial responses occurred in 15.7% and 5.5% of patients respectively, to produce an overall response in 22.9% and 8.3% of patients respectively ($p = 0.03$). Response rates observed in a trial comparing intensive-course 5-FU plus low-dose LV (425 mg/m^2 5-FU and 20 mg/m^2 LV by i.v. push daily for 5 days) to weekly high-dose LV (500 mg/m^2 as a 2-hour infusion) plus 5-FU (600 mg/m^2 as an i.v. push) were 35% and 31% respectively.[22] Both high- and low-dose LV regimens were superior to single-agent 5-FU with respect to time to disease progression ($p = 0.03$ and 0.01 respectively).[23,24] High-dose LV plus 5-FU was superior to 5-FU alone for time to disease progression ($p = 0.045$).[20] When high-dose LV plus 5-FU was compared with low-dose LV plus 5-FU, no significant difference in disease-free survival was noted. The median time to tumor progression among responding patients was greater in the weekly high-dose LV arm than in the intensive low-dose LV arm (9.1 and 7.3 months).[22] The median time to progression was longer in the high-dose LV plus 5-FU arm (5 months) versus the 5-FU arm (3 months), but this difference was not statistically significant.[21]

The fact that higher response rates can be achieved with 5-FU + (6R, S)-LV demonstrate the need for further laboratory and clinical investigations, with the hope of a greater impact on overall survival time. This may best be approached with combination therapy of a thymidylate synthase inhibitor with inhibitors of topoisomerase I, e.g. CPT-11,[25-27] or by modulation of high-dose 5-FU by low-dose MTX.[28-30]

TOXICITY OF THE 5-FU/LV COMBINATION

A phase I trial of high-dose 5-FU/LV in patients with metastatic colorectal carcinoma has been completed.[14] The dose-limiting toxicities associated with this treatment were leukopenia and gastrointestinal toxicity, mainly diarrhea. Six of 18 patients who received 5-FU 600 mg/m^2 and LV 500 mg/m^2 developed diarrhea, and 3 of these individuals required intravenous hydration. Three of 18 patients also experienced leukopenia of 600, 2700 and 3100/mm^3. All patients recovered completely within one week when the dose of 5-FU was decreased to 500 mg/m^2. Eight of 11 patients who received 5-FU 750 mg/m^2 and LV 500 mg/m^2 developed a WBC nadir at less than 3000/mm^3, and 6 of 11 patients treated with this regimen experienced severe diarrhea of 5–7 days duration. All of these patients except one recovered completely within 7–10 days, and subsequent treatment was continued at 5-FU doses of 500–600 mg/m^2. Maximum toxicity was usually seen at the end of the first course at 600 mg/m^2 of 5-FU or after the third dose of the first course at 750 mg/m^2 of 5-FU. In a subsequent phase III study of high-dose 5-FU/LV,[31] patients received LV (500 mg/m^2/2-h infusion) and 5-FU (600 mg/m^2 i.v. push) (Table 21.4). The dose-limiting toxicity was again predominantly gastrointestinal, specifically diarrhea. There were no instances of thrombocytopenia. Three of 30 patients (10%) treated with this regimen developed stomatitis grade >2. A total of 3 of the 30 patients (10%) developed leukopenia grade >2 on this regimen.

Thirteen of 30 patients (43%) required a dose reduction of 5-FU to 500, 400 or 300 mg/m^2 because of diarrhea (Table 21.4); however, LV was maintained at 500 mg/m^2. Eight of the 13 patients (62%) who developed diarrhea required hospitalization for intravenous hydration. Two demonstrated a partial response to treatment, whereas the other individual showed evidence of disease stabilization. Thus the recommended dose of 5-FU for future clinical trials with the weekly schedule was 500 mg/m^2/weekly × 6 with LV at 500 mg/m^2.

Table 21.4 Toxicity requiring a dose reduction of chemotherapy

Regimen (No. of patients)	Stomatitis (%)	Diarrhea (%)	Leukopenia (%)	Thrombocytopenia (%)
5-FU (22)	2 (10)	8 (36)	0	0
5-FU + MTX (22)	2 (10)	0	9 (41)	1 (5)
5-FU + LV (30)	3 (10)	13 (43)	3 (10)	0

CONCLUSIONS AND FUTURE PROSPECTS

In conclusion, the 5-FU/LV regimen possesses antitumor activity against colorectal carcinoma (and other tumors such as breast carcinoma and squamous cell head and neck cancers). Recent phase III trials demonstrated that the antitumor activity of the 5-FU/LV modulation against colorectal carcinomas is significantly greater than the response rates obtained with 5-FU administered as a single agent at the maximally tolerated dose. The high-dose LV ($500\,mg/m^2$) weekly schedule with 5-FU ($500\,mg/m^2$) demonstrated a higher overall response rate than the low-dose LV ($25\,mg/m^2$) with 5-FU in advanced colorectal cancer. The overall response rate with the daily × 5 schedule, however, was similar for both high ($200\,mg/m^2$) and low ($20\,mg/m^2$) doses of LV with corresponding doses of 5-FU. From the results obtained to date, this treatment modality has not impacted on the overall survival of patients with advanced colorectal cancer, regardless of the dose or schedule of 5-FU/LV. In an adjuvant setting, however, clear improvement in disease-free survival and overall survival have been demonstrated. The dose-limiting toxicity for 5-FU/LV modulation in advanced and adjuvant colorectal cancer is diarrhea with the weekly schedule, and stomatitis, leukopenia and diarrhea for the daily × 5 schedule, independently of the LV dose.

Future studies should include

(1) evaluation of the therapeutic efficacy of this modulation using higher doses of 5-FU by 24-hour infusion and compared with protracted continuous i.v. infusion of low-dose 5-FU;
(2) studies to determine whether the therapeutic activity of the 5-FU/LV regimen can be enhanced by the addition of other agents with alternative mechanisms of action (i.e. platinum, CPT-11, MTX and other antifolates);
(3) the combined use of modulators that interfere with the anabolic and catabolic pathways of 5-FU (e.g. S-1, UFT and EU);
(4) identification of biochemical and molecular markers associated with response to 5-FU/LV modulation (e.g. p53, TS level and topoisomerase I level) for the purpose of identification of drug combinations with greater therapeutic index.

ACKNOWLEDGEMENTS

This work was supported in part by DHP 147 from The American Cancer Society, Atlanta, GA and CA 65761 from the National Cancer Institute, Bethesda, MD.

REFERENCES

1. Au JL-S, Rustum YM, Ledesma EJ et al, Clinical pharmacologic studies of concurrent infusion of 5-fluorouracil and thymidine in treatment of colorectal carcinomas. *Cancer Res* 1982; **42**: 2930–7.

2. Aull JL, Lyon JP, Dunlap RB, Gel-electrophoresis as a means of detecting ternary complex formation of thymidylate synthase. *Microchem J* 1974; **19**: 210–18.

3. Berger SH, Hakala MT, Relationship of dUMP and free FdUMP pools to inhibition of thymidylate synthetase by 5-fluorouracil. *Mol Pharmacol* 1984; **25**: 303–9.

4. Bertino JR, Mini E, Does modulation of 5-fluorouracil by metabolites or antimetabolites work in the clinic? In: *New Avenues in Developmental Cancer Chemotherapy* (Harrop, KR, Connors TA, eds). Orlando: Academic Press, 1987; 163–84.

5. Danenberg PV, Thymidylate synthetase – a target enzyme in cancer chemotherapy. *Biochem Biophys Acta* 1977; **473**: 73–92.

6. Danenberg PV, Locksin A, Fluorinated pyrimidines as tight-binding inhibitors of thymidylate synthetase. *Pharmacol Ther* 1981; **13**: 69–90.

7. Danenberg PV, Heidelberger C, Mulkins M et al, Incorporation of 5-fluoro-2'-deoxyuridine into DNA of mammalian tumor cells. *Biochem Biophys Res Commun* 1981; **102**: 654–8.

8. Danhauser LL, Rustum YM, Chemotherapeutic efficacy of 5-fluorouracil with concurrent thymidine infusion against transplantable colon tumors in rodents. *Cancer Drug Deliv* 1984; **1**: 269–82.

9. Evans RM, Laskin JD, Hakala MT et al, Effect of excess folates and deoxyinosine on the activity and site of action of 5-fluorouracil. *Cancer Res* 1981; **41**: 3288–95.

10. Friedkin M, Thymidylate synthetase. *Adv Enzymol* 1973; **38**: 253–92.

11. Houghton JA, Williams LG, deGraf SSN et al, Selectivity of CF and 5-fluoroacil: critical role of polyglutamation. *Adv Exp Med Biol* 1989; **244**: 85–95.

12. Trave F, Rustum YM, Petrelli N et al, Plasma and tumor tissue pharmacology of high dose intravenous leucovorin calcium in combination with fluorouracil in patients with advanced colorectal carcinoma. *J Clin Oncol* 1988; **6**: 1184–91.

13. Cao S, Frank C, Rustum YM, Role of fluoropyrimidine schedule and (6*R, S*) leucovorin dose in a preclinical animal model of colorectal carcinoma. *J Natl Cancer Inst* 1996; **88**: 430–5.

14. Madajewicz S, Petrelli N, Rustum YM et al, Phase I–II trial of high-dose calcium leucovorin and 5-fluorouracil in advanced colorectal cancer. *Cancer Res* 1984; **44**: 4667–9.

15. Petrelli N, Herrera L, Stulc J et al, A phase III study of 5-fluorouracil (5-FU) versus 5-FU + methotrexate (MTX) versus 5-FU + high-dose leucovorin (CF) in metastatic colorectal adenocarcinoma. *Proc Am Soc Clin Oncol* 1987; **6**: 74.

16. Petrelli NJ, Herrera L, Rustum YM et al, A prospective randomized trial of 5-fluorouracil versus 5-fluorouracil and high dose leucovorin versus 5-fluorouracil and methotrexate in previously untreated patients with advanced colorectal carcinoma. *J Clin Oncol* 1987; **5**: 1559–65.

17. Petrelli NJ, Madajewicz S, Herrera L et al, Biologic modulation of 5-fluorouracil with high-dose leucovorin and combination chemotherapy of 5-fluorouracil and cisplatin in metastatic colorectal adenocarcinoma. *NCI Monographs* 1987; **5**: 189–92.

18. Hines JD, Zakem M, Adelstein D et al, Treatment of advanced-stage colorectal adenocarcinoma with fluorouracil and high-dose leucovorin calcium: a pilot study. *J Clin Oncol* 1987; **6**: 142–6.

19. Piedbois P, Buyse M, Rustum YM et al, Modulation of fluorouracil by leucovorin patients with advanced colorectal cancer: evidence in terms of response rates. *J Clin Oncol* 1992; **10**: 896–903.

20. Doroshow JH, Multhauf P, Leong L et al, Prospective randomized comparison of fluorouracil and high-dose continuous infusion leucovorin calcium for the treatment of advanced measurable colorectal cancer in patients previously unexposed to chemotherapy. *J Clin Oncol* 1990; **8**: 491–501.

21. Nobile MT, Rosso R, Sertoli MR et al, Randomized comparison of weekly bolus 5-fluorouracil with or without leucovorin in metastatic colorectal carcinoma. *Eur J Cancer* 1992; **28A**: 1823–7.

22. Buroker TR, O'Connell MJ, Wieand HS et al, Randomized comparison of two schedules of fluorouracil and leucovorin in the treatment of advanced colorectal cancer. *J Clin Oncol* 1994; **12**: 14–20.

23. O'Connell MJ, A Phase III trial of 5-fluorouracil and leucovorin in the treatment of advanced colorectal cancer. *Cancer* 1989; **63**: 1026–30.

24. Poon MA, O'Connell MJ, Wieand HS et al, Biochemical modulation of fluorouracil with leu-

covorin: confirmatory evidence of improved therapeutic efficacy in advanced colorectal cancer. *J Clin Oncol* 1991; **9**: 1967–72.

25. Armond JP, In: *The Camptothecins: From Discovery to the Patient. A New York Academy of Sciences Conference, Bethesda, MD, 1996*: abst 32.

26. Saltz LB, Kanowitz J, Kemeny NE et al, Phase I clinical and pharmacokinetic study of ironotecan, fluorouracil and leucovorin in patients with advanced solid tumors. *J Clin Oncol* 1996; **14**: 2959–67.

27. Creemers GJ, Gerrits CJH, Schellens JHM et al, Phase II and pharmacologic study of topotecan administered as a 21-day continuous infusion to patients with colorectal cancer. *J Clin Oncol* 1996; **14**: 2540–5.

28. Blijham G, Wagener T, Wils T et al, Modulation of high dose infusional fluorouracil by low-dose MTX in patients with advanced or metastatic colorectal cancer: final result of a randomized European organizations for research and treatment of cancer study. *J Clin Oncol* 1996; **14**: 2266–73.

29. Piedbois P, Buyse M, Blijham G et al, Meta-analysis of randomized trials testing the biochemical modulation of fluorouracil by methotrexate in metastatic colorectal cancer. *J Clin Oncol* 1994; **12**: 960–9.

30. Conti JA, Kemeny N, Seiter K et al, Trial of sequential trimetrexate, fluorouracil, and high-dose leucovorin in previously treated patients with gastrointestinal carcinoma. *J Clin Oncol* 1994; **12**: 695–700.

31. Petrelli N, Herrera L, Rustum YM et al, A prospective randomized trial of 5-fluorouracil and high-dose leucovorin versus 5-fluorouracil and methotrexate in previously untreated patients with advanced colorectal carcinoma. *J Clin Oncol* 1987; **5**: 1559–65.

22

Modulation of 5-fluorouracil with folinic acid: High or low dose?

Roberto Labianca, M Adelaide Pessi, Gianfranco Pancera, Gino Luporini

CONTENTS • Introduction • Experimental basis • Clinical studies • Conclusions

INTRODUCTION

The optimal chemotherapy for advanced colorectal cancer has not yet been defined: for many years, 5-fluorouracil (5-FU) has been the most common treatment, but the response rate to this drug administered by bolus infusion is only 10%, and median overall survival does not exceed one year.[1] Of the various attempts made over the last few years to increase 5-FU activity by modifying the administration schedule, the most convincing one seems to be the use of short- or long-term continuous infusion.[2] Another interesting approach has been that of so-called 'biochemical modulation', i.e. the association of 5-FU with agents capable of increasing the activity and/or reducing the toxicity of the drug through an interaction with its metabolic pathways. Although several innovative compounds are now available for the treatment of this disease, modulated 5-FU remains the reference chemotherapy in both clinical research and practice.

Among the various agents evaluated in clinical trials, leucovorin or folinic acid (FA) is of particular interest. The rationale for the association between FA and 5-FU is that the administration of folic coenzymes, precursors of N^5,N^{10}-methylenetetrahydrofolic acid, is able to increase the intracellular levels of this cofactor and to enhance the formation and retention of the ternary complex with 5-fluorodeoxyuridine monophosphate (5-FdUMP) and thymidylate synthase (TS), with subsequent increase of DNA synthesis inhibition. This kind of biochemical modulation was detected in experimental models, both in vitro and in vivo in mice, and then confirmed in several clinical trials. As is well known, there are two main schedules for the administration of 5-FU + FA: the daily-times-five regimen, developed by Machover at Villejuif (France) in 1982,[3] and the weekly regimen developed by Madajewicz and Rustum at the Roswell Park Memorial Institute (RPMI), Buffalo (USA) in 1994.[4] In Table 22.1 these two regimens are outlined: in the original reports their activity appeared very similar (complete + partial responses, CR + PRs = 30–40%), while there was a sharp difference in the dose-limiting toxicity, represented by mucositis for the daily-times-five regimen and diarrhoea for the weekly schedule. Other studies employed continuous infusion of FA or oral administration of the drug: this latter way of administration should have been able, according to some experiences,[5]

Table 22.1 Main schedules of folinic acid + 5-fluorouracil

Daily-times-five regimen[3]

Folinic acid 200 mg/m² i.v. bolus;
immediately followed by
5-fluorouracil 370 mg/m² i.v. in 15-minute infusion.
Repeat for 5 consecutive days every 4 weeks

Weekly regimen[4]

Folinic acid 500 mg/m² in 2-hour infusion;
5-fluorouracil 600 mg/m² i.v. bolus at mid-infusion.
Repeat weekly for 6 times; then 2 weeks rest

---

to produce a selective absorption of the laevorotatory stereoisomer, which is fully responsible for the activity of the drug. The clinical results, however, were quite disappointing, and did not justify an extensive use of these last regimens.

At least 730 patients, in 22 phase II published studies, were treated with FA + 5-FU according to the above-reported schedule:[6] in 177 of them an objective response (CR or PR) was reported. The response rate was superior (30%) in patients not previously exposed to 5-FU in comparison with those pretreated with the fluoropyrimidine (13%).

On the basis of these promising results, in the late 1980s several phase III trials were performed in order to compare FA + 5-FU with 5-FU alone and to evaluate if the combination of the two drugs was a real step ahead in the treatment of this disease. At least 10 clinical studies were performed, both in Northern America and in Europe,[7–16] with a response rate for the combination fluctuating from 15% to 48% and a superiority over the single-drug therapy in all but two trials. As far as the effect on overall survival is concerned, a significant advantage for FA + 5-FU was reported only in the NCCTG study,[13] while in the Canadian trial[15] the initial advantage was lost with the increase of follow-up. In Table 22.2 an outline of the most important comparative studies is reported. In 1992 nine trials (the NCCTG declined to participate) were included in a strict meta-analysis:[17] in 1381 patients there was a significant advantage of FA + 5-FU versus 5-FU alone in terms of objective response rate (odds ratio = 0.44), with a slight superiority of weekly compared with monthly regimens (odds ratio = 0.31 and 0.58 respectively): however, no difference was detected for overall survival (odds ratio = 0.97).

The superiority of FA-modulated 5-FU over 5-FU alone, even though detectable only in terms of response rate and with a still-limited level of activity, stimulated great interest among medical oncologists on both sides of the Atlantic, and prompted the vast majority of them to consider this particular kind of biochemical modulation as the reference or 'standard' treatment of advanced colorectal cancer. However, the lack of homogeneity among the various trials made it difficult to establish the best treatment schedule: factors related to the selection of cases, the criteria and methods to assess the activity of chemotherapy, the dosage of the two drugs and the modality of treatment (i.e. the duration of infusion, the interval between the two drugs, etc.) had a potentially relevant influence on the outcome of treatment.

One of the key questions concerns the definition of the dose of FA needed for optimal modulation of 5-FU: the meta-analysis failed to identify the best doses and schedules of administration of both drugs, since only indirect comparisons could be made from the data at hand at that time. From the survey of the phase III studies, it had been suggested that the weekly schedule of administration required a high dose of FA, whereas in the daily-times-five regimen low doses were at least equally effective in terms of tumour response, symptomatic relief and overall survival. In particular, the Mayo Clinic regimen (FA 20 mg/m²/day i.v. immediately followed by 5-FU 425 mg/m²/day, with both drugs given by bolus administration for 5 days every 4–5 weeks) became very popular

Table 22.2 Randomized clinical trials of FA + 5-FU versus 5-FU

No. of patients	Schedule	% CR + PR	Survival	Ref
82	5-FU 600 mg/m² + FA 500 mg/m² weekly versus 5-FU 600 mg/m² weekly	16% versus 5% ($p = 0.05$)	No significant difference	9
318	5-FU 600 mg/m² + FA 500 or 25 mg/m² 6 out of 8 weeks versus 5-FU 500 mg/m² × 5 every 4 weeks	30.3% versus 18.8% versus 12.1% ($p < 0.01$)	55 versus 45 versus 46 weeks ($p = 0.08$)	8
41	5-FU 600 mg/m² + FA 500 mg/m² 6 out of 8 weeks versus 5-FU 450 mg/m² × 5	48% versus 11% ($p = 0.0009$)	No significant difference ($p = 0.6$)	7
153[a]	5-FU 400 mg/m² × 5 + FA 200 mg/m² × 5 every 4 weeks versus 5-FU 480 mg/m² followed by 600 mg/m²/week	18.8% versus 17.3% ($p = 0.4$)	24 versus 20 weeks ($p = 0.4$)	10
181	5-FU 400 mg/m² × 5 + FA 200 mg/m² × 5 every 4 weeks versus 5-FU 540 mg/m² × 5	15% versus 16%	25 versus 21 weeks	11
182	5-FU 400 mg/m² × 5 + FA 200 mg/m² × 5 every 4 weeks versus 5-FU 400 mg/m² × 5 every 4 weeks	20.6% versus 10% ($p = 0.046$)	46 versus 44 weeks	12
208	5-FU 370 mg/m² × 5 + FA 20 or 200 mg/m² × 5 versus 5-FU 500 mg/m² × 5	43% versus 26% versus 10% ($p = 0.001$)	53 versus 52 versus 34 weeks ($p = 0.05$)	13
74	5-FU 370 mg/m² × 5 + FA 500 mg/m² × 5 every 4 weeks versus 5-FU 370 mg/m² × 5	44% versus 13% ($p = 0.0019$)	63 versus 55 weeks ($p = 0.25$)	14
124	5-FU 370 mg/m² × 5 + FA 200 mg/m² × 5 versus 5-FU 370 mg/m² × 5	33% versus 7% ($p < 0.0005$)	54 versus 41 weeks ($p = 0.05$)[b]	15

[a] Randomization 2 : 1.
[b] Not confirmed in a further analysis.

both in Northern America (where it is regarded as a kind of 'standard' treatment for advanced colorectal cancer) and in Europe: this regimen is now probably the most widely used, also for practical and economical reasons.

In spite of the wide popularity of the low-dose monthly regimen, the debate about the optimal FA dosage is still open for several reasons: the real evaluation of the financial costs may be more difficult than considered before, the equiactivity of the low doses has been questioned in recent experimental and clinical studies, and the introduction, both in research and in practice, of the laevorotatory stereoisomer of FA ((6S)-FA) has added another issue to the discussion.

In this chapter a short reappraisal will be made of the experimental basis and the clinical results of the FA low-dose treatment (overall, more than 2000 patients have been included to date in trials comparing different doses and schedules of administration of the combination of FA and 5-FU).

EXPERIMENTAL BASIS

The concentration of FA needed for optimal potentiation of 5-FU is different according to the specific experimental model: while Rustum et al,[18] studying murine sarcoma 180, human carcinoma Hep-2 and murine leukemia L1210, suggested that optimal stabilization of the ternary complex and potentiation of 5-FU cytotoxicity could only be achieved with a total FA concentration of 20 µmol/l (thus providing a preclinical rationale for the use of high doses of FA combined with 5-FU in clinical studies), Mehta et al[19] and Keyomarsi and Moran[20] observed that FA at a concentration of 1 µmol/l could produce maximal growth-inhibitory potency against a variety of murine and human leukemia cell lines exposed to 5-FU or 5-fluorodeoxyuridine in vitro. According to these authors, therefore, a dose of 10–20 mg/m^2 (capable of giving 1 µmol/l serum levels of FA) should be enough in the clinical field.

Another method to study the effect of FA on 5-FU cytotoxicity is the evaluation of TS inhibi-

tion in biopsy specimens: Peters et al observed that high-dose weekly FA increased TS inhibition when compared with the results obtained in biopsies from patients treated with 5-FU alone,[21] whereas patients receiving a lower (25 mg/m^2) FA dose had reduced TS inhibition in comparison with those treated with the higher (500 mg/m^2) weekly dose.[22] On the other hand, Jolivet[23] demonstrated that FA dose is not the only factor influencing activity and toxicity of the biochemical modulation of 5-FU: he observed that the FA length of administration and the 5-FU duration of exposure are also important parameters in optimizing FA + 5-FU therapy, and concluded that prolonged cellular exposure (>24 hours) to relatively low FA concentrations simultaneously with prolonged 5-FU administration is a strategy deserving further clinical investigation.

Recently Etienne et al[24] reviewed the preclinical and clinical data dealing with prediction of sensitivity to FA + 5-FU and optimization of the schedule of these two drugs. On the basis of the clinical data (which, as will be reported below, do not indicate a clear consensus about the need of administering high doses of FA), they surveyed experimental studies of human cell lines and confirmed a wide variability among them: the laevorotatory FA concentration required for maximal 5-FU potentiation ranged from 0.05 or 200 µmol. Moreover, pharmacokinetic studies reported a significant variability of active folates in plasma after administration of 'standard-dose' FA. They concluded that these observations, taken altogether, favour a high-dose FA administration in order to achieve high folate concentrations in plasma and to counteract the variability of required concentrations. Another conclusion of their survey, in agreement with Jolivet's opinion, is that increasing the duration of exposure to FA enhances 5-FU cytotoxicity and that therefore a schedule of prolonged administration of both 5-FU and FA should be considered preferable.

More recently again, Cao et al[25] developed a new experimental model capable of detecting the importance of FA dose in the biochemical modulation of 5-FU: they studied three clinically relevant schedules in rats bearing advanced Ward colorectal carcinomas, and observed that there is a strong experimental support for the clinical observation of a relation between the optimal FA dose required and the schedule of administration: their data confirm that for the weekly regimen high doses are needed, whereas the daily-times-five schedule seems to be active also with low doses.

The experimental data reported above, considered altogether, indicate that

- FA dose is one of the critical factors influencing the activity of this kind of biochemical modulation of 5-FU;
- there is a wide variability according to the specific cell line studied and also (pharmacokinetic data) according to the individual patient treated;
- high doses are better in the weekly regimen;
- low doses seem to be equiactive in the daily-times-five schedule;
- other factors, such as the length of administration of both drugs, have an influence on FA + 5-FU activity, and can potentially interfere with the effect of FA dose.

It is interesting to observe that these experimental researches were not always performed *before* the clinical studies, but, in many cases, were activated *after* the results of large clinical trials. Therefore, the relation between preclinical and clinical studies should be considered a dynamic process, and medical oncologists should have a deep knowledge of both these fields of investigation.

CLINICAL STUDIES

Only a few trials have addressed, in the clinical field, the question of the optimal FA dose in the biochemical modulation of 5-FU.[26] A synopsis of the most prominent studies is reported in Table 22.3, and a short presentation of the results and a brief comment will be given here.

Petrelli et al,[8] on behalf of the Gastrointestinal Tumour Study Group (GITSG), performed a study on 318 patients,[8] randomized between 5-FU alone (500 mg/m² for 5 days every 4 weeks) and the same drug given weekly for 6 or 8 weeks at a dose of 600 mg/m² bolus i.v. and modulated by 2-hour FA infusion at high (500 mg/m²) or 10-minute FA infusion at low (25 mg/m²) dosage. The high-dose FA arm demonstrated a superior activity in terms of response rate in comparison both with the low-dose FA and with the single-drug arm (% CR + PR = 30.3, 18.8 and 12.1 respectively, with $p < 0.01$); in contrast, no significant difference in survival was detected, even though there was a trend ($p = 0.08$) in favour of high-dose FA + 5-FU. This trial is in agreement with the preclinical observations indicating the need for high doses of FA in the biochemical modulation of 5-FU administered with the weekly schedule.

Jaeger and other members of the German PALL I Study Group presented at the 1994 ASCO Meeting results of a trial[27] in which patients were randomized to receive weekly 5-FU 500 mg/m² bolus i.v. combined with high-dose (500 mg/m²) or low-dose (20 mg/m²) FA in 2-hour infusions. Treatment was continued for 4 weeks beyond the best achieved remission. On 298 evaluable patients they observed 28.6% CR + PR in the high-dose group and 17.3% CR + PR in the low-dose arm. Median duration of response and median time to progression were similar in the two groups, whereas median survival had not yet been reached at the time of the report. Serious diarrhoea occurred significantly more frequently in the high-dose FA arm, whereas the other side-effects were similar in the two groups. Also the requirement of dose and schedule adjustment was much more frequent in the first arm. The authors concluded that, despite the higher response rate observed with high-dose FA, there was no superior overall benefit for the patients, even though survival data were still pending: the recent publication of this study as a full paper confirmed these data.[27a]

Poon et al[13] reported the results of a study performed by the North Central Cancer Treatment Group (NCCTG): 429 patients were randomized among six different regimens: two of these schedules included FA, given at high

Table 22.3 Randomized clinical trials comparing low-dose with high-dose FA as modulator of 5-FU in advanced colorectal cancer

Institution	Low-dose FA + 5-FU		High-dose FA + 5-FU	
GITSG[8]	FA 25 mg/m² (10-min infusion) 5-FU 600 mg/m² i.v.	Weekly (6/8)	FA 500 mg/m² (2-h infusion) 5-FU 600 mg/m² i.v.	Weekly (6/8)
PALL I Study Group[27]	FA 20 mg/m² (2-h infusion) 5-FU 500 mg/m² i.v.	Weekly	FA 500 mg/m² (2-h infusion) 5-FU 500 mg/m² i.v.	Weekly
NCCTG[13,28]	FA 20 mg/m² i.v. 5-FU 370–425 mg/m² i.v.	× 5 days every 4–5 weeks	FA 200 mg/m² i.v. 5-FU 370 mg/m² i.v.	× 5 days every 4–5 weeks
GISCAD[32]	L-FA 10 mg/m² i.v. 5-FU 370 mg/m² (15 minute infusion)	× 5 days every 4 weeks	L-FA 100 mg/m² i.v. 5-FU 370 mg/m² (15-min infusion)	× 5 days every 4 weeks
NCCTG[29]	FA 20 mg/m² i.v. 5-FU 425 mg/m² i.v.	× 5 days every 4–5 weeks	FA 500 mg/m² (2-h infusion) 5-FU 600 mg/m² i.v.	Weekly (6/8)
FFCD/GERCOD/SFNMI[35]	FA 20 mg/m² i.v. 5-FU 425 mg/m² i.v.	× 5 days every 4 weeks	FA 200 mg/m² (2-h infusion) 5-FU 400 mg/m² i.v. + 600 mg/m² (22-h infusion)	Days 1–2 every 2 weeks
SWOG[36]	• FA 20 mg/m² i.v. 5-FU 425 mg/m² i.v. • FA 20 mg/m² i.v. every week 5-FU 200 mg/m² continuous infusion, days 1–28, every 5 weeks	× 5 days every 4–5 weeks	FA 500 mg/m² (2-h infusion) 5-FU 600 mg/m² i.v.	Weekly (6/8)

(200 mg/m^2/day) or low (20 mg/m^2/day) doses, immediately followed by 5-FU at 370–425 mg/m^2/day. Both drugs were given by rapid i.v. injection daily for 5 consecutive days. Courses were repeated at 4 weeks, 8 weeks, and every 5 weeks thereafter. The median survivals achieved with these two regimens were identical (12.2 and 12 months), and were significantly superior (7.7 months) to that obtained with 5-FU alone, administered by rapid i.v. push at 500 mg/m^2/day for 5 consecutive days, with courses repeated every 5 weeks. A subset analysis according to measurable disease status indicated that the major benefit was obtained with each of the FA regimens in patients with non-measurable metastatic disease, but not in those with measurable neoplastic lesions. As far as the objective response is concerned, 5-FU + low-dose FA was associated with the highest response rate (CR + PR = 43%), and was significantly superior to 5-FU alone ($p = 0.001$); 5-FU + high-dose FA yielded 26% response rate, and also this value was statistically superior to 5-FU alone ($p = 0.04$). Only the low-dose FA regimen was associated with significant superiority ($p < 0.05$) to 5-FU in each of the parameters related to quality of life: improvement of performance status (PS), weight gain and symptomatic relief. The toxicity profile of the two FA-containing regimens was very similar, with the dose-limiting side-effect represented by ulcerative stomatitis, which occurred in one-quarter to one-third of patients. The authors conclude that for economic reasons, tolerable toxicity and survival benefit, the low-dose FA + 5-FU regimen should be preferred in advanced disease and should be evaluated in the adjuvant setting. Although the design and the results of this study should be criticized for several reasons (the number of included patients is relatively small, about half of the cases do not present evaluable disease, the survival in the 5-FU alone group appears particularly short, among others), since the publication of these data, the low-dose FA daily-times-five regimen has become a kind of 'standard' regimen in USA, and has also been widely used in the rest of the world.

Two years later, NCCTG presented an update of the results:[28] both low- and high-dose FA proved to be more efficacious than methotrexate + 5-FU in the biochemical modulation of 5-FU (in all, 457 patients were randomly assigned to one of these three regimens), and it was confirmed that it was not necessary to use high doses of FA to achieve an increase in survival, objective response rate and symptomatic relief: the respective values are nearly identical to those reported in the first part of the study.

Therefore the low-dose FA regimen was confirmed to be at least as effective as the high-dose schedule, even though the authors observed a higher rate of hospitalization for chemotherapy toxicity (15% versus 5.4%), perhaps because of the 11–15% higher dose of 5-FU allowed.

Buroker et al,[29] again on behalf of NCCTG, published the results of a large phase III trial, in which 372 patients were randomized to receive the daily-times-five low-dose FA regimen or the weekly high-dose FA combination. There were no significant differences in therapeutic efficacy between the two regimens (objective response 35% versus 31%, median survival 9.3 versus 10.7 months, palliative effects identical on PS and weight gain, not significantly in favour of the low-dose regimen for symptom relief). A significant difference was observed in toxicity, with more leukopenia and stomatitis seen with the daily-times-five regimen, and more diarrhoea and requirement for hospitalization to manage toxicity with the weekly regimen. Also financial costs were higher for the weekly regimen. The authors concluded that the low-dose FA daily-times-five regimen has, for the reasons reported above, a superior therapeutic index in comparison with the high-dose FA weekly schedule.

The publication of these results stimulated a lively debate about the relative merits of these two regimens,[30,31] and about the need for further confirmatory trials and better methods to evaluate the economic aspects of cancer chemotherapy.

Our group (GISCAD, the Italian Group for the Study of Digestive Tract Cancer) performed a comparative study in which the laevorotatory stereoisomer of FA ((6S)-FA) was employed.[32] Recent data by NCCTG[33] confirmed the phase II data that this formulation is as effective as the racemic compound in the biochemical modulation of 5-FU, so, given that pure (6S)-FA is the only formulation of the drug now available in various European countries, it seemed to be of interest to evaluate two dose levels of this agent in a large-scale pragmatic trial. Between November 1991 and June 1994, 422 patients (all with measurable disease previously untreated with chemotherapy) were randomized to (6S)-FA (100 mg/m^2 i.v.) + 5-FU (370 mg/m^2/15 min i.v. infusion), both administered for 5 days every 28 (arm A), or to (6S)-FA (10 mg/m^2 i.v.) + 5-FU (doses as above), also given for 5 days every 28 (arm B). In analogy with the NCCTG trials, the low-dose of FA used in our study was 10% of the high one, and the reference schedule was exactly that developed at Villejuif[3] in order to be able to make a comparison with the regimen considered 'standard' in Europe at the beginning of the 1990s. The primary endpoint of the study was the comparison of response rates, and the secondary ones the assessment of survival and tolerability. In this trial no evaluation of the quality of life or the symptomatic effect of treatment was planned. The response rates were similar in the two arms (9.3% and 10.7%), such as the median times to progression (8 months in both groups) and median overall survival (11 months in each arm). Toxicity mainly consisted of gastrointestinal side-effects (mucositis and diarrhoea), which were rarely severe (WHO grade 3–4: 5–10% of patients) and were similar in the two groups.

We conclude that the low and high doses of (6S)-FA (in agreement with what is reported for the racemic compound) are also equivalent in the biochemical modulation of 5-FU when employed in the daily-times-five regimen. The response rate is lower than those reported previously: this can be related to the strict evaluation of response, the high number of patients with unfavourable prognostic factors, the multi-institutional nature of the study and perhaps the specific modality of 5-FU administration (short infusion instead of true bolus).[34]

Given the sharp difference in economic cost between the two dosages, the use of high-dose (6S)-FA in the daily-times-five regimen is not recommended in clinical practice.

A French study[35] compared two regimens in which FA is administered at different dosages; even though another important difference between the two arms is represented by the administration of 5-FU (bolus or continuous infusion), this study deserves a comment in this chapter. A large number of patients (437) were randomized between the low-dose Mayo Clinic regimen (arm A) and FA 200 mg/m^2 2-hour infusion followed by 5-FU 400 mg/m^2 i.v. bolus and then a 22-hour infusion of 600 mg/m^2, both drugs given on days 1 and 2 every 2 weeks (arm B). The response rate was significantly higher in arm B (34% versus 17%, with $p = 0.002$), and also toxicity was in favour of arm B ($p = 0.0004$). No difference was detected in terms of progression-free and overall survival. In this trial the high-dose-containing regimen seems more active (even though the modality of administration could also have played a role), and the response rate obtained with the Mayo regimen is much lower than previously reported.

A large randomized phase II trial performed by SWOG (Southwest Oncology Group)[36] included seven arms: three of them included FA + 5-FU, two with low-dose FA (the Mayo regimen and FA + continuous-infusion 5-FU) and one with the Roswell Park regimen. The response rates of these three arms were similar (27%, 26% and 21%), suggesting a lack of influence of the dose of FA with these schedules.

CONCLUSIONS

The influence of FA dose on the biochemical modulation of 5-FU in advanced colorectal cancer is not yet clear. Although a wide consensus, based on both experimental and clinical studies, exists about the need to use a high dose with the weekly regimen, the data strongly supporting the administration of low doses in the daily-times-five regimen are not always confirmed in more recent studies. Moreover, the lower response rates reported in the last trials, the introduction in many countries of the laevorotatory stereoisomer of FA and the wider use of 5-FU continuous infusion seem to complicate the situation.

In order to clarify the question, a meta-analysis comparing all patients randomized between the two dose levels of FA could be warranted. An important point of this meta-analysis should be a strict cost–effectiveness analysis.

REFERENCES

1. Moertel CG, Chemotherapy for colorectal cancer. *N Engl J Med* 1994; **330:** 1136–42.
2. Anderson N, Lokich JJ, Controversial issues in 5-fluorouracil infusion use. *Cancer* 1992; **70:** 998–1002.
3. Machover D, Schwarzenberg L, Goldschmidt E et al, Treatment of advanced colorectal and gastric adenocarcinomas with 5FU combined with high-dose folinic acid: a pilot study. *Cancer Treat Rep* 1982; **66:** 1803–7.
4. Madajewicz P, Phase I/II trial of high-dose calcium leucovorin and 5-fluorouracil in advanced colorectal cancer. *Cancer Res* 1984; **44:** 4667–9.
5. Schilsky RL, Clinical pharmacokinetics of high-dose leucovorin calcium after intravenous and oral administration. *J Natl Cancer Inst* 1990; **82:** 1411–12.
6. Luporini G, Labianca R, Pancera G, Treatment of metastatic colorectal cancer: improvement of 5-fluorouracil activity with modulating agents. *Forum* 1991; **1:** 246–56.
7. Petrelli N, Herrera L, Rustum Y et al, A prospective randomized trial of 5-fluorouracil versus 5-fluorouracil and leucovorin in previously untreated patients with advanced colorectal carcinoma. *J Clin Oncol* 1987; **5:** 1559–65.
8. Petrelli N, Douglass HD, Herrera L et al, The modulation of fluorouracil with leucovorin in metastatic colorectal carcinoma. A perspective randomized phase III trial. *J Clin Oncol* 1989; **7:** 1419–26.
9. Nobile MT, Vidili MG, Sobrero A et al, 5-Fluorouracil alone or combined with high-dose folinic acid in advanced colorectal cancer patients: a randomized trial. *Proc Am Soc Clin Oncol* 1988; **7:** 97.
10. Valone FH, Friedman MA, Wittingler PS et al, Treatment of patients with advanced colorectal carcinomas with fluorouracil alone, high-dose leucovorin plus fluorouracil or sequential methotrexate, fluorouracil, leucovorin: a randomized trial of the Northern California Oncology Group. *J Clin Oncol* 1989; **7:** 1427–35.
11. Di Costanzo F, Bartolucci R, Sofra M et al, 5-Fluorouracil alone versus high-dose folinic acid and 5-FU in advanced colorectal cancer. A randomized trial of the Italian Oncology Group for Clinical Research. *Proc Am Soc Clin Oncol* 1989; **8:** 410.
12. Labianca R, Pancera G, Aitini E et al, Folinic acid + 5-fluorouracil (5-FU) versus equidose 5-FU in advanced colorectal cancer. Phase III study of GISCAD (Italian Group for the Study of Digestive Tract Cancer). *Ann Oncol* 1991; **2:** 673–9.
13. Poon MA, O'Connell MJ, Moertel CG et al, Biochemical modulation of fluorouracil. Evidence of significant improvement of survival and quality of life in patients with advanced colorectal carcinoma. *J Clin Oncol* 1989; **7:** 1407–17.
14. Doroshow JH, Multauf P, Leong L et al, Prospective randomized comparison of fluorouracil versus fluorouracil and high-dose continuous infusion leucovorin calcium for the treatment of advanced measurable colorectal cancer in patients previously unexposed to chemotherapy. *J Clin Oncol* 1990; **8:** 491–501.
15. Erlichman C, Fine S, Wong A et al, A randomized trial of fluorouracil and folinic acid in patients with metastatic colorectal carcinoma. *J Clin Oncol* 1988; **6:** 469–75.
16. Cricca A, Martoni A, Guaraldi M et al, Randomized clinical trial of 5-FU + folinic acid versus 5-FU in advanced gastrointestinal cancers. *Proc Eur Soc Med Oncol* 1988; **13:** 427.
17. Advanced Colorectal Cancer Meta-Analysis Project, Modulation of fluorouracil by leucovorin in patients with colorectal cancer: evidence in terms of response rate. *J Clin Oncol* 1982; **10:** 896–903.
18. Rustum W, Trave F, Zakrzewski SF et al, Biochemical and pharmacologic basis for potentiation of 5-fluorouracil action by leucovorin. *NCI Monogr* 1987; **5:** 165–70.
19. Mehta BM, Gisolfi AL, Hutchison DJ et al, Serum distribution of citrovorum factor and 5-methyl-

tetrahydrofolate following oral and i.v. administration of calcium leucovorin in normal adults. *Cancer Treat Rep* 1978; **62**: 345–50.

20. Keyomarsi K, Moran RG, Folinic acid augmentation of the effect of fluoropyrimidines on murine and human leukemic cells. *Cancer Res* 1986; **46**: 5229–35.

21. Peters GJ, Vanderwilt CL, Vangroeningen CJ et al, Thymidylate synthase inhibition after administration of fluorouracil with or without leucovorin in colon cancer patients: implications for treatment with fluorouracil. *J Clin Oncol* 1994; **12**: 2035–42.

22. Peters GJ, Hoekman K, Vangroeningen CJ et al, Potentiation of 5-fluorouracil induced inhibition of thymidylate synthase in human colon tumors by leucovorin is dose dependent. *Adv Exp Med Biol* 1993; **338**: 613–16.

23. Jolivet J, Role of leucovorin dosing and administration schedule. *Eur J Cancer* 1995; **31A**: 1311–15.

24. Etienne MC, Guillot T, Milano G, Critical factors for optimizing the 5-fluorouracil/folinic acid association in cancer chemotherapy. *Ann Oncol* 1996; **7**: 283–9.

25. Cao C, Frank C, Rustum Y, Role of fluoropyrimidine schedule and (6R, S) leucovorin dose in a preclinical animal model of colorectal carcinoma. *J Natl Cancer Inst* 1996; **88**: 430–6.

26. Doroshow JH, Biochemical modulation of fluoropyrimidines: is there an optimal (6R, S) leucovorin schedule? *J Natl Cancer Inst* 1996; **88**: 393–5.

27. Jaeger E, Klein O, Bernhard H et al, Weekly high-dose folinic acid (FA)/5-fluorouracil (FU) versus low dose FA/FU in advanced colorectal cancer. Result of a randomized multicenter trial. *Proc Am Soc Clin Oncol* 1994; **13**: 556.

27a. Jaeger E, Heike M, Bernhard H et al, Weekly high-dose leucovorin versus low-dose leucovorin combined with fluorouracil in advanced colorectal cancer. *J Clin Oncol* 1996; **14**: 2274–9.

28. Poon MA, O'Connell MJ, Wieand HS et al, Biochemical modulation of fluorouracil with leucovorin: confirmatory evidence of improved therapeutic efficacy in advanced colorectal cancer. *J Clin Oncol* 1991; **9**: 1967–72.

29. Buroker TR, O'Connell MJ, Wieand HS, Randomized comparison of two schedules of fluorouracil and leucovorin in the treatment of advanced colorectal cancer. *J Clin Oncol* 1994; **12**: 14–20.

30. Borner MN, Sartor O, More is not always better: a case for the low-dose leucovorin. *J Clin Oncol* 1993; **11**: 382.

31. Petrelli N, Rustum Y, Fluorouracil and leucovorin: there is a choice. *J Clin Oncol* 1993; **11**: 1434.

32. Valsecchi R, Labianca R, Cascinu S et al, High-dose versus low-dose L-leucovorin as a modulator of 5 days 5-fluorouracil in advanced colorectal cancer: a GISCAD phase III study. *Proc Am Soc Clin Oncol* 1995; **14**: 457.

33. Goldberg RM, O'Connell MJ, Wieand HS et al, A prospective randomized trial of intensive course 5-FU combined with A) The *l*-isomer of intravenous leucovorin, B) Oral (*d*, *l*) leucovorin or C) intravenous (*d*, *l*) leucovorin for the treatment of advanced colorectal cancer: a North Central Cancer Treatment Group study. *Proc Am Soc Clin Oncol* 1996; **15**: 471.

34. Glimelius B, Hoffman K, Graf W, Quality of life during chemotherapy in patients with symptomatic advanced colorectal cancer. *Cancer* 1994; **73**: 556–62.

35. de Gramont A, Bosset JF, Milan C et al, A prospective randomized trial comparing 5FU bolus with low-dose folinc acid (FUFOLld) and 5FU bolus plus continuous infusion with high-dose folinic acid (LV5FU2) for advanced colorectal cancer. *Proc Am Soc Clin Oncol* 1995; **14**: 455.

36. Leichman CG, Fleming TR, Muggia FM et al, Phase II study of fluorouracil and its modulation in advanced colorectal cancer: a Southwest Oncology Group study. *J Clin Oncol* 1995; **13**: 1303–11.

23

Protracted infusion of 5-FU for colorectal cancer

Paul J Ross, David Cunningham

CONTENTS • **Introduction** • **Randomized trials of PVI 5-FU** • **Other continuous-infusion schedules** • **Chronomodulation of 5-FU** • **Conclusions**

INTRODUCTION

5-Fluorouracil (5-FU) has been the standard cytotoxic agent used in advanced colorectal cancer since it was first synthesized in 1957. However, the optimal dosing schedule and method of administration are yet to be established. Response rates of 10–25% have been reported with single-agent bolus 5-FU. The drug has been delivered according to a variety of treatment schedules, either as a single agent or in combination with biochemical modulators or other cytotoxic drugs. Technological advances (venous-access devices and portable infusion pumps) have rendered infusional administration of cytotoxic agents (particularly 5-FU) feasible, and such delivery has become common and even standard practice in some oncology centres. A range of infusional 5-FU regimens have been administered, including 2600 mg/m^2 over 24 hours given weekly, 1000 mg/m^2 per day over 5 days every 3 weeks, and 300 mg/m^2 per day by protracted venous infusion (PVI) for several weeks or months. Infusional 5-FU regimens have demonstrated improved response rates with favourable toxicity profiles compared with bolus 5-FU schedules, but no significant survival benefits have been demonstrated for the infusional regimens. More recently, the use of chronomodulated infusional regimens has been evaluated. There is, however, no consensus as to the optimal duration or dose rate of the infusion.

5-FU is an antimetabolite that acts during the S phase of the cell cycle, and has a short plasma half-life (10–12 minutes), although the cytotoxic metabolite 5-fluorodeoxyuridine monophosphate (5-FdUMP) binds to thymidylate synthase (thereby inhibiting pyrimidine synthesis) for up to 6 hours at physiological concentrations of reduced folate.[1] At any time, only 3% of cells are in S phase, and therefore susceptible to the cytotoxic effect of 5-FU. A further feature of 5-FU favouring its administration as an infusion is the observation that an increased duration of exposure to 5-FU results in significantly increased cellular toxicity as measured by increased cell kill.[2] Administration as a continuous infusion is aimed to enhance the effectiveness of 5-FU by prolonging the binding to thymidylate synthase.

In 1981 Lokich et al[3] reported on the results of a phase I study. Seventeen patients with advanced solid tumours were administered 19 courses of PVI 5-FU at doses ranging from 200 to 600 mg/m^2 per day, with treatment suspended at the onset of mucositis. At doses of less than 300 mg/m^2 per day, the treatment did not require interruption for up to 60 days, whereas at higher doses virtually all patients developed mucositis. This study also demonstrated that serious (common toxicity criteria, CTC, grade 3/4) myelosuppression did not occur with PVI 5-FU. No other non-haematological toxicity was observed in this study.[3] Pharmacokinetic studies of continuous infusion have demonstrated a reduced distribution to the bone marrow, explaining the lower incidence of myelosuppression.[4]

Numerous phase II trials were conducted to determine the clinical efficacy of PVI 5-FU in the treatment of advanced colorectal cancer. A total of 284 patients were treated in 6 of these studies (Table 23.1).[5–10] Response rates for these trials are between 31% and 53%. This is significantly higher than the reported response rates for single-agent bolus 5-FU. The toxicity observed was substantially lower than with bolus 5-FU. The most frequently observed toxicity was plantar–palmar erythema, with an incidence between 39% and 98%.[8–10] Pyridoxine (vitamin B$_6$, 150 mg daily), commenced at the onset of plantar–palmar erythema, was demonstrated to reduce its severity and enable patients to continue treatment uninterrupted for a median time of 6 months compared with 2.5 months for patients who did not receive pyridoxine.[7] No neutropenia was recorded, and consequently there was no neutropenic sepsis.

In a randomized phase II study the Southwest Oncology Group (SWOG) evaluated the efficacy and toxicity of seven regimens of 5-FU.[11] The regimens (treatment arms) were as follows:

(1) 5-FU 500 mg/m^2 intravenous bolus on days 1 to 5 every 5 weeks;

(2) 5-FU 425 mg/m^2 intravenous bolus plus folinic acid 20 mg/m^2 intravenous bolus every 4 weeks for 2 cycles, then every 5 weeks;

(3) folinic acid 300 mg/m^2 as a 3-hour intravenous infusion, followed by 5-FU 600 mg/m^2 intravenous bolus weekly for 6 weeks every 8 weeks;

(4) PVI 5-FU 300 mg/m^2 on days 1–28 every 5 weeks;

(5) PVI 5-FU 200 mg/m^2 on days 1–28, with folinic acid 20 mg/m^2 on days 1, 8, 15 and 22 of a 5-week cycle;

(6) 5-FU 2600 mg/m^2 24-hour intravenous infusion weekly;

(7) N-phosphonoacetyl-L-aspartate (PALA) 250 mg/m^2 given over 15 minutes prior to 5-FU 2600 mg/m^2 24-hour intravenous infusion weekly.

Table 23.1 Phase II trials of PVI 5-FU in colorectal cancer

Regimen	Ref	Patients	Response rate (%)
5-FU 200 mg/m^2/d	5	16	31
5-FU 200–300 mg/m^2/d	6	26	39
5-FU 200 mg/m^2/d	7	25	44
5-FU 170–300 mg/m^2/d	8	100	53
5-FU 300 mg/m^2/d	9	91	33
5-FU 250–300 mg/m^2/d	10	26	42
TOTAL		**284**	**42**

Table 23.2 Response and survival in the Southwest Oncology Group randomized phase II study[11]

	5-FU IVB	5-FU IVB + LD FA	5-FU IVB + HD FA	PVI 5-FU	PVI 5-FU + LD FA	24-h 5-FU	24-h 5-FU + PALA
Number of evaluable patients	88	85	86	85	84	85	86
Response rate (%)	24	17	14	18	19	13	15
Median survival (months)	14	14	13	15	14	15	11

Abbreviations: IVB, intravenous bolus; LD, low-dose; HD, high-dose; FA, folinic acid; PALA, N-phosphonoacetyl-L-aspartate.

Table 23.3 CTC grade 3/4 toxicity in the Southwest Oncology Group randomized phase II study[11]

	5-FU IVB	5-FU IVB + LD FA	5-FU IVB + HD FA	PVI 5-FU	PVI 5-FU + LD FA	24-h 5-FU	24-h 5-FU + PALA
% with							
Diarrhoea	9	10	23	5	9	9	8
Stomatitis	4	12	1	5	9	1	6
Vomiting	2	5	5	3	4	3	3
Neutropenia	41	40	7	0	0	0	3

Abbreviations: IVB, intravenous bolus; LD, low-dose; HD, high-dose; FA, folinic acid; PALA, N-phosphonoacetyl-L-aspartate.

In this study, 620 patients were randomized, of whom 599 were evaluable. The confirmed response rates were similar in all of the treatment groups (Table 23.2). With a median follow-up of 37 months at the time of reporting, there was a survival advantage with PVI 5-FU and 24-hour 5-FU infusion compared with the other regimens. However, because of the design of the study, this lacked power to achieve statistical significance. CTC grade 3/4 neutropenia occurred more frequently with bolus regimens than with infusional regimens. CTC grade 3/4 diarrhoea was most frequent with bolus 5-FU modulated by high-dose folinic acid, with a much lower incidence in all of the infusion groups: 6% in arm 4, 11% in arms 5 and 6, and 10% in arm 7 (Table 23.3).[11]

RANDOMIZED TRIALS OF PVI 5-FU

Lokich et al[12] reported the first randomized study of PVI 5-FU (300 mg/m²/day) in a comparison with bolus 5-FU (500 mg/m²) on 5 consecutive days every 35 days. In this study, 174 patients (87 on each treatment regimen) were randomized and evaluable for response. The radiological response rate was significantly higher for the group treated with PVI 5-FU 29% (26/87) compared with 7% (6/87) for the bolus arm ($p < 0.001$). Four patients treated with PVI 5-FU achieved a complete response compared with none treated with bolus 5-FU. Despite the higher response rate, no survival advantage was detected (median survival time 10 months versus 11 months).

There was significantly less CTC grade 3/4 leucopenia in patients treated with PVI 5-FU (1% versus 20%; $p < 0.001$). Four patients treated with bolus 5-FU died of neutropenic sepsis, whilst there were no toxic deaths in patients treated with PVI 5-FU. Stomatitis was also observed more frequently in the group treated with bolus 5-FU. Thirteen percent experienced severe stomatitis with bolus 5-FU compared with 4% with PVI 5-FU. There was a 24% incidence of plantar–palmar erythema with PVI 5-FU.[12]

The Eastern Cooperative Oncology Group (ECOG) randomized trial comparing PVI 5-FU (300 mg/m^2/day) with single-agent bolus 5-FU (500 mg/m^2 for 5 days followed in 2 weeks by weekly 5-FU 600 mg/m^2) demonstrated a higher response rate for PVI 5-FU (28% versus 18%; $p = 0.045$).[13] An analysis comparing survival for the 312 patients treated with PVI 5-FU (with or without cisplatin) with the 153 patients treated with bolus 5-FU (with or without cisplatin) showed a significant improvement in progression-free survival ($p = 0.003$). However, there was no significant difference in overall survival ($p = 0.307$). Toxicity analysis is similar to the earlier study, with leucopenia following the 5-day loading course being the major toxicity for the cohort treated with bolus 5-FU, and plantar–palmar erythema being the most common toxicity with PVI 5-FU.[13]

Biochemical modulation of 5-FU with folinic acid (FA) provides an excess of reduced folate, stabilizing the 5-FdUMP/thymidylate synthase complex, and enhancing efficacy and increasing toxicity. Consequently, FA-modulated 5-FU regimens are the most widely used in the treatment of colorectal cancer. However, there are no published results of phase III trials comparing PVI 5-FU with FA-modulated 5-FU. The SWOG study discussed earlier in this chapter and summarized in Tables 23.2 and 23.3 demonstrated similar efficacy for PVI 5-FU with lower toxicity than 5-FU modulated by either low or high doses of FA.[11] An analysis comparing published reports of 173 patients treated with FA-modulated 5-FU with 255 patients treated with PVI 5-FU demonstrated similar survival in the two groups (11.5 months versus 11.1 months).[14] There was less toxicity reported

Table 23.4 Common toxicity criteria grade 3/4 toxicity in a randomized trial of PVI 5-FU compared with bolus 5-FU FA as adjuvant treatment in colorectal cancer (unpublished data)

Percentage with	PVI 5-FU	5-FU + FA	p
Stomatitis	4.2	30.6	<0.0001
Diarrhoea	3.2	23.5	0.0001
Nausea	0	4.1	0.05
Alopecia	0	15.3	<0.0001
Plantar–palmar	7.4	4.1	<0.0001
Neutropenia	1.1	53.1	<0.0001
Anaemia	0	1.0	Not significant
Infection	2.1	9.2	0.03

with PVI 5-FU, particularly the absence of severe myelosuppression. These toxicity advantages have been observed in a planned interim analysis of a randomized study of adjuvant chemotherapy for colorectal cancer comparing 5-FU (425 mg/m^2) with FA (20 mg/m^2) on days 1–5 every 4 weeks for 6 cycles with PVI 5-FU (300 mg/m^2/day) for 12 weeks (unpublished data) (Table 23.4).

The role of biochemical modulation of PVI 5-FU with FA has been evaluated in a phase II study of 41 patients. The regimen comprised FA-modulated PVI 5-FU (200 mg/m^2/day) for four weeks followed by a two-week rest and then by monthly cycles of three weeks of treatment followed by a one-week rest and FA (20 mg/m^2) by intravenous bolus at the start of each treatment week.[15] There was a 46% response rate, with the median duration of survival being 16 months. It appeared in this study that the duration of 5-FU infusion was shortened owing to the earlier onset of dose-limiting toxicity, mucositis and plantar–palmar erythema. The SWOG randomized phase II study demonstrated similar efficacy to the regimen used in the earlier phase II study of PVI 5-FU alone.[11] The incidence of severe diarrhoea and mucositis was more frequent with the modulated schedule. Furthermore, the frequency of dose-limiting toxicity was higher than in the original phase II trial. On the basis of these studies, there is no benefit from the biochemical modulation of PVI 5-FU with folinic acid.

Interferon-α is a second agent that has been used as a modulator of 5-FU. This was based on in vitro evidence that it increases the formation of active metabolites, enhances incorporation into DNA, and inhibits upregulation of thymidylate synthase and thymidine salvage pathways.[16–19] Initial phase II trials with bolus 5-FU suggested that this synergy could enhance efficacy, and consequently The Royal Marsden Hospital evaluated its combination with PVI 5-FU. A phase II study demonstrated increased activity when interferon-α was given concurrently, with reversal of 5-FU resistance.[20] Subsequently The Royal Marsden Hospital conducted a prospective, randomized study of 180 patients who were treated with PVI 5-FU

(300 mg/m^2/day) with or without interferon-α 5 MU subcutaneously three times weekly.[21] The radiological response rate was 28%, with no significant difference between the two groups. There was no improvement in failure-free duration (median 161 versus 193 days) or overall survival duration (median 328 versus 357 days) from the addition of interferon-α. Symptomatic improvement occurred equally in the two treatment groups, with response rates between 61% and 80%, depending on the symptom (Table 23.5). For PVI 5-FU, improvements in pain were seen in 68%, improvements in weight loss in 85% and improvements in anorexia in 78%. There were no measurable differences in quality of life between the two groups using the EORTC QLQ C-30 questionnaire. Toxicity was significantly greater with the addition of interferon-α, with increased leucopenia (24% versus 5%; $p = 0.001$), neutropenia (13% versus 4%; $p = 0.04$), mucositis (61% versus 39%; $p = 0.008$) and alopecia (69% versus 21%; $p = 0.0002$). This study confirmed that PVI 5-FU is an effective palliative chemotherapy regimen for the treatment of metastatic colorectal cancer, with only mild to moderate toxicity and maintenance of quality of life. However, interferon-α results in a higher incidence of toxicity with no response or survival benefit. This finding was consistent with other trials evaluating the role of interferon-α as a biochemical modulator of 5-FU.[22–24] Consequently, with currently used doses and schedules, there is no role for interferon-α in the palliative treatment of colorectal cancer.

Table 23.5 Symptomatic response with PVI 5-FU[21]

Symptom	Patients	%
Weight loss	49/61	80
Anorexia	28/43	65
Oesophageal reflux	13/20	65
Nausea	18/28	64
Pain	57/93	61

Combinations of cisplatin and 5-FU are widely used in the treatment of oesophagogastric cancer and head and neck cancers. The Mid Atlantic Oncology Programme evaluated the addition of cisplatin to PVI 5-FU using $20 \, mg/m^2/week$ of cisplatin, and found no improvement beyond that obtained with PVI 5-FU alone.[25] The ECOG study comparing infusional and bolus 5-FU also randomized patients between 5-FU alone or the addition of cisplatin $20 \, mg/m^2$ weekly.[13] Again there was no further improvement in response or progression-free survival. Severe vomiting and diarrhoea were more frequent with the addition of cisplatin, whilst the incidence of mucositis, palmar–plantar erythema and myelosuppression were similar.

The results of the randomized studies evaluating PVI 5-FU confirm that it is effective in treating the symptoms of metastatic colorectal cancer. A dose of 5-FU $(300 \, mg/m^2/day)$ causes acceptable levels of toxicity when treatment is continued for up to six months. Treatment can continue with CTC grade I toxicity and appropriate symptomatic measures instituted for diarrhoea, mucositis and plantar–palmar erythema. For more severe toxicity, the infusion of 5-FU should be suspended until resolution of the toxicity and subsequently recommenced with a reduction in dose. Complications with skin-tunnelled central venous catheters requiring removal is relatively low; the reported removal rate in one study was 11%.[21] At The Royal Marsden Hospital, 832 patients have been treated in the ambulatory chemotherapy programme. Clinically significant complications on insertion were rare. All patients receive prophylactic antibiotics prior to insertion, and warfarin 1 mg daily commencing on the day of insertion. Eighteen percent of catheters were removed because of complications, including thrombosis (4.7%), infection (5.7%), migration (3.6%), pain (2.5%) and damage (2.0%). Complications were significantly more frequent in those catheters with their tips in the superior vena cava than in the right atrium ($p = 0.003$). A further 15% developed complications not requiring removal, the majority of which were infections treated with antibi-otics. Quality-of-life issues were significantly affected in 10–23% of patients.

OTHER CONTINUOUS-INFUSION SCHEDULES

In efforts to develop the optimal regimen for the treatment of colorectal cancer, the duration of infusion ranged from 24 hours to 14 days. The maximum tolerated dose of continuous-infusion 5-FU over 24 hours was found to be $2.6 \, g/m^2$ once weekly, with dose-limiting toxicity being non-haematological.[26] In a phase II study a 45% (10/22) response rate was demonstrated from 5-FU $(2600 \, mg/m^2)$ infused concurrently with folinic acid $(500 \, mg/m^2)$ over 24 hours.[27]

The Spanish Cooperative Group for Gastrointestinal Tumor Therapy has developed a regimen of 5-FU given over 48 hours each week combined with oral folinic acid. In phase I and II studies the maximum tolerated dose of weekly 4-hour continuous infusion of 5-FU was established[28,29] as $3.5 \, mg/m^2$. Dose-limiting toxicity was diarrhoea and mucositis, and the overall response rate in the multicentre phase II study was 38.5%. Aranda et al[30] evaluated modulated continuous-infusion high-dose 5-FU $(3.0 \, mg/m^2)$ with oral FA in an effort to increase efficacy, but the high incidence of toxicity (diarrhoea and mucositis) with this schedule necessitated a reduction in the dose of 5-FU.[30] In a subsequent trial, weekly 48-hour continuous infusion of 5-FU $(2 \, mg/m^2)$ combined with oral FA (60 mg every 6 hours) during the infusion achieved a 37.5% response rate, with a median survival of 14.5 months.[31] Toxicity was evaluated according to the World Health Organisation (WHO) criteria, with grade 3 diarrhoea occurring in 24.5%, grade 3/4 vomiting in 12.6% and grade 3/4 mucositis in 9%. The incidence of diarrhoea and vomiting with this regimen is higher than we have experienced with PVI 5-FU.

Another schedule principally used in the United Kingdom and France is the 'de Gramont' regimen, which combines bolus $(200 \, mg/m^2)$ and infusional $(600 \, mg/m^2)$ 5-FU with a 2-hour infusion of high-dose FA $(200 \, mg/m^2)$ daily for 2 days every 2 weeks. In a randomized trial, this schedule produced a significantly higher response rate than the FA-modulated bolus 5-FU given according to the Mayo schedule (34% versus 17%; $p = 0.002$). Furthermore, progression-free and overall survival were significantly improved ($p = 0.008$ and $p = 0.006$).[32]

CHRONOMODULATION OF 5-FLUOROURACIL

There is some evidence that cancer cells have abnormal circadian rhythms. This has been exploited by chronomodulating the administration schedule of 5-FU. In ambulatory patients, 5-FU (600 mg/m^2/day), FA (300 mg/m^2/day) and oxaliplatin (20 mg/m^2/day) for 5 days were administered every 21 days with the use of a programmable-in-time pump.[33] Ninety-two patients were randomized to receive either fixed rate or chronomodulated infusion (maximum delivery of 5-FU and FA at 04:00 and maximum delivery of oxaliplatin at 16:00). The response rate was significantly higher for patients treated with the chronomodulated schedule (53% versus 32%; $p = 0.038$), and there was a corresponding improvement in survival (19 months versus 14.9 months; $p = 0.03$). WHO grade 3/4 mucositis was significantly more frequent with fixed-rate infusion (89% versus 18%; $p < 0.001$).

CONCLUSIONS

The activity of 5-FU during the S phase of the cell cycle and the pharmacokinetics of 5-FU favour its administration as an infusion. Continuous infusions of 5-FU, including protracted venous infusions and chronomodulated infusions, have become feasible with the development of venous access devices, with acceptable complication rates, and modern portable pumps. These regimens are well tolerated, with lower frequencies of severe toxicity than bolus regimens – in particular, significant myelosuppression occurs rarely. PVI 5-FU is effective in palliating the symptoms of metastatic colorectal cancer, and in randomized studies achieved higher objective response rates than bolus regimens. In addition, the ECOG study showed a significant improvement in progression-free survival with PVI 5-FU compared with bolus 5-FU.[13] Three shorter infusional schedules have been the subject of particular interest: 24-hour weekly high-dose 5-FU and weekly 48-hour continuous infusion 5-FU have both demonstrated encouraging response rates in phase II studies. The de Gramont regimen has demonstrated response, progression-free advantages compared with the Mayo schedule of 5-FU and folinic acid.[32] In Europe, in larger centres these infusional regimens are gradually being adopted as standard therapy on the basis of the data demonstrating higher response rates with less toxicity than bolus 5-FU regimens. Chronomodulation may further enhance efficacy and improve toxicity profiles compared with infusional regimens currently used.

REFERENCES

1. Macmillan WE, Wolberg WH, Welling PG, Pharmacokinetics of 5-fluorouracil in humans. *Cancer Res* 1978; **38:** 3479–82.
2. Drewinko B, Yang L, Cellular basis for the inefficiency of 5-fluorouracil in human colon carcinoma. *Cancer Treat Rep* 1985; **69:** 1391–8.
3. Lokich J, Bothe A, Fine N, Perri J, Phase I study of protracted venous infusion of 5-fluorouracil. *Cancer* 1981; **48:** 2565–8.
4. Fraile RJ, Baker LH, Buroker TR et al, Pharmacokinetics of 5-fluorouracil administered orally, by rapid intravenous and by slow infusion. *Cancer Res* 1980; **40:** 2223–8.
5. Leichman L, Leichman C, Kinzie J et al, Long term low dose 5-fluorouracil in advanced measurable colon cancer: no correlation between toxicity and efficacy. *Proc Am Soc Clin Oncol* 1985; **4:** 86.
6. Belt RJ, Davidner ML, Lyron MC et al, Continuous low dose 5-fluorouracil for adenocarcinoma: confirmation of activity. *Proc Am Soc Clin Oncol* 1985; **4:** 90.

7. Molina R, Fabian C, Slavik M et al, Reversal of palmar–plantar erythrodysaesthesia by B6 without loss of response in colon cancer patients receiving 200 mg/m sq/day continuous 5-FU. *Proc Am Soc Clin Oncol* 1987; **6:** 74.

8. Wade JL, Herbst S, Greenberg A, Prolonged venous infusion of 5-fluorouracil for metastatic colon cancer: a follow-up report. *Proc Am Soc Clin Oncol* 1988; **7:** 94.

9. Hansen R, Quebberman E, Ausman R et al, Continuous systemic 5-fluorouracil chemotherapy in advanced colorectal cancer: results in 91 patients. *J Surg Oncol* 1989; **40:** 177–81.

10. Kuo S, Finck S, Cho J et al, Continuous ambulatory infusion 5-fluorouracil chemotherapy in advanced colorectal cancer: a single institution retrospective study. *Proc Am Soc Clin Oncol* 1989; **8:** 126.

11. Leichman CG, Fleming TR, Muggia F et al, Phase II study of fluorouracil and its modulation in advanced colorectal cancer: a Southwest Oncology Group study. *J Clin Oncol* 1995; **13:** 1303–11.

12. Lokich JJ, Ahlgren JD, Gullo JJ et al, A prospective randomized comparison of continuous infusion fluorouracil with a conventional bolus schedule in metastatic colorectal carcinoma: a Mid-Atlantic Oncology Program study. *J Clin Oncol* 1989; **7:** 425–32.

13. Hansen RM, Ryan L, Anderson T et al, Phase III study of bolus versus infusion fluorouracil with or without cisplatin in advanced colorectal cancer. *J Natl Cancer Inst* 1996; **88:** 668–74.

14. Ahlgren J, Protracted infusional schedules of fluorouracil in colorectal cancer versus fluorouracil with modulators: differences in similarities. *J Infus Chemother* 1992; **2:** 128–37.

15. Leichman CG, Leichman L, Spears P et al, Prolonged continuous infusion of fluorouracil with weekly bolus leucovorin: a phase II study in patients with disseminated colorectal cancer. *J Natl Cancer Inst* 1993; **85:** 41–4.

16. Elias L, Sandoval JM, Interferon effects upon fluorouracil metabolism by HL-60 cells. *Biochem Biophys Res Commun* 1989; **163:** 867–74.

17. Houghton JA, Morton C, Adkins D et al, Locus of the interaction among 5-fluorouracil, leucovorin, and interferon-α2a in colon carcinoma cells. *Cancer Res* 1993; **53:** 4243–50.

18. Chu E, Zinn S, Boarman D et al, Interaction of gamma interferon and 5-fluorouracil in H630 human colon carcinoma cell lines. *Cancer Res* 1993; **50:** 5834–40.

19. Pfeffer LM, Tamm I, Interferon inhibition of thymidine incorporation into DNA through effects on thymidine transport and uptake. *J Cell Physiol* 1984; **121:** 431–6.

20. Findlay M, Hill A, Cunningham D et al, Protracted venous infusion 5-fluorouracil and interferon-α in advanced and refractory colorectal cancer. *Ann Oncol* 1994; **5:** 239–43.

21. Hill M, Norman A, Cunningham D et al, Impact of protracted venous infusion fluorouracil with or without interferon alfa-2b on tumour response, survival, and quality of life in advanced colorectal cancer. *J Clin Oncol* 1995; **13:** 2317–23.

22. York M, Greco FA, Figlin RA et al, A randomised phase III trial comparing 5-FU with or without interferon alfa 2a for advanced colorectal cancer. *Proc Am Soc Clin Oncol* 1993; **12:** 590 (abst).

23. Dufour P, Husseini F, Dreyfuss B et al, Randomised study of 5-fluorouracil (5-FU) vs 5-FU + alpha 2a interferon (IFN) for metastatic colorectal carcinoma (MCRC). *Ann Oncol* 1994; **5:** 220 (abst).

24. Hill M, Norman A, Cunningham D et al, Royal Marsden phase III trial of fluorouracil with or without interferon alfa-2b in advanced colorectal cancer. *J Clin Oncol* 1995; **13:** 1297–302.

25. Lokich JJ, Ahlgren JD, Cantrell J et al, A prospective randomised comparison of protracted infusion 5FU with or without weekly bolus cisplatin in metastatic colorectal carcinoma. A Mid Atlantic Oncology Programme Study. *Cancer* 1991; **67:** 4–19.

26. Ardalan B, Singh G, Sieberman H, A randomised phase I and II study of short-term infusion of high dose fluorouracil with and without N-(phosphonoacetyl)-L-aspartic acid in patients with advanced pancreatic and colorectal cancers. *J Clin Oncol* 1988; **6:** 1053–8.

27. Ardalan B, Chua L, Tian E-M et al, A phase II study of weekly 24-hour infusion with high dose fluorouracil with leucovorin in colorectal carcinoma. *J Clin Oncol* 1991; **9:** 625–30.

28. Diaz-Rubio E, Aranda E, Martin M et al, Weekly high-dose infusion of 5-fluorouracil in advanced colorectal cancer. *Eur J Cancer* 1990; **26:** 727–9.

29. Diaz-Rubio E, Aranda E, Camps C et al, A phase II study of weekly 48-hour infusion with high-dose fluorouracil in advanced colorectal cancer: an alternative to biochemical modulation. *J Infus Chemother* 1994; **4:** 58–61.

30. Aranda E, Cervantes A, Dorta J et al, A phase II

trial of weekly high-dose continuous-infusion 5-fluorouracil plus oral leucovorin in patients with advanced colorectal cancer. *Cancer* 1995; **76:** 559–63.

31. Aranda E, Cervantes A, Carrato A et al, Outpatient weekly high-dose continuous-infusion 5-fluorouracil plus oral leucovorin in advanced colorectal cancer. A phase II trial. *Ann Oncol* 1996; **7:** 581–5.

32. de Gramont A, Bosset JF, Milan C et al, A prospectively randomized trial comparing 5-fluorouracil bolus with low dose folinic acid (FUFOld) and 5-fluorouracil bolus plus continuous infusion with high dose folinic acid (L-V5FU2) for advanced colorectal cancer. *Proc Am Soc Clin Oncol* 1995; **14:** 455 (abst).

33. Levi FA, Zidani R, Vannetzel J-M et al, Chronomodulated versus fixed-infusion-rate delivery of ambulatory chemotherapy with oxaliplatin, fluorouracil, and folinic acid (leucovorin) in patients with colorectal cancer metastases: a randomized multi-institutional trial. *J Natl Cancer Inst* 1994; **86:** 1608–17.

24

High-dose 24- or 48-hour infusion of 5-fluorouracil plus/minus folinic acid in the treatment of metastatic colorectal cancer

Andrés Cervantes, Eduardo Díaz-Rubio, Enrique Aranda, on behalf of the Spanish Group for Gastrointestinal Tumor Therapy (TTD)

INTRODUCTION

Since its introduction in clinical oncology 40 years ago, 5-fluorouracil (5-FU) remains the most useful drug in the treatment of patients with advanced colorectal cancer. Many schedules, dosages and routes of administration have been used for 5-FU, not only as a single agent, but also in combination with modulating compounds such as folinic acid, methotrexate, N-(phosphonoacetyl)-L-aspartic acid (PALA), interferon, dipyridamole and hydroxyurea, among others. Randomized trials using strict response criteria showed that the objective response rate that may be achieved with 5-FU, given as an intravenous push, ranges around 10–15%. Despite some advances in the understanding of the metabolic pathways by which 5-FU may eventually produce tumor cell death, the impact of biomodulation on the natural history of the disease is limited, with some improvement in response rate, but without any significant effect on survival.[1] However, improvement in tumor-related symptoms is frequently seen, and for this reason, palliative chemotherapy of metastatic colorectal has a major role.

Although intravenous administration of 5-FU is the most widely accepted way to give the drug, the optimal schedule is still not settled. There are tumor cell kinetics as well as pharmacological considerations that may explain the low response rates observed in colorectal cancer when 5-FU is administered as a rapid bolus injection.

As with other antimetabolites, 5-FU is most effective against tumor cells that are in active cell division. Colorectal cancer is a slowly growing tumor with most tumor cells in G0 or resting phase and only a small proportion in the susceptible S phase. This may be one of the reasons why 5-FU, when given by rapid push injection, will only kill a small proportion of malignant cells. On the other hand, owing to its rapid catabolism, the serum half-life of 5-FU is very short, not exceeding 11 minutes; therefore tumor cells are exposed to the drug only for a short period of time.

Prolonged intravenous infusion may circumvent these disadvantages. However, low serum concentrations of a drug may induce drug-resistant cell clones.

WEEKLY HIGH-DOSE 24- OR 48-HOUR INFUSION OF 5-FU: HIGHER DOSE INTENSITY WITH BETTER THERAPEUTIC INDEX

To develop a theoretically optimal approach to the use of 5-FU in metastatic colorectal cancer, several factors have to be taken into account: high dose and appropriate dose intensity, prolonged exposure, limiting toxicity and ways of effective biomodulation. A dose–response relationship has been suggested for 5-FU in colorectal cancer,[2] and it is clear that, by employing a continuous-infusion schedule, a much higher dose intensity can be obtained. However, data supporting the concept of a dose–response relationship are mainly derived from retrospective analysis of a study or from a comparison of different trials. This means of analysis may be misleading because a supposed dose–response relation can simply reflect the fact that patients with better prognostic factors can tolerate higher doses of chemotherapy. Comparisons of different trials have many flaws because of widely varying selection criteria and means of assessing the response. Despite these problems, the collected data suggest that there is a dose–response relation, and they underline the impact of the dose intensity of 5-FU. This applies not only for bolus injection of 5-FU, but also for continuous-infusion schedules.[3]

Investigators in Vancouver pioneered a number of ways to administer 5-FU in continuous infusions of short duration but at frequent intervals.[4] The best results, with an overall response rate of 30%, were achieved with a 48-hour infusion of 60 mg/kg 5-FU given weekly. The dose intensity of this schedule reached approximately 2500 mg/m²/week, which was at that time considerably higher than with any other schedule. In a phase I–II trial design, it was shown that, when administered weekly in such a 48-hour infusion schedule, the maximum tolerated dose of 5-FU was 3500 mg/m²/week, with a good toxicity profile and a response rate of 43% in non-pretreated patients.[5] When different ways of giving 5-FU are compared in order to define dose intensity (Table 24.1), it is found that bolus injection of 5-FU may reach a maximum dose intensity of 500–750 mg/m²/week, with myelosuppression as the limiting toxicity.[6,7] When the duration of the infusion is prolonged to five days, the dose

Table 24.1 A dose-intensity comparison of different routes of 5-FU administration

Dose (mg)	Infusion duration	Schedule	Dose intensity (mg/m²/week)	Limiting toxicity	Reference
500 × 5	i.v. push	5 weeks	500	Myelosuppression	6
750	i.v. push	Weekly	750	Myelosuppression	7
5000	120 hours	Monthly	1250	Muscositis	8, 9
300	Protracted	Daily	2100	Hand–foot	6
2600	24 hours	Weekly alone	2600	Diarrhea	10
		+LV			11, 13
		+PALA			12
3500	48 hours	Weekly	3500	Diarrhea	14

Abbreviations: LV, leucovorin; PALA, N-(phosphonoacetyl)-L-aspartic acid.

intensity achieved is almost doubled, but mucositis appears as the limiting toxic effect, and three to four weeks are needed for recovery before the next dose may be administered.[8,9] When 5-FU is given as a protracted infusion of at least five weeks, the daily dose goes down to 300 mg/m², but the dose intensity increases to 2100 mg/m²/week. This indicates a threefold increase in dose intensity over bolus injection, with a significant improvement in response rate (30% versus 7%) in a randomized study.[6] The therapeutic index is also better, with fewer episodes of grade 3 or 4 toxicity, and evidence of the hand–foot syndrome as a prominent feature. However, no survival benefit could be found.[6]

Prolonged continuous infusion of 5-FU produces relatively low plasma levels of 5-FU during a long time. Theoretically, this may facilitate development of resistance, although there is no clinical evidence of this phenomenon. Some other schedules with weekly short-term infusions of 24- or 48-hour duration have been studied, in order to allow the delivery of higher dose intensity. With those schedules, the tumor is exposed every week to higher plasma concentrations than with the protracted infusion, leading to a higher dose intensity. This is particularly clear with the weekly 48-hour schedule, which achieves the highest dose intensity ever achieved with 5-FU, allowing the administration of 3500 mg/m²/week.[5] A summary of several published studies of weekly high-dose 5-FU in 24- or 48-hour infusion is presented in Table 24.2.

A weekly 24-hour infusion of 5-FU in escalating doses up to 3400 mg/m² with or without PALA in patients with colorectal and pancreatic cancer yielded a 40% response rate among a total of 30 patients with colorectal cancer, while only four patients out of eleven receiving 5-FU alone responded in this small phase I–II trial. The maximum tolerated dose for 5-FU in this weekly schedule appeared to be 2600 mg/m².[10] Other authors modulated the same schedule with PALA, leucovorin or interferon, with response rates ranging from 80% to 19%.[11–13] Limiting toxicity was mainly diarrhea. However, these results raised the question whether they were due to the weekly high-dose schedule of 5-FU or to the addition of the modulating agents.

Table 24.2 Data from phase I–II or III trials of weekly 24- or 48-hour continuous infusions of 5-FU as single agent in advanced colorectal cancer patients

Phase	Dose	Infusion duration (hours)	Dose intensity (mg/m²/week)	Number of patients	Response rate (%)	Toxicity: WHO grade 3 + 4 (%)	Reference
I–II	2600 mg/m²	24	2600	11	21	12	10
III	2600 mg/m²	24	2600	63	13	19	16
III	2600 mg/m²	24	2600	132	n.s.	11[a]	17
II	60 mg/kg	48	2500	30	30	14	4
III	60 mg/kg	48	1600	110	10	5	15
II	3500 mg/m²	48	3500	83	39	21	14

Abbreviation: n.s., not stated.
[a] Only grade 4 toxicity.

Data on the 48-hour weekly schedule have been developed by the Spanish Group for Gastrointestinal Tumor Therapy (TTD) and by the Gastrointestinal Tract Cooperative Group of the European Organization for Research and Treatment of Cancer (EORTC).[14,15] The European study tried to confirm the activity observed by Shah et al[4] in a randomized trial comparing weekly high-dose infusional 5-FU (60 mg/kg) over a 48-hour period plus/minus methotrexate.[15] The addition of low-dose methotrexate led to a doubling of the response rate from 10% to 21% without any significant effect on survival. It may be important to consider that in this schedule the dose intensity of 5-FU was approximately 1600 mg/m^2/week, which is below the maximum of 3500 mg/m^2/week intended by the Spanish trial. The suboptimal dose intensity administered may explain the low response rate obtained with infusional 5-FU alone.

However, in an extended multicenter phase II trial,[14] the Spanish Group confirmed the results previously achieved in the early phase I–II study.[5] The response rate was 38.5% in 83 patients with a median administered dose intensity of 3000 mg/m^2/week, ranging from 1800 to 3500 mg/m^2/week. Grade 3 and 4 diarrhea and mucositis were only observed in 12% and 11% of cases respectively. Weekly 48-hour continuous infusion of 5-FU permits a dose intensity and a maximum tolerated dose superior to all other schedules, with an activity that is superior to bolus 5-FU and comparable to the combination with leucovorin. Another point of interest is the low toxicity observed and the excellent tolerance of the treatment.

When the response rates obtained by different schedules of continuous infusion of 5-FU in several randomized and non-randomized trials are plotted against the planned dose intensity, there seems to be a linear relationship (Figure 24.1). However, the analysis of dose intensity and response is mainly based on retrospective studies. Data from randomized studies to support the hypothesis of a relationship between dose intensity and response are lacking. A seven-arm trial with a screening design, including 620 patients with advanced colorectal

cancer, was not able to detect any differences in survival or response rate.[16] Four infusional regimens were included in this Southwest Oncology Group (SWOG) study: protracted infusion of 5-FU alone or modulated by leucovorin, and 24-hour infusion of high-dose 5-FU alone with or without PALA modulation. None of these schedules provided substantial improvement over the classical 5-FU bolus. While screening trials are a useful approach in clinical trials, especially in the setting of assessing multiple schedules of dosing, delivery or modulation, it is important to remember that such trials are not designed to provide definitive evidence about a regimen's clinical efficacy. Thus the lack of positive survival trends in a screening trial does not usually provide evidence against benefit.

When protracted infusional studies of 5-FU were analyzed in terms of toxicity, myelosuppression was virtually absent and the hand–foot syndrome was the most prominent toxic effect.[6] Despite the high dose intensity achieved, the toxicity profile of weekly high doses of 5-FU in 24- or 48-hour infusion schedules indicates excellent tolerance. In the EORTC trial, only 5% of the patients receiving 5-FU alone showed a grade 3–4 toxicity,[15] none of

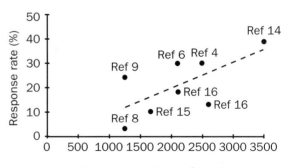

Figure 24.1 Relation between planned dose intensity and response rate observed in several randomized[6,8,9,15,16] and non-randomized[4,14] trials of continuous infusion of 5-FU given without biomodulation in advanced measurable colorectal cancer patients.

them having the hand–foot syndrome. The toxicity observed in the SWOG for the 24-hour infusional arm without PALA modulation was generally mild.[16] Twenty percent of patients suffered from severe toxicity – mainly diarrhea (11%). This observation was confirmed in a recently published randomized study of the same 24-hour schedule plus or minus modulation with leucovorin, interferon or PALA.[17] The single-agent 5-FU was the better-tolerated arm, with only 11% of grade 4 toxicity, particularly diarrhea. As previously stated, the Spanish phase II trial achieved the highest dose intensity of 5-FU as a weekly infusion.[14] However, grade 4 toxicity was seen in only 10% of patients. The most frequently observed toxic effects were diarrhea (12%) and mucositis (11%). It is important to stress that almost half of the patients treated did not require a dose reduction because of toxicity, and the median dose intensity that could be given was 3000 mg/m^2/week. Overall, weekly 24- or 48-hour infusions of 5-FU offer the possibility of achieving a high dose intensity of 5-FU, with a response rate in the same range of that observed for the modulation of bolus 5-FU plus leucovorin and with an improved toxicity profile.

BIOMODULATION OF WEEKLY HIGH-DOSE 24- OR 48-HOUR INFUSION OF 5-FU

It is reasonable to try to improve the therapeutic activity of weekly high-dose continuous-infusion schedules of 5-FU by the addition of modulating agents, and several phase II and III studies have addressed this particular issue. Table 24.3 shows a summary of the studies using 24-hour infusion. An ECOG/CALGB phase III trial randomized 1118 patients with advanced colorectal cancer to five different arms.[17] The first consisted of a weekly 24-hour infusion of 2600 mg/m^2 of 5-FU. The second added 250 mg/m^2 of PALA to the previous schedule of 5-FU. The other arms included the classical Roswell Park protocol with weekly high-dose leucovorin plus bolus 5-FU, weekly high-dose leucovorin given orally plus bolus 5-FU, and a continuous infusion of 5-FU during 120 hours modulated by interferon. No significant differences in survival were observed between these arms. Although mature data from this trial are still lacking, it was reported that the weekly infusional regimens of 5-FU were equally active, but significantly less toxic than bolus 5-FU modulated by leucovorin or interferon. No data have been reported so far

Table 24.3 Phase II–III trials of weekly 24-hour continuous infusion of biomodulated 5-FU (2600 mg/m^2) in advanced colorectal cancer patients

Phase	Biomodulating agent	Dose intensity (mg/m^2/week)	Number of patients	Response rate (%)	Toxicity: WHO grade 3 + 4 (%)	Reference
II	i.v. LV + PALA	2600	26	43	n.s.	12
III	i.v. LV	2600	91	44	25	11
III	IFN	2600	90	18	11	11
III	i.v. LV + IFN	2600	49	27	23	11
III	i.v. PALA	2600	132	n.s.	11*	17

Abbreviations: LV, leucovorin; PALA, *N*-(phosphonoacetyl)-L-aspartic acid; IFN, interferon; n.s., not stated.
[a] Only grade 4 toxicity.

on the comparison between the single-agent infusional 5-FU and the PALA-modulated arm. A small phase II trial combined weekly low-dose bolus PALA with a 24-hour infusion of 5-FU (2600 mg/m²) together with an infusional high dose of leucovorin (500 mg/m²).[12] Out of 26 patients included in the trial, 11 (42%) had an objective response. Ten patients required a 5-FU dose reduction to 2100 mg/m² due to several instances of toxicity. Mild fatigue and hand–foot syndrome were observed in almost half of the patients.

A German multicenter trial included 236 patients with three different arms.[11] Patients were randomized to receive a weekly 24-hour infusion of 5-FU at a dose of 2600 mg/m² with an infusion of 500 mg/m² of leucovorin given over two hours, or the same dose of infusional 5-FU modulated with three million units of α-interferon three times weekly. A third arm considered a double modulation with leucovorin and interferon, but was closed at the first interim analysis owing to similar activity to the leucovorin-modulated arm and a high incidence of severe toxicity, with a 10% incidence of toxic deaths. The leucovorin-modulated arm showed a significant increase in response rate (44% versus 18%), a prolonged time to progression (7 versus 4 months) and a better survival (17 versus 13 months) compared with the inter-

feron-modulated arm. However, this trial did not have a 5-FU-alone control arm; therefore it is not possible to conclude if those results are really due to the modulation of 5-FU.

It is concluded from these trials that weekly 5-FU (2600 mg/m²) in infusions over 24 hours may be safely given in combination with leucovorin, PALA or both with a tolerable incidence of reversible toxicity. Modulation of this schedule with α-interferon led to lower activity. Definite data on the need for leucovorin modulation to increase the activity of these 24-hour infusion schedules may come from mature data of the previously mentioned ECOG/CALGB phase III trial.

Some European investigators have developed several forms of modulation for the 48-hour schedule (Table 24.4). So far, the EORTC trial is the only randomized study that has shown that a small dose of 40 mg/m² of methotrexate was able to increase the activity of infusional 5-FU over 48 hours versus 5-FU alone.[15] The response rate was 21% in the modulated arm, compared with 11% in the 5-FU-alone arm. Severe toxicity was also double in the modulated arm, rising to a 24% incidence of grade 3 and 4 episodes, mainly stomatitis, compared with a 5% incidence in the control arm. A point to underline in this study is the low dose intensity of 5-FU. In the beginning, four courses

Table 24.4 Phase II–III trials of weekly or biweekly 48-hour continuous infusions of biomodulated 5-FU in advanced colorectal cancer patients

Phase	Dose	Biomodulating agent	Dose intensity (mg/m²/week)		Number of patients	Response rate (%)	Toxicity: WHO grade 3 + 4 (%)	Reference
			Planned	Achieved				
III	60 mg/kg	Methotrexate	1600	n.s.	106	21	24	15
III	2000 mg/m² a	i.v. LV	1000	n.s.	159	34	9	18
II	3000 mg/m²	Oral LV	3000	2200	43	29	78	20
II	2000 mg/m²	Oral LV	2000	1600	110	37	40	21

Abbreviations: LV, leucovorin; n.s., not stated.
[a]A combination of bolus 5-FU (400 mg/m²) and 22-hour infusion (600 mg/m²) on days 1 and 2, every two weeks, is used in this schedule.

were given on a weekly basis. Thereafter, four more courses were given biweekly, meaning a total of 8 courses in 12 weeks. This implies a dose intensity of 1600 mg/m^2/week. As can be seen from other studies of short-term infusional therapy, when 5-FU is modulated, the dose intensity of the drug goes down. In other words, 5-FU can be modulated only if a lower dose intensity of the drug is given.

A multicenter French phase III trial compared the low-dose leucovorin plus 5-FU schedule of the Mayo Clinic against an infusional arm.[18] The experimental arm of the trial consisted of a combination of bolus and continuous infusion of 5-FU modulated by high-dose leucovorin. This schedule was based on the lack of cross-resistance of these two forms of administration of the drug.[19] After a 2-hour infusion of leucovorin, a bolus injection of 5-FU (400 mg/m^2) was given, followed by a 22-hour infusion of 5-FU (600 mg/m^2). This treatment was repeated for two days every two weeks. The infusional arm showed a significantly superior response rate (34% versus 17%) and a prolonged time to progression (29.5 versus 22.8 weeks) compared with the bolus 5-FU plus leucovorin arm. No significant difference in overall survival was observed. A lower incidence of grade 3–4 toxicity (9.2% versus 21.5%) also favored the infusional arm. Despite the lower dose intensity administered in this modulated biweekly schedule (1000 mg/m^2/week), its activity is similar to other infusional therapies.

In two consecutive phase II trials, the Spanish group showed that when very high-dose infusional 5-FU over 48 hours is modulated by oral leucovorin there is a higher incidence of severe toxicity, while activity does not seem to increase.[20,21] In the first TTD study with 3000 mg/m^2 of 5-FU plus oral leucovorin, 78% of patients suffered from severe toxicity. In many of them, dose reductions had to be made and the actual dose intensity went down to 2000 mg/m^2/week. When in a second trial, also with oral leucovorin, the dose of 5-FU was reduced to 2000 mg/m^2/week, a lower incidence of severe toxicity without loss of antitumor activity was observed, despite a reduction in the real dose intensity to 1600 mg/m^2/week.

In summary, oral modulation with leucovorin is not useful when weekly 5-FU is given over 48 hours at doses of 5-FU higher than 3000 mg/m^2, owing to the appearance of intolerable toxicity without any evidence of increasing activity. A similar observation was also made from the meta-analysis of nine studies of leucovorin modulation. If high doses of 5-FU were used in the control arm, leucovorin was not able to improve the results.[1]

When the intended dose intensity of several biomodulated infusional programs of 5-FU given over 24 or 48 hours is plotted against antitumor activity observed in different phase II or III trials, a linear relationship is not seen (Figure 24.2). This finding reinforces the concept that when short-term 5-FU is given alone without any modulating drug, it is critical to give an adequate dose intensity. This approach will yield a response rate superior to 30%, with a tolerable toxicity. However, if the concept of modulation is applied, dose intensity is not of such critical importance. When effective modulation of infusional 5-FU schedules with leucovorin, PALA or methotrexate is used, a similar antitumor activity is usually observed, despite a clear dose-intensity reduction and a slightly worse toxicity profile.

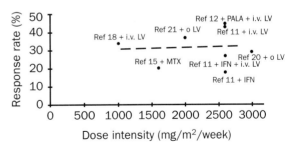

Figure 24.2 Lack of relationship between planned dose intensity and response rate observed in several randomized[11,15,18] and non-randomized[12,20,21] trials of continuous infusion with different forms of biomodulation of 5-FU in advanced measurable colorectal cancer patients. o LV, oral leucovorin; i.v. LV, intravenous leucovorin; PALA, N-(phosphonoacetyl)-L-aspartic acid; IFN, interferon; MTX, methotrexate.

The Spanish group has recently completed the accrual of a phase III trial in which the weekly 3500 mg/m^2 continuous infusion over a 48-hour schedule was chosen as experimental arm against the 'standard' Mayo Clinic program. The results of this trial will help in answering the practical question of whether to use an infusional treatment with the highest dose intensity ever reached or a classical-program bolus 5-FU modulated by a low dose of leucovorin. The advantage of one treatment over the other should be measured in terms of response rate, time to progression, tolerance, overall survival and quality of life.

REFERENCES

1. Advanced Colorectal Cancer Meta-Analysis Project, Modulation of fluorouracil by leucovorin in patients with advanced colorectal cancer: evidence in terms of response rate. *J Clin Oncol* 1992; **10**: 896–903.
2. Hryniuk WM, Figueredo A, Goodyear M, Applications of dose intensity to problems in chemotherapy of breast and colorectal cancer. *Semin Oncol* 1987; **14**(Suppl 4): 3–11.
3. Wils J, High dose fluorouracil: a new perspective in the treatment of colorectal cancer. *Semin Oncol* 1992; **19**(Suppl 3): 126–30.
4. Shah A, MacDonald W, Goldie J et al, 5-FU infusion in advanced colorectal cancer: a comparison of three dose schedules. *Cancer Treat Rep* 1985: **69**: 739–42.
5. Díaz-Rubio E, Aranda E, Martín et al, Weekly high-dose infusion of 5-fluorouracil in advanced colorectal cancer. *Eur J Cancer* 1990; **26**: 727–9.
6. Lokich JJ, Ahlgren JD, Gullo JJ et al, A prospective randomized comparison of continuous infusion fluorouracil with a conventional bolus schedule in metastatic colorectal carcinoma. A Mid-Atlantic Oncology Program study. *J Clin Oncol* 1989; **7**: 425–33.
7. Ansfield F, Klots J, Nealon T et al, A phase III study comparing the clinical utility of four regimens of 5-fluorouracil. *Cancer* 1977; **39**: 34–40.
8. Kemeny N, Israel K, Niedzwiecki D et al, Randomized study of continuous infusion fluorouracil versus fluorouracil plus cisplatin in patients with metastatic colorectal cancer. *J Clin Oncol* 1990; **8**: 313–18.
9. Díaz-Rubio E, Jimeno J, Antón A et al, A prospective randomized trial of continuous infusion 5-fluorouracil (5-FU) versus 5-FU plus cisplatin in patients with advanced colorectal cancer. *Am J Clin Oncol* 1992; **15**: 56–60.
10. Ardalan B, Singh G, Silberman H, A randomized phase I and II study of short term infusion of high dose fluorouracil with or without N-(phosphonacetyl)-L-aspartic acid in patients with advanced pancreatic and colorectal cancer. *J Clin Oncol* 1988; **6**: 1053–8.
11. Köhne CH, Wilke H, Schöffski P et al, High dose infusional 5-FU (HDFU) plus folinic acid is superior compared to HDFU plus interferon. Final results of a multicenter randomized trial of the AIO. *Ann Oncol* 1996; **7**(Suppl 5): 2110.
12. Ardalan B, Donofrio K, Livingstone A et al, A phase II study of weekly low dose bolus phosphonacetyl-L-aspartic acid (PALA) and 24-hour infusion with high dose 5-fluorouracil with leucovorin in advanced colorectal cancer. *Proc Am Soc Clin Oncol* 1995; **14**: 558.
13. O'Dwyer PJ, Paul AR, Walczak J et al, Phase II study of biochemical modulation of fluorouracil by low-dose PALA in patients with colorectal cancer. *J Clin Oncol* 1990; **8**: 1497–503.
14. Díaz-Rubio E, Aranda E, Camps C et al, A phase II study of weekly 48-hour infusion with high dose 5-fluorouracil in advanced colorectal cancer: an alternative to biochemical modulation. *J Infus Chemother* 1994; **4**: 58–61.
15. Blijham G, Wagener T, Wils J et al, Modulation of high-dose infusional fluorouracil by low dose methotrexate in patients with advanced colorectal cancer: final results of a randomized European Organization for Research and Treatment of Cancer study. *J Clin Oncol* 1996; **14**: 2266–73.
16. Leichman CG, Fleming TR, Muggia FM et al, Phase II study of fluorouracil and its modulation in advanced colorectal cancer: a Southwest Oncology Group study. *J Clin Oncol* 1995; **13**: 1303–11.
17. O'Dwyer PJ, Ryan LM, Valone FH et al, Phase III trial of biochemical modulation of 5-fluorouracil by iv or oral leucovorin or by interferon in advanced colorectal cancer. An ECOG/CALGB phase III trial. *Proc Am Soc Clin Oncol* 1996; **15**: 469.
18. De Gramont A, Bosset JF, Milan C et al, Randomized trial comparing monthly low-dose

leucovorin and fluorouracil bolus with bimonthly high dose leucovorin and fluorouracil bolus plus continuous infusion for advanced colorectal cancer. *J Clin Oncol* 1997; **15**: 808–15.

19. Sobrero AF, Ashele C, Guglielmi AP et al, Synergism and lack of cross-resistance between short-term and continuous exposure to fluorouracil in human colon adenocarcinoma cells. *J Natl Cancer Inst* 1993; **85**: 1937–44.

20. Aranda E, Cervantes A, Dorta J et al, A phase II trial of weekly high dose continuous infusion 5-fluorouracil plus oral leucovorin in patients with advanced colorectal cancer. *Cancer* 1995; **76**: 559–63.

21. Aranda E, Cervantes A, Carrato A et al, Outpatient weekly high-dose continuous infusion 5-fluorouracil plus oral leucovorin in advanced colorectal cancer. A phase II trial. *Ann Oncol* 1996; **7**: 581–5.

25

5-Fluorouracil and methotrexate in metastatic colorectal cancer

Geert H Blijham

INTRODUCTION

As early as the late 1970s it was discovered in experimental systems that methotrexate (MTX) can enhance the cytotoxic activity of 5-fluorouracil (5-FU).[1-3] Soon after the publication of these findings, phase I and II studies were initiated,[4,5] followed by a number of phase III studies comparing MTX + 5-FU with 5-FU alone or 5-FU plus other modulators, including reduced folates such as leucovorin (LV).[6,7] Now, after 20 years of experimental and clinical research, we are in a position to determine the usefulness of the MTX + 5-FU approach for daily practice. In this chapter data on the mechanism of interaction, efficacy and toxicity will be summarized.

MECHANISM OF INTERACTION (Table 25.1)

5-Fluorouracil induces cell death by inhibiting, after conversation to the nucleotide 5-fluorodeoxyuridine monophosphate (5-FdUMP), the enzyme thymidylate synthase (TS). This enzyme is a key enzyme in the synthesis of DNA. Also, 5-FU may be converted to the nucleotide 5-fluoruridine triphosphate (5-FUTP), which will be incorporated into RNA. The resulting fraudulent RNA has adverse effects on cell function.[8] Recent evidence suggests that the mode of administration of 5-FU may influence its biochemical effect. In

---

Table 25.1 MTX and 5-FU: mechanisms of modulation

- Increased levels of the phosphate donor PRPP
    Enhanced anabolism of 5-FU to the nucleotide 5-FUTP
      + damage to RNA function
    Enhanced anabolism of 5-FU to the nucleotide 5-FdUMP
      + inhibition of thymidylate synthase →
      inhibition of DNA synthesis
- Increased levels of polyglutamated MTX
    Inhibition of thymidylate synthase →
      + inhibition of DNA synthesis

particular, bolus administration may favour RNA incorporation and inhibition, whereas continuous infusions favour inhibition of TS.[9,10]

Methotrexate inhibits the enzyme dihydrofolate reductase (DHFR). This leads, among other things, to an inhibition of purine synthesis and thereby to increased levels of the cellular phosphate donor phosphoribosyl pyrophosphate (PRPP). This donor may provide the phosphate groups necessary for the anabolism of 5-FU to the nucleotides 5-FdUMP and 5-FUTP. The addition of MTX to 5-FU may therefore enhance the ability of 5-FU to inhibit DNA synthesis as well as RNA function.[2] Furthermore, polyglutamated MTX may act as a cofactor for the formation of the covalent bond between TS and 5-FdUMP and thereby enhance the inhibition of DNA synthesis by 5-FU.[11] In experimental systems the positive modulation of 5-FU by MTX is dose- and schedule-dependent. Enhanced 5-FU-induced cytotoxicity was mostly obtained with MTX levels between 1 and 10 μmol/l and with MTX given 18–24 hours before 5-FU.[1,3] These data were used to design phase I and phase II studies in patients with metastatic colorectal cancer.

PHASE II STUDIES

Kemeny et al,[4] Hermann et al[5] and Bruckner and Cohen[12] summarized the phase II studies of MTX–5-FU combinations in colorectal cancer carried out before 1984. In these trials response rates of around 30% (ranging from 5% to 50%) were obtained. MTX was given in a variety of doses ranging from 40 mg/m^2 to 250 mg/m^2; the interval between MTX and 5-FU varied between 0 and 24 hours. Since none of those studies compared doses or intervals directly, it is rather difficult to determine the optimal schedule of the MTX–5-FU combination. Taken together, however, the results suggest an increased response rate if MTX precedes 5-FU by at least 4 hours and is given in a dose of at least 40 mg/m^2.

PHASE III STUDIES

The Advanced Colorectal Cancer Meta-Analysis Project identified eight randomized trials comparing 5-FU alone with MTX–5-FU, including a total of 1178 patients[6] (Table 25.2). In three of these trials the response rate was significantly higher in the MTX–5-FU arm; the overall survival was significantly longer in one study. The meta-analysis revealed a highly significant superiority of MTX–5-FU for response rate (odds ratio 0.51, 95% confidence interval 0.37–0.70, $p < 10^{-4}$) and a moderately significant superiority of MTX–5-FU for survival (odds ratio 0.87, 95% confidence interval 0.77–0.98, $p = 0.02$). The results did not change if, by making use of a Cox regression model, prognostic information was taken into account.

The main contributor to the meta-analysis of MTX–5-FU was the EORTC 40872 study.[7] In this study 310 patients were randomized between receiving high-dose infusional FU (60 mg/kg over 48 hours) given weekly × 4 and thereafter every 2 (×4) and 3 weeks, or the same schedule with low-dose MTX (40 mg/m^2) at the start of the infusion. The addition of MTX lead to a doubling of the response rate from 10% to 21% ($p = 0.02$). In the meta-analysis of all eight randomized trials the RR also doubled from 10% to 19% ($p < 10^{-4}$). In the EORTC study the median survival time increased by 3 months from 9.3 to 12.5 months. This difference was not significant ($p = 0.1$); in the meta-analysis the prolongation of median survival was a somewhat smaller 1.6 months, which was now significant ($p = 0.02$), because of greater patient numbers. It appears that the EORTC data are very much in line with those obtained in the other studies. The improvements are often too small, however, to be detected in trials with a size of 300 patients or less.

DOSE, SCHEDULE AND THE ROLE OF LEUCOVORIN RESCUE

Most phase III studies used MTX doses in the intermediate range (200–250 mg/m^2). These doses should provide the necessary in vitro

Table 25.2 Meta-analysis of 5-FU modulation in colorectal cancer[6,13]

	Response rate (%)		Survival (median in months)	
	5-FU	Modulated 5-FU	5-FU	Modulated 5-FU
MTX–5-FU modulation				
All trials	10	19[a]	9.1	10.7[a]
Trials with higher 5-FU dose in control arm	13	19		No difference
5-FU–LV modulation				
All trials	11	23[a]	10	10.5
Trials with higher 5-FU dose in control arm	17	17		No difference

[a] $p < 0.05$.

concentrations of 1–10 µmol/l. The results of the EORTC study show, however, that doses as low as 40 mg/m^2 may be sufficient to obtain clinical modulation. This confirms data from the phase II study reported by Kemeny et al.[4] Because of this low MTX dose, rescue with leucovorin (LV) was given in less than 5% of the patients.

In some other trials included in the meta-analysis, LV rescue was routinely given. Therefore some contribution of LV to the results of the MTX–5-FU combination in these studies cannot be excluded. However, the EORTC data clearly show that MTX does modulate 5-FU activity also in the absence of leucovorin. Moreover, recent in vitro data indicate that MTX–5-FU–LV combinations are often not superior to the combination without LV.[14] This may be partly due to the competition of MTX and LV for the same cellular membrane carriers or polyglutamation reactions.[15]

Virtually all phase III studies of MTX–5-FU allowed for some time to elapse between the administration of MTX and 5-FU. In the EORTC study MTX was given simultaneously with the start of the 5-FU infusion. This should lead to peak cellular PRPP levels in the middle of the 48-hour infusion time, thus allowing maximal modulation through this mechanism. Only one study has addressed the interval question in a randomized fashion. Marsh et al[16] compared a 1-hour with a 24-hour interval, and found the longer interval to be superior for response rate (29% versus 15%) and survival (15 versus 11 months).

Trials using the same dose of 5-FU in both arms provide a real test of the modulation of 5-FU by MTX. This requirement was fulfilled in three trials submitted to the meta-analysis, including the EORTC study. In these studies the benefit of adding MTX to 5-FU was larger than in the overall analysis, with an odds ratio of 0.40 for response rate and 0.78 for survival. The clinical relevance of this modulation however, depends partly on whether a similar efficacy can be reached with higher doses of 5-FU.

When the five trials using a higher dose of 5-FU in the 5-FU-alone arm were analysed separately, a benefit from the addition of MTX could no longer be demonstrated. The choice between a modulated lower dose or a higher unmodulated dose of 5-FU would then depend on the toxicity of both regimens.

TOXICITY

In the EORTC study a low dose of MTX was added to infusional 5-FU; in the Nordic Gastrointestinal Tumor Adjuvant Therapy Group (NGTATG) trial, intermediate-dose MTX ($250\,mg/m^2$) with LV rescue was added to bolus 5-FU.[17] The doses of 5-FU in both arms were virtually identical. Grade 3 or 4 toxicities are given in Table 25.2, and show the excellent tolerance of the modulated regimens. Different results were obtained in the trials with higher 5-FU doses in the 5-FU-alone arm. In the German study the overall toxicity in the 5-FU-alone arm was higher, although the four patients with a toxic death occurred in the MTX–5-FU arm and the deaths were apparently due to the classical MTX toxicity syndrome consisting of mucositis, diarrhoea and renal failure.[18] Also, the NCOG trial with bolus injections of two different doses of 5-FU showed considerably higher toxicity in the high-dose 5-FU-alone arm.[19] It therefore appears justified to conclude that MTX modulates 5-FU to higher efficacy at the expense of relatively little added toxicity, when MTX is given in doses in the intermediate range.

MTX OR LV MODULATION OF 5-FU?

The currently most widely used modulator of 5-FU is LV. Is MTX a better modulator? Both modulators have been subjected to a methodologically similar meta-analysis; the results suggest that two modulators are quite comparable as far as efficacy is concerned (Table 25.2).[6,13] In the overall analysis the response rates appear to double from 10–11% to 19–23%; a small survival benefit was only observed in the MTX

trials. Three studies were part of both meta-analyses, since they contained three arms: 5-FU-alone, 5-FU–LV and MTX–5-FU. A separate analysis on the 429 patients in these three trials did not show a trend in favour of either 5-FU–LV or MTX–5-FU. The NGTATG performed a head-to-head comparison of the two modulated regimens; neither response rates (21% versus 17%) nor survival (9 months versus 7.5 months) were significantly different.[20]

An exception to these results is the data from the NCCTG study comparing weekly 5-FU with high-dose LV, daily-times-five 5-FU with low-dose LV and 3–4 weekly 5-FU with intermediate-dose MTX.[21] This extension of their prior six-arm trial showed an inferior response rate (13% as opposed to 31% and 42%) and median survival (8.4 months versus 12.7 months) for the MTX–5-FU combination. This is also the only trial comparing MTX and LV modulation that used a lower dose of 5-FU in the MTX–5-FU arm. The dose intensity of 5-FU in the 5-FU–LV arms was about 30% higher. The difference in efficacy may therefore be at least partly due to differences in the dose intensity of 5-FU. It can be concluded that MTX and LV are equally effective modulators of 5-FU in patients with metastatic colorectal cancer. Toxicity data from trials comparing MTX–5-FU or 5-FU–LV with 5-FU alone suggest that the therapeutic index of the former combination may be more favourable (Table 25.3). In particular, severe stomatitis and diarrhoea are more common with the most often used 5-FU–LV combinations.

If MTX and LV each modulate 5-FU activity but through different mechanisms, would it be useful to combine both agents to obtain double modulation? Results from experimental models have suggested that three-drug combinations of 5-FU, MTX and LV are not superior to two-drug combinations, and may even be antagonistic.[14,22] One reason may be that MTX and LV compete for the same reduced folate transport mechanism to enter the cell.[15] Trimetrexate, a MTX analogue, can enter the cell by simple diffusion and may be more suitable for combination with LV.[15,23–25] A phase I trial with this combination in patients with metastatic colorec-

Table 25.3 Toxicity of selected MTX–5-FU (LV) regimens

Study group	Treatment	Percentage of patients with severe			Toxic deaths (%)
		leucopenia (%)	stomatitis (%)	diarrhoea (%)	
NGTATG[17]	5-FU[a]	2	2	0	0
	MTX–5-FU (LV)	3	5	0	0
EORTC[7]	5-FU[a]	0	1	1	
	MTX–5-FU	0	10	3	
AIO[18]	5-FU[b]	18	3	0	0
	MTX–5-FU (LV)	9	9	5	5
NCOG[19]	5-FU[b]	19	12	14	2
	MTX–5-FU (LV)	2	7	3	0
	5-FU-LV	12	16	14	2
NCCTG[21]	MTX–5-FU (LV)	14	n.a.	n.a.	1
	5-FU–HDLV	15	28	19	1
	5-FU–LDLV	22	28	16	1
NGTATG[20]	MTX–5-FU (LV)	4	4	4	3
	5-FU–LV	6	5	5	1

n.a., not available.
[a] 5-FU dose identical in both arms.
[b] 5-FU dose higher in control arms.

tal cancer has been performed, with promising results.[26]

CONCLUSIONS

Methotrexate modulates the activity of 5-fluorouracil. With similar 5-FU doses, response rates and median survival times are modestly increased to a level that can also be obtained with more intense single-agent 5-FU treatment, albeit at the cost of more toxicity. Whether this is also true if MTX is added to very dose-intense, short-term (24–48 hours) weekly 5-FU infusions is unclear; in the EORTC study addressing this issue, the maximum tolerated dose of 5-FU was not reached. At present, MTX–5-FU is probably no better treatment than 5-FU–LV combinations or high-dose infusions of 5-FU, nor is it less active; in some schedules (e.g. the EORTC schedule) its low toxicity makes it an attractive alternative. The observed capacity of MTX to modulate 5-FU activity with little added toxicity make this drug or its analogues attractive agents in the development of double or triple modulating therapy schedules.

REFERENCES

1. Bertino JR, Sawicki WL, Linquist CA et al, Schedule-dependent antitumor effects of methotrexate and 5-fluorouracil. *Cancer Res* 1977; **37:** 327–8.

2. Cadman E, Davis L, Heimer R, Enhanced 5-fluorouracil nucleotide formation following methotrexate: biochemical explanation for drug synergism. *Science* 1979; **205:** 1135–7.

3. Benz C, Schoenberg M, Choti M et al, Schedule-dependent cytotoxicity of methotrexate and 5-fluorouracil in human colon and breast tumor cell lines. *J Clin Invest* 1980; **66:** 1162–5.

4. Kemeny NE, Ahmed T, Michaelson RA, Activity of sequential low-dose methotrexate and fluorouracil in advanced colorectal carcinoma: attempt at correlation with tissue and blood levels of phosphoribosylphosphate. *J Clin Oncol* 1984; **2:** 311–15.

5. Hermann R, Spehn J, Beyer JH et al, Sequential methotrexate and 5-fluorouracil: improved response rate in metastatic colorectal cancer. *J Clin Oncol* 1984; **2:** 591–4.

6. Piedbois P, Buyse M, Blijham GH et al, Meta-analysis of randomized trials testing the biochemical modulation of 5-fluorouracil by methotrexate in metastatic colorectal cancer. Advanced Colorectal Cancer Meta-analysis Project. *J Clin Oncol* 1994; **12:** 960–9.

7. Blijham GH, Wagener Th, Wils et al, Modulation of high-dose infusional 5-fluorouracil by low-dose methotrexate in patients with advanced or metastatic colorectal cancer: final results of a randomized EORTC study. *J Clin Oncol* 1996; **14:** 2266–73.

8. Pinedo HM, Peters GF, Fluorouracil: biochemistry and pharmacology. *J Clin Oncol* 1988; **6:** 1653–64.

9. Aschele C, Sobrero A, Faderan MA et al, Novel mechanisms of resistance to 5-fluorouracil in human colon cancer (HCT-8) sublines following exposure to two different clinically relevant dose schedules. *Cancer Res* 1992; **53:** 1855–64.

10. Ahlgren J, Protracted infusional schedules of fluorouracil in colorectal cancer versus fluorouracil with modulators: differences and similarities. *J Infus Chemother* 1992; **2:** 128–37.

11. Fernandes DJ, Bertino JR, 5-Fluorouracil–methotrexate synergy: enhancement of 5-fluorodeoxyuridylate binding to thymidylate synthetase by dihydropteroylglutamates. *Proc Natl Acad Sci USA* 1980; **76:** 5663–7.

12. Bruckner H, Cohen J, MTX/5-FU trials in gastrointestinal and other cancers. *Semin Oncol* 1983; **10:** 32–9.

13. Advanced Colorectal Cancer Meta-Analysis Project, Modulation of fluorouracil by leucovorin in patients with advanced colorectal cancer: evidence in terms of response rate. *J Clin Oncol* 1992; **10:** 896–903.

14. Van der Wilt CL, Braakhuis JM, Pinedo HM et al, Addition of leucovorin in modulation of 5-fluorouracil with methotrexate: potentiating or reversing effect? *Int J Cancer* 1995; **61:** 672–8.

15. Romanini A, Li WW, Colofiore JR et al, Leucovorin enhances cytotoxicity of trimetrexate/fluorouracil, but not methotrexate/fluorouracil, in CCRF/CEM cells. *J Natl Cancer Inst* 1992; **84:** 1033–8.

16. Marsh JC, Bertino JR, Katz KH et al, The influence of drug interval on the effect of methotrexate and fluorouracil in the treatment of advanced colorectal cancer. *J Clin Oncol* 1991; **9:** 371–80.

17. Nordic Gastrointestinal Tumor Adjuvant Therapy Group, Superiority of sequential methotrexate, fluorouracil and leucovorin to fluorouracil alone in advanced symptomatic colorectal carcinoma: a randomized trial. *J Clin Oncol* 1989; **7:** 1437–46.

18. Hermann R, Knuth A, Kleebert U et al, Sequential methotrexate and 5-fluorouracil (FU) vs FU alone in metastatic colorectal cancer. *Ann Oncol* 1992; **3:** 539–43.

19. Valone FH, Friedman MA, Wittlinger PS et al, Treatment of patients with advanced colorectal carcinoma with fluorouracil alone, high-dose leucovorin plus fluorouracil, or sequential methotrexate, fluorouracil, and leucovorin: a randomized trial of the Northern California Oncology Group. *J Clin Oncol* 1989; **7:** 1427–36.

20. Glimelius B et al, Biochemical modulation of 5-fluorouracil: a randomized comparison of sequential methotrexate, 5-fluorouracil and leucovorin versus sequential 5-fluorouracil and leucovorin in patients with advanced symptomatic colorectal cancer. *Ann Oncol* 1993; **4:** 235–40.

21. Poon MA, O'Connell MJ, Wieand HS et al, Biochemical modulation of fluorouracil with leucovorin: confirmatory evidence of improved therapeutic efficacy in advanced colorectal cancer. *J Clin Oncol* 1991; **9:** 1967–72.

22. Danhauser LL, Heimer R, Cadman E, Lack of

enhanced cytotoxicity of cultured L1210 cells using folinic acid in combination with sequential methotrexate and fluorouracil. *Cancer Chemother Pharmacol* 1985; **15:** 214–19.

23. Sobrero A, Romanini A, Russello O et al, Sequence-dependent enhancement of HCT-8 cell kill by trimetrexate and fluoropyrimidines: implications for the mechanism of their interaction. *Eur J Clin Oncol* 1989; **25:** 977–82.

24. Kamen BA, Eibl B, Cashmore AR et al, Uptake and efficacy of trimetrexate (TMQ, 2,4-diamino-5-methyl-6[(3,4,5-trimethylanilino)quinazoline]), a non-classical antifolate in methotrexate-resis-tant leukemia cells in vitro. *Biochem Pharmacol* 1984; **33:** 1697–9.

25. Fry DW, Wasserman TH, Characterization of trimetrexate transport in human lymphoblastoid cells and development of impaired influx as a mechanism of resistance to lipophilic antifolates. *Cancer Res* 1988; **48:** 6986–91.

26. Conti JA, Kemeny N, Goker E et al, A phase I trial of sequential trimetrexate (MTX), fluorouracil (FU) and high-dose leucovorin (LV) in previously treated patients (pts) with gastrointestinal (GI) carcinoma (Ca). *Proc Am Soc Clin Oncol* 1993; **12:** 567 (abst).

26

The role of second-line chemotherapy in colorectal cancer

Hans-Joachim Schmoll, Thomas Büchele, Christoph Schöber

CONTENTS • **Introduction** • **Prolonged administration of fluoropyrimidines ± folinic acid** • **Oxaliplatin ± 5-FU/FA** • **Irinotecan** • **Results of trials showing no activity in refractory colorectal cancer** • **Predictive factors for response** • **Time to response, treatment duration and dose intensity** • **Conclusions**

INTRODUCTION

Some years ago, it was still a controversial issue whether advanced colorectal cancer should be treated by palliative chemotherapy at all because of a low remission rate and a marginal gain in survival. However, despite a low objective response rate, about 50% of patients have some benefit from 5-fluorouracil (5-FU)/folinic acid (FA) chemotherapy in terms of improvement of quality of life and a significant prolongation of disease- and progression-free lifetime, as well as the potential improvement of the individual residual lifespan;[1] however, this improvement should be achieved with as minimal toxicity and time-consuming procedures as possible and necessary.[2] These considerations for the choice of palliative chemotherapy and the selection of a specific protocol are particularly relevant for the salvage situation when the first-line 5-FU-based chemotherapy has failed, since the patients are in a worse performance status compared with the first-line palliative treatment, might suffer from more tumor-related symptoms than before, and have a somewhat reduced tolerability of chemotherapy-related side-effects.

In the last two years several phase II studies have appeared indicating that there might be several effective second-line treatment options for patients pretreated with or refractory to 5-FU ± FA. However, in the absence of the results of prospective randomized trials comparing one option with another or best supportive care, it is difficult to evaluate the definitive value of the different options, since the above-mentioned parameters for a 'good' palliative treatment (e.g. quality-of-life investigations, number of MR or NC in previously progressing patients, as well as length of progression-free and overall survival) are poorly reported. More importantly, the patient populations in phase II or III studies differ from a general patient population in clinical practice because of stringent exclusion criteria (e.g. of patients with poor performance status, short expected survival or impaired liver function). Furthermore, the study populations are very heterogeneous with respect to the following parameters, which might be associated with a different outcome of salvage chemotherapy:

- degree of 5-FU resistance;
- duration of previous chemotherapy (e.g. treatment until best response or until progression);

- length of treatment-free interval;
- type and dose intensity of previous chemotherapy (bolus or infusion schedules; 5-FU alone or plus biochemical modulation with folinic acid, interferon or methotrexate);
- quality and duration of response to previous chemotherapy;
- number of previous salvage chemotherapies.

A small but very important study[3] demonstrated that retreatment with a 5-FU/FA bolus protocol after a median of 9 months without chemotherapy – with the identical protocol as used for the first-line chemotherapy – resulted in an objective remission rate of 25%, including 5% CR and further 20% MR/NC for a duration of 5 months and a survival of 7 months. This result indicates that any type of 5-FU-based salvage chemotherapy should at least be effective in about 50% of patients and capable of inducing objective remissions in 25%. This result, however, cannot be expected in patients who had proven resistance to prior 5-FU-based chemotherapy and clearly defined progressive disease while on treatment before the initiation of the salvage protocol. However, resistance to a 5-FU ± FA regimen with 5-FU given as a bolus or short infusion indicates a lower level of 5-FU resistance in comparison with 5-FU resistance that developed under prolonged 5-FU (continuous or 24/48 hours) exposure,[4,5] owing to different mechanisms of activity and resistance.[6]

Another problem for the evaluation of the best salvage treatment is that we presently have no conclusive data about the level of cross-resistance between novel agents (e.g. oxaliplatin or irinotecan) and 5-FU ± FA infusion schedules; therefore it is not clear whether a specific sequence should be preferred. Despite these difficulties and the lack of definitive data, in the light of many presently available reports about 'effective' salvage treatments in refractory colorectal cancer, our patients deserve a preliminary evaluation. It is clear, however, that we shall have (if any) not just *one* 'standard' salvage treatment but different 'adequate' options, depending on the type and duration of the previous (first-line) treatment protocol. These options will be discussed below, followed by a suggestion for the optimal choice of salvage treatment in an individual patient.

PROLONGED ADMINISTRATION OF FLUOROPYRIMIDINES ± FOLINIC ACID

Various phase II studies have investigated different infusion schedules of 5-FU (continuously over 5 days, 14 days, 21 days, 24 hours weekly) without or with FA (bolus; short infusion), or of 5-FU prodrugs. The results are shown in Tables 26.1 and 26.2. A comparison of the different studies is of no value, because of the heterogeneity discussed above; however, it appears that any type of prolonged 5-FU administration is able to induce an objective remission rate of 20–30% and an overall antitumor activity (including PR, MR and NC) in 65–85%, for a duration of 5–7 months, resulting in a overall survival of 8–12 months. The role of chronomodulation is very unclear in this setting, although of great interest and of possible relevance for first-line treatment.

Most consistent are the data from four different groups investigating weekly 24-hour 5-FU infusion plus FA (Table 27.2). However, it is not clear whether this type of prolonged 5-FU administration would be superior to a 5- or 21-day schedule, and whether FA is required to achieve that result. Responses have been observed in all metastatic sites, including liver, lung, lymph nodes and ascites.[18,19] More important than objective remissions or the rate of tumor control (PR + MR + NC) is the effect on the quality of life. Jaeger et al[19] reported significant and clinically relevant pain relief in 33/38 patients (89%). However, 8–15% developed grade III diarrhea and 5–10% grade III mucositis and/or hand–foot syndrome, whereas bone-marrow toxicity and infections were low and negligible; in comparison with protracted continuous infusion of 5-FU, the toxicity seems to be somewhat higher.[7,22]

In particular, the results of the study by Jaeger et al[19] are of interest because all patients had documented progression on 5-FU

Table 26.1 Various 5-FU ± FA-based salvage regimens with prolonged 5-FU (or oral prodrug) administration in colorectal cancer refractory to bolus-5-FU ± FA

Ref	Salvage regimen	Route[a]	No. of patients	CR (%)	PR (%)	CR + PR + MR/NC (%)	Response duration (months)	Survival
7	5-FU 250 mg/m² daily (7 weeks)	c.i.	57	—	5	50	11	n.a.
8	5-FU 300–400 mg/m² daily until progression	c.i.	23	—	—	9	n.a.	12% 1 year
9	5-FU 200 mg/m² d1–21 + FA 20 mg/m²	c.i.	11	—	n.a.	50	6	n.a.
10, 11	5-FU 800–1800 mg/m² d1–5, q d22	c.i. (chm)	15	—	20	73	n.a.	12 months
12	5-FU 650 mg/m² + FA 200 mg/m² d1–5, q d22	c.i.	10	10	—	30	n.a.	n.a.
13	5-FU 600–1100 mg/m² d1–5, q d22	c.i. (chm)	17	—	18	n.a.	n.a.	n.a.
14	5-FU 250 mg/m² + FA 20 mg/m² d1–14, q d29	c.i. (chm)	19	—	11	37	n.a.	n.a.
15	5-dFUR (doxifluridine) 3000 mg + FA	i.v. bolus	14	—	29	n.a.	5	n.a.
	6000 mg + FA d1–5 q d15	Orally	34	—	12	n.a.	6	n.a.
18	FUdR (fluorodeoxyuridine) 130–150 mg/kg d1, weekly	24 h c.i.	9	—	56	n.a.	n.a.	n.a.

[a] c.i., continuous infusion; chm, chronomodulated.

bolus ± FA; in the case of progression during a treatment-free interval the patient had been retreated with a 5-FU/FA bolus protocol, and referred to the infusional 5-FU/FA salvage protocol only in the case of progression under retreatment. In 65 refractory patients a 25% PR rate (no CR) with a duration of 7 months and a 86% PR + MR + NC rate have been achieved.

Of interest also is the oral protocol of Bajetta et al,[15] with a 5-day schedule every 10 days of

Table 26.2 5-FU 24-h infusion + FA weekly in refractory colorectal cancer

Ref	No. of patients	CR	PR (%)	PR + MR + NC (%)	Duration (median; months)	Survival (months)
17	10	—	30	n.a.	n.a.	10
18	57	—	9	65	3	8
19	69	—	25	86	7	9
20	55	—	35	81	n.a.	n.a.
21	38	—	32	77	n.a.	n.a.

Table 26.3 Salvage treatment with 5-FU + FA plus further agents in refractory colorectal cancer

Ref	Protocol	No. of patients	CR/PR (%)	MR/NC (%)	Survival (months)	Comments
23	5-FU bolus + IFN-α	34	3	48	5	—
24	Continuous infusion of 5-FU + epirubicin + cisplatin	16	—	31	7	Very toxic
25	5-FU bolus + FA + cisplatin weekly	30	23	n.a.	n.a.	Toxic

the 5-FU prodrug doxifluridine (5-dFUR) (6000 mg p.o. per day) plus oral FA; 12% responded for a median of 6 months, with grade III diarrhea in 15%. Because of the practicability of this full oral protocol, further investigation is of interest for this group of patients.

The combinations of 5-FU continuous infusion with cisplatin or cisplatin/epirubicin (Table 26.3) do not seem not to offer any advantage over protocols with infusional 5-FU ± FA, but add more toxicity.

In summary, protracted continuous infusion of 5-FU and weekly 24-hour infusions of 5-FU/FA are effective salvage treatments, which

differ in the degree of mucositis and diarrhea and practical management (a pump every day versus only once a week). The choice between them will depend on institutional factors.

OXALIPLATIN ± 5-FU/FA

Oxaliplatin is an interesting cisplatin analogue with very little bone-marrow toxicity but more pronounced and dose-limiting peripheral sensitive neuropathy. In vitro, oxaliplatin exerts antitumor activity against cisplatin-resistant and colon carcinoma cell lines.[26–28] This is reflected

Table 26.4 Single-agent activity of oxaliplatin in colorectal cancer

Ref	No. of patients	Pretreatment characteristics	Route	CR	PR (%)	MR/NC (%)	CR + PR + MR + NC (%)	PR duration (median; months)	Survival (months)
29	14	Untreated	2-h infusion	—	21	43	64	n.a.	n.a.
30	55	Refractory	2-h infusion	—	11	42	53	6	8.3
30	51	Refractory	2-h infusion	—	10	31	41	5	n.a.
31	29	Refractory	Chrono-modulated 24-h infusion	—	10	24	34	6	9

by an antitumor activity (Table 26.4) in untreated colorectal cancer of 21% PR and 43% MR/NC, which compares to single-agent 5-FU if confirmed in larger studies.[29] Moreover, in patients refractory to 5-FU/FA bolus protocols a PR rate of 10–11% and an MR/NC rate of 24–42% for an overall antitumor activity of 34–64% have been reported. The PRs lasted 5–6 months, and the survival was 8.2 and 9 months. The toxicity included paresthesia/dysesthesia in over 90% of patients and grade III in 14–23%, and caused functional impairment in 4–8%. This peripheral neuropathy was strongly related to the cumulative dose, and disappearance or improvement of these symptoms are generally observed after 3–6 months.[30] Bone-marrow toxicity or mucositis is uncommon; 50% of patients have diarrhea, with 10% having grade III. For palliative treatment, it is of relevance that oxaliplatin has no nephrotoxicity or ototoxicity and does not produce alopecia. In summary, oxaliplatin has a marginal but definitive activity in refractory colorectal cancer with a favourable toxicity profile.

The preclinically demonstrated synergism of oxaliplatin[26] with 5-FU also seems to be clinically relevant (Table 26.5). In four phase II studies and a further patient population treated on a com-passionate-use program with oxaliplatin plus 5-FU/FA, the partial remission rate was 25–58% plus 0.5–3% CR; including MR/NC, the overall antitumor activity in patients refractory to and progressing on bolus 5-FU/FA was 67–92%.[32,37] A median survival of 12–17 months reported in three studies is impressive. The contribution of a true synergy of oxaliplatin and 5-FU/FA is obvious from the studies of de Gramont et al[32] as well as those of Garufi et al,[34] who, in the case of progressive disease under a 5-FU/FA infusional protocol (48-hour infusion at constant rate,[32] or 5-day infusion, chrono-modulated rate[34]) proceeded with the same 5-FU/FA regimen plus the addition of oxali-platin. In the case of only additive activity, an objective remission rate of 10% should be expected; actually, the achieved PR rate was 46% in 22 refractory patients[32] and 29% in 25 refractory patients,[34] indicating that oxaliplatin can partially reverse resistance to infusional 5-FU/FA. The 'FOLFOX-2' regimen of de Gramont and colleagues consists of oxaliplatin 100 mg/m^2 as a 2-hour infusion on day 1, and FA 500 mg/m^2 as a 2-hour infusion on day 1, followed by a 24-hour infusion of 5-FU 1.5–2 g/m^2 on days 1 and 2, repeated every 2 weeks. The side-effects with the FOLFOX-2 protocol were

Table 26.5 5-FU/FA plus oxaliplatin in refractory colorectal cancer

Ref	No. of patients	Comments	CR (%)	PR (%)	CR + PR + MR/NC (%)	Duration (median; months)	Survival (months)
32	22	Refractory to 5-FU 24-h continuous infusion + FA	—	46	n.a.	n.a.	n.a.
	46	pretreated plus refractory	3	43	96	n.a.	17
33	19	Refractory to bolus 5-FU/FA; chronomodulated	—	58	n.a.	n.a.	n.a.
34	25	Chronomodulated	—	29	67	n.a.	12
35 36	206	± Chronomodulation; compassionate use	0.5	25	n.a.	n.a.	n.a.
37	27	Chronomodulated; intensive biweekly schedule	—	41	92	n.a.	17

pronounced but tolerable, and induced the following grade III/IV toxicities: peripheral neuropathy (9%), diarrhea (9%), mucositis (13%), neutropenia (39%), thrombocytopenia (11%), alopecia (9%) and allergic reaction (2%).

The chronomodulated protocols are associated with comparable side-effects, but much lower bone-marrow toxicity and perhaps more hand–foot syndrome. However, the contribution of the chronomodulation to the overall result is unclear,[35] since the FOLFOX-2 regimen exerts comparable efficacy without chronomodulation; chronomodulation seems to be of importance to further increase the dose intensity of oxaliplatin and 5-FU.[37] With an intensified biweekly program of oxaliplatin plus 5-FU/FA, Bertheault-Cvitkovic et al reported in 27 patients refractory to 5-FU/FA a 3% CR rate, 41% PR, an overall antitumor activity including MR/NC in 92% and a median survival of 17 months. Responders with metastases accessible for surgical removal even underwent complete resection of residual tumor mass as a 'curative' treatment attempt.

IRINOTECAN

The topoisomerase I inhibitor irinotecan (CPT-11) has the highest efficacy in colorectal cancer in comparison with other topo-I inhibitors. In pretreated patients a PR rate of 15–22% with a duration of 7–8 months has been observed (Table 26.6), and in patients with proven resistance to 5-FU ± FA a CR rate of 1%, a PR rate of 11.2–16%, with a mean of 13%, and a CR + PR + MR/NC rate of 43–64% have been observed.

Quality-of-life data from the four European studies indicate a substantial clinical benefit for patients, with improvement or stabilization of performance status for more than two cycles in 91%, a gain in body weight in 79% and resolution of pain in 57%. This benefit is perhaps

Table 26.6 Irinotecan (CPT-11) in pretreated or refractory colorectal cancer

Ref	No. of patients	CR (%)	PR (%)	CR + PR + MR/NC (%)	Duration (median; months)	Survival (months)
Pretreated						
38	88	—	15	n.a.	8	8
39	43	2	21	n.a.	6	10
40	46	—	22	n.a.	7	n.a.
41	58	2	21	72	9	10
Refractory to 5-FU + FA						
41	57	2	16	44	9	10
42	95	—	14	58	8	10
43	99	—	12	64	7	n.a.
43	107	1	9	53	8	n.a.

more important than objective responses, particularly because it is observed despite toxicities, with grade III–IV neutropenia in 41% of patients and 17% of cycles, associated with fever or infection in 8% of patients, grade III–IV cholinergic syndrome in 2% of patients, grade III/IV diarrhea in 26% of patients and 8% of cycles, and complete alopecia in 59% of patients. Cholinergic syndrome, nausea/vomiting and severe sequels of diarrhea must consequently be managed by prophylactic and interventional treatment with atropine, loperamide, and quinolone antibiotics and antiemetics; these supportive means make irinotecan a relatively safe drug (350 mg/m^2 as a 30-minute infusion every 3 weeks), particularly in the hands of experienced oncologists. However, particularly for female patients, the high risk of complete alopecia is a disadvantage of this agent.

RESULTS OF TRIALS SHOWING NO ACTIVITY IN REFRACTORY COLORECTAL CANCER

Several phase I and II studies looked at further agents alone or in combination, as well as immunomodulation (Table 26.7). None of these trials have shown any clinically relevant results beyond the discussed options for salvage treatment in colorectal cancer; this also includes Tomudex.

PREDICTIVE FACTORS FOR RESPONSE

Basically all patients could achieve an objective remission to a salvage treatment protocol. However, patients could be selected for salvage chemotherapy based on several pretreatment characteristics. Weh et al[18] found a PR/MR/NC rate of 81% in patients who had achieved an NC or PR with previous chemotherapy, but also 44% with previous progression on bolus 5-FU had PR or MR/NC to a weekly 24-hour infusion of 5-FU/FA; another significant predictor for a better chance to respond was a PS >80%. In the integrated analysis of the four European studies with irinotecan, the following factors were predicted for response: low tumor burden, no peritoneal involvement, and a longer interval (>45 days) between progression on 5-FU and start of irinotecan.[51]

Table 26.7 Recent salvage treatments without relevance in refractory colorectal cancer

Ref	Treatment	No. of patients	Comments
44	MTX + VCR + MeCCNU	41	5% PR, 10% MR/NC; no improvement of symptoms
45	Ara-C + cisplatin	17	18% NC; toxic
46	Oral etoposide	21	23% NC; short
47	Oral etoposide + cisplatin	14	No response; toxic
48	IL-2 + melatonin	25	12% PR (?)
49	125-J-A33-MoAB	20	15% MR, short
50	Immunotoxin LMB1	n.a.	1 PR, 2 MR

TIME TO RESPONSE, TREATMENT DURATION AND DOSE INTENSITY

Because of the very palliative nature of salvage chemotherapy in refractory colorectal cancer, the aim of treatment is rather to control progressive disease and reduce tumor-related symptoms than to achieve an objective remission; in most of the reported series, particularly with irinotecan and oxaliplatin, the PRs were achieved after 3–6 cycles, or after 1 or 2 cycles in the case of further treatment because an antitumor effect had initially been observed. Therefore the treatment should be given for a minimum of 6 weeks, and prolonged in the case of any relevant antitumor effect as well as tolerable side-effects until progression. A tight adherence to the protocol schedule does not seem to be indicated in this situation; the objective toxicity and subjective tolerance of the patients should play the main roles in determining for dose and time schedule in this palliative situation.

CONCLUSIONS

Although the data are premature, there is clear evidence that several treatment options are available for refractory colorectal cancer. With respect to the published data on pretreatment characteristics within different trials, antitumor efficacy and toxicity, these options should be offered to patients who failed after first-line chemotherapy, if they have a good to intermediate performance status and progressive disease. It is too early to define a standard protocol or a specific treatment sequence; all patients with refractory colorectal cancer should be treated within prospective comparative clinical trials.

The following recommendations might help to find a protocol suitable for patients who are not candidates for one of the ongoing trials.

- In cases of >2–3 months from the end of the first-line (or previous) 5-FU ± FA-based chemotherapy and previous response (PR or MR), patients should be retreated with the same regimen
- In cases of progression under retreatment or shortly after a first-line 5-FU/FA, there are several options.
  - if previous 5-FU treatment was given as a bolus or short infusion, one could try any type of protracted 5-FU infusion ± FA (e.g. 5-FU continuously

until progression or weekly 24-hour infusions of 5-FU/FA). An alternative is irinotecan as a single agent, which is easier to apply but more toxic (particularly with respect to diarrhea and alopecia).

- If previous 5-FU treatment was given as prolonged high-dose infusion, one could proceed with an infusional 5-FU regimen plus FA plus oxaliplatin, either weekly or biweekly (e.g. the FOLFOX2 protocol) or a 5-day chronomodulated infusion every 3 weeks. The alternative is irinotecan as a single agent every 3 weeks; this protocol avoids the neuropathy induced by oxaliplatin.

- In cases of progression after high-dose infusions of 5-FU/FA plus oxaliplatin and no previous exposure to irinotecan, the latter agent is the last available option, which yielded a 12% RR in one study.[52]

- If the bulk of the disease is located in the liver, besides all the above options one should always consider locoregional treatment via hepatic artery (by femoral catheterization).

REFERENCES

1. Scheithauer W, Rosen H, Kornek G et al, Randomised comparison of combination chemotherapy plus supportive care with supportive care alone in patients with metastatic colorectal cancer. *Br J Cancer* 1993; **306:** 752–5.
2. Köhne-Wömpner CH, Schmoll HJ, Harstick A, Rustum Y, Chemotherapeutic strategies in metastatic colorectal cancer. An overview of current clinical trials. *Semin Oncol* 1992; **19:** 105–25.
3. Hejna M, Kornek G, Weinländer G et al, Reinduction therapy with the same cytostatic regimen in patients with advanced colorectal cancer. *Acta Chir Austriaca* 1995; **115:** 21 (Abst 52).
4. Hastrick A, Gonzales A, Hoffmann A et al, Development and characterisation of human gastric, colon and breast carcinoma cell lines resistant to 5-FU using various, clinically relevant application schedules. *Proc Am Soc Clin Oncol* 1995; **14:** Abst 1989.
5. Aschele C, Sobrero A, Faderan A, Bertino JR, Novel mechanism(s) of resistance to 5-fluorouracil in human colon cancer (HCT-8) sublines following exposure to two different clinically relevant dose schedules. *Cancer Res* 1992; **52:** 1855–64.
6. Wang FS, Aschele C, Sobrero A et al, Decreased folypolyglutamate synthetase expression: a novel mechanism of fluorouracil resistance. *Cancer Res* 1993; **53:** 3677–80.
7. Ducreux M, Rougier Ph, Voni R et al, Lack of relationship between plasma concentration and clinical parameters in patients with metastatic colorectal cancer treated with prolonged infusion of 5-fluorouracil and oral leucovorin. *Proc Am Assoc Cancer Res* 1996; **37:** 408 (abst 2782).
8. Logue JP, Kiltie AE, James RD, Wilkinson PM, Continuous infusion of 5-fluorouracil in patients with progressive metastatic colorectal carcinoma following intermittent 5FU based chemotherapy. *Proc Am Soc Clin Oncol* 1995; **14:** Abst 571.
9. Lim HL, Wong JE, Wang TL, Kong HL, Salvage chemotherapy in previously treated metastatic colorectal cancer. *Proc Am Soc Clin Oncol* 1995; **14:** Abst 505.
10. Lévi F, Soussan A, Adam R et al, A phase I–II trial of five-day continuous intravenous infusion of 5-fluorouracil delivered at circadian rhythm modulated rate in patients with metastatic colorectal cancer. *J Inf Chemother* 1995; **5**(Suppl 1): 153–8.
11. Lévi F, Giacchetti S, Adam R et al, Chronomodulation of chemotherapy against metastatic colorectal cancer. International Organization for Cancer Chronotherapy. *Eur J Cancer* 1995; **31A:** 1264–70.
12. Streit M, Stemetzne S, Jaehde U et al, A multicenter phase II clinical and pharmacokinetic trial of prolonged continuous infusion of 5-fluorouracil and folinic acid in patients with advanced colorectal carcinoma. *Proc Am Soc Clin Oncol* 1996; **15:** Abst 554.
13. Curé H, Garufi C, Focan C et al, A phase I–II assessment of five-day chronomodulated 5-fluorouracil–leucovorin against metastatic colorectal cancer. *Proc Am Soc Clin Oncol* 1996; **15:** Abst 1708.
14. Bjarnason GA, Marsh R, Chu NM et al, Phase II study of 5-fluorouracil and leucovorin by a

14-day circadian infusion in patients with metastatic colorectal cancer. *Proc Am Soc Clin Oncol* 1996; **15**: Abst 543.

15. Bajetta E, Di Bartolomeo M, Somma L et al, Doxifluridine in patients with 5-FU resistant colorectal cancer. In: *Abstract Book, 8th European Cancer Conf (ECCO), Paris*, 1995; Abst 705.

16. Ardalan B, Restrepo A, Deng Z et al, Phase I–III study of high dose 24-hour infusion of fluorodeoxyuridine (FldR) in patients with colorectal cancers (previously failed 5-fluorouracil). *Proc Am Soc Clin Oncol* 1996; **15**: Abst 450.

17. Ardalan B, Chua L, Tian EM et al, A phase II study of weekly 24-hour infusion with high-dose fluorouracil with leucovorin in colorectal carcinoma. *J Clin Oncol* 1991; **9**: 625–30.

18. Weh HJ, Wilke HJ, Dierlamm J et al, Weekly therapy with folinic acid and high-dose 5-fluorouracil 24-hour infusion in pretreated patients with metastatic colorectal carcinoma. *Ann Oncol* 1994; **5**: 233–7.

19. Jaeger E, Klein O, Wächter B et al, Second line treatment with high-dose 5-fluorouracil and folinic acid in advanced colorectal cancer refractory to standard-dose 5-fluorouracil treatment. *Oncology* 1995; **52**: 470–3.

20. Loeffler TM, Huck L, Hausamen TU, Weekly high-dose continuous infusion fluorouracil, leucovorin and interferon-alpha (LIF) as second-line chemotherapy in metastatic colorectal cancer. In: *Abstract Book, 19th Annual Meeting, European Society of Medical Oncology, Lisbon*, 1994; 55, Abst 275.

21. Lorenz M, Staib-Sebler E, Gog C et al, Intravenous weekly high-dose infusion of 5-fluorouracil and folinic acid in pretreated patients with metastatic colorectal cancer. *Onkologie* 1997; **20**: 222–5.

22. Izzo J, Fandi A, Villalobos W et al, Low-dose protracted continuous 5-fluorouracil infusion in solid tumors. *J Inf Chemother* 1995; **4**: 135–9.

23. Pérez J, Lacava J, Sabatini C et al, Interferon and 5-fluorouracil as second line therapy in advanced colorectal cancer: phase II study. *Proc Am Soc Clin Oncol* 1996; **15**: Abst 529.

24. Penel N, Adenis A, Fournier C et al, ECF regimen as salvage treatment in patients with progressive metastatic colorectal carcinoma. *Proc Am Soc Clin Oncol* 1996; **15**: Abst 533.

25. Tsavaris N, Tentas K, Bacoyiannis C et al, 5-fluorouracil, folinic acid and cisplatin in advanced colorectal cancer: a pilot study. *Anticancer Drugs* 1995; **6**: 599–603.

26. Mathé G, Kidani Y, Segiguchi M, Oxalato-platinum or L-OHP, a third generation platinum complex: an experimental and clinical appraisal and preliminary comparison with cis-platinum and carboplatinum. *Biomed Pharmacother* 1989; **43**: 237–50.

27. Pendyala L, Creaven PJ, Shah G et al, In vitro cytotoxicity studies of oxaliplatin in human tumor cell lines. *Proc Am Assoc Cancer Res* 1991; **32**: Abst 410.

28. Fojo T, Myers T, Tanimura H, Phenotypic aspects of platinum resistance. In: *Abstract Book 7th International Symp on Platinum and Other Metal Coordination Compounds in Cancer Chemotherapy (ISPCC '95)*, 1995; Abst 171.

29. Diaz-Rubio E, Zaniboni A, Gastiaburu J et al, Phase II multicentric trial of oxaliplatin as first line chemotherapy in metastatic colorectal carcinoma. *Proc Am Soc Clin Oncol* 1996; **15**: Abst 468.

30. Machover D, Diaz-Rubio E, de Gramont A et al, Two consecutive phase II studies of oxaliplatin for treatment of patients with advanced colorectal carcinoma who were resistant to previous treatment with fluoropyrimidines. *Ann Oncol* 1996; **7**: 95–8.

31. Lévi F, Perpoint B, Garufi C et al, Oxaliplatin activity against metastatic colorectal cancer. A phase II study of 5-day continuous venous infusion at circadian rhythm modulated rate. *Eur J Cancer* 1993; **29A**(Suppl 9): 1280–4.

32. de Gramont A, Vignoud J, Tournigand C et al, Oxaliplatin with high-dose folinic acid and 5-fluorouracil 48 h infusion in pretreated metastatic colorectal cancer. In: *Abstract Book, 8th European Cancer Conf (ECCO), Paris*, 1995; Abst 716.

33. Lévi F, Misset JL, Brienza S et al, A chronopharmacologic phase II clinical trial with 5-fluorouracil, folinic acid, and oxaliplatin using an ambulatory multichannel programmable pump. High antitumor effectiveness against metastatic colorectal cancer. *Cancer* 1992; **69**: 893–900.

34. Garufi C, Brienza S, Bensmain MA et al, Addition of oxaliplatin to chronomodulated 5-fluorouracil and folinic acid for reversal of acquired chemoresistance in patients with advanced colorectal cancer. *Proc Am Soc Clin Oncol* 1995; **14**: Abst 446 .

35. Louvet C, Bleiberg H, Gamelin E et al, Oxaliplatin (L-OHP) synergistic clinical activity with 5-fluorouracil in FU resistant colorectal cancer patients is independent of FU ± folinic acid. *Proc Am Soc Clin Oncol* 1996; **15**: Abst 467.

36. Soulié P, Raymond E, Misset JL, Cvitkovic E,

Oxaliplatin: update on a active and safe DACH platinum complex. In: *Platinum and Other Metal Coordination Compounds in Cancer Chemotherapy 2* (Pinedo HM, Schornagel JH, eds). New York: Plenum Press, 1996; 165–74.

37. Bertheault-Cvitkovic F, Jami A, Ithzaki M et al, Biweekly intensified ambulatory chronomodulated chemotherapy with oxaliplatin, 5-fluorouracil and folinic acid in patients with metastatic colorectal cancer. *J Clin Oncol* 1996; **14:** 2950–8.

38. Pitot HC, Wender D, O'Connell MJ et al, A phase II trial of CPT-11 (irinotecan) in patients with metastatic colorectal carcinoma: a North Central Cancer Treatment Group study. *Proc Am Soc Clin Oncol* 1994; **13:** Abst 573.

39. Rothenberg ML, Eckardt JR, Kuhn JG et al, Phase II trial of irinotecan in patients with progressive or rapidly recurrent colorectal cancer. *J Clin Oncol* 1996; **14:** 1128–35.

40. Shimada Y et al, Phase II study of CPT-11, a new camptothecin derivate, in metastatic colorectal cancer. CPT-11 Gastrointestinal Cancer Study Group. *J Clin Oncol* 1993; **11:** 909–13.

41. Rougier R, Bugat R, Douillard JY et al, Phase II study of irinotecan in the treatment of advanced colorectal cancer in chemotherapy-naive patients and patients pretreated with fluorouracil-based chemotherapy. *J Clin Oncol* 1997; **15:** 251–60.

42. Van Cutsem E, Cunningham W, Ten Bokkel Huinink W et al, Irinotecan (CPT-11) multicenter phase II study in colorectal cancer patients with documented progressive disease on prior 5-FU: preliminary results. *Proc Am Soc Clin Oncol* 1996; **15:** Abst 230.

43. Droz JP, Marty M, Douillard JY et al, CPT-11 in 5-FU-resistant colorectal cancer: management of delayed diarrhea (ENG). In: *Abstract Book, 21st Annual Meeting, European Society of Medical Oncology, Vienna*, 1996; Abst 223.

44. Cascinu S, Fedeli A, Luzi-Fedeli S, Catalano G, Salvage chemotherapy in colorectal cancer patients with good performance status and young age after failure of 5-fluorouracil/leucovorin combination. *J Chemother* 1992; **4:** 46–9.

45. Adenis A, Carlier D, Darloy F et al, Cytarabine and cisplatin as salvage therapy in patients with metastatic colorectal cancer who failed 5-fluorouracil + folinic acid regimen. French Northern Oncology Group. *Am J Clin Oncol* 1995; **18:** 158–60.

46. Zaniboni A, Labianca R, Pancera G et al, Oral etoposide as second-line chemotherapy for colorectal cancer: a GISCAD study. Gruppo Italiano Studio Carcinomi Apparato Digerente. *J Chemother* 1995; **7:** 246–8.

47. Stuart K, Posner M, Campbell K, Huberman M, Cisplatin and chronic oral etoposide as salvage therapy for advanced colorectal carcinoma. *Am J Clin Oncol* 1995; **18:** 300–2.

48. Barni S, Lissoni P, Cazzaniga M et al, A randomized study of low-dose subcutaneous interleukin-2 plus melatonin versus supportive care alone in metastatic colorectal cancer patients progressing under 5-fluorouracil and folates. *Oncology* 1995; **52:** 243–5.

49. Welt S, Scott AM, Divgi CR, Phase I–II study of iodine 125-labeled monoclonal antibody A33 in patients with advanced colon cancer. *J Clin Oncol* 1996; **14:** 1787–97.

50. Pai LH, Wittes RE, Setser A et al, Phase I study of the immunotoxin LMB-1, an anti-cancer murine Mab B3, coupled to a recombinant form of pseudomonas exotoxin PE38. *Proc Am Soc Clin Oncol* 1996; **15:** Abst 1528.

51. Data on file at Rhone-Poulenc Rorer.

52. Saliba F, Magipattelli R, Misset JL et al, Pathophysiology and therapy of irinotecan (CPTII) induced delayed onset diarrhoea. A prospective assessment. Data on file at Rhone-Poulenc Rorer.

27

Chronomodulation of chemotherapy against metastatic colorectal cancer

Francis Lévi, Sylvie Giacchetti

INTRODUCTION

The adaptation of chemotherapy delivery to circadian rhythms has shown improved tolerability and antitumor efficacy against metastases from colorectal cancer. This strategy has been based primarily upon the ability to increase dose intensity through an adjustment of drug delivery to 24-hour rhythms in tolerability. The new active but toxic drug oxaliplatin benefited from this approach at a time when it was about to be dropped. Therefore it should not be surprising that the high activity of a novel three-drug combination combining oxaliplatin with the standard treatment consisting of 5-fluorouracil and folinic acid was developed first as a chronomodulated schedule. The selection of peak times of drug delivery was based upon

- chronopharmacological studies in rodents (experimental prerequisites);
- the demonstration of rhythms in normal host tissues that may be damaged by chemotherapy (clinical prerequisites);
- the occurrence of dosing-time dependence in drug pharmacokinetics (clinical prerequisites).

A specific technology (programmable-in-time injectors) was required in order to achieve both sufficient quality and adequate chronomodulated drug-delivery profiles and to allow the administration of chronotherapy to ambulatory patients. This chapter will review the experimental and clinical rationale of cancer chronotherapy, summarize our knowledge of the drug-delivery systems needed for its implementation, and review the clinical data available in patients with metastatic colorectal cancer.

RATIONALE FOR CHRONOMODULATION OF CHEMOTHERAPY

Circadian system physiology

Biological functions of living beings are organized on a 24-hour time scale. These circadian rhythms are endogenous, since they persist in constant conditions in laboratory rodents and in humans. Genes responsible for circadian periodicity have been demonstrated and/or cloned in *Drosophila*, hamsters and mice.[1-3]

Studies performed on homozygous or heterozygous twins support a genetic background for these rhythms in humans. Biological clocks can display circadian rhythms in vitro, irrespective of environmental temperature, and can be reset by physical or chemical stimuli. This is notably the case of the suprachiasmatic nucleus, which coordinates most circadian rhythms in mammals, including both the rest–activity cycle and body-temperature rhythm.[4] The regular alternation of light and darkness over 24 hours calibrates the endogenous circadian period at precisely 24 hours through its resetting effects on this clock. Under such synchronization conditions, the times of peaks and troughs of circadian rhythms in cellular metabolism and proliferation can be predicted, the amplitudes of these rhythms can be estimated, and their implications for anticancer drug pharmacology can be assessed.[5]

Chronopharmacology of relevant anticancer drugs

Toxicity rhythms

Circadian dosing time influences the extent of toxicity of about 30 anticancer drugs, including cytostatics and cytokines, in mice or rats.[6] This effect characterizes the agents that are active against colorectal cancer, both long-standing ones such as 5-fluorouracil (5-FU), floxuridine (FUDR), methotrexate (MTX) and mitomycin-C (MIT), as well as recent drugs such as oxaliplatin (L-OHP) and irinotecan (CPT-11) (E Filipski, F Lévi, unpublished work) (Figure 27.1).[7–13]

For all these drugs, the difference in survival rate varied by two- to eightfold, depending on the dosing time of a potentially lethal dose. Thus the same dose could either kill 80% of mice or spare 90% of them. The least-toxic time was located in the first half of the rest span of

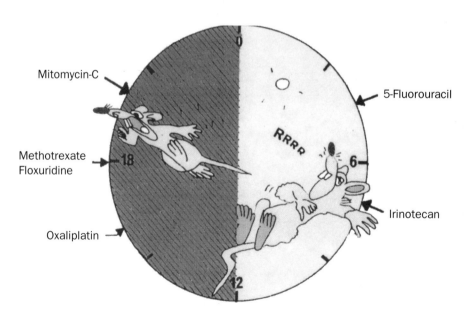

Figure 27.1 Circadian rhythms in tolerability of anticancer drugs in mice or rats. Only those agents that are known to be active against colorectal cancer are shown. Survival rate was two to eight times larger if a potentially lethal dose of a drug was injected at the circadian time indicated with an arrow, as compared with an administration 12 hours earlier or later. These drug-tolerability rhythms are coupled to the rest–activity cycle of these animals, synchronized with a regular alternation of 12 hours of light and 12 hours of darkness. Time is expressed in hours after light onset (HALO).

mice (day) for 5-FU,[7] in the second half of the rest span for CPT-11 (E Filipski, unpublished work), and in the second half of the activity span (night) for MTX, MIT and L-OHP.[10–13] The lethal toxicity of these drugs mainly involved cellular damage to both bone marrow and intestinal mucosa. These tissues usually display synchronous rhythms in their susceptibility to the same agent.

Chronopharmacological mechanisms involve circadian changes in drug pharmacokinetics and/or susceptibility rhythms of target tissues.

Drug disposition

Times of high toxicity corresponded to the longest plasma-elimination half-life for MTX.[10] This was not the case for 5-FU or for L-OHP.[14,15] Conversely, platinum concentration in spleen and gut mucosa was least following L-OHP dosing, at its least-toxic time.[13] These and other results suggest that toxicity rhythms may more closely match cellular changes in drug uptake or efflux than circadian plasma pharmacokinetics (reviewed in reference 6).

Cellular mechanisms

Circadian changes in cellular enzymatic activities by two- to eightfold appear to contribute to the chronopharmacology of antimetabolites. This has been shown for dihydrofolate reductase (a target enzyme for MTX cytotoxicity), dehydropyrimidine dehydrogenase (DPDase – the rate-limiting catabolic enzyme of fluoropyrimidines), and uridine phosphorylase (URDPase), orotate phophoribosyltransferase (OPRTase) and deoxythymidine kinase (TKase) – all three of which are involved in the anabolism of the cytotoxic forms of fluoropyrimidines, 5-fluorodeoxyuridylate (5-FdUMP) and 5-fluorouridylate (5-FUMP).[8,16–18]

Cellular resistance to many cytostatics involves reduced glutathione. Its concentration in liver cells doubles along the 24-hour time scale: lowest and highest values respectively occur near dark onset and near light onset.[19,20]

Finally, O^6-alkylguanine-DNA alkyltransferase (AGTase), a DNA repair enzyme of alkylated DNA, was about sixfold higher at 19 hours after light onset (HALO) (second half of activity span) as compared with 7 HALO (second half of rest span) in mouse liver.[21]

These data point towards an essential role for rhythmic enzymatic mechanisms in the cellular detoxification of chemotherapy damage to healthy cells.

Antitumor efficacy

Dosing time not only affects drug tolerability, but may also modify anticancer efficacy, as was shown first with arabinosylcytosine (Ara-C) against mouse L1210 leukemia.[22,23] Similarly, 5-FU displayed increased efficacy against murine colon tumors (CO36 and CO38) following dosing in the early rest span, when it was less toxic.[24] Thus most experimental data support a link between the rhythm in drug tolerability and anticancer efficacy, through an increase in tolerable dose (reviewed in reference 6). This principle led to incremental approaches in chronopharmacological combination of drugs, which documented that the rate of tumor cures could be brought up from 25% to 80% or more with adequately circadian-scheduled chemotherapy involving up to five cytostatics.[25]

Rhythms in relevant human tissues

Proliferative activity (DNA synthesis) in hematopoietic or oral mucosa progenitor cells varies by 50% or more along the 24-hour time scale in healthy subjects. This is also the case for ex vivo DNA synthetic activity in human rectal mucosa or skin. For these four tissues, lower mean values in DNA synthesis occurred between midnight and 04.00 h at night, while higher mean values occurred between 08.00 h and 20.00 h.[26–33] Reduced glutathione also varied rhythmically in human bone marrow, yet intersubject variability appeared to be larger than that of proliferative indices.[34] The activity of DPDase in human mononuclear cells increased by almost 50% between 10.00 h and midnight, both in healthy subjects and in cancer patients (Figure 27.2).[35,36]

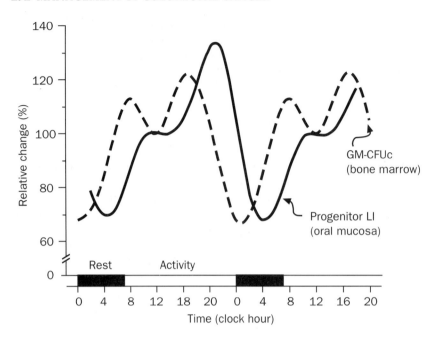

Figure 27.2 Twenty-four-hour changes in human normal tissues. The proliferative ability of bone-marrow granulomonocytic precursors was assessed from seven 4-hourly bone-marrow aspirations in 19 healthy volunteers;[30] that of oral mucosa progenitors was documented with a similar sampling scheme in 11 healthy subjects.[33] A 4-hour span, located between midnight and 04.00 h, corresponds to a low point in the DNA-synthetic activity of both of these tissues, as well as skin and rectal mucosa in humans.[26,32]

Mitotic index and/or DNA synthesis have been used to evaluate the proliferative activity of many experimental and human breast, ovarian or lymphomatous tumors. Data suggest that well-differentiated, slowly growing tumors retain a circadian time structure, whereas poorly differentiated, rapidly growing tumors tend to lose it[37,38] (reviewed in reference 39).

Drug chronopharmacokinetics

Short intravenous infusions of 5-FU or MTX were associated with modifications of plasma and/or urinary pharmacokinetics according to dosing time. Physiological rhythms in urinary excretion or plasma proteins contributed to MTX chronopharmacokinetics.[40,41]

However, the most striking results stemmed from flat intravenous infusion of chemotherapeutic agents. To the best of our knowledge, five such clinical investigations were reported for 5-FU. In four of them, 5-FU was infused at a flat rate for 24 hours or 4 or 5 days.[42–45] Mean plasma 5-FU nearly doubled from around midday to around 01.00 h or 04.00 h at night.

This circadian pattern was similar on all infusional days tested in patients with bladder or gastrointestinal metastatic cancer and in those receiving prior cisplatin, concurrent flat infusion of FA alone or associated with L-OHP. However, after a 14-day venous infusion of 5-FU, the plasma 5-FU rhythm peaked near noon in 9 patients with gastrointestinal malignancy; furthermore, DPDase activity in circulating mononuclear cells also displayed a circadian rhythm, with a peak occurring near 01.00 h at night, i.e. about 12 hours out of phase of the 5-FU rhythm.[35] This rhythm remained unaffected by 5-FU infusion. We hypothesize that high-dose flat infusion or bolus injection of 5-FU saturates DPDase activity, which no longer represents a relevant mechanism in such experimental conditions. In both of these cases, 5-FU clearance is least near 01.00 h at night, while this parameter is highest near 13.00 h when 5-FU is infused for 14 days at a lower dose, and its 24-hour mean plasma level is about $\frac{1}{20}$ that observed during a

4- or 5-day infusion (16 versus 340 ng/ml).[35,42,43] Thus either infusion duration or daily dose of 5-FU may influence the peak time location of the circadian rhythm in drug plasma level.

Similarly, circadian changes also characterized flat infusion of folinic acid, although with a lower amplitude (10%) than for 5-FU.[43]

DRUG-DELIVERY DEVICES FOR CHRONOMODULATING CHEMOTHERAPY

Technology, first- and second-generation injectors

The availability of programmable-in-time ambulatory pumps was indispensable for testing the relevance of chronotherapy principles. Programmable-in-time single-reservoir pump prototypes (AS 20C-Chronopump, Autosyringe, Baxter Travenol, Hooksett, USA; Zyklomat, Ferring, Germany) were first used for pilot or phase I–II trials of single-drug chronomodulated regimens. A multichannel programmable pump (IntelliJect, Aguettant, Lyon, France) has been mostly used for chronotherapy delivery since 1987.

This pump is equipped with four 30-ml disposable syringes. In the case of chemical incompatibilities between drugs, one, two or three of the reservoirs (each corresponding to a different drug solution) can be connected to a single central venous line by a manifold. The remaining channel(s) can be connected to a second separate central venous line. This system allows different reservoirs to contain incompatible drug solutions and to be connected to different central venous lines.

A second generation of multiple programmable-in-time pumps has now completed testing in Europe. Two devices have been approved for clinical use. Both have extended versatility in programmability, and offer much better comfort to the patient than IntelliJect. The Z-pump (Zambon-Inphardial, Antibes, France) is a two-channel injector that can be equipped with one or two 100-ml reservoirs, and thus appears to be appropriate for chronomodulated delivery of 5-FU and FA. The Mélodie pump (Aguettant-Santé, Lyon, France) is a four-channel device, which can be programmed with user-friendly software under Windows on a PC, and can accommodate any reservoir volume and delivery profile (Table 27.1). These new systems

Table 27.1 Approved drug-delivery devices used for multiple drug chronotherapy in gastrointestinal malignancies

Model	Manufacturer	Main characteristics	Main drugs
Z-pump	Zambon-Inphardial (Antibes, France)	Two 100 ml-reservoirs programmable on PC, or pump or via code-bar (laser printer)	5-FU–FA
IntelliJect	Aguettant-Santé (Lyon, France)	Four 30 ml-reservoirs programmable on PC	5-FU–FA ± L-OHP
Mélodie	Aguettant-Santé (Lyon, France)	Four reservoirs of any capacity programmable on PC computer	5-FU–FA ± L-OHP

should prove as suitable for extended applications of fully ambulatory cancer chronotherapy.

Drug pharmacokinetics during chronomodulated infusions

Plasma concentrations of 5-FU, active folates and L-OHP have been studied along the course of chronomodulated infusions.

It was verified that circadian changes in 5-FU plasma levels matched rather well the sinusoidal delivery waveform over the 4 or 5 infusional days (Figure 27.3).[36,43,45] Interestingly, chronomodulated delivery with a peak flow rate at 4.00 h was associated with markedly reduced interpatient variability in plasma levels as compared with constant-rate infusions or with chronomodulated administrations with peak flow rate at 13.00 h or 19.00 h.[36,43] We should emphasize that these three latter sched-

ules displayed increased toxicity compared with the former one.

Chronomodulated delivery of l-folinic acid resulted in 24-hour changes in the plasma concentrations of both l-FA and methyltetrahydro-folate (mTHF), a metabolite that reflects the intracellular active form. Interpatient variability was reduced if FA delivery peak was set at 4.00 h as compared with 13.00 h or 19.00 h.[36] Nevertheless, the peak time of mTHF occurred about 2 hours after l-FA peak delivery (I Assier, P Bargnoux, P Chollet, unpublished work).

Similarly, 'free' platinum plasma concentration reflected the chronomodulated flow rate of L-OHP, yet accumulation was patent from the first to the fourth infusional day (G Metzger, F Lévi, unpublished work).

These pharmacokinetic studies are needed to ensure that the target rhythm in tissue exposure has been adequately achieved with the drug-delivery profile, and may serve to improve it further.

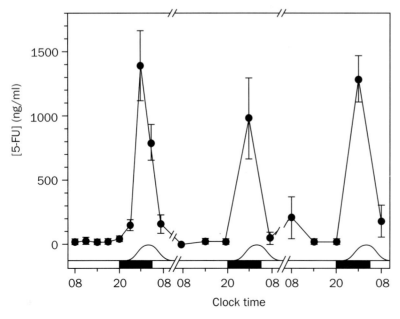

Figure 27.3 Twenty-four-hour changes in 5-FU plasma levels, during a 5-day chronomodulated infusion of 5-FU (600 mg/m^2/day), dl-FA (300 mg/m^2/day) and L-OHP (20 mg/m^2/day) in 6 patients with metastatic colorectal cancer.[43] The drug-delivery scheme is shown in Figure 27.4.

CHRONOTHERAPY TOLERABILITY AND EFFICACY

Overall strategy and hypothesis

To achieve a high dose intensity, we aimed at reducing treatment toxicity as much as possible so that doses could be increased compared with standard chemotherapeutic schedules. For this purpose, we adapted the drug infusion rate to circadian rhythms. The hypothesis was that high doses of all drugs and proper circadian scheduling of drug delivery were needed to achieve clinical synergy.

The main results of phase I, II and III clinical trials will be briefly reviewed in order to define the role of chronotherapy in the medicosurgical management of patients with metastatic colorectal cancer.

Drug delivery in the chronomodulated schedules varied sinusoidally along the 24-hour time scale (cf above). Times of maximum flow rate were extrapolated from murine experiments. For these reasons, peak delivery was scheduled at 4.00 h for 5-FU and FA, and at 16.00 h for L-OHP (reviewed in references 5 and 6) (Figure 27.4).

5-Fluorouracil with or without folinic acid

5-Fluorouracil has remained the main active drug against colorectal cancer. Its efficacy was enhanced by modulating its cytotoxicity with folinic acid (FA) or by administering it as a continuous venous infusion. Both such regimens resulted in a three- to fourfold improvement in tumor response rate in patients with metastatic disease compared with standard 5-FU treatment. A dose–response relationship characterized the antitumor efficacy of 5-FU against colorectal cancer.[46]

The infusion rate of 5-FU alone was chronomodulated along the 24-hour time scale for 5 consecutive days (every 3 weeks), with peak delivery at 04.00 h and no infusion from 16.00 h to 22.00 h. The drug was administered with a single-reservoir external programmable pump (Autosyringe, Baxter Travenol, Hooksett, USA). Thirty-five patients with metastatic colorectal cancer participated in this phase I–II trial, with intrapatient dose escalation according to defined toxicity criteria. As a result of good tolerability (<8% courses with severe (WHO grade 3) toxic symptoms), the recommended dose could be escalated up to

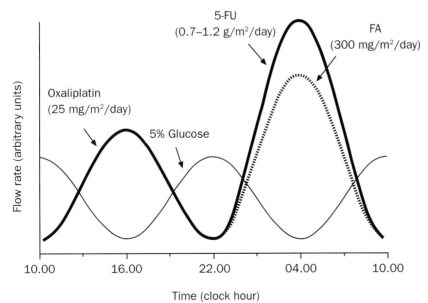

Figure 27.4 Schedule for intravenous chronomodulated infusion of 5-fluorouracil (5-FU), folinic acid (FA) and oxaliplatin (L-OHP). This 24-hour cycle was repeated automatically for 5 consecutive days followed by a 16-day interval,[55–58] or for 4 days followed by a 10-day interval.[59,60] This complex drug-delivery pattern was administered to fully ambulatory patients using a programmable multichannel pump.

1400 mg/m^2/day or more for 5 days in 80% of assessable patients. This represents a 40–100% increase in dose or dose intensity as compared with 5-day flat infusion, for which the recommended dose ranges from 800 to 1000 mg/m^2/day for 5 days every 3–4 weeks.[47]

Three phase I trials have evaluated the tolerability and recommended dose of chronomodulated infusions of various 5-FU–FA combination schedules. In a German study 75% of the 5-FU was given by flat infusion from 24.00 h to 07.00 h, combined with concurrent low-dose FA infusion for 5 consecutive days. The maximum tolerated dose (MTD) of 5-FU was 600 mg/m^2/day (2500 mg/m^2/course), while that of FA was 60 mg/m^2/day (300 mg/m^2/course). As a result, 5-FU dose intensity was 625 mg/m^2/week (with low-dose FA). It was suggested that a sinusoidal shape of 5-FU–FA infusion might be more tolerable and effective.[48] In a Canadian study 5-FU was infused for 14 days, together with low-dose FA. Both drugs were admixed and infused according to a quasi-sinusoidal 24-hour rhythmic chronomodulated pattern with peak flow rate near 04.00 h at night. Each course was followed by a 2-week treatment-free interval. MTD was 250 mg/m^2/day of 5-FU (3500 mg/m^2/course), together with 20 mg/m^2/day of FA. The theoretical dose intensity over 3 courses was 875 mg/m^2/week (with low-dose FA). It was suggested that peak delivery at early night (22.00 h) could further improve tolerance in some patients.[49]

A phase I study established the MTD of the combination of 5-FU and *l*-FA given as a 5-day chronomodulated infusion to ambulatory patients with metastatic colorectal cancer. 5-FU was delivered from 22.00 h to 10.00 h, with peak flow rate at 4.00 h. Courses were repeated after a 16-day interval. Thirty-four patients were included, with six patients per planned dose level. Dose-limiting toxicities were stomatitis and diarrhea. The MTD are 900 mg/m^2/day for 5-FU and 150 mg/m^2/day for *l*-FA. Objective responses were achieved in 8/20 untreated patients and in 1/13 previously treated ones.[50]

The low toxicity profile and the apparently dose-related antitumor activity in chemotherapy-naive patients prompted an attempt at further intensification of this regimen. Both drugs were delivered at MTD as chronomodulated infusions for 4 days instead of 5, each course being repeated after a 10-day rather than a 16-day treatment-free interval. This pilot study was conducted in 22 patients, and allowed a further 20% increase in theoretical dose intensity as compared with the above 5 days on/16 days off 5-FU–FA regimen. The main dose-limiting toxicity was cumulative hand–foot syndrome (H Curé, P Chollet, personal communication).

The antitumor efficacy and tolerability of such an intensified 5-FU–FA schedule (FF4-10) are currently being investigated in a multicenter European phase II trial that plans to register 100 patients with previously untreated metastatic colorectal cancer. While the FA dose remains fixed (150 mg/m^2/day of *l*-FA or 300 mg/m^2/day of *dl*-FA), the 5-FU dose is escalated in the absence of grade 2 or greater toxicity from 900 mg/m^2/day in the first course to 1000 mg/m^2/day in the second course and 1100 mg/m^2/day in the third course (H Curé, P Chollet, personal communication).

Other teams are independently assessing the activity of this schedule (J Jolivet, personal communication).

Oxaliplatin

Oxaliplatin (L-OHP) is 1,2-diaminocyclohexane (*trans-l*) oxalatoplatinum(II), a third-generation platinum complex, which lacks any renal toxicity and displays moderate yet definitive antitumor activity against colorectal cancer. Thus its administration as a single drug achieved 10% objective responses in a total of 150 patients with previously treated metastatic disease.[51,52] The first phase II trial of this drug was conducted using a 5-day chronomodulated delivery schedule, because this infusion modality was shown to display less hematological, gastrointestinal and neurological toxicity than flat infusion in a randomized phase I trial. As a result, the recommended dose per course was

125 mg/m^2 for flat infusion, i.e. close to that recommended for a standard 2- or 6-hour infusion of this drug once every 3 weeks. Conversely, the recommended L-OHP dose for chronotherapy was 175 mg/m^2/course.[53] In the multicenter chronotherapy phase II trial, such a high dose was confirmed to be rather well tolerated in fully ambulatory conditions. No renal and minimal hematological toxic effects were encountered, while dose-limiting toxicities mostly consisted of nausea or vomiting, diarrhea, and cumulative peripheral sensitive neuropathy. In the 29 heavily pretreated patients with metastatic colorectal cancer from this study, L-OHP achieved 10% objective responses.[51]

5-Fluorouracil, folinic acid and oxaliplatin combination

Because oxaliplatin exhibits in vivo synergistic antitumor activity with 5-FU against transplantable tumor models,[54] and because it is not associated with renal toxicity and has minimal hematological toxicity, we considered it to be a good candidate for further platinum modulation of 5-FU and FA cytotoxicity. Since single-drug solutions of 5-FU, FA or L-OHP remained stable at ambient temperature and under normal lighting conditions for 5 days or more, this three-drug combination chemotherapy was further amenable to continuous ambulatory infusion.

In a pilot randomized trial, involving nine patients, we first compared the tolerability of a chronomodulated infusion to that of a flat delivery of 5-FU (600 mg/m^2/day), FA (300 mg/m^2/day) and L-OHP (20 mg/m^2/day). Severe oral mucositis (WHO grade 3 or 4) was encountered in 3/4 patients receiving the flat infusion, as compared with 0/5 patients treated with the chronomodulated schedule.[43]

From April 1988 to May 1990, a phase II study of a 5-day schedule of chronomodulated chemotherapy with 5-FU, FA and L-OHP (chronoFFL) was performed in 93 patients with unresectable colorectal metastases. Of these patients, 46 had received previous chemother-

apy. Courses were repeated every 21 days. A 58% objective response rate was obtained. Moreover, all treatments were administered on an outpatient basis, and less than 10% of the 784 courses given were associated with severe toxicity. Median overall survival was 16 months, irrespective of prior chemotherapy, with a 17% three-year survival rate in chemotherapy-naive patients. These results appeared largely superior to those achieved with standard 5-FU–FA combination chemotherapy, the reference treatment for this disease. We related the high antitumor efficacy of chronoFFL both to L-OHP, a new active agent against colorectal cancer, and to chronomodulation, which allowed safe delivery of high drug doses.[55]

The role of this latter factor was investigated in two consecutive European multicenter phase III studies, which compared flat versus chronomodulated infusion of the same three-drug combination in patients with previously untreated metastatic colorectal cancer.

A first randomized trial was then undertaken in 92 patients. Patient characteristics were similar in both groups. The proportion of patients experiencing grade 3 or 4 toxicity was five times higher with the flat infusion than with chronotherapy for stomatitis (89% versus 18%) and 2.5 times higher for hand–foot syndrome (11% versus 4%), despite the delivery of a median dose of 700 mg/m^2/day of 5-FU in the chronotherapy group and 500 mg/m^2/day in the flat infusion group. Thus chronotherapy achieved a 22% increase in 5-FU dose intensity as compared with flat infusion. Response rate, the main judgement criterion, was significantly increased from 32% with flat infusion to 53% with chronotherapy. Median progression-free survival and overall survival of all patients were 8 months and 14.9 months in the flat arm, and 11 months and 19 months in the chronotherapy arm. A risk of partial chemical inactivation of L-OHP with the basic pH of 5-FU in the flat schedule was documented, however, and prompted an early termination of this trial.[56]

A new multicenter trial was undertaken in which any risk of drug chemical interaction was avoided. Accrual of 186 patients to this trial was completed by February 1993. Results supported the above main findings and conclusions. Severe stomatitis was incurred by 76% on the flat infusion regimen as compared with 14% of those on chronotherapy. Cumulative peripheral sensitive neuropathy with functional impairment was reported in 31% patients on constant delivery and in 16% patients on chronotherapy. This latter schedule allowed administration of a higher dose of 5-FU (700 mg/m²/day) than flat infusion (500 mg/m²/day) and a 22% larger dose intensity. Objective response rate was 51% on chronotherapy and 29% on flat delivery. Median overall survival was 16 months in both modalities, possibly because 24% of the patients crossed over from the flat schedule to chronotherapy.[57]

Thus both of these trials, involving a total of 278 patients with metastatic colorectal cancer, have confirmed that a 5-day chronomodulated infusion of 5-FU, FA and L-OHP produced about twice as many objective responses as current chemotherapeutic schedules or flat three-drug infusion. Furthermore, in this European multicenter randomized setting, the most active chronomodulated schedule was also the least toxic.[58]

The high efficacy, together with the good tolerability of this chronomodulated three-drug regimen, prompted us to attempt to intensify it further. As a first step, this schedule was administered for 4 days every 2 weeks (10-day interval, chronoFFL4-10), rather than for 5 days every 3 weeks (16-day interval, chronoFFL5-16). Respective daily doses (mg/m²/day) of 5-FU, FA and L-OHP remained similar (e.g. 700, 300 and 25). This trial, which involved 54 patients, demonstrated the feasibility of a 20% increase in dose intensity.[59]

A subsequent step consisted of an intrapatient 5-FU dose escalation scheme in this chronoFFL4-10. The goals of this trial were to determine whether this 3-drug chronomodulated regimen could be further intensified in ambulatory outpatients and to estimate antitumor efficacy. Fifty patients with metastatic colorectal cancer (37 previously treated and 13 chemotherapy-naive) were enrolled in this

study. The first treatment course consisted of the daily administration of 5-FU (700 mg/m²/day), FA (300 mg/m²/day) and L-OHP (25 mg/m²/day) for 4 days. Courses were repeated every 14 days (10-day intermission) in ambulatory patients, 5-FU being escalated by 100 mg/m²/day in each patient, following each course if toxicity was <grade 2.

Median 5-FU and L-OHP dose intensities were increased by 32% and 18% respectively, as compared with our previous 5 days on/16 days off phase II protocol. Objective response rate was 40% (24–57%) in previously treated patients and 69% (48–90%) in chemotherapy-naive ones. Furthermore, the response rate was about twice as high in those patients receiving higher cumulative 5-FU dose or dose intensity over the first four courses, irrespective of prior chemotherapy administration. A complete surgical removal of residual metastases was performed in 13 patients (26%), 12 of them being unresectable before treatment onset. Median progression-free survival was 9.3 months (95% CI 6.6–11.2). Median survival was 16.9 months in previously treated patients and 20.7 months in chemotherapy-naive patients.[60] This highly effective fully ambulatory outpatient regimen was subsequently confirmed in a multicenter European phase II trial.[61] Figure 27.5 summarizes the relationship between 5-FU dose intensity and objective response rate in those trials that involved chemotherapy-naive patients.

The main characteristics and results from these trials are summarized in Table 27.2.

SURGERY OF METASTASES AFTER CHRONOTHERAPY: A NEW STRATEGY WITH CURATIVE INTENT

Rationale

The achievement of a 50% or greater objective response rate with the three-drug chronomodulated regimen allowed surgical resection of metastases in a substantial proportion of patients. In a retrospective study we examined the outcome of those patients with initially unresectable colorectal metastases who under-

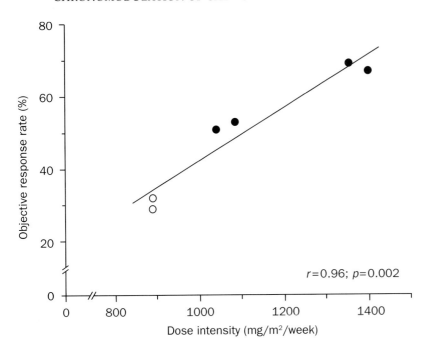

Figure 27.5 Relationship between 5-FU dose intensity and objective response rate in 381 patients with previously untreated metastatic colorectal cancer. All these patients received 5-FU, FA and L-OHP as a 5 days on/16 days off regimen (FFL 5-16) or as a 4 days on/10 days off regimen (FFL 4-10). Drug delivery was either constant (○) or chronomodulated over 24 hours (●). Results from two randomized phase III trials[56–58] and from two phase II trials.[60,61]

went infusional L-OHP/5-FU/FA chemotherapy followed by surgery between 1988 and 1993. The cohort involves patients with a median follow-up of 4 years and a minimum follow-up of 2 years. The goal of this investigation was to assess any survival benefit of performing surgery of metastases in patients with initially unresectable metastases.

Clinical results

From March 1988 to July 1993, 301 patients with unresectable colorectal metastases received ambulatory infusional chemotherapy with 5-FU, FA and L-OHP at our institution. Chronomodulated infusion was administered to 248/301 patients (86.3%), and flat infusion was administered to 53 chemotherapy-naive patients (phase III trials). Out of 301 patients, 124 had unresectable liver-only metastases, and

have been analyzed. Fifty-eight patients (47%) underwent liver surgery with curative intent. Thirty-seven patients had a complete resection. A complete histological response was documented in four patients. With a median and a minimum follow-up of respectively 4 years and 2 years, the median overall survival of the 124 patients with liver-only metastases was 23 months. Forty-seven percent of patients were alive at 2 years and 33% at 3 years (Figure 27.6). With regard to the 58 patients operated upon, median progression-free survival (PFS) was 18 months, and median overall survival has not yet been reached. Seventy-two percent of the patients were alive at 2 years, and the estimated 3-year survival is 58%.[62] Surgery-related morbidity was <10%, i.e. it was comparable to that observed in patients with primary resection of metastases, and was not apparently increased by chemotherapy.[63]

Thus, combining effective and safe chemotherapy and surgery altered the natural

Table 27.2 Summary of main clinical trials of chronomodulated venous infusions of cancer chemotherapy

Phase	Trial design	Drug	Dose, schedule	Tumor type, no. of patients (no. pretreated)	Main conclusions	Ref
I–II	Intrapatient dose escalation if toxicity <grade 2	5-FU	800–1900 mg/m²/d (peak at 4.00 h) × 5 d 21 d	Colorectal, 35 (15)	• Dose-limiting toxicities: mucositis, diarrhea, hand-foot syndrome • Recommended dose: 1400 mg/m²/d × 5 d q 21 d • Objective responses: 3/15 pretreated (20%) 7/20 naive (35%)	47
I	Inter- and intrapatient dose escalation if toxicity <grade 2	5-FU and lFA	600–1100 mg/m²/d 150 mg/m²/d (peak at 4.00 h) × 5 d q 21 d	Colorectal, 34 (13)	• Dose-limiting toxicities: mucositis, diarrhea • Recommended dose of 5-FU: 900 mg/m²/d × 5 d q 21 d • Objective responses 1/13 pretreated (8%), 8/20 naive (40%)	50
I	Interpatient dose escalation	5-FU and dlFA	200–300 mg/m²/d 5–20 mg/m²/d (peak at 4.00 h) × 14 d q 28 d	Solid tumors, 14 (7)	• Dose-limiting toxicities: mucositis, hand–foot synd. • MTD: 250 mg/m²/d of 5-FU and 20 mg/m²/d of FA	49
I	Randomized intrapatient dose escalation	L-OHP	25–40 mg/m²/d flat vs chrono (peak at 16.00 h) × 5 d q 21 d	Breast or liver, 23 (16)	• Dose-limiting toxicities: neutropenia, vomiting, peripheral sensitive neuropathy (cumulative) • Recommended dose: chronomodulated 35 mg/m²/d × 5 d; flat 25 mg/m²/d × 5 d	53
I	Randomized intrapatient dose escalation	FUDR	0.15 mg/m²/d flat vs chrono (peak from 15.00 h to 21.00 h) × 14 d q 28 d	Solid tumors, 36	• Dose-limiting toxicity: diarrhea; none with chrono • Dose intensity +45% with chrono • Recommended dose: chronomodulated 0.23 mg/kg/d × 14 d flat 0.15 mg/kg/d × 14 d	68
I–II	Two-center	5-FU i.v.	1000–1400 mg/m²/d (peak at 04.00 h)	Colon cancer (liver metastases), 56 (16)	• Chrono less toxic than flat • Response rate similar: 48% vs 38% • Marked center effect for long-term outcome	69
		FUDR i.a.	80–120 mg/m²/d (peak at 16.00 h) × 5 d q 21 d			

Phase	Setting	Drugs	Dose	Cancer (patients)	Results	Ref
II	Multicenter (France 2, Belgium 1, (Italy 1))	5-FU and *dl*-FA	600–800 mg/m²/d 300 mg/m²/d (peaks at 4.00 h) × 5 d q 21 d	Colorectal, 36 (17)	• No toxicity > grade 2 • Objective responses: 1/17 pretreated 6/19 naive (35%)	70
II	Multicenter (France 3, Belgium 1, Italy 1)	L-OHP	30–40 mg/m²/d (peak at 16.00 h) × 5 d q 21 d	Colorectal, 29 (26)	• Median dose: 35 mg/m²/d × 5 d • Objective responses: 3 (10%)	51
II	Single-institution	5-FU *dl*-FA L-OHP	700 mg/m²/d 300 mg/m²/d (peaks at 4.00 h) 25 mg/m²/d (peak at 16.00 h) × 5 d q 21 d	Colorectal, 93 (46)	• Dose-limiting toxicities: diarrhea, vomiting, peripheral sensitive neuropathy (cumulative) • Objective responses: 54 (58%)	55
II	Single-institution	5-FU *dl*-FA L-OHP	700 mg/m²/d 300 mg/m²/d 25 mg/m²/d × 4 d q 14 d	Colorectal, 54 (46)	• Objective responses: 38% • Median survival: 13 months	59
II	Single-institution intrapatient dose escalation	5-FU *dl*-FA L-OHP	700–1200 mg/m²/d 300 mg/m²/d 25 mg/m²/d × 4 d q 14 d	Colorectal, 50 (37)	• Objective responses: 15/37 pretreated (40%) 9/13 naive (69%) • Median survival: 18 months	60
II	Multicenter	5-FU FA L-OHP	850 mg/m²/d 300 mg/m²/d 25 mg/m²/d × 4 d q 14 d	Colorectal, 90	• Objective responses: 67% • Median survival: 19 months	61
II	Multicenter	5-FU *dl*-FA	900 mg/m²/d 300 mg/m²/d × 4 d q 14 d	Colorectal, 100	Ongoing	70
III	Multicenter randomized 8 institutions	5-FU *dl*-FA L-OHP	600 mg/m²/d 300 mg/m²/d 25 mg/m²/d × 5 d q 21 d	Colorectal, 92 (flat 45 patients, chrono 47 patients)	Chrono > flat • Objective responses: 53% vs 32% • Grade 3–4 mucositis: 89% vs 16% • Median survival: 19 vs 15 months	56
II	Multicenter randomized 9 institutions	idem	idem	Colorectal, 186 (flat 93 patients chrono 93 patients)	Chrono > flat • Objective responses: 51% vs 29% • Grade 3–4 mucositis: 76% vs 14% • Grade 2–3 neuropathy: 31% vs 16% • Median survival: 16 months (similar)	57,58
II	Multicenter randomized 14 institutions	5-FU *dl*-FA L-OHP	700 mg/m²/d 300 mg/m²/d × 5 d q 21 d 125 mg/m²/d 6 h infusion d q 21 d	Colorectal, 200 (5-FU–FA: 100 patients L-OHP–5-FU–FA: 100 patients)	Ongoing	71

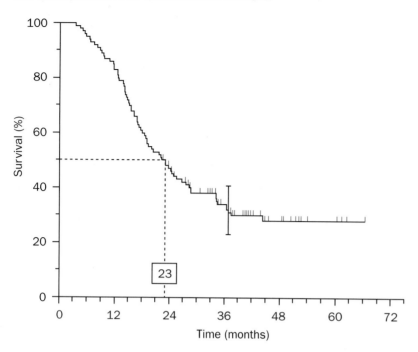

Figure 27.6 Survival curve of 124 patients with previously unresectable liver-only metastases from colorectal cancer. All patients were treated at Paul Brousse Hospital with 5-FU, FA and L-OHP between March 1988 and July 1993, and 47% of them could undergo secondary surgical resection of liver metastases. (After reference 62.)

history of primary unresectable colorectal cancer metastases. This study further emphasizes the need for active collaboration between surgeons and oncologists.[62]

CONCLUSIONS AND PERSPECTIVES

The extrapolation of the least-toxic times of chemotherapy from mice to human beings has been validated in patients with metastatic colorectal cancer using clinical phase III trial methodology. It has led to the recognition of the activity of a new active drug, oxaliplatin, against colorectal cancer, and has given rise to a new curative intent management of patients with metastatic disease.

Survival or quality of life as endpoints

Chronomodulated delivery of 5-FU–FA and L-OHP decreased toxicity, increased dose intensity, and improved efficacy in terms of response rate. The next task for chronotherapy trials will be to further assess any survival and/or quality-of-life improvement as compared with standard administration schedules. Intensified chronotherapy regimens seem to produce even better patient outcome. Nevertheless, the relevance of dose intensification of the three-drug schedule needs to be further evaluated with regard to survival and quality of life within a prospective randomized trial.

The combination of chronotherapy with surgery permitted long-term survival in patients with unresectable metastases. The role of this efficient and well-tolerated chemotherapy regimen does, however, need to be assessed as a neoadjuvant treatment in these patients within randomized trials. Chronotherapy also deserves to be evaluated as an adjuvant chemotherapy in patients with Dukes C colon cancer.

New drugs and combinations

Irinotecan (CPT-11) is a new active drug in colorectal cancer. Several phase II studies in Japan, Europe and USA showed objective response rates of 17–27% in chemotherapy-naive or pre-treated patients. The limiting toxicity of this drug is digestive (delayed diarrhea) and hematological. A dose–response relationship characterized CPT-11 activity, but toxicity limited the administration of the most-effective dose levels (>500 mg/m^2).[64] Since the toxicity of this drug varied according to the time of administration in mice, a proper circadian scheduling of CPT-11 delivery could well decrease its toxicity and allow a safe dose increase in tolerable dose.

Over the last few years, two new drugs, CPT-11 and L-OHP, have both demonstrated an activity against colorectal cancers that is modest and comparable to that of 5-FU. Our experience makes it clear that combinations of these agents should largely benefit from a chronopharmacological optimization. Because chronomodulated infusions are usually better tolerated than standard administration modalities, early phase II combination trials should permit safe and optimal exploration of the antitumor efficacy potential of a new regimen.

Prognostic factors

Prognostic factors influencing the natural history of colorectal liver metastases were reported in three prospective studies. The combination of these factors led to median survival times that could vary from 3.8 to 21.3 months in the absence of specific therapy.[65–67] The prognostic factors of outcome in patients receiving chronotherapy need to consider cancer-associated alterations of the circadian system.

Thus the 'group chronotherapy' approach, where all patients receive the same chronomodulated chemotherapy regimen, relies on the fact that groups of cancer patients who enter clinical trials do exhibit significant circadian rhythms in almost every variable that has been investigated. Nevertheless, investigations of rhythms in individual patients and/or in subgroups of cancer patients with very advanced disease and/or with a poor performance status have shown marked alterations in circadian rhythms (reviewed in reference 39). Their incidence and relevance for the outcome of patients with metastatic colorectal cancer receiving chronotherapy are under active investigation at present. The results may warrant the administration of specific supportive care for treating circadian-system dysfunctions in some patients prior to chronotherapy delivery.

ACKNOWLEDGEMENTS

We are indebted to all our colleagues and friends from the Paul Brousse Hospital and from the actual Chronotherapy Study Group of the European Organization for Research and Treatment of Cancer. This chapter could not have been written without their active scientific contribution and exciting discussions throughout the past few years.

We thank M Lévi for fine editorial assistance and the Association pour la Recherche sur le Temps Biologique et la Chronothérapie, Hôpital Paul Brousse, Villejuif, for supporting these research activities.

REFERENCES

1. Touitou Y, Haus E (eds), *Biologic Rhythms in Clinical and Laboratory Medicine.* Berlin: Springer-Verlag, 1992.
2. Redfern PH, Lemmer B (eds), *Handbook of Experimental Pharmacology.* Vol 125: *Physiology and Pharmacology of Biological Rhythms.* Berlin: Springer-Verlag, 1997.
3. Hall JC, Genetics of circadian rhythms. *Annu Rev Genet* 1990; **24:** 659–97.
4. Klein DC, Moore RY, Reppert SM, *Suprachiasmatic Nucleus. The Mind's Clock.* Oxford: Oxford University Press, 1991.
5. Levi F, Chronotherapy for gastrointestinal cancers. *Curr Opin Oncol* 1996; **8:** 334–41.

6. Levi F, Chronopharmacology of anticancer agents. In: *Handbook of Experimental Pharmacology*. Vol 125: *Physiology and Pharmacology of Biological Rhythms*. Chap 11: *Cancer Chemotherapy* (Redfern PH, Lemmer B, eds). Berlin: Springer-Verlag, 1997; 229–331.

7. Burns ER, Beland SS, Effect of biological time on the determination of the LD50 of 5-fluorouracil in mice. *Pharmacology* 1984; **28**: 296–300.

8. Zhang R, Lu Z, Liu T et al, Relationship between circadian-dependent toxicity of 5-fluorodeoxyuridine and circadian rhythms of pyrimidine enzymes: possible relevance to fluoropyrimidine chemotherapy. *Cancer Res* 1993; **53**: 2816–22.

9. Von Roemeling R, Hrushesky WJM, Determination of the therapeutic index of floxuridine by its circadian infusion pattern. *J Natl Cancer Inst* 1990; **82**: 386–93.

10. English J, Aherne GW, Marks V, The effect of timing of a single injection on the toxicity of methotrexate in the rat. *Cancer Chemother Pharmacol* 1982; **9**: 114–17.

11. Klein F, Danober L, Roulon A et al, Circadian rhythms in murine tolerance for the anticancer agent mitomycin-C (Mit-C). *Annu Rev Chronopharmacol* 1989; **5**: 367–70.

12. Sothern RB, Haus R, Langevin TR et al, Profound circadian stage dependence of mitomycin-C toxicity. *Annu Rev Chronopharmacol* 1989; **5**: 389–92.

13. Boughattas N, Levi F, Fournier C et al, Circadian rhythm in toxicities and tissue uptake of 1,2-diaminocyclohexane (*trans-l*) oxalatoplatinum(II) in mice. *Cancer Res* 1989; **49**: 3362–8.

14. Codacci-Pisanelli G, Van Der Wilt C, Pinedo H et al, Antitumor activity, toxicity and inhibition of thymidilate synthase of prolonged administration of 5-fluorouracil in mice. *Eur J Cancer* 1995; **31A**: 1517–25.

15. Boughattas NA, Hecquet H, Fournier C et al, Comparative pharmacokinetics of oxaliplatin (L-OHP) and carboplatin (CBDCA) in mice with reference to circadian dosing time. *Biopharm Drug Disp* 1994; **15**(864): 1–13.

16. Malmary-Nebot M, Labat C, Casanovas A et al, Aspect chronobiologique de l'action du methotréxate sur la dihydrofolate réductase. *Ann Pharm Fr* 1985; **43**: 337–43.

17. El Kouni MH, Naguib FNM, Park KS et al, Circadian rhythm of hepatic uridine phosphorylase activity and plasma concentration of uridine in mice. *Biochem Pharmacol* 1990; **40**: 2479–85.

18. Naguib FNM, Soong SJ, El Kouni MH, Circadian rhythm of orotate phosphoribosyltransferase, pyrimidine nucleoside phosphorylases and dihydrouracil dehydrogenase in mouse liver. *Biochem Pharmacol* 1993; **45**: 667–73.

19. Belanger PM, Labrecque G, Biological rhythms in hepatic drug metabolism and biliary systems. In: *Biologic Rhythms in Clinical and Laboratory Medicine* (Touitou Y, Haus E, eds). Berlin: Springer-Verlag, 1992; 403–9.

20. Li XM, Metzger G, Filipski E et al, Pharmacologic modulation of reduced glutathione (GSH) circadian rhythms by tuthionine sulfoximine (BSO): relationship with cisplatin (CDDP) toxicity in mice. *Toxicol Appl Pharmacol* 1997; **143**: 281–90.

21. Martineau-Pivoteau N, Cussac-Buchdahl C, Chollet P et al, Circadian variation in O6-methylguanine–DNA methyltransferase activity in mouse liver. *Anticancer Drugs* 1996; **7**: 1–7.

22. Haus E, Halberg F, Scheving L et al, Increased tolerance of leukemic mice to arabinosylcytosine with schedule-adjusted to circadian system. *Science* 1972; **177**: 80–2.

23. Scheving LE, Haus E, Kuhl JFW et al, Different laboratories closely reproduce characteristics of circadian rhythm in tolerance of mice for arabinofuranosylcytosine. *Cancer Res* 1976; **36**: 1133–7.

24. Peters GJ, Van Dijk J, Nadal JC et al, Diurnal variation in the therapeutic efficacy of 5-fluorouracil against murine colon cancer. *In Vivo* 1987; **1**: 113–18.

25. Scheving LE, Burns ER, Halberg F et al, Combined chronochemotherapy of L1210 leukemic mice using β-D-arabinofuranosylcytosine, cyclophosphamide, vincristine, methylprednisolone and *cis*-diamminedichloroplatinum. *Chronobiologia* 1980; **17**: 33–40.

26. Buchi KN, Moore JG, Hrushesky WJM et al, Circadian rhythm of cellular proliferation in the human rectal mucosa. *Gastroenterology* 1991; **101**: 410–15.

27. Killman SA, Cronkite ZEP, Fliedner TM et al, Mitotic indices of human bone marrow cells. 1. Number and cytologic distribution of mitoses. *Blood* 1962; **19**: 743–50.

28. Mauer AM, Diurnal variation of proliferative activity in the human bone marrow. *Blood* 1965; **26**: 1–7.

29. Smaaland R, Laerum OD, Lote K et al, DNA synthesis in human bone marrow is circadian stage dependent. *Blood* 1991; **77**: 2603–11.

30. Smaaland R, Laerum OD, Sothern RB et al, Colony-forming unit–granulocyte–macrophage

and DNA synthesis of human bone marrow are circadian stage-dependent and show covariation. *Blood* 1992; **79**: 2281–7.

31. Smaaland R, Abrahamsen JF, Svardal AM, DNA cell cycle distribution and glutathione (GSH) content according to circadian stage in bone marrow of cancer patients. *Br J Cancer* 1992; **66**: 39–45.

32. Brown WR, A review and mathematical analysis of circadian rhythms in cell proliferation in mouse, rat and human epidermis. *J Invest Dermatol* 1991; **97**: 273–80.

33. Warnakulasuriya KAAS, MacDonald DG, Diurnal variation in labelling index in human buccal epithelium. *Arch Oral Biol* 1993; **38**: 1107–11.

34. Smaaland R, Svardal AM, Lote K et al, Glutathione content in human bone marrow and circadian stage relation to DNA synthesis. *J Natl Cancer Inst* 1991; **83**: 1092–8.

35. Harris B, Song R, Soong S et al, Relationship between dihydropyrimidine dehydrogenase activity and plasma 5-fluorouracil levels: evidence for circadian variation of plasma drug levels in cancer patients receiving 5-fluorouracil by protracted continuous infusion. *Cancer Res* 1990; **50**: 197–201.

36. Langouet AM, Metzger G, Comisso M et al, Plasma drug concentration control through time-programmed administration. *Proc Am Assoc Cancer Res* 1996; **37**: 183 (abst 1253).

37. Klevecz R, Shymko R, Braly P, Circadian gating of S phase in human ovarian cancer. *Cancer Res* 1987; **47**: 6267–71.

38. Smaaland R, Lote K, Sothern RB et al, DNA synthesis and ploidy in non-Hodgkin's lymphomas demonstrate variation depending on circadian stage of cell sampling. *Cancer Res* 1993; **53**: 3129–38.

39. Mormont MC, Lévi F, Circadian system alterations during cancer processes: a review. *Int J Cancer* 1997; **70**: 241–7.

40. Koren G, Ferrazini G, Sohl H et al, Chronopharmacology of methotrexate pharmacokinetics in childhood leukemia. *Chronobiol Int* 1992; **9**: 434–8.

41. Nowakowska-Dulawa E, Circadian rhythm in 5-fluorouracil (FU) pharmacokinetics and tolerance. *Chronobiologia* 1990; **17**: 27–35.

42. Petit E, Milano G, Lévi F et al, Circadian varying plasma concentration of 5-FU during 5-day continuous venous infusion at constant rate in cancer patients. *Cancer Res* 1988; **48**: 1676–9.

43. Metzger G, Massari C, Etienne MC et al, Spontaneous or imposed circadian changes in plasma concentrations of 5-fluorouracil coadministered with folinic acid and oxaliplatin: relationship with mucosal toxicity in cancer patients. *Clin Pharmacol Ther* 1994; **56**: 190–201.

44. Fleming GF, Schilsky RL, Mick R et al, Circadian variation of 5-fluorouracil (5-FU) and cortisol plasma levels during continuous-infusion 5-FU and leucovorin (LV) in patients with hepatic or renal dysfunction. *Proc Am Soc Clin Oncol* 1994; **13**: 139 (abst 352).

45. Assier I, Leger-Enreille A, Bargnoux PJ et al, Relationship of dose-limiting toxicity (DLT) with plasma 5-fluorouracil (5-FU) accumulation during chronomodulated (CM) infusion of 5-FU and *l*-folinic acid (FA). *Proc Am Assoc Cancer Res* 1996; **37**: 180 (abst 1232).

46. Hryniuk WM, The importance of dose intensity in the outcome of chemotherapy. In: *Important Advances in Oncology* (De Vita VT, Holman S, Rosenberg SA, eds). Philadelphia: JB Lippincott, 1988; 121–42.

47. Lévi F, Soussan A, Adam R et al, A phase I–II trial of five-day continuous intravenous infusion of 5-fluorouracil delivered at circadian rhythm modulated rate in patients with metastatic colorectal cancer. *J Infus Chemother* 1995; **5**: 153–8.

48. Adler S, Lang S, Langenmayer I et al, Chronotherapy with 5-fluorouracil and folinic acid in advanced colorectal carcinoma. Results of a chronopharmacologic phase I trial. *Cancer* 1994; **73**: 2905–12.

49. Bjarnason GA, Kerr IG, Doyle N et al, Phase I study of 5-fluorouracil and leucovorin by a 14-day circadian infusion in metastatic adenocarcinoma patients. *Cancer Chemother Pharmacol* 1993; **33**: 221–8.

50. Garufi C, Lévi F, Aschelter AM et al, A phase I trial of five day chronomodulated infusion of 5-fluorouracil and *l*-folinic acid in patients with metastatic colorectal cancer. *Eur J Cancer* 1997; in press.

51. Lévi F, Perpoint B, Garufi C et al, Oxaliplatin activity against metastatic colorectal cancer. A Phase II study of 5-day continuous venous infusion at circadian rhythm modulated rate. *Eur J Cancer* 1993; **29**: 1280–4.

52. Machover D, Diaz-Rubio E, De Gramont A et al, Two consecutive phase II studies of oxaliplatin (L-OHP) for treatment of patients with advanced colorectal carcinoma who were resistant to previous treatment with fluoropyrimidines. *Ann Oncol* 1996; **7**: 95–8.

53. Caussanel JP, Lévi F, Brienza S et al, Phase I trial of 5-day continuous infusion of oxaliplatinum at

circadian-modulated vs constant rate. *J Natl Cancer Inst* 1990; **82**: 1046–50.

54. Mathe G, Kidani Y, Segiguchi M, Oxalato-platinum or L-OHP, a third-generation platinum complex: an experimental and clinical appraisal and preliminary comparison with *cis*-platinum and carboplatinum. *Biomed Pharmacother* 1989; **43**: 237–50.

55. Lévi F, Misset JL, Brienza S et al, A chronopharmacologic phase II clinical trial with 5-fluorouracil, folinic acid and oxaliplatin using an ambulatory multichannel programmable pump. High antitumor effectiveness against metastatic colorectal cancer. *Cancer* 1992; **69**: 893–900.

56. Lévi F, Zidani R, Vannetzel JM et al, Chronomodulated versus fixed infusion rate delivery of ambulatory chemotherapy with oxaliplatin, 5-fluorouracil and folinic acid in patients with colorectal cancer metastases. A randomized multiinstitutional trial. *J Natl Cancer Inst* 1994; **86**: 1608–17.

57. Lévi F, Zidani R, Di Palma M et al, for the International Organisation for Cancer Chronotherapy (IOCC), Improved therapeutic index through ambulatory circadian rhythmic delivery (CRD) of high dose 3-drug chemotherapy in a randomized phase III multicenter trial. *Proc Am Soc Clin Oncol* 1994; **13**: 197 (abst 574).

58. Lévi F, Zidani R, Vannetzel JM et al, Chronomodulated versus flat infusion of 5-fluorouracil (5-FU), folinic acid (FA) and oxaliplatin (L-OHP) against metastatic colorectal cancer (MCC) in 2 consecutive European randomized multicenter trials (T). *Proc Am Soc Clin Oncol* 1995; **14**: 204 (abst 493).

59. Brienza S, Lévi F, Valori V et al, Intensified (every 2 weeks) chronotherapy with 5-fluorouracil (5-FU), folinic acid (FA) and oxaliplatin (L-OHP) in previously treated patients with metastatic colorectal cancer. *Proc Am Soc Clin Oncol* 1993; **12**: 197 (abst 577).

60. Bertheault-Cvitkovic F, Jami A, Ithzaki M et al, Biweekly dose intensification of circadian chronotherapy with 5-fluorouracil, folinic acid and oxaliplatin in patients with metastatic colorectal cancer. *J Clin Oncol* 1996; **14**: 2950–8.

61. Lévi F, Dogliotti L, Perpoint B et al, A multicenter phase II trial of intensified chronotherapy with oxaliplatin (L-OHP), 5-fluorouracil (5-FU) and folinic acid (FA) in patients (pts) with previously untreated metastatic colorectal cancer (MCC). *Proc Am Soc Clin Oncol* 1997; **16**: abst 945.

62. Giacchetti S, Itzhaki M, Adam R et al, Long term survival of patients (pts) with unresectable colorectal liver metastases, following infusional chronotherapy with 5-fluorouracil (5-FU), folinic acid (FA), oxaliplatin (L-OHP) and surgery. *Ann Oncol* 1996; **7**(Suppl 5): 34 (abst 153 O).

63. Bismuth H, Adam R, Lévi F et al, Resection of nonresectable liver metastases from colorectal cancer after neoadjuvant chemotherapy. *Ann Surg* 1996; **224**: 509–22.

64. Abigerges D, Chabot GG, Armand JP et al, Phase I and pharmacologic studies of the camptothecin analog irinotecan administered every 3 weeks in cancer patients. *J Clin Oncol* 1995; **13**: 210–21.

65. Stangl R, Altendorf-Hofmann A, Charnley RM, Scheele J, Factors influencing the natural history of colorectal liver metastases. *Lancet* 1994; **343**: 1405–10.

66. Rougier Ph, Milan C, Lazorthes F et al, Prospective study of prognostic factors in patients with unresected hepatic metastases from colorectal cancer. *Br J Surg* 1995; **82**: 1397–400.

67. Lahr CJ, Soong SJ, Cloud G et al, A multifactorial analysis of prognostic factors in patients with liver metastases from colorectal carcinoma. *J Clin Oncol* 1983; **11**: 720.

68. Roemeling RV, Hrushesky WM, Circadian patterning of continuous floxuridine infusion reduces toxicity and allows higher dose intensity in patients with widespread cancer. *J Clin Oncol* 1989; **7**: 1710–19.

69. Focan C, Kreutz F, Focan-Henrard D et al, Treatment of hepatic metastases from colorectal cancer with continuous delivery of venous 5-fluorouracil (5-FU) and arterial 5-fluorodesoxyuridine (FUDR). A randomized evaluation comparing combined flat versus chronomodulated infusion. *Proc 19th ESMO Congress, Lisbon, Portugal, 18–22 November, Ann Oncol* 1994; **5** (Suppl 8): (abst 0215).

70. Chollet Ph, Cure H, Garufi C et al, Phase II trial with chronomodulated 5-fluorouracil (5-FU) and folinic acid (FA) in metastatic colorectal cancer. *Proc 6th Int Conf Chronopharm Chronother, Amelia Island, FL, 5–9 July,* 1994; abst VIIIb-4.

71. Giacchetti S, Zidani R, Perpoint B et al., Phase III trial of 5-fluorouracil (5-FU), folinic acid (FA), with or without oxaliplatin (OXA) in previously untreated patients (pts) with metastatic colorectal cancer (MCC). *Proc Am Soc Clin Oncol* 1997; **16**: abst 805.

28

Pharmacokinetic adjustment of chemotherapy

Erick Gamelin, Michele Boisdron-Celle

INTRODUCTION

After over 30 years use, recent advances in both basic and clinical research have improved the therapeutic efficacy of 5-fluorouracil (5-FU) in advanced colorectal carcinomas through biochemical modulation.[1,2] In addition, certain retrospective analyses have strongly suggested a relationship between 5-FU dose and response, and have emphasized the impact of 5-FU dose intensity on the response rate.[3–5] However, high-dose 5-FU treatment can generate severe side-effects, which are sometimes life-threatening. Leucovorin (LV), often used in 5-FU biomodulation, potentiates its efficiency, but also increases its toxicity and leads to a reduction of the maximum tolerated dose.[2]

5-Fluorouracil has a narrow therapeutic index, i.e. a small ratio of the theoretical minimum effective dose to the maximum tolerated dose. There is also a marked variability in drug handling, i.e. pharmacokinetics, between individual patients. It has been demonstrated that, for a given standard dose, systemic clearance of 5-FU exhibits wide interpatient variability, regardless of schedule.[6–10] This contributes to variability in the pharmacodynamic effects of a given dose of the drug. Consequently, some

interpatient differences, in terms of toxicity and efficacy, can be expected from this variability in systemic exposure to 5-FU. Therefore an identical dose of 5-FU given to three different patients may result in a therapeutic response with acceptable toxicity in one patient, unacceptable and possibly life-threatening toxicity in the second, and no response or toxicity in the third. The concept of dose intensity, the low response rate to 5-FU of colon cancer, the increasing risk of both hematological and extrahematological side-effects with the dose, and the wide interpatient variability of systemic clearance are strong arguments for individual 5-FU dose-monitoring. Dose adjustment with pharmacokinetic follow-up requires some conditions to be assessed for justifying its usefulness. The therapeutic index – representing the difference between the efficacy and the toxicity plasma thresholds – must be determined. The drug kinetics in plasma must permit dose adjustment.[11] Several authors have demonstrated a significant link between systemic exposure to 5-FU and the risk of developing 5-FU-related toxicities.[12,13] Individual adaptation of 5-FU dose based on pharmacokinetics has already significantly proved its clinical usefulness for reducing toxicity.[14] An even more interesting approach is to analyse the link between systemic exposure to 5-FU and treatment efficacy, even though the weak relationship between extratumoral and intratumoral drug concentrations and the need for intracellular drug activation of the prodrug 5-FU can lead to difficulties in demonstrating such a pharmacodynamic relationship.[8] So far, this relationship has been poorly studied in advanced colon cancer, whereas some results are available for head and neck tumors.[12-15]

The major pharmacokinetic parameter for quantifying systemic exposure in pharmacodynamic studies of a drug is the *area under the curve (AUC)*. This takes into account both the plasma concentration of the drug and the time of exposure to it. It is better correlated with the intensity of pharmacodynamic effects than is the absolute dose, which suffers from a combination of physiological variables and genetic characteristics that influences the outcome of the drug.[11]

The definition of the relationship between the AUC and the drug's pharmacodynamic endpoints – both toxicity and tumor response – may allow the administration of the optimum drug dosage.[16,17] The goal is to maximize the likelihood of response and simultaneously minimize the likelihood of toxicity. For some drugs, like carboplatin, the optimum dosage can be defined for an individual patient from measurable physiological variables, such as renal function. For 5-FU, the problem is more complex, and the determination of the dosage requires pharmacokinetic data obtained from an initial dose and often from subsequent doses of 5-FU in the individual patient.

In this chapter, we shall develop the concept of dose intensity of 5-FU in colorectal cancer, the analysis of the link between 5-FU exposure, and both the toxicity and the efficacy of the treatment. Then we shall describe the pharmacokinetics of 5-FU in plasma and approaches for individual dosage adjustment.

CONCEPT OF DOSE INTENSITY IN COLORECTAL CANCER

A relationship between 5-FU dose and response in metastatic colorectal cancer has been strongly suggested by retrospective analyses, but, until now, dose-limiting hematologic and mucosal toxicity hindered both the application and the development of intensive dosage strategies.[3-5,18] Hryniuk et al[3] and then Arbuck,[4] in meta-analyses, showed a clear relationship between 5-FU dose, in mg/m^2/week, and response. More recently, in a multivariate analysis of the response rates in studies dealing with patients treated with 5-FU ± LV, Brohee[2] found that the most important variables delineated were cumulative dose of 5-FU, weekly schedule and LV use. She suggested that 5-FU should be titrated to the highest tolerable doses.

RELATIONSHIP BETWEEN TOXICITY AND 5-FU PLASMA LEVELS

A close relationship has been described between exposure to 5-FU and hematological toxicity (Table 29.1). Yoshida et al[19] noted that for patients with colorectal cancer treated by continuous infusion of 5-FU, the 5-FU concentrations at the steady state and the AUC over 72 hours were higher in the group who had a toxicity than in the group with no toxicity, for the same 5-FU dosage according to body area. Au et al[20] found equivalent results with 5-day continuous infusions of 5-FU plus thymidine. A threshold of 1.5 µmol/l for 5-FU steady-state plasma concentrations was associated with a high risk of leucopenia. In addition, Trump et al[9] reported equivalent results for patients treated by 3-day continuous infusion of 5-FU, showing a close relationship between steady-state 5-FU plasma concentration and the risk of leucopenia and mucositis.

Similar relationships have been found for non-hematological toxicities (Table 28.1). In spite of quite different 5-FU schedules, the same AUC toxic threshold was found in several studies.[12-15] However, toxicity profile depends on 5-FU schedule: leucopenia is more frequent

Table 28.1 Studies of the relationships between hematological toxicity, non-hematological toxicity, response and pharmacokinetics of 5-FU in different administration schedules

Relationship between hematological toxicity and pharmacokinetic variables

Pharmacokinetic variable, threshold	Type of toxicity	Administration schedule, tumor type	Ref
$C_{ss} > 1.5$ µmol/l	Leucopenia	5-day CVI, CCR	20
C_{ss}	Leucopenia	3-day CVI, CCR	9
AUC	Leucopenia	5-day CVI, CCR	19
AUC	Leucopenia	Weekly, IVB, CCR	22
AUC > 30 mg/h per liter	Leucopenia	5-day, HNC	13

Relationship between non-hematological toxicity and pharmacokinetic variables

AUC > 30 mg/h per liter	Stomatitis, diarrhea	5-day CVI + CP, HNC	13
AUC > 30 mg/h per liter	Stomatitis, diarrhea	5-day CVI, CCR	12
AUC > 30 mg/h per liter	Stomatitis, diarrhea	5-day CVI, HNC	14
AUC	Stomatitis	Weekly, IVB, CCR	22
C_{ss}	Stomatitis	3-day CVI, CCR	9
AUC > 24 mg/h per liter	Diarrhea, hand–foot	Weekly 8-hour	21
$C_{ss} > 3000$ µg/l	syndrome	CVI + LV	

Relationship between response and pharmacokinetic variables

AUC		5-day CVI, DTC	23
AUC		Weekly IVB	24
AUC > 16 mg/h per liter ($C_{ss} > 2000$ µg/l)		Weekly 8-hour CVI	21

Abbreviations: AUC, area under the curve; C_{ss}, steady-state concentration; CVI, continuous venous infusion; IVB, i.v. bolus; CCR, colorectal cancer; HNC, head and neck cancer; DTC, digestive tract cancer.

with bolus administration,[1] mucositis and diarrhea with 5-day infusion,[12] and hand–foot syndrome and diarrhea with weekly 8- or 24-hour administration.[5,21] Thyss et al[13] have demonstrated a relationship between an elevated AUC of 5-FU over 30 mg/h per liter and the frequency of cycles with leucopenia, mucositis and diarrhea for patients with head and neck cancer, treated by chemotherapy combining cisplatin and 5-day continuous infusion of 5-FU.[13] Milano et al[15] found the same AUC threshold value for patients with metastatic colorectal cancer treated by 5-day continuous infusion of

5-FU without cisplatin. Thus cisplatin did not influence the maximum tolerated AUC of 5-FU.

We found the same relationship in a prospective clinical trial carried out in metastatic colorectal cancer.[21] Forty patients were treated with weekly high doses of 5-FU and LV. 5-Fluorouracil was administered as weekly 8-hour infusions at a starting dose of 1000 mg/m². Every 3 weeks, the dose was escalated by 250 mg/m² steps until dose-limiting toxicity was observed. A weekly pharmacokinetic follow-up of 5-FU in plasma was performed. We looked for a relationship between the individual pharmacokinetic parameters of 5-FU and both toxicity and treatment efficacy. The duration of infusion was much longer than four times the half-life of 5-FU, 15–20 minutes, i.e. the time considered as necessary to reach the steady state. Thus we could use steady-state 5-FU plasma concentrations (C_{ss}) for the pharmacodynamic study.

5-FU plasma concentrations varied widely between patients for each dose step. Thus the same dose administered after adjustment for body surface led to very variable therapeutic intensities. This had important consequences for the 5-FU maximum tolerated dose, which varied from 900 to 6000 mg/week. There was a close link between the acute toxicity and the steady-state 5-FU plasma levels. Over 3000 µg/l, diarrhea or a hand–foot syndrome appeared, the grade of toxicity being linked with the levels in plasma. The toxicity was not related to the dose of 5-FU calculated with body area. It is important to note that three patients who had previously undergone pelvic radiotherapy for rectal tumor had diarrhea with 5-FU levels lower than 3000 µg/l. Thus previous irradiation of the pelvis needs to be taken into account in this pharmacodynamic study.

The 5-FU toxic plasma threshold of 3000 µg/l corresponded to a value of AUC over 24 mg/h per liter, which was very close to the above-mentioned results (30 mg/h per liter), in spite of a very different administration schedule.[12–14] The slightly lower value of AUC that we found in our regimen (24 versus 30) could be explained by the addition of LV, which is known to potentiate 5-FU toxicity.

Van Groeningen et al[22] described mathematically the relationship between toxicity and plasma levels, with a 5-FU bolus schedule. The use of a logistic regression method showed that clinical toxicity was correlated with the AUC.

RELATIONSHIP BETWEEN TUMOR RESPONSE AND 5-FU PLASMA LEVELS

The next step for defining a therapeutic index is the determination of the therapeutic threshold. However, the relationship between 5-FU pharmacokinetics and treatment response has been less extensively explored than toxicity. Other mechanisms, such as intrinsic cellular resistance and tumor kinetics can be involved in treatment failure. Hillcoat et al[23] were the first to show that for patients with digestive tract cancer and treated by 5-day continuous infusion of 5-FU, AUC values were significantly higher when objective response or stabilization were observed. Seitz et al[24] reported equivalent results later with 5-FU bolus in colorectal cancer.

In the above-mentioned phase I study that we carried out for 40 patients treated for advanced colorectal cancer, a close link has been found between 5-FU concentrations in plasma and therapeutic outcome.[21] The patients who had plasma levels over the mean levels of the overall population had better chances of an objective response than patients who had lower levels (14/17 versus 3/21) ($p < 0.01$). On the other hand, patients who experienced an objective response had significantly higher levels, whatever the dose, than patients who failed to respond. Notably, they rapidly reached levels of 2000 µg/l with dose escalation; consequently, they were soon in a narrow range, close to the toxic levels. In contrast, patients whose treatment failed had very low initial concentrations, which increased more slowly with the dose. They later reached equivalent levels, with a higher dose. Our hypothesis was that for patients whose 5-FU clearance was elevated, the dose of 5-FU was initially too low and the patients had insufficient doses of 5-FU for the major part of the treatment. This result can explain some primary treatment failures, which would not be due to a real tumor cell resistance but to an insufficient dose of 5-FU. We studied the survival according to 5-FU plasma levels. The overall survival at one year and later was better for patients who had plasma levels over the mean concentrations, but the difference was not significant ($p < 0.2$). The lack of statistical difference may be due in part to the small number of patients.

5-FU METABOLISM

These results indicate the problem of the genetic polymorphism of 5-FU metabolism.[25,26] 5-Fluorouracil is metabolized to dihydrofluorouracil by dihydropyrimidine dehydrogenase (DPD), the key enzyme of pyrimidine catabolism, which is widespread in the organism, mainly in liver, lung, kidney and lymphocytes. A few cases of patients with a complete deficiency in DPD activity have been reported.[27] Extremely high and prolonged levels of 5-FU were measured after a low dose of 5-FU, and the subsequent toxicity was severe, sometimes fatal. The consequences are multiple.

Firstly, there is a wide polymorphism of 5-FU metabolism. A large range of degrees of DPD activity, with a Gaussian distribution, has been shown among a large population of patients.[26,27] Some patients had very low DPD activity. In a population of 185 unselected cancer patients, DPD activity was on average 15% lower in women than in men.[28] Age did not modify 5-FU clearance. On the other side of the Gaussian distribution, some patients had a high DPD activity. These patients are potentially underdosed with standard doses in conventional regimens.

Secondly, the polymorphism of 5-FU metabolism and the link between 5-FU plasma levels and both toxicity and response to treatment again beg the question of the individual adjustment of the 5-FU dose. The method of the test dose appears difficult to put into practice, since the plasma kinetics of 5-FU are complex. Pretreatment DPD activity determination by a radioenzymatic technique would be an elegant solution. A relationship between DPD activity in lymphocytes and 5-FU plasma levels has been reported in certain studies.[26,29] Fleming et al[29] found a significant linear correlation between DPD activity in peripheral blood mononuclear cells (PBMC) and 5-FU plasma clearance. Thus this method seems to be of great interest for the detection of DPD deficiency. However, it remains insufficient for the prediction of 5-FU plasma concentrations in practice, since the correlation coefficient between PBMC DPD activity and 5-FU plasma

clearance is only 0.31. Other sites of catabolism are involved, and modifications of 5-FU metabolism can occur throughout a prolonged treatment. Moreover, a circadian variation of DPD activity has been shown,[30] and the rhythm presents an interindividual variability. It must be also kept in mind that the degree of DPD activity in tumor cell lines plays a major role in resistance to 5-FU.[31] Thus the determination of DPD activity cannot be a useful indicator for improving 5-FU dose adaptation strategy.[29,30] Individual dose adjustment with a pharmacokinetic follow-up appears to be actually more interesting and practicable.

INDIVIDUAL 5-FU DOSE ADJUSTMENT

The last step for individual dose adjustment in practice is to show that it is possible to predict what the blood concentration of 5-FU will be for a given dose administered. 5-Fluorouracil is primarily eliminated by a dihydrogenation process, depending on DPD activity, which is genetically determined and saturable.[10,32] The first metabolite, dihydrofluorouracil, has no activity. In parallel, 5-FU undergoes a metabolic activation in the cell and is transformed into 5-FdUMP and FUTP. These anabolites are in the cell, and seem to be less interesting in pharmacodynamic studies.

The pharmacokinetics of 5-FU have been extensively studied.[10,32] It quickly disappears from plasma, and its half-life is 10–20 minutes. Its total body clearance varies according to the administration schedule. From 0.5 to 1.5 l/min with i.v. bolus, it reaches 5–58 l/min with continuous infusion.[6,10,22,32] The elevated plasma clearance of 5-FU with continuous infusion is due to the addition of other sites of catabolism to the liver, such as lung and kidney. This explains why continuous infusion makes it possible to administer higher doses of 5-FU than bolus schedules, and implies that it is not possible to compare dose intensities in continuous and bolus administrations. With bolus schedules, the clearance is lower than the hepatic blood flow, owing to a saturable metabolic process that leads to a nonlinear relationship between the 5-FU dose and its plasma levels. In practice, relatively low dose increments are followed by disproportionate and variable increases of 5-FU plasma levels. Van Groeningen et al[22] showed a decrease in plasma clearance with increasing 5-FU dose in bolus administration. 5-FU plasma concentrations rose much more steeply than expected under linear pharmacokinetics after a 20% increase in dose. Thus, with 5-FU bolus, it appears impossible to predict 5-FU plasma levels for a given dose.

In contrast, the predictability of 5-FU concentrations is possible with infusions. Continuous-infusion chemotherapy is an excellent model for the study of anticancer drug pharmacodynamics, especially if the duration of the infusion is long enough to approximate a steady-state plasma concentration (C_{ss}). The C_{ss} can then be used for pharmacodynamic modelling, rather than the AUC, because it is simpler. Furthermore, if the drug has linear pharmacokinetics then AUC = C_{ss} × infusion duration, and thus pharmacodynamic models for C_{ss} and AUC are potentially interchangeable. Spicer et al[18] found a linear correlation between the dose of 5-FU and the plasma concentration at the steady state for patients treated by very prolonged continuous infusion of 300–500 mg/m^2 5-FU. Erlichman et al,[32] Milano et al[12] and Thyss et al[13] made similar observations with 5-day continuous infusion schedules at 1.25–2.25 g/m^2/day, and concluded that under these conditions, 5-FU concentrations proportionally followed 5-FU dose modifications.[12,13,32] They found that 5-FU clearance was globally constant at around 2 liters/min per m^2.

We found equivalent results with weekly 8-hour infusions, namely a simple relation between plasma levels and 5-FU dose. We established a simple dose adjustment table, to reach within 3 weekly cycles the optimal therapeutic range we have determined. The predictability of 5-FU concentrations was reliable and very efficient. Actually, since we wanted to test the dose-intensity concept, we administered very high 5-FU doses, and we observed that 5-FU plasma clearance diminished progressively with the dose and slumped when plasma levels were close to the toxic levels. The linear

relationship between blood levels and dose disappeared when the 5-FU plasma levels were getting near 3000 µg/l.[21] The metabolic process was saturated, and a low dose increase led to important rise of plasma levels. This loss of linearity was taken into account in the table for 5-FU dose adjustments. The follow-up of the plasma concentrations had to be very careful in that high range of 5-FU plasma levels.

RESULTS OF 5-FU DOSE ADJUSTMENT

Dose adjustment has been poorly investigated in advanced colorectal cancer, though the concept of dose intensity has been reported and 5-FU kinetics permits a dose predictability. Some studies have been carried out on head and neck tumors. Certain authors attempted to adjust 5-FU dose individually, principally for reducing the incidence of toxicity.[14] They controlled AUC in the middle of a 5-day infusion, and then adjusted the dose of 5-FU with a nomogram to maintain the total AUC below the toxic value. This approach permitted a significant decrease in toxicity when compared with a historical group treated with a constant dose of 5-FU. More recently, in a randomized study comparing monitoring to a standard dose of 5-FU in a 5-day continuous infusion, combined with cisplatin, it was shown that pharmacologically guided dosing was feasible and provided an improved hematological tolerance.[33] We must emphasize that these trials attempted first to decrease the toxicity. Their purpose was not an intensification.

Since we found from our experience in colorectal cancer that a large proportion of patients had insufficient doses of 5-FU and that this could be responsible for treatment failure, we looked for an intensification with control of the risk of toxicity by individual dose adjustment. We carried out a large prospective multicentric phase II study to prove the interest of this approach in terms of efficacy, tolerance and survival.[34] We adapted the 5-FU dose weekly from one administration to the next, according to steady-state 5-FU plasma concentrations. We used the dose-adjustment table previously established for reaching the optimal therapeutic range we have determined.[21] The trial, carried out on 130 patients, with a median follow-up of 3 years, confirmed the results of our previous study, and proved that this kind of treatment could be performed in clinical routine. Fifty-six percent objective responses (17% complete responses) were observed. These results were higher than, or at least equivalent to, those previously reported with weekly high doses of 5-FU in much more toxic schedules.[5,35,36] The median duration of complete or partial response was 16 months. The incidence of toxicity was inferior to 5% of all the courses (mean duration of treatment 1 year), and the toxicity was mild (≤grade II); none of the toxic events was life-threatening or led to total interruption of the treatment. The weekly 5-FU doses we reached with this pharmacokinetic follow-up (3000 mg total dose) were higher than those usually administered with a conventional regimen (Figure 28.1). They were a little lower than those reported by Ardalan et al[5] in a 24-hour weekly regimen. However, they reported a very high incidence of toxicity, which required a treatment interruption every 6 weeks. In contrast, we treated patients every week, with no interruption. Overall and event-free survival rates were 68% and 46.6% at one year and 38% and 17.5% at 2 years respectively. The median survival was 16 months.

We found a wide variability in 5-FU metabo-

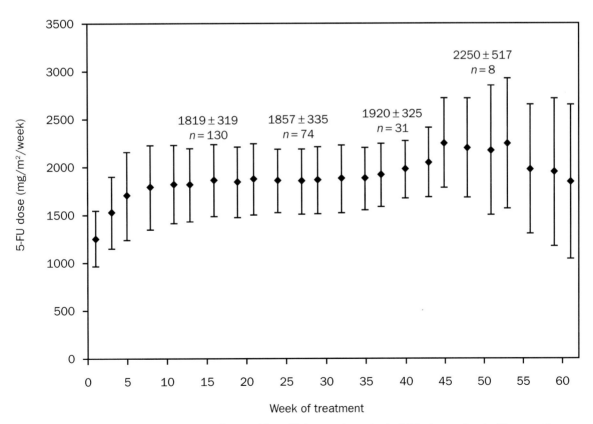

Figure 28.1 Mean optimum 5-FU doses for reaching efficient and non-toxic 5-FU plasma levels (therapeutic index); vertical lines show standard deviation.

lism, and the 5-FU optimal dose differed greatly within the population of patients for identical therapeutic plasma range. The mean optimal total dose was 3000 mg/week at the beginning of the treatment (range 900 and 4000 mg/week) (Figure 28.1). Five patients were in the toxic zone with the first dose. This required a marked reduction of the dose: down to 900 mg. With no dose adjustment, these patients, who presented a DPD deficiency, would have been at high risk of toxicity with a conventional regimen.

The dose necessary for optimal plasma levels changed throughout the treatment for some patients. The optimal dose increased to 3500 mg/week after 6 months of treatment, higher than after 3 months, and the range was between 1300 and 7000 mg. An induction of 5-FU metabolism could be hypothesized.

CONCLUSIONS

The ultimate goal of pharmacokinetic and pharmacodynamic studies is to optimize the therapeutic index of cytotoxic agents that exhibit substantial pharmacokinetic variability and have a narrow therapeutic index, such as 5-FU. A therapeutic drug monitoring would be of value in maintaining a precise level of systemic exposure, while avoiding overtreatment.

The challenge in practice now is to manage 5-FU continuous infusion to optimize therapy on an individual basis. So far, 5-FU dose adaptation based on pharmacokinetics has been mainly focused on controlling 5-FU-related toxicity. However, a clear relationship has been shown between 5-FU plasma levels and response. The therapeutic index, close to the maximum-tolerated AUC, should be reached to improve response rate and, it is hoped, survival. Individual dose adjustment can help to intensify the treatment and improve the outcome, and a pharmacokinetic follow-up with plasma measurement appears to be the best method. It helps to detect DPD deficiencies and prevent toxicity. On the other hand, it permits an increased 5-FU dose for patients with high levels of DPD activity that can lead to underdosage. It enables therapeutic 5-FU plasma levels to be reached much more quickly and safely than a clinical dose adjustment; it enables the 5-FU dose to be adapted throughout prolonged treatments, and could help to prolong remission durations. Its impact on overall and disease-free survival remains to be proven. Controlled randomized trials are in progress to assess its reliability. Once developed and validated, these approaches of individual dosage adjustment will have to be easily accessible to busy practising clinicians. Simple formulas have already been developed. With such a goal in mind, the benefit of pharmacodynamic research will reach the level of common practice.

REFERENCES

1. Machover D, Goldschmidt E, Chollet P, Treatment of advanced colorectal and gastric adenocarcinoma with 5-fluorouracil and high dose folinic acid. *J Clin Oncol* 1986; **4:** 685–96.
2. Brohee D, 5-Fluorouracil with or without folinic acid in human colorectal cancer? Multivariate meta-analysis of the literature. *Med Oncol Tumor Pharmacother* 1991; **8:** 271–80.
3. Hryniuk WM, Figueredo A, Goodyear M, Applications of dose intensity to problems in chemotherapy of breast and colorectal cancer. *Semin Oncol* 1987; **14:** 3–11.
4. Arbuck SG, Overview of clinical trials using 5-fluorouracil and leucovorin for the treatment of colorectal cancer. *Cancer* 1989; **63:** 1036–44.
5. Ardalan B, Chua L, Tian E et al, A phase II study of weekly 24 hour infusion with high dose fluorouracil with leucovorin in colorectal carcinoma. *J Clin Oncol* 1991; **9:** 625–30.
6. Hull WE, Port RE, Herrmann R et al, Metabolites

of 5-fluorouracil in plasma and urine, as monitored by ^{19}F nuclear magnetic resonance spectroscopy, for patients receiving chemotherapy with or without methotrexate pretreatment. *Cancer Res* 1988; **48**: 1680–8.

7. McDermott BJ, Van den Berg HW, Murphy RF, Non linear pharmacokinetics for the elimination of 5-fluorouracil after intravenous administration in cancer patients. *Cancer Chemother Pharmacol* 1982; **9**: 173–8.

8. Pinedo HM, Peters GFJ, Fluorouracil: biochemistry and pharmacology. *J Clin Oncol* 1988; **6**: 1653–64.

9. Trump DL, Egorin MJ, Forrest A et al, Pharmacokinetic and pharmacodynamic analysis of fluorouracil during 72-hour continuous infusion with and without dipyridamole. *J Clin Oncol* 1991; **9**: 2027–35.

10. Wagner JG, Gyves JW, Stetson PL et al, Steady state non linear pharmacokinetics of 5-fluorouracil during hepatic arterial and intravenous infusions in cancer patients. *Cancer Res* 1986; **46**: 1499–506.

11. Ratain MJ, Schilsky RLR, Conley BA et al, Pharmacodynamics in cancer therapy. *J Clin Oncol* 1990; **8**: 1739–53.

12. Milano G, Roman P, Khater P et al, Dose versus pharmacokinetics for predicting tolerance to 5-day continuous infusion of 5-FU. *Int J Cancer* 1988; **41**: 537–41.

13. Thyss A, Milano G, Renee et al, Clinical pharmacokinetic study of 5-FU in continuous 5-day infusions for head and neck cancer. *Cancer Chemother Pharmacol* 1986; **16**: 64–6.

14. Santini J, Milano G, Thyss A et al, 5-FU therapeutic monitoring with dose adjustment leads to an improved therapeutic index in head and neck cancer. *Br J Cancer* 1989; **59**: 287–90.

15. Milano G, Etienne MC, Renee N et al, Relationship between fluorouracil systemic exposure and tumor response and patient survival. *J Clin Oncol* 1994; **12**: 291–5.

16. Jusko WJ, A pharmacodynamic model for cell-cycle-specific chemotherapeutic agents. *J Pharmacokinetics Biopharmacol* 1973; **1**: 175–200.

17. Sheiner LB, Population pharmacokinetics/pharmacodynamics. *Annu Rev Pharmacol Toxicol* 1993; **32**: 185–200.

18. Spicer DV, Ardalen B, Daniels JR et al, Reevaluation of the maximum tolerated dose of continuous venous infusion of 5-fluorouracil with pharmacokinetics. *Cancer Res* 1988; **48**: 459–61.

19. Yoshida T, Araki E, Ligo M et al, Clinical significance of monitoring serum levels of 5-fluorouracil by continuous infusion in patients with advanced colonic cancer. *Cancer Chemother Pharmacol* 1990; **26**: 352–4.

20. Au JLS, Rustum YM, Lederma EJ et al, Clinical pharmacological studies of concurrent infusion of 5-fluorouracil and thymidine in the treatment of colorectal carcinoma. *Cancer Res* 1982; **42**: 2903–37.

21. Gamelin EC, Danquechin-Dorval EM, Dumesnil et al, Relationship between 5-fluorouracil dose-intensity and therapeutic response in patients with advanced colorectal cancer receiving 5-FU containing infusional therapy. *Cancer* 1996; **77**: 441–51.

22. Van Groeningen CJ, Pinedo HM, Heddes J et al, Pharmacokinetics of 5-fluorouracil assessed with a sensitive mass spectrometric method in patients on a dose escalation schedule. *Cancer Res* 1988; **48**: 6956–61.

23. Hillcoat BL, McCulloch PB, Figueredo AT et al, Clinical response and plasma levels of 5-fluorouracil in patients with colonic cancer treated by drug infusion. *Br J Cancer* 1978; **38**: 719–24.

24. Seitz JF, Cano JP, Rigault JP et al, Chimiothérapie des cancers digestifs étendus par le 5-fluorouracile: relations entre la réponse clinique et la clairance plasmatique du médicament. *Gastroentérol Clin Biol* 1989; **7**: 374–80.

25. Etienne MC, Lagrange JL, Dassonville O et al, Population study of dihydropyrimidine dehydrogenase in cancer patients. *J Clin Oncol* 1994; **12**: 2248–53.

26. Lu Z, Zhang R, Diasio RB, Dihydropyrimidine dehydrogenase activity in human peripheral blood mononuclear cells and liver: population characteristics, newly identified deficient patients, and clinical implication in 5-fluorouracil chemotherapy. *Cancer Res* 1993; **53**: 5433–8.

27. Harris BE, Carpenter JT, Diasio RB, Severe 5-fluorouracil toxicity secondary to dihydropyrimidine dehydrogenase deficiency: a potentially more common pharmacogenetic syndrome. *Cancer* 1991; **68**: 499–501.

28. Milano G, Etienne MC, Cassuto-Viguier E et al, Influence of sex and age on fluorouracile clearance. *J Clin Oncol* 1992; **10**: 1171–5.

29. Fleming R, Milano G, Thyss A et al, Correlation between dihydropyrimidine dehydrogenase activity in peripheral mononuclear cells and systemic clearance of fluorouracil in cancer patients. *Cancer Res* 1992; **52**: 2899–902.

30. Harris BE, Song R, Soong SJ, Diasio RB, Relationship between dihydropyrimidine dehydrogenase activity and plasma 5-fluorouracil levels with evidence for circadian variation of enzyme activity and plasma drug levels in cancer patients receiving 5-fluorouracil by protracted continuous infusion. *Cancer Res* 1990; **50:** 197–201.

31. Etienne MC, Cheradame S, Fischel JL et al, Response to fluorouracil therapy in cancer patients: the role of tumoral dihydropyrimidine dehydrogenase activity. *J Clin Oncol* 1995; **13:** 1663–70.

32. Erlichman C, Fine S, Elhakim T, Plasma pharmacokinetics of 5FU given by continuous infusion with allopurinol. *Cancer Treat Rep* 1986; **70:** 903–4.

33. Fety R, Rolland F, Barberi-Heyob M et al, Clinical randomized study of 5-FU monitoring versus standard dose in patients with head and neck cancer: preliminary results. *Anticancer Res* 1994; **14:** 2347–52.

34. Gamelin E, Maillart P, Dumesnil Y et al, Intensified chemotherapy of metastatic colorectal cancer with individual adaptation of 5-FU dose. Results of a 2 year multicentric prospective study. *Proc Am Assoc Cancer Res* 1994; **35:** 2448.

35. Diaz-Rubio E, Aranda E, Martin M et al, Weekly high dose infusion of 5-fluorouracil in advanced colorectal cancer. *Eur J Cancer* 1990; **26:** 727–9.

36. Wils JA, High dose fluorouracil: a new perspective in the treatment of colorectal cancer? *Semin Oncol* 1992; **19**(Suppl 3): 126–30.

29

Intrahepatic (locoregional) chemotherapy for liver metastases from colorectal cancer

Philippe Rougier, Michel Ducreux

CONTENTS • **Introduction** • **Rationale for intra-arterial hepatic chemotherapy** • **Results of IAHC** • **Drawbacks of IAHC** • **Other locoregional therapy** • **Conclusions and indications**

INTRODUCTION

Liver metastases are frequent in colorectal cancer, and are the cause of death in about 20% of cases. They are confined to the liver in about 10–20%, and are operable in approximately half these cases. When they are not operable, liver metastases of colorectal cancer (LMCRC) have a poor prognosis, even when restricted to the liver: the one-year survival ranges from 13% for patients with performance status (PS) > 0 and elevated alkaline phosphatase (AP) to 47% if PS is 0 and AP normal.[1] Locoregional therapy, especially intra-arterial hepatic chemotherapy (IAHC), was developed 15 years ago, when no efficient systemic chemotherapy was available. Since then, the efficacy of IAHC has been demonstrated in many trials,[2–7] but its value compared with modern systemic chemotherapy has never been well established,[8–11] nor has that of combining IAHC and systemic chemotherapy. This chapter emphasizes the place of IAHC and other locoregional therapy in the management of LMCRC.

RATIONALE FOR INTRA-ARTERIAL HEPATIC CHEMOTHERAPY

IAHC is a logical approach for two main reasons:

(1) most liver metastases are irrigated by the hepatic arterial blood flow;[12]
(2) the healthy liver's high extraction rate of drugs infused via the hepatic arterial route decreases their systemic concentration.[13]

These two properties result in an increase in drug concentration at the tumor level. The concentration of fluoropyrimidines in the liver and the metastases is higher with 5-fluoro-2′-deoxyuridine (FUDR), which has a very high hepatic clearance, than with 5-FU,[14] and is higher after hepatic arterial infusion than after portal infusion.

RESULTS OF IAHC

Phase II trials of IAHC initially used 5-FU, with an exteriorized catheter and an external electric pump. They gave interesting results, with a 30–80% response rate, but complications were common. Subsequently, the development of totally implantable pumps using FUDR, requiring an external refill only every 2 weeks, made IAHC more feasible. This system gave encouraging results in many phase II trials, with a response rate between 30% and 60%, which prompted the initiation of randomized trials.

Phase III trials have been performed using an implanted pump (Infusaid 400) for the intra-arterial administration of FUDR (between 0.2 and 0.3 mg/kg/d for 14d q 28d). Six randomized trials compared IAHC using this technique against a control arm without IAHC.[2-7] In three of these trials, IV FUDR via the same type of implanted pump was the treatment chosen for the control group.[3-5] In another trial the monthly schedule of IV bolus 5-FU administered on 5 consecutive days was the treatment of the control groups,[6] and in the last two trials IAHC was tested against ad libitum treatment (symptomatic or IV 5-FU).[2,7]

Results in terms of response rate and survival are reported in Table 29.1.

In the four trials comparing IA with IV FUDR or IV 5-FU, there was a two- to threefold increase in response rate, which was highly significant in all trials (Table 29.1). This has been fully confirmed in a meta-analysis by the Meta-Analysis Group in Cancer, which reports a response rate of 41% (CR 3%, PR 38%) for the patients receiving IA treatment versus 14% (CR 2%, PR 12%) for the patients receiving IV chemotherapy ($p < 0.0001$).[15]

Results for survival are more difficult to interpret. In four trials comparing IA with IV chemotherapy there was no significant increase in survival; but in two of these trials the number of entered patients and the number of eligible patients were so small that these studies lack power.[3,6] In two other trials[4,5] it was possible for the patients allocated to the IV group to

Table 29.1 Results of randomized trials comparing intra-arterial hepatic chemotherapy with other, non-intra-arterial, treatments

Study	No. of patients (eligible)	IAHC	IV	Response rate	Survival IA/IV (months)
Kemeny (1987)[5]	163 (99)	FUDR	FUDR	53%/21%[a]	17/12 NS[b]
Hohn (1988)[4]	43 (117)	FUDR	FUDR	42%/10%[a]	17/16 NS[b]
Chang (1987)[3]	64 (50)	FUDR	FUDR	62%/17%[a]	NS
Martin (1990)[6]	69	FUDR	5-FU	48%/21%[a]	12.6/10.5 NS
Rougier (1992)[7]	166 (163)	FUDR	(5-FU) ad libitum	49%/13%[a]	15/11 $p = 0.02$
Allen-Mersh (1994)[2]	100	FUDR	ad libitum	—	13/7.5 $p = 0.03$
Meta-analysis (1996)[15]	654	FUDR	FUDR or 5-FU or 0	41%/14% $p < 10^{-10}$	AHC > control $p = 0.0009$

[a] $p < 0.05$.
[b] Crossover.

crossover and to receive IAHC in the case of tumor progression in the liver: this occurred in 31% and 60% of the cases, preventing survival comparisons between the IAHC group and the control group. In contrast, the two European trials[2,7] specifically addressed the survival issue compared with symptomatic treatment or IV bolus 5-FU, which was the standard chemotherapy 10 years ago, as endpoint. These two studies entered a larger number of patients (166 and 100), and demonstrated that IAHC significantly improved the overall survival ($p = 0.02$ and $p = 0.03$ respectively) and improved the survival without progression (Table 29.1).

Thus these studies have clearly established that IAHC is an effective treatment that prolongs overall survival compared with symptomatic treatment or bolus 5-FU. Indeed, the relative value of IAHC compared with the more recent and efficient systemic chemotherapies (i.e. combinations of 5-FU and leucovorin and/or methotrexate, or high-dose 5-FU in weekly or biweekly 24–48-hour infusions, etc.) is still unknown.

In these trials many factors influenced the survival. We conducted a prognostic-factor analysis using the Cox model for multivariate analysis (Table 29.2), and demonstrated that the survival rate was significantly influenced by two main factors: (i) the degree of hepatic involvement by the tumor (worse if it was greater than 50%), and (ii) the level of CEA (worse if it was greater than 100 ng/ml).[16] Technical expertise is also an important factor influencing the results. In the French trial the survival was significantly better for patients treated in centers that had included more than 10 patients.[7]

Thus these results demonstrate that IAHC is an effective treatment, especially for well-selected patients, but this method has some drawbacks that must be investigated and debated. These problems are presently the subject of ongoing trials aiming to improve IAHC results.

DRAWBACKS OF IAHC

Toxicity

Tolerance has long been a limiting factor for IAHC. It generally takes the form of hepatic, digestive and systemic toxicity.

Table 29.2 Prognostic-factor analysis for patients treated by IAHC: results of an analysis performed on 148 patients treated at IGR (1984–92)

Variable	Median survival (months)	p
Hepatomegaly	24/12	<0.00001
Replacement < 50%	21/11	<0.00001[a]
CEA < 100 ng/ml	25/12	<0.0001[a]
Alkaline phosphatase < 200 U/ml	23/14	<0.0001
Adequate arterial perfusion	25/15	0.006

- 20% of patients with good prognostic factors are alive at 3 years.
- Treatment protocols (5-FU, FUDR, THP adriamycin and MMC) did not influence survival (NS).

[a] This factor was significantly predictive of a good prognostic when using the Cox model.

Hepatic and biliary toxicity is clearly dependent on the drug and its administration schedule. It occurs with FUDR continuous administration over a 14-day period every 28 days via implanted pumps, and seems to be cumulative. Its frequency increases with the duration of IAHC. For instance, in the French randomized trial, chemical hepatitis was noted in about 35% of cases at one year and sclerosing cholangitis in about 25%.[7] This toxicity is probably due to a direct and toxic effect of the continuous FUDR infusion in the biliary arteries inducing a chemical arteriolitis in these small terminal vessels. Many efforts have been made to reduce this toxicity. For instance, careful biological follow-up with IAHC interruption if alkaline phosphatase increases, or addition of dexamethasone[17] and/or shortening of the IA perfusion from 14 to 7 days every 28 days,[10] have resulted in a significant decrease in the rate of sclerosing cholangitis. In contrast, IAHC using short 5-FU infusions has no (or a very low rate of) hepatic toxicity,[16] and other drugs like mitomycin C and TEP-rubicin, used in short infusions, seem to have no hepatic toxicity.[18]

Gastrointestinal toxicity has been reported in 20–40% of cases. These are mainly gastroduodenal inflammation or ulceration, and may occasionally lead to duodenal perforation. This digestive toxicity is mainly due to extrahepatic perfusion, especially through unligated pyloric arteries, and can be partly prevented by a careful dissection of the first part of the common hepatic artery at the time of the catheter placement.[19]

Arterial and/or catheter thrombosis occurs in IAHC when subcutaneous access and discontinuous arterial perfusions are used. It is clearly related to the team's experience, and in our practice the median lifespan of a functional catheter has increased from 6.5 months 5 years ago[15] to 12 months most recently.[20]

Extrahepatic progression

In all the phase II and III trials, this is reported to occur in about 50% of patients when hepatic metastases are controlled by IAHC. Many authors have noticed the unusual location of some extrahepatic metastases (e.g. the brain or the adrenal gland). This suggests a possibility for the combination of intra-arterial and intravenous chemotherapies. At present there has been only one randomized trial that compared IAHC alone with IAHC plus IV 5-FU. It demonstrated an advantage in terms of survival without progression.[21] However, other trials using a more active systemic regimen are clearly necessary.

Technical expertise

When possible, surgical placement of the catheter seems preferable to catheterization under radiological control, because it allows a careful dissection of the gastroduodenal artery and common hepatic artery, a cholecystectomy, a ligation of the distal gastroduodenal artery, a direct verification of the perfusion quality, and if necessary the ligation of abnormal hepatic arteries.[22] In our experience, it seems that the quality of perfusion and the rate of digestive complications and probably of catheter thrombosis are dependent on the quality of surgical catheterization. In the French randomized trial the experience of participating centers (separated into those including more than 10 patients, and the others) influenced significantly (and independently of other prognostic factors) the overall survival.[7] It is also interesting to note that in the UK study 90% of the catheters were placed by the same surgeon, and no failures of catheterization were reported,[2] compared with 11% in our multicentric study, in which 17 centers were involved.[7] This is consistent with the results reported by Campbell on 70 patients: 37% technical complication rate for inexperienced versus 7% for experienced surgeons. If we consider patients with a standard anatomy, the difference is greater: 42% for inexperienced surgeons and 0% technical complications for experienced surgeons.[23]

Cost

The cost of IAHC is high when we consider the cost of equipment, especially for implantable pumps, and the cost of the surgical implantation of the pump and the catheter. However, the cost of hospitalization must also be considered. In fact, when we compared patients treated with the implanted pump with classical IV chemotherapies administered weekly or 5 times per month, the cost was equivalent after 6 months of treatment without complications, because, with implanted pumps, patients needed only two outpatient visits per month.[10] Thus IAHC appears affordable when performed by an experienced team in patients with favorable prognostic factors.

PROSPECTS FOR IAHC

New drugs and new protocols

Most previous studies used fluoropyrimidines that have favorable pharmacokinetic properties. Other products, such as mitomycin C (MMC) and cisplatin, also have a favorable pharmacokinetic profile, and some studies have reported almost 30% response rates using monthly IA injection of MMC after failure of IAHC using FUDR.

Recently we reported the pharmacokinetic and experimental interest of THP–adriamycin (Teprubicin, Bellon Oncologie Laboratory, Neuilly S/S, France), which is an anthracycline. Its intra-arterial hepatic administration in a rabbit model bearing VX2 tumors implanted in the liver resulted in a 20-fold increase in intratumoral concentration of the drug compared with its intravenous administration. After these preclinical studies, a phase I study was conducted in patients with LMCRC, and demonstrated that this product was well tolerated by the liver and has a hematological limiting toxicity. The recommended dose for IA administration was 75 mg/m² in 30-minute IAH infusion every 3 weeks.[18] Thirdly, a phase II trial was conducted in patients with LMCRC, and a 30% response rate was observed – which was outstanding considering the classical and well-established resistance of CRC to anthracyclines. This high response probably reflects the very high intra-

cellular concentration, which perhaps has overcome MDR-related resistance.

Another approach is that of IAHC polychemotherapy. Kemeny has reported interesting results using the FUDR + leucovorin combination, but with a high toxicity rate. She has also reported, in a randomized trial conducted in pretreated patients,[24] the superiority of IAHC using the FUDR + MMC + BCNU combination over the use of FUDR alone in terms of response rate (47% versus 25%) and survival (median 19 months versus 14).

Combination of IAHC with effective systemic chemotherapy

As IAHC using fluoropyrimidines has very little systemic toxicity, and IV chemotherapy has demonstrated its efficacy in patients suffering from colorectal cancer metastases, the combined approach was logical and is presently being explored. Safi et al[21] have reported a significant increase in survival without progression, combining IA FUDR and IV 5-FU. We have reported a phase II study exploring the combination of IA THP–adriamycin and IV 5-FU + leucovorin with good results.[25] We have also studied the efficacy and tolerance of the combination of IA MMC and IV 5-FU + leucovorin IV,[26] and also of IA continuous infusion of high-dose 5-FU for 4 days combined with IV 5-FU + leucovorin.[20] Recently Kemeny has reported interesting results combining intra-arterial FUDR and IV 5-FU + leucovorin.[27] These combinations of IAH and IV chemotherapy are well tolerated and effective in our experience,[20,26] but it is too early to know their impact on survival, and so extrahepatic progression must be investigated further in randomized trials.

OTHER LOCOREGIONAL THERAPY

Intraportal chemotherapy (IPC)

The portal blood flow irrigates most of the healthy liver, but also any small liver metastases from CRC. This is because cancer cells reach the liver via the portal system. However, once they attain a diameter of 1 mm, these metastases are mainly irrigated by the hepatic arteries, and the portal blood is only involved in vascularization of their peripheral rim. IPC has been tested in two studies: a first randomized trial, comparing IPC chemotherapy and hepatic-artery ligation with hepatic-artery ligation alone, was conducted by Gerard et al,[28] and no difference in overall or survival without progression was demonstrated. A second study using a similar protocol compared with no treatment reported a significant increase in survival.[29] This technique seems more suitable as an adjuvant treatment in colorectal cancer after complete surgery. In this indication, it does decrease the relative risk of mortality by about 13%, as reported in a recent meta-analysis.[30] In some studies, it has decreased the rate of liver metastasis.

Chemoembolization

The combination of intra-arterial chemotherapy with hepatic arterial embolization seems interesting in the case of hypervascularized metastases, approximately 30% of LMCRC. EORTC studies using repeated embolization with microspheres combined with chemotherapy reported a 30% response rate. A randomized trial was conducted in the UK, and demonstrated a small but non-significant advantage in

favor of chemoembolization opposed to systemic chemotherapy. Thus, at the present time, chemoembolizations have no demonstrated place in the therapeutic arsenal for the treatment of LMCRC. However, some trials are still ongoing, and further improvements in embolization technique are highly probable.

CONCLUSIONS AND INDICATIONS

Locoregional chemotherapy is an active and useful technique in highly selected cases of LMCRC. The best indication is for patients with inoperable isolated liver metastases involving less than 50% of the liver. These represent about 5–10% of cases. Using these indications and with optimal techniques, we can hope for a 50% 2-year survival and 5–14% 5-year survival. In some cases IAHC efficacy permits secondary resection, which was impossible prior to IAHC.[31] However, this secondary surgery is difficult because of changes in the healthy liver caused by the IAHC, which must be as short and as light as possible.

Further developments combining IAHC and more active IV chemotherapy warrant careful evaluation, since IAHC has demonstrated its ability to control the progression of liver metastases and systemic chemotherapies have shown their efficacy on microscopic extrahepatic metastases. Only randomized trials will be able to demonstrate the value of such a sophisticated approach.

REFERENCES

1. Rougier P, Milan C, Lazorthes F et al, Unresected hepatic metastases from colorectal cancer: prognostic factor analysis from a prospective study on 544 cases from the Fondation Francaise de Cancerologie Digestive (FFCD). *Br J Surg* 1995; **82:** 1397–400.
2. Allen-Mersh TG, Earlam S, Fordy C et al, Quality of life and survival with continuous hepatic-artery floxuridine infusion for colorectal liver metastases. *Lancet* 1994; **344:** 1255–60.
3. Chang AE, Schneider PD, Sugarbaker PH et al, A prospective randomized trial of regional versus systemic continuous 5-fluorodeoxyuridine chemotherapy in the treatment of colorectal liver metastases. *Ann Surg* 1987; **206:** 685–93.
4. Hohn DC, Stagg RJ, Friedman MA et al, A randomized trial of continuous intravenous versus hepatic intraarterial floxuridine in patients with colorectal cancer metastatic to the liver: the Northern California Oncology Group trial. *J Clin Oncol* 1989; **7:** 1646–54.
5. Kemeny N, Daly J, Riechman B et al,

Intrahepatic or systemic infusion of fluo-rodeoxyuridine in patients with liver metastases from colorectal carcinoma. *Ann Intern Med* 1987; **107:** 459–65.

6. Martin JK, O'Connell MJ, Wieand HS et al, Intra-arterial floxuridine vs systemic fluorouracil for hepatic metastases from colorectal cancer. A randomized trial. *Arch Surg* 1990; **125:** 1022–7.

7. Rougier P, Laplanche A, Huguier M et al, Hepatic arterial infusion of floxuridine in patients with liver metastases from colorectal carcinoma: long-term results of a prospective randomized trial. *J Clin Oncol* 1992; **10:** 1112–18.

8. Kemeny N, Is hepatic infusion of chemotherapy effective treatment for liver metastases? Yes. In: *Important Advances in Oncology* (DeVita VT, Hellman S, Rosenberg SA, eds). Philadelphia: JB Lippincott, 1992; 207–28.

9. O'Connell MJ, Is hepatic infusion of chemotherapy effective treatment for liver metastases? No. In: *Important Advances in Oncology* (DeVita VT, Hellman S, Rosenberg SA, eds). Philadelphia: JB Lippincott, 1992; 229–34.

10. Patt Y, Regional hepatic arterial chemotherapy for colorectal cancer metastatic to the liver: the controversy continues. *J Clin Oncol* 1993; **11:** 815–19.

11. Patt Y, Hepatic artery chemotherapy for colorectal liver metastases: yet more controversy. *J Clin Oncol* 1993; **11:** 2053–4.

12. Breedis C, Young C, The blood supply of neoplasm in the liver. *Am J Pathol* 1954; **30:** 969–74.

13. Chen GHG, Gross JF, Intra-arterial infusion of anticancer drugs: theoretic aspects of drug delivery and review of responses. *Cancer Treat Rep* 1980; **64:** 31–40.

14. Ensminger WD, Gyves JW, Regional chemotherapy of neoplastic diseases. *Pharmacol Ther* 1983; **21:** 277–93.

15. Meta-Analysis Group in Cancer, Reappraisal of arterial infusion in the treatment of non resectable liver metastases from colorectal cancer. *J Natl Cancer Inst* 1996; **88:** 252–8.

16. Elias D, Ducreux M, Rougier P et al, Chimiothérapie intra-artérielle hépatique: Expérience de 200 cas. *Gastroentérol Clin Biol* 1994; **18:** 975–82.

17. Kemeny N, Conti JA, Cohen A et al, Phase II study of hepatic arterial floxuridine, leucovorin, and dexamethasone for unresectable liver metastases from colorectal carcinoma. *J Clin Oncol* 1994; **12:** 2288–95.

18. Munck JN, Riggi M, Rougier P et al, Pharmacokinetic and pharmacodynamic advantages of pirarubicin over adriamycin after intraarterial hepatic administration in the rabbit VX2 tumor model. *Cancer Res* 1993; **53:** 1550–4.

19. Hohn DC, Rayner AA, Economou JS et al, Toxicities and complications of implanted pump hepatic arterial and intravenous floxuridine infusion. *Cancer* 1986; **57:** 465–70.

20. Rougier Ph, Ducreux M, Ychou M et al, Intra-arterial chemotherapy (IAHC) using mitomycin C (MMC) combined to intra-venous chemotherapy (IVC) using 5FU + folinic acid (FA) for hepatic metastases from colorectal cancer (HMCRC). *Proc Am Soc Clin Oncol* 1996; **15:** 206.

21. Safi F, Hepp G, Link KH, Beger HG, Simultaneous adjuvant regional and systemic chemotherapy after resection of liver metastases of colorectal cancer. *Proc Am Soc Clin Oncol* 1995; **14:** 217.

22. Elias D, Lasser P, Rougier P, A simplified surgical technical procedure for intra-arterial chemotherapy in secondary liver cancer. Experience in 50 patients. *Eur J Surg Oncol* 1987; **13:** 441–8.

23. Campbell KA, Burns RC, Sitzmann JV et al, Regional chemotherapy devices: effect of experience and anatomy on complications. *J Clin Oncol* 1993; **11:** 822–6.

24. Kemeny N, Cohen A, Seiter K et al, Randomized trial of hepatic floxuridine, mitomycin, and carmustine versus floxuridine alone in previously treated patients with liver metastases from colorectal cancer. *J Clin Oncol* 1993; **11:** 330–5.

25. Mahjoubi R, Ychou M, Ducreux M et al, Multicentric phase II trial of intrahepatic arterial (HAI) pirarubicin (P) and systemic 5 fluorouracil (5FU) + leucovorin (LV) for liver metastases (LM) from colorectal cancer (CRC). *Proc Am Soc Clin Oncol* 1994; **13:** 223 (abst).

26. Villanova G, Ducreux M, Samelis G et al, Chimiothérapie intraartérielle hépatique (CIAH) par 5-fluorouracile (5-FU) en perfusion continue (PC) associé à un traitement intraveineux (IV) par 5-FU et acide folinique. *Bull Cancer* 1996; **83:** 439.

27. Kemeny N, Conti JA, Sigurdson E et al, A pilot study of hepatic artery floxuridine combined with systemic 5-fluorouracil and leucovorin. *Cancer* 1993; **71:** 1964–71.

28. Gerard A, Buyse M, Pector JC et al, Hepatic artery ligation with and without portal infusion of 5-FU. A randomized study in patients with unresectable liver metastases from colorectal carcinoma. *Eur J Surg Oncol* 1991; **17:** 289–94.

29. Hafström L, Engaras B, Holmberg SB et al, Treatment of liver metastases from colorectal cancer with hepatic artery occlusion, intraportal 5-fluorouracil infusion, and oral allopurinol. A randomized clinical trial. *Cancer* 1994; **74:** 2749–56.

30. Piedbois P, Buyse M, Gray R et al, Portal vein infusion is an effective adjuvant treatment for patients with colorectal cancer. *Proc Am Soc Clin Oncol* 1995; **14:** 192 (abst).

31. Elias D, Lasser P, Rougier P et al, Frequency, technical aspects, results and indications of major hepatectomy after prolonged intra-arterial hepatic chemotherapy for initially unresectable hepatic tumors. *J Am Coll Surg* 1995; **180:** 213–219.

30

New agents in the treatment of advanced colorectal cancer: Irinotecan, Tomudex and Oxaliplatin

Harry Bleiberg

CONTENTS • **Introduction** • **Irinotecan** • **Tomudex** • **Oxaliplatin** • **Conclusions**

INTRODUCTION

The non-specific thymidylate synthase (TS) inhibitor 5-fluorouracil (5-FU) has remained the mainstay of chemotherapy for the treatment of advanced colorectal cancer since its introduction into clinical practice in the 1950s. Response rates achieved with 5-FU bolus monotherapy are approximately 10–15%.[1] Alternative 5-FU-based therapeutic strategies have been investigated, including the combination of 5-FU with the biochemical modulating agent folinic acid (leucovorin), the biochemical modulation of 5-FU by methotrexate, high doses of 5-FU by continuous infusion, and the combination of 5-FU with other cytotoxic agents.[2,3] Although an improvement in response rate has been demonstrated with continuous versus bolus therapy,[4,5] there is a lack of conclusive data to suggest that any of the combination regimens of 5-FU with, for example, cisplatin[6] or methyl-CCNU plus vincristine[7] are superior to 5-FU alone.

Locoregional therapy in the treatment of colorectal hepatic metastases has also been investigated. Although promising results have been reported in terms of response rate (42–50%)[8,9] and survival (median survival 13.5–15 months),[9,10] no definite advantage over systemic treatment could be demonstrated,[11] and this procedure should remain investigational.

Thus, although advances have been made in the treatment of advanced colorectal cancer with 5-FU-based treatments, the achieved survival benefit is typically modest, and for this reason clinical studies are still ongoing to identify more effective treatment regimens. Major research has been conducted to identify agents with novel mechanisms of action distinct from that of 5-FU. Numerous examples of such agents are in various stages of development for the treatment of colorectal cancer, and the remit of this chapter is to provide an overview of the main compounds that are entering daily practice and that should have a considerable impact on the treatment of that disease.

IRONOTECAN

The nuclear enzyme topoisomerase I is essential for relaxing supercoiled double-stranded DNA, thus enabling DNA transcription and translation to proceed. This is achieved by forming a covalent adduct between topoisomerase I and

DNA, termed a cleavable complex. This covalent topoisomerase I–DNA complex induces a transient single-strand break in the DNA backbone through which the intact strand can pass, facilitating the transcription and translation of the genetic material, and the nicked strand is subsequently resealed. Topoisomerase I inhibitors reversibly stabilize this cleavable complex, and the resulting collision between this cleavable complex and the moving DNA replication fork is the principal cause of their cellular cytotoxicity. This results in the formation of double-strand DNA breaks and leads to the arrest of the cell cycle, predominantly in the S phase.[12,13] The high intracellular levels of topoisomerase I in some tumour cells (e.g. colon cancer cells) compared with normal tissue[14] makes this enzyme a rational target for the development of novel anticancer agents.

Camptothecin, an alkaloid extract of the plant *Camptotheca acuminata*, was the first topoisomerase I inhibitor to be isolated. In the early 1970s the efficacy of camptothecin was evaluated. However, despite promising activity against several experimental tumour models, camptothecin was found to be associated with excessive toxicity, including myelosuppression and haemorrhagic cystitis. This led to the cessation of further development of the drug. An investigational programme was subsequently pursued to develop structurally related compounds with greater antitumour activity and reduced toxicity, and this resulted in the identification of a number of active analogues, the most investigated being irinotecan (Campto).

Irinotecan is a semisynthetic water-soluble derivative of camptothecin, which is converted by the carboxylesterase enzyme in vivo to the active metabolite 7-ethyl-10-hydroxycamptothecin (SN-38).[12] The efficacy of single-agent irinotecan has been evaluated as both first- and second-line treatment for advanced colorectal cancer in phase II studies in over 300 patients. Four phase II studies have been conducted in Japan and the USA using a variety of administration schedules: 100 mg/m^2 once weekly or 150 mg/m^2 once every 2 weeks in Japan,[15] and 125 mg/m^2 weekly for 4 weeks followed by a 2-week rest in the USA.[15–17] Response rates of

15–32% and 22–25% were reported in chemotherapy-naive and pretreated patients respectively.

The pivotal phase II study conducted in France evaluated an irinotecan dose of 350 mg/m^2 administered once every 3 weeks. Response rates were comparable in both the chemotherapy-naive ($n = 48$) and pretreated ($n = 130$) eligible patient groups: 18.8% (95% CI 8.9–32.6) and 17.7% (95% CI 11.5–25.5) respectively.[18] A response rate of 16.1% (95% CI 8–27.6) reported for 62 eligible patients who had progressed whilst on a previous 5-FU-based chemotherapy was suggestive of a lack of cross-resistance between 5-FU and irinotecan. In both the pretreated and chemotherapy-naive patient groups, the median duration of response was 9.1 months (range 1.6–17).

Although not cumulative, 47% of patients experienced a grade 3/4 neutropenia in the French study, and febrile neutropenia was reported in 15% of the patients.[19] The administration of irinotecan is also frequently associated with the development of two different types of diarrhoea; an early type, which can be controlled by anticholinergic therapy, and a delayed type, which appears to be predominantly secretory[20] and can lead to severe dehydration if not promptly treated. In the French phase II study, delayed diarrhoea developed in 87% of patients (grade 3/4 in 39%),[20] and high-dose loperamide was reported to be the best supportive treatment.[21] Preventive treatment with the enkephalinase inhibitor acetorphan alone,[22] has not demonstrated any utility in this setting. In a recent confirmatory European phase II study, special care was taken regarding the need for prompt measures after any episode of diarrhoea. Guidelines for the management of diarrhoea were clearly established before the study started. The treatment was initiated after the first soft or liquid stool, and continued for 12 hours after the last episode of diarrhoea, and the patients were to receive oral broad-spectrum antibiotics for the next 7 days if diarrhoea persisted for more than 24 hours despite loperamide therapy. Comparison with the French study indicates that although the incidence of diarrhoea was similar in both studies (87% versus 86%), severe (grade 3 and 4) delayed diarrhoea has been observed in only 26% of patients as compared with 39% in the French study, with an even greater decrease in the incidence of grade 4 diarrhoea from 8% to 2.5%.[23] In Europe, irinotecan was used to treat a total of 455 patients with documented 5-FU-resistant colorectal cancers involved in four phase II trials. All had documented progressive disease at study entry, and 44.5% had tumour-related pain. The overall response rate in 363 eligible patients was 12.9%, and an additional 42% had a stabilization of their disease. The median duration of response was 33 weeks, and 22 weeks for stabilized patients. The median time to progression was 18 weeks. The median survival time was 41 weeks. Six- and nine-month survival was 72% and 53% respectively. Sixty-one percent of patients with response or stabilization had pain relief attributable to irinotecan.[24] In order to develop therapeutic options as first-line treatment, phase I combinations of irinotecan with 5-FU, Tomudex and oxaliplatin are underway. Two phase III trials, comparing irinotecan as second-line treatment with best supportive care and with any 5-FU-containing regimen, are ongoing and will establish the benefit of irinotecan in this setting.

TOMUDEX

The quinazoline folate analogue Tomudex (raltitrexed, ZD1694) is a direct, specific TS inhibitor currently undergoing phase III evaluation as single-agent, first-line therapy for advanced colorectal cancer. Tomudex is taken up into the cells via the reduced folate membrane carrier system and then extensively polyglutamated to more potent forms. Polyglutamation extends the intracellular retention of Tomudex and prolongs TS inhibition, permitting the use of a single-dose schedule once every 3 weeks.[25]

To date, Tomudex has demonstrated clinical activity in the treatment of advanced colorectal cancer in phase II and phase III studies.[26,27] Tomudex, 3 mg/m², was administered as a 15-minute intravenous infusion once every 3 weeks in patients with advanced or metastatic disease.

In the phase II studies, 176 patients were enrolled and objective responses (4 complete and 41 partial responses) were reported in 26% of patients (95% CI 19–33%), with a median duration of 5.7 months.[26] Median time to disease progression was 4.2 months, and median survival time was 9.6 months. The subsequent phase III study compared the efficacy and tolerability of Tomudex with the Mayo Clinic regimen of 5-FU (425 mg/m²) plus low-dose folinic acid (20 mg/m²) for 5 consecutive days every 4–5 weeks.[27] A total of 439 patients were randomized, and objective response rates of 20% and 13% were reported in the Tomudex and 5-FU/folinic acid cohorts respectively (odds ratio 1.7; 95% CI 0.98–2.81; $p = 0.059$). There was no statistically significant difference in time to disease progression between the two treatment groups.

Both groups experienced an improvement in terms of emotional function, sleep disturbance, pain and global quality of life. Tomudex also demonstrated palliative benefits (improved performance status (34 versus 25%) and weight gain (15 versus 12%) at least as frequently as the comparative Mayo regimen.

In the phase III study, Tomudex was associated with a significantly lower incidence of both severe (grade 3/4) leucopenia (10% versus 26%) and mucositis (2% versus 22%) ($p < 0.001$) compared with treatment with 5-FU/folinic acid. The incidence of increased liver transaminases was significantly higher in the Tomudex cohort (10% versus 0%, $p < 0.001$), but this effect was generally self-limiting and asymptomatic. Other frequent adverse effects included diarrhoea developing in 13% and 11% and nausea and vomiting developing in 12% and 9% of Tomudex and 5-FU/folinic acid-treated patients respectively. Of note, 74% of patients receiving Tomudex and 52% of those receiving 5-FU/folinic acid were able to receive their treatment on time without significant dose reduction or delay. The administration of Tomudex was not associated with the development of severe delayed diarrhoea.[27]

Two other phase III studies were performed

in Europe (versus the Machover schedule) and in the USA (versus the Mayo schedule). The results should bring more information on the real place of Tomudex in the treatment of advanced colorectal cancer.

OXALIPLATIN

Oxaliplatin (1,2-diaminocyclohexane (*trans-l*) oxalatoplatinum(II), L-OHP) is a non-nephrotoxic third-generation platinum complex under clinical development. The recommended dose for phase II studies is 130 mg/m^2 given i.v. over 2 hours in 5% glucose every 3 weeks. It causes minimal haematological toxicity, no ototoxicity and no hair loss. The dose-limiting toxicity of the drug is a peripheral dysaesthesia and/or pharyngo-laryngeal paresia caused and aggravated by the cold. This effect is dose-dependent in terms of duration and intensity, and may in some cases cause functional impairment that is generally reversible after discontinuation of the treatment.[28]

As a single agent in first- or second-line treatment, the response rate is about 20% and 10% respectively.[29,30] Adverse events were peripheral sensory neuropathy (84% of courses), mild nausea and vomiting (61%), which in 81% of the courses required no antiemetic medication, and diarrhoea (43%). No renal or audiotoxicity developed, and haematological toxicity was minimal.[31]

Oxaliplatin has demonstrated promising activity in combination with 5-FU. Studies have been conducted using a combination of 5-FU, folinic acid and oxaliplatin, administered using a chronomodulated or a constant-rate continuous-infusion schedule. Response rates of 50% and 28% have been reported for first- and second-line treatment respectively, with an overall median survival time of between 16 and 12 months.[31-35] Between 20% and 30% of patients with liver or lung metastases could be reoperated with a curative aim.[36] In one of these series, median survival time, including the patients submitted to surgery, was not reached at 37 months.[37]

Two hundred and six patients refractory to 5-FU or progressing after 5-FU therapy were treated in a compassionate-need program using various combinations of oxaliplatin with the same or a different 5-FU regimen. Depending on the schedule administered, the response rate varied from 14% to 32%. The number of previous chemotherapy treatments was also important, with 30.5%, 19%, 12.5% objective response rates after one, two or three previous chemotherapies respectively.[38]

Further studies trying to better define the role of oxaliplatin in first- and second-line therapy are underway.

CONCLUSIONS

Past efforts to introduce new agents and thus replace the standard chemotherapeutic agent, 5-FU, have proved unsuccessful. However, the 1990s have heralded a new era in drug development for colorectal cancer, with intensive research efforts directed at designing novel chemotherapeutic agents with improved efficacy and tolerability profiles compared with standard 5-FU-based regimens. Although many of these agents are currently in the early stages of development, their profusion and varied mechanisms of action provide grounds for optimism regarding the management of patients with advanced disease. The three agents anticipated to have the greatest impact on treatment in the near future are Tomudex, irinotecan and oxaliplatin, and it is hoped that the benefits of these and other drugs will ultimately improve the prognosis and further increase the survival of patients with advanced colorectal cancer.

REFERENCES

1. Advanced Colorectal Cancer Meta-Analysis Project, Modulation of fluorouracil by leucovorin in patients with advanced colorectal cancer: evidence in terms of response rate. *J Clin Oncol* 1992; **10**: 896–903.
2. Moertel CG, Chemotherapy for colorectal cancer. *N Engl J Med* 1994; **330**: 1136–42.
3. Advanced Colorectal Cancer Meta-Analysis Project, Meta-analysis of randomized trials testing the biochemical modulation of fluorouracil by methotrexate in metastatic colorectal cancer. *J Clin Oncol* 1994; **12**: 960–9.
4. Seifert P, Baker LH, Reed ML, Vankevicivo VK, Comparison of continuously infused 5-fluorouracil with bolus injection in treatment of patients with colorectal adenocarcinoma. *Cancer* 1975; **36**: 123–8.
5. Lokich JJ, Ahlgren JD, Gullo JJ et al, A prospective randomized comparison of continuous infusion fluorouracil with a conventional bolus schedule in metastatic colorectal carcinoma: a Mid-Atlantic Oncology Program study. *J Clin Oncol* 1989; **7**: 425–32.
6. Bleiberg H, Vanderlinden B, Buyse M et al, Randomized phase II study of a combination of cisplatin (DDP), 5-fluorouracil (5-FU) and allopurinol (HHP) versus 5-fluorouracil in colorectal cancer. An EORTC Gastrointestinal Tract Cancer Cooperative Group Study. *Cancer Invest* 1990; **8**: 471–5.
7. Moertel CG, Schutt AJ, Hahn RG, Reitemeier RJ, Therapy of advanced colorectal cancer with a combination of 5-fluorouracil, methyl-1,3-*cis*-(2-chloroethyl)-1-nitrosourea and vincristine. *J Natl Cancer Inst* 1975; **54**: 69–71.
8. Kemeny N, Daly J, Reichman B et al, Intrahepatic or systemic infusion of fluorodeoxyuridine in patients with liver metastases from colorectal carcinoma. *Ann Intern Med* 1987; **107**: 459–65.
9. Rougier P, Laplanche A, Huguier M et al, Hepatic arterial infusion of floxuridine in patients with liver metastases from colorectal carcinoma: long-term results of a prospective randomized trial. *J Clin Oncol* 1992; **10**: 1112–18.
10. Allen-Mersch TG, Earlam S, Fordy C et al, Quality of life and survival with continuous hepatic-artery floxuridine infusion for colorectal liver metastases. *Lancet* 1994; **344**: 1255–60.
11. Meta-Analysis Group in Cancer, Reappraisal of hepatic arterial infusion in the treatment of non-resectable liver metastases from colorectal cancer. *J Natl Cancer Inst* 1996; **88**: 252–8.
12. Creemers GJ, Lund B, Verweij J, Topoisomerase I inhibitors: topotecan and irinotecan. *Cancer Treat Rev* 1994; **20**: 73–96.
13. Hsiang YH, Lihou MG, Liu LF, Arrest of replication forks by drug-stabilised topoisomerase I–DNA cleavable complexes as a mechanism of cell killing by camptothecin. *Cancer Res* 1989; **49**: 5077–82.
14. Giovanella BC, Stehlin JS, Wall ME et al, DNA topoisomerase I targeted chemotherapy of human colon cancer in xenografts. *Science* 1989; **246**: 1046–8.
15. Shimada Y, Yashino M, Wakui A et al, Phase II study of CPT-11, a new camptothecin derivative, in metastatic colorectal cancer. *J Clin Oncol* 1993; **11**: 909–13.
16. Conti JA, Kemen N, Saltz L et al, Irinotecan (CPT-11) is an active agent in untreated patients with metastatic colorectal cancer (CRC). *Proc Am Soc Clin Oncol* 1994; **13**: 565 (abst).
17. Pitot HC, Wender D, O'Connell MJ et al, A phase II trial of CPT-11 (irinotecan) in patients with metastatic colorectal carcinoma: a North Central Cancer Treatment Group (NCCTG) study. *Proc Am Soc Clin Oncol* 1994; **13**: 573 (abst).
18. Rothenberg ML, Eckardt JR, Burris III HA et al, Irinotecan (CPT-11) as second line therapy for PTS with 5-FU-refractory colorectal cancer *Proc Am Soc Clin Oncol* 1994; **13**: 578 (abst).
19. Rougier P, Bugat R, Douillard JY et al, Phase II study of irinotecan in the treatment of advanced colorectal cancer in chemotherapy-naive patients and patients pretreated with fluorouracil-based chemotherapy. *J Clin Oncol* 1997; **15**: 251–60.
20. Bugat R, CPT-11 in the treatment of colorectal cancer (CRC): safety profile. In: *Proc 5th International Congress of Anti-Cancer Chemotherapy, Paris, France, 31 January–3 February 1995*; S778 (abst).
21. Abigerges D, Armand JP, Chabot G et al, Irinotecan (CPT-11) high-dose escalation using intensive high-dose loperamide to control diarrhea. *J Natl Cancer Inst* 1994; **86**: 446–9.
22. Goncalves E, da Costa L, Abigerges D, Armand JP, A new enkephalinase inhibitor as an alternative to loperamide in the prevention of diarrhea induced by CPT-11. *J Clin Oncol* 1995; **13**: 2144–6.
23. Hagipantelli R, Saliba F, Misset JL et al, Pathophysiology and therapy of irinotecan

(CPT-11) induced delayed diarrhea (DD). A prospective assessment. *Proc Am Soc Clin Oncol, Los Angeles, CA, 20–23 May 1995* (poster presentation).

24. Van Cutsem E, Cunningham D, Ten Bokkel Huinink W et al, Irinotecan (CPT-11) multicenter phase II study in colorectal cancer patients with documented progressive disease on prior 5-FU: preliminary results. *Proc Am Soc Clin Oncol* 1996; **15:** 230.

25. Van Cutsem E, Rougier Ph, Droz JP et al, Clinical benefit of irinotecan (CPT-11) in metastatic colorectal cancer (CRC) resistant to 5-FU. *Proc Am Soc Clin Oncol* 1997; **16:** 268 (abst).

26. Jackman AL, Gibson W, Brown M et al, The role of the reduced-folate carrier and metabolism to intracellular polyglutamates for the activity of CIC D1694. *Adv Exp Med Biol* 1993; **339:** 265–76.

27. Zalcberg JR, Cunningham D, Van Cutsem E et al, Tomudex (ZD1694), a novel thymidylate synthase inhibitor has substantial activity in the treatment of patients with advanced colorectal cancer. *J Clin Oncol* 1996; **14:** 716–21.

28. Cunningham D, Zalberg JR, Rath U et al, Tomudex (ZD1694): results of a randomised trial in advanced colorectal cancer demonstrate efficacy and reduced mucositis and leucopenia. *Eur J Cancer* 1995; **31A:** 1945–54.

29. Brienza S, Fandi A, Hugret F et al, Neurotoxicity of long run oxaliplatin (L-OHP) therapy. *Proc Am Assoc Cancer Res* 1993; **34:** A2421 (abst).

30. Diaz-Rubio E, Zaniboni A, Gastaburu J et al, Phase II multicentric trial of oxaliplatin (L-OHP) as first line chemotherapy in metastatic colorectal carcinoma (MCRC). *Proc Am Soc Clin Oncol* 1996; **15:** 207.

31. Machover D, Diaz-Rubio E, de Grammont A et al, Two consecutive studies of oxaliplatin (L-OHP) for treatment of patients with advanced colorectal carcinoma who were resistant to previous treatment with fluoropyrimidines. *Ann Oncol* 1996; **7:** 95–8.

32. Garufi C, Brienza S, Bensmaine MA et al, Addition of oxaliplatin (L-OHP) to chronomodulated (CM) 5-fluorouracil and folinic acid (FA) for reversal of acquired chemoresistance in patients with advanced colorectal cancer (ACC). *Proc Am Soc Clin Oncol* 1995; **14:** 192 (abst).

33. Levi F, Perpoint B, Garufi C et al, Oxaliplatin activity against metastatic colorectal cancer. A phase II study of 5-day continuous venous infusion at circadian rhythm modulated rate. *Eur J Cancer* 1993; **29A:** 1280–4.

34. Lévi F, Misset JL, Brienza S et al, A chronopharmacologic phase II clinical trial with 5-fluorouracil, folinic acid, and oxaliplatin using an ambulatory multichannel programmable pump. *Cancer* 1992; **69:** 893–900.

35. Lévi F, Zidani R, Vannetzel JM et al, Chronomodulated versus fixed-infusion-rate delivery of ambulatory chemotherapy with oxaliplatin, fluorouracil, and folinic acid (leucovorin) in patients with colorectal cancer metastases: a randomized multi-institutional trial. *J Natl Cancer Inst* 1994; **86:** 1608–17.

36. de Gramont A, Tournigand C, Louvet C et al, High-dose folinic acid, 5-fluorouracil 48H-infusion and oxaliplatin in metastatic colorectal cancer. In: *Proc 5th International Congress of Anti-Cancer Chemotherapy, Paris, France, 31 January–3 February 1995;* O269 (abst).

37. Bismuth H, Adam R, Lévi F et al, Resection of nonresectable liver metastases from colorectal cancer after neoadjuvant chemotherapy. *Ann Surg* 1996; **224:** 509–22.

38. Giachetty S, Itzhaki M, Adam R et al, Long term survival of patients with unresectable colorectal cancer liver metastases, following infusional chronotherapy with 5-fluorouracil (5-FU), folinic acid (FA), oxaliplatin (L-OHP). *Ann Oncol* 1996; **7**(Suppl 5): 34.

31

New chemotherapy approaches in colon cancer

Richard M Goldberg, Charles Erlichman

INTRODUCTION

In this chapter we shall touch upon new pharmacologic approaches to the treatment of colon cancer. Novel uses of 5-fluorouracil (5-FU), new agents that target thymidylate synthase, and new therapeutic targets identified through the better understanding of tumor biology (specifically matrix metalloproteinase, farnesyltransferase and angiogenesis) will be discussed.

IMPROVEMENTS IN THE EFFICACY OF 5-FU

One strategy for improving the efficacy of 5-FU has centered on biochemical modulation of its catabolism. The goal of this approach is to prolong the drug's half-life to maximize exposure of tumor cells to high levels of 5-FU in a comparable manner to the pharmacokinetic pattern achieved by continuous intravenous infusion. In the three formulations of 5-FU to be discussed – namely UFT (uracil, U, with ftorafur, FT), 5-FU plus 776C85, and S-1 – a 5-FU prodrug or 5-FU is given with an additional drug that interferes with 5-FU breakdown. All three preparations are orally administered to obviate the requirement for long-term intravenous access or infusion pumps. This tactic has the potential to both allow prolonged exposure of tumor cells to the drug and increase the therapeutic index of 5-FU.

The first step in the degradation of 5-FU is catalyzed by the enzyme dihydropyrimidine dehydrogenase (DPD). The administration of exogenous uracil, or of two types of inhibitors – 776C85 (also known as ethynyluracil), which covalently binds to DPD, and 5-chloro-2,4-dihydroxypyridine (CDHP) – have been three approaches exhibiting sufficient promise in vitro and in human tumor xenografts to engender clinical trials in humans. A compound in early clinical testing, known as S-1, combines UFT with CDHP and oxonic acid, the latter being added to ameliorate GI toxicity.

UFT

UFT, an oral formulation in which uracil and tegafur (ftorafur, FT) are combined, has been the subject of clinical trials for over 15 years. Tegafur, 1-(2-tetrahydrofuryl)-5-fluorouracil, is a 5-FU prodrug, which is hydroxylated and converted to 5-FU by hepatic microsomal enzymes.[1] Uracil potentiates 5-FU through interference with hepatic DPD. In vivo, UFT increases intratumoral 5-FU concentration, and has been reported to result in augmented antitumor activity in comparison to tegafur alone.[2] In AH-130 human tumor xenografts the ratio of 4:1 uracil to tegafur resulted in the highest tumor tissue-to-blood partition coefficient, and it is that formulation which has been clinically evaluated.[3] Pazdur has shown that peak plasma levels of 5-FU that resulted from UFT administration at a tegafur dose of 370 mg/m^2 in three divided doses exceeded those achieved by continuous intravenous infusion of 5-FU at a dose of 250 mg/m^2/day.[4]

UFT has been most thoroughly evaluated in Japan, where it is approved for treatment of colorectal cancer. Clinical studies in Japan and the United Kingdom in which patients ingested 300–600 mg per day of UFT for four-week intervals followed by a two-week rest have indicated a modest level of activity, with a 15–25% response rate in patients with previously untreated colorectal cancer.[5a,b,6]

Attempts have been made to employ an all-oral means of double modulation of 5-FU through the addition of leucovorin to UFT. Saltz et al[7] have reported a 25% response rate with moderate toxicity, principally mucositis and diarrhea, in a phase II trial of oral UFT at 350 mg/m^2/day plus oral leucovorin at 5 mg every 8 hours in 20 patients with advanced colorectal cancer. Pazdur et al[8] administered an oral regimen of 300–350 mg/m^2/day of UFT plus 150 mg/m^2/day of leucovorin in divided doses thrice daily for 28 days to patients who had been previously treated with chemotherapy or biologic therapy for advanced colorectal cancer. The response rate reported was 42% (95% confidence interval 28–58%). Toxicity included diarrhea, abdominal pain, rash and mucositis. This report indicated that a randomized trial of intravenous 5-FU plus leucovorin and UFT plus leucovorin was planned by these investigators.

A trial reporting the use of a different dose and schedule of UFT plus leucovorin in previously treated patients with rectal cancer indicated a similar response rate of 43%.[9] Nogue et al[10] presented results from a 33-patient trial of

tegafur 0.75 g/m^2/day for 21 days and oral leucovorin 15 mg every 8 hours for 28 days. Limiting side-effects were mucositis, diarrhea, and nausea and vomiting. A 30% response rate was noted, with median survival time of 14 months.

776C85

The half-life of intravenously administered 5-FU is approximately 14 minutes.[11] 5-FU is rapidly reduced by DPD to α-fluoro-β-alanine, which has no cytotoxic activity but has been associated with neurotoxicity.[12] Patients with inherited DPD deficiency eliminate 5-FU over hours rather than minutes, and eliminate 90% of unmetabolized 5-FU in their urine.[13] 776C85 is a potent, covalently bound, inhibitor of DPD, and is capable of inactivating 99% of endogenous DPD without producing intrinsic toxicity.[14]

When 5-FU and 776C85 are coadministered, the half-life of the 5-FU is prolonged to approximately 5 hours.[15] Additionally, the therapeutic index and activity of 5-FU in human tumor xenograft models is increased by two- to six-fold. 776C85 was noted to be a more potent modulator of 5-FU than either leucovorin or N-(phosphonoacetyl)-L-aspartate (PALA).[16,17]

In phase I testing, oral 5-FU has been combined with oral 776C85 in 7-day and 28-day schedules.[18,19] The double modulation of 5-FU with 776C85 plus leucovorin has also been tested in the phase I setting.[20] Optimal dose and scheduling remain to be determined. However, maximal tolerated 5-FU doses are an order of magnitude smaller than those that can be safely administered without coadministration of 776C85, ranging from 10 to 25 mg/m^2/day. Principal toxicities have included myelosuppression with sepsis and gastrointestinal toxicities, including stomatitis, nausea, diarrhea and bleeding. Responses have been seen in previously treated patients with colorectal cancer, and phase II testing of the two-drug and three-drug regimens is expected to begin shortly.

S-1

S-1 is a new oral antitumor agent that combines three agents: tegafur (FT), 5-chloro-2,4-dihydroxypyridine (CDHP) – a potent inhibitor of DPD – and oxonic acid (Oxo) – an inhibitor of the phosphorylation of 5-FU to form 5-fluorouridine monophosphate (5-FUMP) (5-FUMP is toxic to gastrointestinal mucosa). The combination was created because CDHP with tegafur exhibited enhanced antitumor activity and Oxo inhibited 5-FU-induced GI toxicity without loss of antitumor efficacy.[21,22] The formulation consists of molar ratios of 1:0.4:1 of FT:CDHP:Oxo, and was developed on the basis of activity and toxicity profiles in rodents bearing Yoshida sarcomas.[23] When FT + CDHP without Oxo was administered to dogs, the incidence of vomiting (7/11 animals) and diarrhea (10/11 animals) was markedly higher than when the three-drug preparation was used (vomiting 1/11 and diarrhea 1/11).

Phase II evaluations of two doses (50 mg and 75 mg/m^2/day FT given twice daily for 28 days followed by a 14-day respite) are in progress.[24] Overall efficacy in 30 previously treated patients with colorectal cancer is 17%. The principal side-effects included stomatitis, anorexia, diarrhea and myelosuppression.

NOVEL THYMIDYLATE-SYNTHASE INHIBITORS

5-FU combined with leucovorin effectively improves the cure rate in the adjuvant setting for patients with stage III colon cancer over surgery alone, and can result in clinically meaningful remissions in patients with advanced disease.[25,26] One potential means of improving response rates in GI malignancies is the discovery of more potent and specific inhibitors of thymidylate synthase (TS) that do not require cofactors.

New agents have been synthesized by modification at the pteridine ring, the p-aminobenzoic acid moiety, and/or the glutamate end of the folate molecule. These compounds have then been screened for antitumor activity. Novel TS inhibitors have also been designed utilizing the X-ray crystallographic structure of TS, and can occupy the reduced folate-binding site. The initial compound is varied and optimized in a process involving co-crystallization and structure determination of the protein–ligand complexes. This innovative approach results in compounds that are not based on modification of folate structure but can inhibit thymidylate synthase.

Quinazoline (5,8-dideaza) analogs of folic acid were demonstrated to inhibit TS in the 1970s. Jones synthesized and his colleagues at the Institute for Cancer Research performed clinical testing of an N^{10}-propargylfolic acid analog designated CB3717, which had promising in vitro and in vivo activity.[27] This drug had modest activity, but was found to have too high renal, dermatologic and hepatic toxicities for further use after phase I testing.[28] In order to overcome the renal toxicity, new analogs were developed and tested, which led to the discovery of ICI D1694 (Tomudex). This agent is more soluble, is extensively polyglutamated and thus retained intracellularly, has antitumor activity in 10 human tumor xenografts of diverse histology, and is not nephrotoxic.[29]

Phase I testing of Tomudex was completed in two studies, which found the maximum tolerated dose to be 3.5 and 4.0 mg/m^2 every three weeks. Dose-limiting toxicity was myelosuppression and mucositis. Diarrhea, rash and elevation of liver-associated enzymes were lesser side-effects.[30,31] Phase II testing at a dose of 3.0 mg/m^2 every three weeks in 176 patients with metastatic colorectal cancer and no prior chemotherapy for advanced disease was encouraging, with a 26% (19–33% CI) response rate observed.[32] Diarrhea and myelotoxicity were dose-limiting.

A report has been given (in abstract form)[33] of a phase III study in which patients with no prior chemotherapy exposure for advanced colorectal cancer were randomized to 5-FU 425 mg/m^2 and leucovorin 20 mg/m^2 daily for five days every 4–5 weeks or to Tomudex 3 mg/m^2 every three weeks. The median follow-up time for the 434 entered patients was 18 months. Response rates (20% versus 16%), times to progression (4.9 versus 3.6 months) and median survival time (10.3 versus 10.5 months) were comparable for Tomudex and for 5-FU plus leucovorin. Mucositis was more frequent in the 5-FU arm of the study. However, ice-chip oral prophylaxis was not employed in either arm of the study, which raises the question of whether patients were treated with intensive doses of either regimen. Response rates and survivals for the 5-FU arm are somewhat inferior to the medians suggested in the meta-analysis of 5-FU and leucovorin.[26] Nevertheless, the activity profile is comparable to that of 5-FU plus leucovorin.

Two other classical folate analogs are currently in the process of clinical testing. BW1843U89 is a 3-methylbenzoquinazoline folate analog, with glutaric acid replacing the glutamate found in folates.[34] This leads to the addition of only one glutamate intracellularly. The compound is in the process of undergoing phase I testing, since it has shown promising activity in vitro and in vivo. Principal side-effects have included asthenia, rash, stomatitis and neutropenia. Clinical activity in colon cancer has been noted.[35]

LY231514 is a compound in which a pyrrole ring replaces the pyrazine portion of the pterine present in folic acid, and a methylene group replaces the benzylic nitrogen in the bridging portion of folic acid.[36] Promising in vitro and in vivo activity in colon cancer have led to two phase I clinical trials. Neutropenia, thrombocytopenia and fatigue have been dose-limiting, and some activity was noted in patients with colon cancer.[37] A dose of 600 mg/m^2 has been recommended for phase II testing, which is now underway in patients with colorectal cancer.[38]

The first two compounds to reach clinical trials that were designed to interact with the crystal structure of TS are AG-331 (N^6-[4-(N-morpholinosulfonyl)benzyl]-N^6-methyl-2,6-diaminobenz[cd]indole glucuronate) and AG-337 (3,4-dihydro-2-amino-6-methyl-4-oxo-5-(4pyridylthio)quinazoline dihydrochloride). These molecules lack the N-terminal glutamate of classical TS inhibitors, and are able to enter cells via passive diffusion rather than carrier-mediated transport. Both compounds result in cell-cycle arrest at the G1/S boundary.[39,40] While AG-331 is more potent both in vitro and in vivo, AG-337 is 90% bioavailable after oral absorption, and it has been brought forward for further clinical evaluation.

AG-337 has been subjected to phase I study in its oral and intravenous formulations for 5-day and 10-day periods of administration.[41] The phase II recommended intravenous dose was 1000 mg/m^2/day for 5 days. Neutropenia and stomatitis were dose-limiting. Local complications require central line placement for drug administration. A single response was noted in a patient with colon cancer. A phase II dose for oral administration of AG-337 is currently underway.[42] Phase II studies using a 5-day continuous-infusion schedule have been accruing patients, but data are not yet reported on trial outcomes.

MATRIX-METALLOPROTEINASE INHIBITORS

Matrix metalloproteinases (MMP) are enzymes that degrade proteins and tissue extracellular matrix. These proteins exhibit specific well-defined properties, and are classified into a family of enzymes consisting of at least 14 members. Historically, the enzymes have been subcategorized into collagenases, gelatinases, stromelysins and others. The individual enzymes have been assigned a number ranging from MMP 1 to 14.[43–45] Table 31.1 lists some of these MMPs, including the enzyme name, the MMP number and the substrate. The MMPs are secreted as proenzymes, which undergo auto-proteolytic cleavage leading to the active moiety. A series of membrane-type matrix metalloproteinases[46] (MT-MMP) that are over-expressed in malignant tissue have also been identified. On binding extracellular MMP, these MT-MMPs will activate the MMP. Tissue inhibitors of metalloproteinases (TIMP) can bind to these MT-MMPs such that they inhibit the activation of the MMP. Regulation of this complex system has not been fully elucidated. However, different MMPs may be positively or negatively affected by cytokines such as TGF-β, IL-1, TNF-α, IFN-γ, EGF, PDGF and bFGF.[47] The MMPs are produced by both tumor cells and normal cells such as monocytes or macrophages, connective-tissue cells and endothelial cells. The enzymes are involved in tumor invasion through normal epithelium, leading to breakdown of tissue architecture, invasion of blood vessels to enter the circulation, and extravasation from the vascular system at distant sites, which is necessary for the development of metastatic lesions. Tumor angiogenesis is dependent on both proliferation of endothelial cells (see below) and the invasion of endothelial cells into stroma to form blood vessels. MMPs appear to play a role in this latter step. Hence this complex system may contribute to tumor invasion, tumor metastasis and tumor angiogenesis. These major roles make MMPs a very attractive target for antitumor therapy.

Studies have been done in clinical material demonstrating high levels of MMPs in colorectal cancer,[48–62] and there appears to be a correlation between tumor growth and MMP activity.

Table 31.1 Matrix metalloproteinases

MMP No.	Name	Substrate	Tissue localization
1	Interstitial collagenase	Collagens (I, II, III, V, VII, X)	Connective-tissue cells, monocytes/macrophages, endothelial cells
2	Gelatinase A	Gelatin, elastin, collagens (IV, V, VII, X, XI), fibronectin	Most cell types, tumor cells
3	Stromelysin-1	Proteoglycans, gelatins, fibronectin, laminins, collagens (III, IV, V, IX)	Connective-tissue cells, monocytes/macrophages, endothelial cells, tumor cells
7	Matrilysin	Gelatins, fibronectin, elastin, proteoglycans	Monocytes, tumor cells, connective-tissue cells
8	Neutrophil collagenase	Collagens (I, II, III), gelatin	Neutrophils
9	Gelatinase B	Gelatin, elastin, collagens (IV, V, VII, X, XI), fibronectin	Connective-tissue cells, monocytes/macrophages, tumor cells
10	Stromelysin-2	Proteoglycans, gelatins, fibronectin, laminins, collagens (III, IV, V, IX)	Macrophages, tumor cells

These results support the rationale for design of MMP inhibitors to complement the classic cytotoxic agents. Clinical development of MMP inhibitors (MMPI) is currently underway.[63,64] Batimastat,[65-70] Marimastat,[71] AG 3319 and 3340[72] are four compounds that have undergone preclinical evaluation. The results are encouraging, with tumor regression when combined with chemotherapy, inhibition of tumor growth when started shortly after tumor inoculation in vivo, and growth inhibition of tumor when started after tumor establishment. Initial clinical trials of Batimistat were abandoned because of difficulties with solubility, formulation and hence administration. Ongoing studies of Marimastat have demonstrated that this is a tolerable oral treatment. Further work is in progress to determine whether any clinical activity can be observed.

FARNESYLTRANSFERASE INHIBITORS

RAS is a small guanine triphosphate-binding protein that is an important component of a signal-transduction pathway used by a variety of growth factors to initiate cell proliferation.[71-75] Mutation of the RAS oncogene, which occurs in approximately 50% of all colorectal cancers, leads to a constitutive expression of this oncogene and stimulates tumor proliferation. In most colon cancers in which RAS is not mutated and constitutively expressed, growth-factor (GF) stimulation by insulin (IGF) and epidermal growth factor (EGF) may contribute significantly to the proliferative component of colon carcinogenesis. RAS can be activated[76] by IGF or EGF binding to their respective receptors. RAS normally exists in an inactive guanine diphosphate membrane-bound state, and, when activated by GF binding to its respective receptor or as a consequence of mutation, becomes a guanine triphosphate membrane-bound form.[77] The addition of a farnesyl group to a cysteine residue on the RAS protein is catalyzed by the enzyme farnesyltransferase (FT). This step is required for the RAS protein to become activated. Insertion of mutated RAS has been associated with transformation to the malignant phenotype both in vitro and in vivo. An understanding of this biochemical process has identified the FT enzyme as a potential target for antitumor effects. Investigations have focused on developing inhibitors of the tetrapeptide-binding site of FT, and series of such compounds (FTIs) – some pepidomimetic – have been developed. These agents are potent inhibitors of FT in the nanomolar range.[78-93] Inhibition of FT has resulted in growth inhibition in RAS-transformed cells, both in vitro and in vivo.[94-104] The treatment in vivo requires long-term administration of the FTI. Cessation of the inhibitor administration leads to regrowth of the tumors in vivo. A recent report suggests that resistance to FT inhibition may develop.[105] Questions still remain to be addressed in regard to these compounds before clinical utility can be defined. Among these is whether inhibition of this pathway, which is important in the farnesylation of other intracellular proteins, will result in novel toxicities or side-effects.[106] Another question is whether farnesyltransferase of RAS is necessary for RAS processing.[107] Can the downstream proliferative effects of RAS be mediated by other pathways when the RAS pathway is inhibited? Since the preclinical data indicate that long-term administration of the FTI is necessary to suppress tumor growth, the mechanism of action appears to be cytostatic rather than cytotoxic. This suggests that combinations of FTIs with cytotoxic agents or radiation[108] might result in a more potent therapeutic effect than either alone.

ANGIOGENESIS INHIBITORS

Angiogenesis is a fundamental step in the growth and metastasis of tumors.[45,109-112] Without neurovascularization, tumors rarely grow larger than 2–3 mm³. Angiogenesis is a tightly controlled process between positive and negative regulators of microvascular growth. Tumors may overexpress one or more of the positive regulators of angiogenesis or stimulate normal cells such as macrophages to produce angiogenic substances. The most commonly found angiogenic factors in tumors are basic

Table 31.2 Angiogenesis inhibitors

Endogenous inhibitors

Platelet factor 4

Thrombospondin-1

Tissue inhibitors of metallproteinases: TIMP-1, TIMP-2, TIMP-3

Prolactin

Angiostatin

bFGF soluble receptor

TGF-β

IFN-γ

Natural products

Minocycline

AGM-1470

Herbamycin A

Tecogalan

Taxol

Hormones and vitamins

Corticosteroids

Medroxyprogesterone

Estrogens

Antiestrogens

Vitamin D analogs

Retinoids

Polysulfated and glycosylated compounds

Suramin

Pentosan polysulfate

Protamine

Cartilage-derived factors

Vitreous extract

Heparin analogs

Sulfated polysaccharide peptidoglycans

Miscellaneous agents

D-Penicillamine

Inhibitors of prostaglandin synthesis

Gold salts

Anti-bFGF monoclonal antibodies

fibroblast growth factor (bFGF) and vascular endothelial growth factor (VEGF). In addition to growth-promoting angiogenic factor, there are negative regulators of endothelial cell proliferation that normally balance the effect of the angiogenic factors. For example, bFGF soluble receptor will act to bind bFGF, thereby inhibiting the effect of bFGF. When this balance of positive and negative regulation is tilted towards the positive regulatory factors, uncontrolled angiogenesis may occur. The importance of angiogenesis in colorectal cancer[113–116] has been documented in a variety of studies that have looked at markers of angiogenesis using immunohistochemical techniques and correlated these findings with patient outcome. Furthermore, in vivo preclinical studies have demonstrated that the use of antiangiogenesis compounds in transplanted xenograft tumors of colon cancer decreased metastasis and increased the survival of animals treated with the antiangiogenesis compounds.[117–119] It should be recognized that endothelial cells will produce angiogenic factors in themselves. Furthermore, hypoxia, which is commonly found in solid tumors, can stimulate VEGF production.[120] As previously noted, RAS mutations resulting in constitutive expression of the RAS protein is associated with colorectal cancer in approximately 50% of cases. It has been reported [121] that such an RAS mutation will increase VEGF expression, which would lead to an angiogenic effect.

The central role of angiogenesis in tumor growth and metastasis has led to the development of antiangiogenesis compounds that may interfere with this process. A variety of compounds[122–144] that can interfere with angiogenesis have been identified. These may be categorized as endogenous inhibitors of angiogenesis, which include angiostatin and platelet factor 4, natural products such as minocycline and AGM 1470, hormones and vitamins such as steroids and retinoids, polysulfated and glycosylated compounds like suramin, and miscellaneous agents (see Table 31.2). It should be noted that MMPIs, as discussed previously, may act, in part, by inhibiting angiogenesis. While studies of many of these agents are still in a preliminary stage, some have undergone phase I testing. The utility of these compounds – either alone or in combination with therapeutic agents – is currently unknown. Preliminary studies[145,146] have explored the feasibility of combining angiogenesis inhibitors with cytotoxic agents. The use of an inhibitor of angiogenesis in combination with classical anticancer drugs will have to be carefully evaluated, since

adequate vascular access to tumor cells is critical for drug delivery.

With the variety of new approaches that are currently being investigated will come many opportunities for clinical trials in patients with colorectal cancer.

REFERENCES

1. Au JL, Freidman MA, Sadeed W, Pharmacokinetics and metabolism of Ftorafur in man. *Cancer Treat Rep* 1979; **63:** 343–50.
2. Ikenaka K, Shirasaka T, Kitano S, Effect of uracil on metabolism of 5-fluorouracil in vitro. *Gann* 1979; **70:** 353–9.
3. Fujii S, Ikenaka M, Fukushima M et al, Effect of coadministration of uracil or cytosine on the antitumor activity of clinical doses of 1-(2-tetrahydro-furyl)-5-fluorouracil and level of 5-fluorouracil in rodents. *Gann* 1979; **70:** 209–14.
4. Pazdur R, Covington WP, Brown NS et al, Comparative steady state pharmacokinetics of oral UFT versus protracted intravenous 5-fluorouracil. *Proc Am Soc Clin Oncol* 1996; **15:** 474.
5a. Watanabe H, Yamamoto S, Naito T, Clinical results of oral UFT therapy under cooperative study. *Jpn J Cancer Chemother* 1988; **7:** 1588–96.
5b. Ota K, Taguchi T, Kumura K, Report on nation-wide pooled data and cohort investigation in UFT phase II study. *Cancer Chemother Pharmacol* 1988; **22:** 333–8.
6. Malik STA, Talbot D, Clarke PI et al, Phase II trial of UFT in advanced colorectal and gastric cancer. *Br J Cancer* 1990; **62:** 1023–5.
7. Saltz LB, Leichman CG, Young CW et al, A fixed-ratio combination of uracil and Ftorafur (UFT) with low dose leucovorin. An active regimen for advanced colorectal cancer. *Cancer* 1995; **75:** 782–5.
8. Pazdur R, Lassere Y, Rhodes V et al, Phase II trial of uracil and tegafur plus oral leucovorin: an effective oral regimen in the treatment of metastatic colorectal carcinoma. *J Clin Oncol* 1994; **12:** 2296–300.
9. Sanchez F, Milla A, Tegafur. Uracil (UFT) plus folinic acid in advanced rectal cancer. *Jpn J Clin Oncol* 1994; **24:** 322–6.
10. Nogue M, Segui M, Batiste E et al, Phase II

study of oral tegafur (TF) and low-dose oral leucovorin (LV) in advanced colorectal cancer (ACC). *Proc Am Soc Clin Oncol* 1996; **15:** 200.
11. Grem JL, Fluoridinated pyrimidines. In: *Cancer Chemotherapy Principals and Practice* (Chabner BA, Colloins JA, eds). Philadelphia: Lippincott, 1990; 180–224.
12. Okeda R, Shibutani M, Matsuo T et al, Experimental neurotoxicity of 5-fluorouracil and its derivatives is due to poisoning by the monofluorinated organic metabolites, monofluoroacetic acid and alpha-fluoro-beta-alanine. *Acta Neuropathol* 1990; **81:** 66–73.
13. Fleming RA, Milano G, Gaspard MH et al, Dihydropyrimidine dehydrogenase in cancer patients. *Eur J Cancer* 1993; **29A:** 740–4.
14. Porter DJT, Chestnut WG, Merril BM et al, Mechanism-based inactivation of dihydropyrimidine dehydrogenase by 5-ethinyluracil. *J Biol Chem* 1992; **267:** 5236–42.
15. Khor SP, Lucas S, Schilsky R et al, A phase I/pharmacokinetic study of 5-ethynyluracil plus 5-fluorouracil in cancer patients with solid tumors. *Proc Am Assoc Cancer Res* 1995; **36:** 241.
16. Baccanari DP, Davis ST, Knick VC et al, 5-Ethynyluracil (776C85): a potent modulator of the pharmacokinetics and anti-tumor efficacy of 5-fluorouracil. *Proc Natl Acad Sci USA* 1993; **90:** 11 064–8.
17. Cao S, Rustum YM, Spector T, 5-Ethynyluracil (776C85): modulation of 5-fluorouracil efficacy and therapeutic index in rats bearing advanced colorectal carcinoma. *Cancer Res* 1994; **54:** 1507–10.
18. Adjei AA, Doucette M, Spector T et al, 5-Ethynyluracil (776C85) an inhibitor of dihydropyrimidine dehydrogenase (DPD), permits reliable oral dosing of 5-fluorouracil (5-FU) and

prolongs its half-life. *Proc Am Soc Clin Oncol* 1995; **14**: 459.

19. Baker SD, Diasio R, Lucas VS et al, Phase I and pharmacologic study of oral 5-fluorouracil (5-FU) on a chronic 28-day schedule in combination with the dihydropyrimidine dehydrogenase (DPD) inactivator 776C85. *Proc Am Soc Clin Oncol* 1996; **15**: 486.

20. Schilsky RL, Burris H, Ratain M et al, Phase I clinical and pharmacologic study of 776C85 (776) plus 5-fluorouracil (5-FU) in patients with advanced cancer. *Proc Am Soc Clin Oncol* 1996; **15**: 485.

21. Taguchi T, Shirasaka T, New oral antitumor agent: S-1. Ninth NCI–EORTC Symposium, Amsterdam, Netherlands, 13 March 1996.

22. Houghton JA, Houghton PJ, Wooten RS, Mechanism of induction of gastrointestinal toxicity in the mouse by 5-fluorouracil, 5-fluorouridine, and 5-fluoro-2'-deoxyuridine. *Cancer Res* 1979; **39**: 2406–13.

23. Shirasaka T, Shimamoto Y, Fukushima M, Inhibition by oxonic acid and gastrointestinal toxicity of 5-fluorouracil without loss of its antitumor activity in rats. *Cancer Res* 1993; **53**: 4004–9.

24. Horikoshi N, Mitachi Y, Sakata Y et al, S-1, new oral fluoropyrimidine is very active in patients with advanced gastric cancer (early phase II study). *Proc Am Soc Clin Oncol* 1996; **15**: 206.

25. O'Connell MJ, Maillaird JA, Kahn MJ et al, A controlled trial of 5-fluorouracil and low-dose leucovorin given for 6 months as post operative adjuvant therapy for colon cancer. *J Clin Oncol* 1997; **15**: 246.

26. Anonymous, Modulation of fluorouracil by leucovorin in patients with advanced colon cancer: evidence in terms of response rate. *J Clin Oncol* 1990; **10**: 896–9.

27. Jones TR, Calvert AH, Jackman AL et al, A potent antitumor quinazoline inhibitor of thymidylate synthase: synthesis, biologic properties and therapeutic results in mice. *Eur J Cancer* 1981; **17**: 11–19.

28. Calvert AH, Alison DL, Harland SJ et al, A phase I evaluation of the quinazoline antifol thymidyllate synthase inhibitor N^{10}-propargyl-5,8-dideazafolic acid (CB3717). *J Clin Oncol* 1986; **4**: 1245–52.

29. Jackman AL, Taylor GA, Gibson W et al, ICI D1694, a quinazoline antifol thymidylate synthase inhibitor that is a potent inhibitor of L1210 tumor cell growth in vitro and in vivo: a new agent for clinical study. *Cancer Res* 1991; **51**: 5579–86.

30. Sorenson JM, Jordan E, Grem JL et al, Phase I trial of D1694, a pure thymidylate synthase inhibitor. *Proc Am Soc Clin Oncol* 1993; **12**: 158.

31. Judson I, Clarke S, Ward J et al, Pharmacokinetics (PK) of ICI D1694 following a 15 minute infusion in patients with advanced cancer. *Proc Am Soc Clin Oncol* 1992; **11**: 117.

32. Zalcberg JR, Cunningham D, Van Cutsem E et al, ZD 1694, a novel thymidylate synthase inhibitor with substantial activity in the treatment of patients with advanced colorectal cancer. *J Clin Oncol* 1996; **14**: 716–21.

33. Seitz JF, Cunningham D, Rath U et al, Final results and survival data of a large randomised trial of 'Tomudex' in advanced colorectal cancer (ACC) confirm comparable efficacy to 5-fluorouracil plus leucovorin. *Proc Am Soc Clin Oncol* 1996; **15**: 201.

34. Prendergast W, Dickerson SH, Johnson JV et al, Benzoquinazoline inhibitors of thymidylate synthase: enzyme inhibitory activity and cytotoxicity of some sulfonamidobenzoylglutamate and related derivatives. *J Med Chem* 1993; **36**: 3464–71.

35. Burris HA, Smetzer LA, Eckardt GI et al, A phase I trial of the novel thymidylate synthase inhibitor 1843U89 with and without high dose oral folate. *Proc Am Soc Clin Oncol* 1996; **15**: 490.

36. Grindley GB, Shih C, Barnett CJ et al, LY231514. A novel pyrrolopyrimidine antifolate that inhibits thymidylate synthase. *Proc Am Assoc Canc Res* 1992; **33**: 411.

37. Rinaldi DA, Burris HA, Dorr FA et al, A phase I evaluation of a novel thymidylate synthase inhibitor, LY231514, in patients with advanced solid tumors. *Proc Am So Clin Oncol* 1994; **13**: 159.

38. Rinaldi DA, Burris FA, Dorr FA et al, A phase I evaluation of LY231514, a novel multitargeted antifolate, administered every 21 days. *Proc Am Soc Clin Oncol* 1996; **15**: 489.

39. Jackson RC, Boritzki TK, Johnston Al et al, Design and development of lipophilic inhibitors of thymidylate synthase. *Proc Am Assoc Cancer Res* 1992; **33**: 592–3.

40. Webber S, Johnston A, Shetty B et al, Preclinical studies on AG-337, a novel lipophilic thymidylate synthase inhibitor. *Proc Am Assoc Cancer Res* 1993; **34**: 273.

41. Rafi I, Taylor GA, Calvette JA et al, A phase I clinical study of the novel antifolate AG-337

given by a 5 day continuous infusion. *Proc Am Assoc Cancer Res* 1995; **36:** 240.

42. Calvete JA, Balmanno K, Rafi I et al, Preclinical and clinical studies of the novel thymidylate synthase inhibitor AG-337, given by oral administration. *Proc Am Assoc Cancer Res* 1995; **36:** 380.

43. Ennis BW, Matrisian LM, Matrix degrading metalloproteinases. *J Neuro-Oncol* 1993; **18:** 105–9.

44. Himelstein BP, Canete-Soler R, Bernhard EJ et al, Metalloproteinases in tumor progression: the contribution of MMP-9. *Invasion Metastasis* 1994; **14:** 246–58.

45. Kohn EC, Liotta LA, Molecular insights into cancer invasion: strategies for prevention and intervention. *Cancer Res* 1995; **55:** 1856–62.

46. Sato H, Motoharu S, Membrane-type matrix metalloproteinases (MT-MMPs) in tumor metastases. *J Biochem* 1996; **119:** 209–15.

47. Mauviel A, Cytokine regulation of metalloproteinase gene expression. *J Cell Biochem* 1993; **53:** 288–95.

48. Crawford HC, Matrisian LM, Tumor and stromal expression of matrix metalloproteinases and their role in tumor progression. *Invasion Metastasis* 1994; **14:** 234–45.

49. Itoh F, Hinoda Y, Kakiuchi H et al, In vivo metastatic potential of matrilysin (MMP-7) transfected human colorectal cancer cells. *Proc Annu Meet Am Assoc Cancer Res* 1995; **36:** A617.

50. Heppner KJ, Matrisian LM, Matrix metalloproteinase expression in intestinal tumors from the min mouse model of colorectal cancer. *Proc Annu Meet Am Assoc Cancer Res* 1995; **36:** A599.

51. Itoh F, Hinoda Y, Kakiuchi H et al, In vivo metastatic potential of matrilysin (MMP-7) transfected human colorectal cancer cells. *Proc Annu Meet Am Assoc Cancer Res* 1995; **36:** A617.

52. Itoh F, Hinoda Y, Yamamoto H et al, Regulation of matrilysin (MMP-7) mRNA expression in human colorectal cancers. *Proc Annu Meet Am Assoc Cancer Res* 1994; **35:** A376.

53. Jessup JM, Cathepsin B and other proteases in human colorectal carcinoma. *Am J Pathol* 1994; **145:** 253–62.

54. Liabakk NB, Talbot I, Smith RA et al, Matrix metalloprotease 2 (MMP-2) and matrix metalloprotease 9 (MMP-9) type IV collagenases in colorectal cancer. *Cancer Res* 1996; **56:** 190–6.

55. Newell KJ, Witty JP, Rodgers WH, Matrisian LM, Expression and localization of matrix-degrading metalloproteinases during colorectal

tumorigenesis. *Mol Carcinogen* 1994; **10:** 199–206.

56. Porte H, Chastre E, Prevot S et al, Neoplastic progression of human colorectal cancer is associated with overexpression of the stromelysin-3 and BM-40/SPARC genes. *Int J Cancer* 1995; **64:** 70–5.

57. Poulson R, Pignatelli M, Stetler-Stevenson WG et al, Stromal expression of 72-kD type IV collagenase and TIMP-2 mRNAs in colorectal neoplasia. *J Pathol* 1992; **167:** 150A.

58. Thompson EW, Yu M, Beuno J et al, Collagen induced MMP-2 activation in human breast cancer. *Breast Cancer Res Treat* 1994; **31:** 357–70.

59. Urbanski SJ, Edwards DR, Hershfield N et al, Expression pattern of metalloproteinases and their inhibitors changes with the progression of human sporadic colorectal neoplasia. *Diagnos Mol Pathol* 1993; **2:** 81–9.

60. Yamamoto H, Itoh F, Hinoda Y et al, Expression of matrilysin mRNA in colorectal adenomas and its induction by truncated fibronectin. *Biochem Biophys Res Commun* 1994; **201:** 657–664.

61. Yoshimoto M, Itoh F, Yamamoto H et al, Expression of MMP-7 (PUMP-1) mRNA in human colorectal cancers. *Int J Cancer* 1993; **54:** 614–18.

62. Zeng ZS, Cohen AM, Guillem JG, Secretion of activated matrix metalloproteinases-2 and 9 is associated with metastases in human colorectal cancer. *Proc Annu Meet Am Assoc Cancer Res* 1995; **36:** A465.

63. Roose JP, Van Noorden CJ, Synthetic protease inhibitors: promising compounds to arrest pathobiologic processes. *J Lab Clin Med* 1995; **125:** 433–41.

64. Brown PD, Giavazzi R, Matrix metalloproteinase inhibition – a review of antitumor activity. *Ann Oncol* 1995; **6:** 967–74.

65. Chirivi RG, Garofalo A, Crimmin MJ et al, Inhibition of the metastatic spread and growth of B16-BL6 murine melanoma by a synthetic matrix metalloproteinase inhibitor. *Int J Cancer* 1994; **58:** 460–4.

66. Brown PD, Clinical trials of a low molecular weight matrix metalloproteinase inhibitor in cancer. *Ann NY Acad Sci* 1994; **732:** 217–21.

67. Watson SA, Morris TM, Robinson G et al, Inhibition of organ invasion by the matrix metalloproteinase inhibitor batimastat (BB-94) in two human colon carcinoma metastasis models. *Cancer Res* 1995; **55:** 3629–33.

68. Watson SA, Brown PD, Morris TM et al, The

matrix metalloproteinase inhibitor BB94 inhibits experimental metastasis and ascites formation of the human colorectal tumor, C170HM2. *Br J Cancer* 1994; **69:** 19.

69. Taraboletti G, Garofalo A, Belotti D et al, Inhibition of angiogenesis and murine hemangioma growth by batimastat, a synthetic inhibitor of matrix metalloproteinases. *J Nat Cancer Inst* 1995; **87:** 293–8.

70. Wang X, Fu, X, Brown PD et al, Matrix metalloproteinase inhibitor BB-94 (batimastat) inhibits human colon tumor growth and spread in a patient-like orthotopic model in nude mice. *Cancer Res* 1994; **54:** 4726–8.

71. Drummond AH, Beckett P, Bone EA et al, BB-2516: an orally bioavailable matrix metalloproteinase inhibitor with efficacy in animal cancer models. *Proc Annu Meet Am Assoc Cancer Res* 1995; **36:** A595.

72. Santos O, Daniels R, McDermott C, Appelt K, Anti-tumor studies with the synthetic matrix metalloproteinase inhibitors AG3319 and AG3340. *Proc Annu Meet Am Assoc Cancer Res* 1996; **37:** 90 (abst).

73. Cho KR, Vogelstein B, Genetic alterations in the adenoma–carcinoma sequence. *Cancer* 1992; **70:** 1727–31.

74. Kern SE, Hamilton SR, Vogelstein B, Clinical implications of colorectal tumor mutations. In: *Molecular Foundations of Oncology* (Broder S, ed). Baltimore: Williams and Wilkins, 1991; 381–90.

75. Sidransky D, Tokino T, Hamilton SR et al, Identification of RAS oncogene mutations in the stool of patients with curable colorectal cancer. *Science* 1992; **256:** 102–5.

76. Margolis B, Skolnik EY, Activation of Ras by receptor tyrosine kinases. *J Am Soc Nephrol* 1994; **5:** 1288–99.

77. Gibbs JB, Oliff A, Kohl NE, Farnesyltransferase inhibitors: Ras research yields a potential cancer therapeutic. *Cell* 1994; **77:** 175–8.

78. Cox AD, Garcia AM, Westwick JK et al, The CAAX peptidomimetic compound B581 specifically blocks farnesylated, but not geranylgeranylated or myristylated, oncogenic Ras signaling and transformation. *J Biol Chem* 1994; **260:** 19 203–6.

79. Garcia AM, Rowell C, Ackermann K et al, Peptidomimetic inhibitors of Ras farnesylation and function in whole cells. *J Biol Chem* 1993; **268:** 18 415–18.

80. Graham SL, DeSolms SJ, Giuliani EA et al, Pseudopeptide inhibitors of Ras farnesyl-protein transferase. *J Med Chem* 1994; **37:** 725–32.

81. Hall CC, Watkins JD, Ferguson SB et al, Inhibitors of farnesyltransferase and Ras processing peptidase. *Biochem Biophys Res Commun* 1995; **217:** 728–32.

82. Kang MS, Stemerick DM, Zwolshen JH et al, Farnesyl-derived inhibitors of ras farnesyl transferase. *Biochem Biophys Res Commun* 1995; **217:** 245–9.

83. Nigam M, Seong CM, Qian Y et al, Potent inhibition of human tumor p21ras farnesyltransferase by A1A2-lacking p21ras CA1A2X peptidomimetics. *J Biol Chem* 1993; **268:** 20 695–8.

84. Tamamoi F, Inhibitors of Ras farnesyltransferases. *Trends Biochem Sci* 1993; **18:** 349–53.

85. Gelb MH, Tamanoi F, Yokoyama K et al, The inhibition of protein prenyltransferases by oxygenated metabolites of limonene and perillyl alcohol. *Cancer Lett* 1995; **91:** 169–75.

86. Karlson J, Borgkarlson AK, Unelius R et al, Inhibition of tumor cell growth by monoterpenes in vitro – evidence of a RAS-independent mechanism of action. *Anti-Cancer Drugs* 1996; **7:** 422–9.

87. Bergstrom JD, Kurtz MM, Rew DJ et al, Zaragozic acids: a family of fungal metabolites that are picomolar competitive inhibitors of squalene synthase. *Proc Natl Acad Sci* 1993; **90:** 80–4.

88. Jayasuriya H, Ball RG, Zink DL et al, Barceloneic acid A, a new farnesyl-protein transferase inhibitor from a *Phoma* species. *J Nat Prod* 1995; **58:** 986–91.

89. Sepp-Lorenzino L, Ma ZP, Bands E et al, A peptidomimetic inhibitor of farnesyl:protein transferase blocks the anchorage-dependent and -independent growth of human tumor cell lines. *Cancer Res* 1995; **55:** 5302–9.

90. Lerner EC, Qian Y, Blaskovich MA et al, Ras CAAX peptidomimetic FTI-277 selectively blocks oncogenic Ras signaling by inducing cytoplasmic accumulation of inactive Ras–Raf complexes. *J Biol Chem* 1995; **270:** 802–6.

91. Vogt A, Qian Y, Blaskovich MA et al, A non-peptide mimetic of Ras-CAAX: selective inhibition of farnesyltransferase and Ras processing. *J Biol Chem* 1995; **270:** 660–4.

92. Kohl NE, Mosser SD, DeSolms SJ et al, Selective inhibition of ras-dependent transformation by a farnesyltransferase inhibitor. *Science* 1993; **260:** 1934–7.

93. Ma Y, Gilbert BA, Rando RR, Inhibitors of the isoprenylated protein endoprotease. *Biochemistry* 1993; **32**: 2386–93.

94. Sepp-Lorenzino L, Ma ZP, Rands E et al, A peptidomimetic inhibitor of farnesyl:protein transferase blocks the anchorage-dependent and -independent growth of human tumor cell lines. *Cancer Res* 1995; **55**: 5302–9.

95. Nagase T, Kawata S, Tamura S et al, Inhibition of cell growth of human hepatoma cell line (Hep G2) by a farnesyl protein transferase inhibitor: a preferential suppression of ras farnesylation. *Int J Cancer* 1996; **65**: 620–6.

96. Nagasu T, Yoshimatu K, Rowell C et al, Inhibition of human tumor xenograft growth by treatment with the farnesyl transferase inhibitor B956. *Cancer Res* 1995; **55**: 5310–14

97. Sebti SM, Tkalcevic GT, Jani JP, Lovostatin, a cholesterol biosynthesis inhibitor, inhibits the growth of human h-RAS oncogene transformed cells in nude mice. *Cancer Commun* 1991; **3**: 141–7.

98. Prendergast GC, Davide JP, DeSolms SJ et al, Farnesyltransferase inhibition causes morphological reversion of ras-transformed cells by a complex mechanism that involves regulation of the actin cytoskeleton. *Mol Cell Biol* 1994; **14**: 4193–202.

99. Kohl NE, Omer CA, Conner MW et al, Inhibition of farnesyltransferase induces regression of mammary and salivary carcinomas in ras transgenic mice. *Nature Med* 1995; **1**: 792–7.

100. James GL, Goldstein JL, Brown MS et al, Benzodiazepine peptidomimetics: potent inhibitors of Ras farnesylation in animal cells. *Science* 1993; **260**: 1937–42.

101. Kothapalli R, Guthrie N, Chambers AF, Carroll KK, Farnesylamine: an inhibitor of farnesylation and growth of ras-transformed cells. *Lipids* 1993; **28**: 969–73.

102. Kohl NE, Wilson FR, Mosser SD et al, Protein farnesyltransferase inhibitors block the growth of ras-dependent tumors in nude mice. *Proc Natl Acad Sci USA* 1994; **91**: 9141–5.

103. Gibbs JB, Kohl NE, Pompliano DL et al, Selective inhibition of Ras-dependent cell transformation by a farnesyl-protein transferase inhibitor. *FASEB J* 1993; **7**: A1048.

104. Leftheris K, Kline T, Vite GD et al, Development of highly potent inhibitors of Ras farnesyltransferase possessing cellular and in vivo activity. *J Med Chem* 1996; **39**: 224–36.

105. Prendergast GC, Davide JP, Lebowitz PF et al, Resistance of a variant ras-transformed cell line to phenotypic reversion by farnesyl transferase inhibitors. *Cancer Res* 1996; **56**: 2626–32.

106. Pittler SJ, Fliesler SJ, Fisher PL et al, In vivo requirements of protein prenylation for maintenance of retinal cytoarchitecture and photoreceptor structure. *J Cell Biol* 1995; **130**: 431–9.

107. Dalton MB, Sinensky M, Farnesylation independent processing of p21ras. *FASEB J* 1995; **9**: A1315.

108. Bernhard EJ, Kao G, Cox AD et al, The farnesyltransferase inhibitor FTI-277 radiosensitizes H-ras-transformed rat embryo fibroblasts. *Cancer Res* 1996; **56**: 1727–30.

109. Cockerill GW, Gamble JR, Vadas MA, Angiogenesis: models and modulators. *Int Rev Cytol* 1995; **159**: 113–60.

110. Folkman J, Ingber D, Inhibition of angiogenesis. *Semin Cancer Biol* 1992; **3**: 89–96.

111. Folkman J, Clinical applications of research on angiogenesis. *N Engl J Med* 1995; **333**: 1757–1763.

112. Sipos EP, Tamargo RJ, Weingart JD, Brem H, Inhibition of tumor angiogenesis. *Ann NY Acad Sci* 1994; **732**: 263–72.

113. Bossi P, Viale G, Lee AK et al, Angiogenesis in colorectal tumors: microvessel quantitation in adenomas and carcinomas with clinicopathological correlations. *Cancer Res* 1995; **55**: 5049–53.

114. Frank RE, Saclarides TJ, Leurgans S et al, Tumor angiogenesis as a predictor of recurrence and survival in patients with node-negative colon cancer. *Ann Surg* 1995; **222**: 695–9.

115. Pritchard A, Powe DG, Wilkinson M, Hewitt RE, Tumor vascularity in colorectal carcinoma. *J Pathol* 1992; **168**: 118A.

116. Takebayashi Y, Yamada K, Maruyama I et al, The expression of thymidine phosphorylase and thrombomodulin in human colorectal carcinomas. *Cancer Lett* 1995; **92**: 1–7.

117. Konno H, Tanaka T, Matsuda I et al, Comparison of the inhibitory effect of the angiogenesis inhibitor, TNP-470, and mitomycin C on the growth and liver metastasis of human colon cancer. *Int J Cancer* 1995; **61**: 268–71.

118. Gallegos NC, Smales C, Savage FJ et al, The distribution of matrix metalloproteinases and tissue inhibitor of metalloproteinases in colorectal cancer. *Surg Oncol* 1995; **4**: 111–19.

119. Konno H, Tanaka T, Kanai T et al, Efficacy of an angiogenesis inhibitor, TNP-470, in xenotrans-

planted human colorectal cancer with high metastatic potential. *Cancer* 1996; **77**: 1736–40.

120. Mukhopadhyay D, Tsiokas L, Zhou XM et al, Hypoxic induction of human vascular endothelial growth factor expression through C-SRC activation. *Nature* 1995; **375**: 577–81.

121. Rak J, Mutsuhashi Y, Bayko L et al, Mutant ras oncogenes upregulate VEGF/VPF expression: implications for induction and inhibition of tumor angiogenesis. *Cancer Res* 1995; **55**: 4575–80.

122. Eckhardt SG, Eckardt JR, Weiss G et al, Results of a phase I trial of the novel angiogenesis inhibitor, tecogalan sodium. *Proc Annu Meet Am Assoc Cancer Res* 1995; **36**: A628.

123. Kohn EC, Reed E, Sarosy G et al, Clinical investigation of a cytostatic calcium influx inhibitor in patients with refractory cancers. *Cancer Res* 1996; **56**: 569–73.

124. O'Reilly MS, Holmgren L, Shing Y et al, Angiostatin: a novel angiogenesis inhibitor that mediates the suppression of metastases by a Lewis lung carcinoma. *Cell* 1994; **79**: 315–28.

125. Oktaba AC, Hunter WL, Arsenault AL, Taxol: a potent inhibitor of normal and tumor-induced angiogenesis. *Proc Annu Meet Am Assoc Cancer Res* 1995; **36**: A2707.

126. Belman N, Lipton A, Harvey H et al, rhuPF4: phase I study of an angiogenesis inhibitor in metastatic colon cancer (MCC). *Proc Annu Meet Am Soc Clin Oncol* 1994; **13**: A670.

127. Clapp C, Martial JA, Guzman RC et al, The 16-kilodalton N-terminal fragment of human prolactin is a potent inhibitor of angiogenesis. *Endocrinology* 1993; **133**: 1292–9.

128. Fotsis T, Zhang Y, Pepper MS et al, The endogenous oestrogen metabolite 2-methoxyoestradiol inhibits angiogenesis and suppresses tumour growth. *Nature* 1994; **368**: 237–9.

129. Fotsis T, Pepper M, Adlercreutz H et al, Genistein, a dietary-derived inhibitor of in vitro angiogenesis. *Proc Natl Acad Sci USA* 1993; **90**: 2690–4.

130. Gagliardi A, Collins DC, Inhibition of angiogenesis by antiestrogens. *Cancer Res* 1993; **53**: 533–5.

131. Galardy RE, Grobelny D, Foellmer HG, Fernandez LA, Inhibition of angiogenesis by the matrix metalloprotease inhibitor N-[2R-2-(hydroxamidocarbonylmethyl)-4-methylpentanoyl)]-L-tryptophan methylamide. *Cancer Res* 1994; **54**: 4715–18.

132. Gilbertson-Beadling S, Powers EA, Stamp-Cole M et al, The tetracycline analogs minocycline and doxycycline inhibit angiogenesis in vitro by a non-metalloproteinase-dependent mechanism. *Cancer Chemother Pharmacol* 1995; **36**: 418–24.

133. Hu DE, Fan TP, Suppression of VEGF-induced angiogenesis by the protein tyrosine kinase inhibitor, lavendustin A. *Br J Pharmacol* 1995; **114**: 262–8.

134. Miyadera K, Sumizawa T, Haraguchi M et al, Role of thymidine phosphorylase activity in the angiogenic effect of platelet derived endothelial cell growth factor/thymidine phosphorylase. *Cancer Res* 1995; **55**: 1687–90.

135. Nguyen NM, Lehr JE, Pienta KJ, Pentosan inhibits angiogenesis in vitro and suppresses prostate tumor growth in vivo. *Anticancer Res* 1993; **13**: 2143–7.

136. Pluda JM, Wyvill K, Figg WD et al, A phase I study of an angiogenesis inhibitor, TNP-470 (AGM-1470), administered to patients (pts) with HIV-associated Kaposi's sarcoma (KS). *Proc Annu Meet Am Soc Clin Oncol* 1994; **13**: A8.

137. Pluda JM, Shay LE, Foli A et al, Administration of pentosan polysulfate to patients with human immunodeficiency virus-associated Kaposi's sarcoma. *J Natl Cancer Inst* 1993; **85**: 1585–92.

138. Ray JM, Stetler-Stevenson WG, The role of matrix metalloproteases and their inhibitors in tumour invasion, metastasis and angiogenesis. *Eur Resp J* 1994; **7**: 2062–72.

139. Tamargo RJ, Bok RA, Brem H, Angiogenesis inhibition by minocycline. *Cancer Res* 1991; **51**: 672–5.

140. Yamamoto T, Sudo K, Fujita T, Significant inhibition of endothelial cell growth in tumor vasculature by an angiogenesis inhibitor, TNP-470 (AGM-1470). *Anticancer Res* 1994; **14**: 1–3.

141. Yamaoka M, Yamamoto T, Ikeyama S et al, Angiogenesis inhibitor TNP-470 (AGM-1470) potently inhibits the tumor growth of hormone-independent human breast and prostate carcinoma cell lines. *Cancer Res* 1993; **53**: 5233–6.

142. Yamaoka M, Yamamoto T, Masaki T et al, Inhibition of tumor growth and metastasis of rodent tumors by the angiogenesis inhibitor O-(chloroacetyl-carbamoyl)fumagillol (TNP-470; AGM-1470). *Cancer Res* 1993; **53**: 4262–7.

143. Zukiwski A, Gutterman J, Bui C et al, Phase I trial of the angiogenesis inhibitor TNP-470 (AGM-1470) in patients (pts) with androgen-independent prostate cancer (AI PCa). *Proc Annu Meet Am Soc Clin Oncol* 1994; **13**: A795.

144. Danesi R, Del Bianchi S, Soldani P et al,

Suramin inhibits bFGF-induced endothelial cell proliferation and angiogenesis in the chick chorioallantoic membrane. *Br J Cancer* 1993; **68:** 932–8.

145. Devineni D, Klein-Szanto A, Gallo JM, Uptake of temozolomide in a rat glioma model in the presence and absence of the angiogenesis inhibitor TNP-470. *Cancer Res* 1996; **56:** 1983–7.

146. Kato T, Sato K, Kakinuma H, Matsuda Y, Enhanced suppression of tumor growth by combination of angiogenesis inhibitor *O*-(chloroacetyl-carbamoyl)fumagillol (TNP-470) and cytotoxic agents in mice. *Cancer Res* 1994; **54:** 5143–7.

32

Postoperative treatment of rectal cancer

Jean-François Bosset, Jean-Claude Horiot, Jean-Jacques Pavy

INTRODUCTION

After curative resection, the prognosis of patients with rectal cancer is strongly correlated with the depth of tumour extension through and beyond the bowel wall, the nodal involvement and the number of involved nodes.[1] The 5-year survival drops from 80% in stage I to about 60% in stage II and 40% in stage III.[2] Local recurrence (LR) remains a major site of failure, ranging from 5% in a few selected series to about 40% in most reports.[3,4] Results from the Burgundy tumour registry indicate a 5-year actuarial risk of LR of 24% and 53% in Dukes B and C respectively.[5] Local failure is responsible for major disability and painful clinical syndromes. Therefore improving local control is a major endpoint for radiotherapy in rectal cancer, which, finally, may translate into a survival gain.

POSTOPERATIVE IRRADIATION ALONE

The theoretical advantages of the postoperative approach are mostly linked to a better selection of patients, excluding those with early stages and those with synchronous metastases to focus on patients with a high LR risk. However, there are also some drawbacks:

(1) the postoperative approach is associated with a longer overall treatment duration, mainly in relation to the healing of surgical wounds;

(2) it is also generally admitted that the residual tumour cells scattered within the surgical scar are relatively hypoxic and consequently somewhat less 'radiosensitive', and a radiation-dose increment is often advised in order to deal with this phenomenon;

(3) the potential risk of late toxicity on the small bowel is increased in relation both to the higher total irradiation dose and to the likelihood of bowel fixity related to primary surgery.

Six randomized trials (Table 32.1) compared postoperative pelvic irradiation with surgery alone for selected Dukes B or C patients. A significant reduction in LR was observed in the MRC trial;[6] a non-significant reduction was also noted in the NSABP and GITSG trials,[7,8] and all the other trials were negative.[9–11] None of these demonstrated a benefit in overall survival. In a meta-analysis compiling published and unpublished series, the annual LR rate was significantly reduced, in favour of a definite local benefit for radiotherapy, but no significant survival gain was observed.[12] The compliance with

Table 32.1 Local-control effect of postoperative irradiation in randomized trials; the radiotherapy dose ranged from 40 to 50 Gy

	Number of patients	Local-control increase	p value
Denmark[11]	494	Dukes C = No	0.47
		Dukes B = No	0.40
GITSG[8]	108	No	0.06
NSABP[7]	368	No	0.06
Netherlands[10]	172	No	Not available
EORTC[9]	172	No	0.46
MRC[6]	469	Yes	0.001

the postoperative treatment was disappointing; overall, 12–27% of the patients did not receive the planned dose. Late complications were not increased by irradiation in the MRC trial,[6] contrasting with 20% of the patients suffering chronic diarrhoea in the EORTC study.[9] Finally, lethal treatment-related complications occurred in 1–3%. Altogether, postoperative irradiation alone displays a moderate local effect without survival improvement; this figure has widely been considered insufficient.

POSTOPERATIVE IRRADIATION PLUS CHEMOTHERAPY

Combining chemotherapy with postoperative radiotherapy was a logical treatment evolution. It started in the mid-1970s in the USA. The rationales were

(1) to increase the local effect of radiotherapy by chemotherapy;
(2) to reduce the risk of distant metastasis.

This approach was constructed in two segments. One segment was a concomitant chemoradiotherapy sequence during which 5-

fluorouracil (5-FU) was administered, and the other segment was an adjuvant chemotherapy sequence.

Four randomized trials have been conducted. They demonstrated that this approach was able to significantly decrease LR and distant metastases (DM), and increase overall survival in comparison with surgery alone[13,14] or with postoperative irradiation alone.[15] The addition of semustine to the 5-FU adjuvant chemotherapy did not demonstrate any advantage compared with 5-FU alone.[16] Finally, it is observed that protracted delivery of 5-FU during all the irradiation duration was able to significantly decrease DM and significantly increase overall survival in comparison with a concurrent 5-FU bolus scheme.[17] The main results of the three positive trials are summarized in Table 32.2. At the beginning of this approach, grade 3 or more acute toxicities were observed in up to 60% of the patients, leading to a poor compliance; furthermore, there were about 5% toxic deaths. Decreasing the number of chemotherapy courses, improving the radiotherapy technique, using four fields rather than two, and certainly gaining experience, permitted, in the last study,[17] an improvement in the therapeutic

Table 32.2 Effects of postoperative combined irradiation and chemotherapy in randomized trials

Trial	Scheme[a]	Number of patients	Local-control increase	Distant-metastases decrease	Survival increase
GITSG[8,13,14]	Surgery versus XRT 5-FU + 5-FU semustine (8 courses)	104	No (0.06)	No (0.06)	Yes (0.005)
NCCTG[15]	XRT versus XRT 5-FU + 5-FU semustine (2 courses)	204	Yes (0.03)	Yes (0.01)	Yes (0.02)
Intergroup US trial[17]	XRT 5-FU bolus versus XRT 5-FU PVI	660	No (0.11)	Yes (0.03)	Yes (0.005)

[a] The positive arm of each trial is underlined.

Table 32.3 Acute toxicity and compliance in postoperative combined irradiation chemotherapy trials

Trial[a]	% grade 3 or more toxicity		% treatment stopped	% toxic death
	Haematology	Diarrhoea		
GITSG[8,13,14]	26	35	35	4
NCCTG[15]	33	41	35	2
Intergroup US trial:[17] Bolus	11	14	2	<0.5
PVI	2	24	3	<0.5

[a] In GITSG a two-field treatment technique was used; in the other two trials a four-field technique was used.

ratio. Toxicity has been reduced: toxic deaths are now less than 1%, late small-bowel obstruction in the combined-modality arms is comparable to what is observed after surgery alone (1–3%), and, finally, excellent compliance is obtained (Table 32.3).

RECOMMENDATIONS

In 1990, the published conclusions of the US NIH Consensus Conference stated that postoperative chemoradiotherapy should be recommended as a standard treatment for rectal cancer patients in stages II and III. This attitude can still be advised in patients who were not considered for a preoperative approach. As demonstrated by the history of the US studies, multidisciplinary harmonization, expertise and quality-assurance procedures are required to obtain the best possible therapeutic ratio.

Treatment recommendations will therefore include surgical procedures to avoid small-bowel fixity, to reduce its volume within the pelvis and to shorten healing duration. Pelvic reconstruction/reperitonization, prevention of haemorrhages, and omental pedicle flap are recommended; temporary devices are also considered. For radiotherapy, a four-field technique, treatment in the prone position with full bladder, small-bowel visualization, delineation of limited pelvic volume, and use of customized shielding blocks are all efficient measures.[18-20]

CONCLUSIONS

In conclusion, postoperative combined irradiation and chemotherapy has demonstrated a definitive efficacy in the adjuvant setting or rectal cancer patients. Expertise is required to lower its toxicity. However, this approach possibly alters the residual sphincter function[21] – an aspect that should be considered as a new endpoint in future studies.[22]

REFERENCES

1. Minsky BD, Mies C, Recht A et al, Resectable adenocarcinoma of the rectosigmoid and rectum. I Patterns of failure and survival. *Cancer* 1988; **61:** 1408–16.
2. Malafosse M, Fourtanier G, *Le traitement des cancers du rectum.* Paris: Monographie de l'Association Française de Chirurgie, Doin, 1987.
3. Heald RJ, Ryall RD, Recurrence and survival after total mesorectal excision for rectal cancer. *Lancet* 1986; **i:** 1479–81.
4. Hurst PA, Prout WG, Kelly JM et al, Local recurrence after low anterior resection using the staple gun. *Br J Surg* 1982; **69:** 275–6.
5. Faivre J, Milan C, Meny B, Risque de récidive loco-régionale après exérèse d'un cancer du rectum. *Ann Chir* 1994; **6:** 520–4.
6. Medical Research Council Rectal Cancer Working Party, Randomised trial of surgery alone versus surgery followed by radiotherapy for mobile cancer of the rectum. *Lancet* 1996; **348:** 1610–14.
7. Fisher B, Wolmark N, Rockette H et al, Postoperative adjuvant chemotherapy or radiation therapy for rectal cancer: results from NSABP Protocol R-01. *J Natl Cancer Inst* 1988; **80:** 21–9.
8. Thomas PRM, Lindblad AS, Adjuvant postoperative radiotherapy and chemotherapy in rectal carcinoma: a review of the Gastrointestinal Tumor Study Group Experience. *Radiother Oncol* 1988; **13:** 245–52.
9. Arnaud JP, Nordlinger B, Bosset JF et al, Radical surgery and postoperative radiotherapy as combined treatment in rectal cancer. Final results of a phase III study of the European Organization for Research and Treatment of Cancer. *Br J Surg* 1997; **84:** 352–7.
10. Treurniet-Donket AD, Van Putten LJ, Wereldsma JC et al, Postoperative radiation therapy for rectal cancer. *Cancer* 1991; **67:** 2042–8.
11. Bentzen SM, Balslev I, Pedersen M et al, A regression analysis of prognosis factors after resection of Dukes' B and C carcinoma of the rectum and rectosigmoid. Does postoperative radiotherapy change the prognosis? *Br J Cancer* 1988; **58:** 195–201.
12. Gray R, Adjuvant radiotherapy: a meta-analysis. *Proc Eur Conf Clin Oncol 8* 1995; abst 314.
13. Gastrointestinal Tumor Study Group, Prolongation of the disease-free interval in surgically treated rectal carcinoma. *N Engl J Med* 1985; **312:** 1465–72.
14. Douglas HO, Moertel CG, on behalf of the Gastrointestinal Study Group, Survival after postoperative combination treatment of rectal cancer. *N Engl J Med* 1986; **315:** 1294.
15. Krook JE, Moertel CG, Gunderson LI et al, Effective surgical adjuvant therapy for high-risk rectal carcinoma. *N Engl J Med* 1991; **324:** 709–15.
16. Gastrointestinal Tumor Study Group, Radiation therapy and fluorouracil with or without semus-

tine for the treatment of patients with surgical adjuvant adenocarcinoma of the rectum. *J Clin Oncol* 1992; **10:** 549–57.

17. O'Connel MJ, Martenson JA, Wieand HS et al, Improving adjuvant therapy of rectal cancer by combining protracted-infusion fluorouracil with radiation therapy after curative surgery. *N Engl J Med* 1994; **331:** 502–7.

18. Gunderson L, Russell AH, Lewellyn HJ et al, Treatment planning for colorectal cancer: radiation and surgical techniques and value of small-bowel films. *Int J Radiat Oncol Biol Phys* 1985; **11:** 1379–93.

19. Letschert JGJ, The prevention of radiation-induced small bowel complications. *Eur J Cancer* 1995; **31A:** 1361–5.

20. Martenson JA, Urias R, Smalley M et al, Radiation therapy quality control in a clinical trial of adjuvant treatment for rectal cancer. *Int J Radiat Oncol Biol Phys* 1995; **32:** 51–5.

21. Kollmorgen CF, Meagher AP, Wolff BG et al, The long-term effects of adjuvant postoperative chemoradiotherapy for rectal carcinoma on bowel function. *Ann Surg* 1994; **220:** 676–82.

22. Bosset JF, Mercier M, Pelissier EP et al, Validation of a patient questionnaire testing the functional results after sphincter sparing surgery for rectal cancer with correlation with the EORTC QLQC30. *Proc Eur Soc Therapeut Radiol Oncol* 1994; **32:** 544 (abst).

33

Biological therapies for colorectal cancer

Thierry Velu, Yves Bécouarn

CONTENTS • **Introduction** • **Non-specific agents for immunotherapy** • **Cell therapy** • **Monoclonal antibodies** • **Cytokines** • **Gene therapy** • **Conclusions**

INTRODUCTION

Because chemotherapy of colorectal cancers is still of limited efficacy, major efforts are being made to develop other therapeutic strategies.[1-4] In this chapter, the different strategies of biotherapy used for the treatment of colorectal cancers are reviewed. Most are immunotherapeutic approaches, aiming at stimulating antitumour immune responses.[5-10] The rational basis of each strategy will be discussed each time that this is possible, before summarizing the experience gained from clinical trials. Non-specific immunotherapeutic agents, specific active immunotherapy, monoclonal antibodies, cytokines, and cell and gene therapies will be evaluated successively.

During the last few decades, the huge development of molecular biology, especially in the field of genetics and immunology, has brought an enormous wealth of information that will very likely have major impacts on the diagnosis, prevention and treatment of diseases, including cancers. The treatments emerging from this research are now frequently designated as *biological therapies*, or *biotherapies*. This rapidly expanding field includes not only many strategies of immunotherapy, but also treatments based either on the processing of cells that are injected to the patients (*cell therapy*) or on the ex vivo or in vivo therapeutic transfer of a gene in cells of patients (*gene therapy*). These latter therapies are being developed for almost any category of diseases, from cystic fibrosis to cardiovascular disorders, cancers or AIDS.

Immunotherapy can be divided in two major categories: active and passive.

Active immunotherapy consists in stimulating the antitumoral immunity of the host. This stimulation can be obtained following two different strategies:

- directly (specific immunotherapy), through vaccines elaborated from tumours, with the objective of developing an antitumour response against the tumour antigens; or
- indirectly (non-specific immunotherapy), through the use of products of very different origin, like immunomodulators (BCG or levamisole) or cytokines.

Passive immunotherapy consists in administrating agents with antitumoral properties that are either spontaneous, such as monoclonal antibodies[9-12] or in vitro induced cells such as lymphokine-activated killer (LAK) cells or tumour-infiltrating lymphocytes (TIL). This simplified presentation of immunotherapy has limitations: for example, the monoclonal antibodies can have either an active or a passive mechanism of action; also, when used alone, the TIL can be considered more as a passive immunity, although they are frequently associated with the administration of interleukin-2 (IL-2) or other cytokines.[9,13] Strategies combining immunotherapy (mainly with cytokines) and chemotherapy are also being developed.

Palliative and adjuvant immunotherapies are frequently evaluated similarly to chemotherapy.[16] However, differences may exist, and may have an impact on the design of classical phase I, II or III clinical trials. For example, the evaluation of some immunotherapies may require criteria other than size reduction, because the absence of tumour reduction does not exclude therapeutic efficacy (inflammatory component or change in cellular growth).

The evaluation of the toxicity of an immunotherapy was originally made following the classical criteria of the WHO.[17] The frequency, the importance and the multiplicity of side-effects[18] have rapidly led to the use of other scales of toxicity.[19]

NON-SPECIFIC AGENTS FOR IMMUNOTHERAPY

Various biological products are used in order to restore or increase the immunological potential of the host: Bacille Calmette–Guérin (BCG), levamisole and other agents such as polyadenylic–polyuridylic acid (Poly A–Poly U acid) or PSK (see below).

BCG

Animal studies demonstrated that the live avirulent mycobacterium BCG or its methanolic extract (BCG/ME) may have immunostimulatory properties, increase the efficacy of some chemotherapeutic molecules and improve the survival of rats, when treated in adjuvant settings.[20,21]

Used alone, as adjuvant therapy
Three phase III randomized studies grouping 1941 patients showed that the addition of BCG does not improve the survival of patients treated in an adjuvant situation.[22–24]

Associated with chemotherapy, as adjuvant therapy
The results of four randomized trials are available, including 1203 patients.[22,24,25,26] The association of 5-FU + methyl-CCNU with BCG does not improve survival.[22,24,25] Only the trial of Robinson et al[26] showed an advantage for the association 5-FU + BCG/ME for patients with Dukes C cancer; unfortunately, the number ($n = 56$) of patients is very low, limiting the significance of this study.

Associated with chemotherapy, as palliative therapy
The study of Higgins et al[27] showed that the addition of BCG/ME to 5-FU + methyl-CCNU resulted in a 2-year survival reduction, as compared with patients treated by 5-FU + methyl-CCNU, although this result is not statistically significant.

Thus BCG, used either alone or combined with chemotherapy, has no place in the treatment of colorectal cancers.

Levamisole

The mechanisms of the immunomodulatory and antitumour activities of levamisole are still not entirely clear.[28] There is no cytotoxic action on human colon tumour cell cultures (at relevant concentrations seen in humans), and an additive effect is noted in association with 5-FU at levamisole concentrations nearly 1000 times higher than those obtained in the clinic.[29,30]

Levamisole alone as adjuvant therapy
Four studies comparing levamisole with placebo (a total of 1705 patients) did not demonstrate any improvement in survival.[8,34–36] However, the trial by the Western Cancer Study Group,[34] including a limited number of

patients, has been updated,[37] and showed that the survival of the group without adujuvant treatment is in fact better than that of the group treated by levamisole after the fifteenth year of randomization ($p < 0.03$): this result could be related to a late deleterious effect of the drug.

Levamisole+5-fluorouracil in an adjuvant situation

Two of three studies published in the USA[8,36] quickly demonstrated the efficacy of levamisole (associated with 5-FU), as adjuvant for colon cancer in Dukes stage C. In 1989, Laurie et al[36] reported a significant decrease in the risk of relapse (31%; $p = 0.003$) for 401 patients after surgery for colon cancer (380 patients) or for rectal cancer (21 patients only). A decrease was also found in the risk of death (13%; $p = 0.03$) for patients classified as stage C in the Dukes system and treated during one year with 5-FU (intravenous administration of 450 mg/m^2/day during 5 days, and then weekly), plus levamisole (150 mg per os/day, for 3 consecutive days, every 15 days). A trial coordinated by the National Cancer Institute has been initiated to confirm these results. The study by Moertel et al[8] was done with an average follow-up of 3 years: the results for Dukes stage B2 colon cancer were far too preliminary, and only the results concerning 929 evaluable stage C patients were given. The patients treated with 5-FU + levamisole had a reduction in their relapse risk of 41% ($p <0.0001$) and in the death risk of 33% ($p \approx 0.006$). These results were confirmed 5 years later.[38] The third study was English,[39] included only a few (141) patients, and used a combination of 5-FU per os during 6 months, with levamisole delivered only during the three days following the surgery: the global survival appears to be better for this combination (32% of death within 5 years) than for the control arm (52% of death; $p = 0.04$).

The combination 5-FU + levamisole is used as reference in American adjuvant trials, and also as standard treatment for patients operated upon for stage C colon cancer (if not included in a trial). However, some comments must be made, and temper these results:

(1) the mechanism involved in the improvement of survival after 5-FU + levamisole is not yet clear;[13]
(2) the association is empirical, and the posology is that used for antihelmintic treatment;[8]
(3) the two American trials did not include the control arm '5-FU alone';[10]
(4) although the toxicity of the treatment seems to be acceptable and to be mainly related to 5-FU, 30% of the patients stopped their adjuvant treatment before the end (after 5 months on average) of the trial coordinated by the National Cancer Institute;[8]
(5) a few cases of central neuropathies with demyelinization were linked to levamisole.[40]

Levamisole and chemotherapy in a palliative situation

Three randomized phase III trials showed that the addition of levamisole to 5-FU alone or to an association of 5-FU + methotrexate or of 5-FU + triazinate did not bring any improvement in efficacy or survival.[31–33]

Polyadenylic–polyuridylic (Poly A–Poly U) acid

Poly A–Poly U acid is a complex of two ribonucleotides that can modulate tumoral and/or cellular immunity and stimulate the secretion of cytokines. A negative adjuvant trial, published in 1992 (288 patients) (Dukes stages B and C) was published, and led to a halt to any further investigation.[41]

PSK

PSK has been shown to induce the expression of genes coding for several cytokines: IL-1, IL-6, IL-8 and tumour necrosis factor (TNF). It is an extract from *Basiomycetes* commercialized in Japan since 1977. An adjuvant randomized trial compared mitomycin C (2 consecutive days) + PSK per os given during 'more than 3 years'.[42]

With a follow-up of approximately 4 years, the trial is positive in favour of PSK for tumour-free survival (72.2% versus 67.7%; $p = 0.01$) and for overall survival (85.8% versus 70.2%; $p = 0.01$).

CELL THERAPY

Tumour vaccines

Specific active immunotherapy aims at immunizing the patient against his or her own cancer. As opposed to classical preventive vaccines, the objectives of these 'tumour vaccines' are therapeutic. This strategy is in fact directed against unidentified tumour-associated antigens, and not against well-defined tumour antigens.[9,10] These antigens can be used to generate an immune cytotoxic immune response able to kill tumour cells. This concept starts from the following hypotheses:

(1) the tumour cells express unique antigens that do not exist on normal cells;
(2) these tumour antigens are weakly immunogenic, and so are not detected by the host;
(3) although unable to induce an immune response, a tumour remains sensitive to antitumour immune responses induced through vaccine strategies.[13]

Several mechanisms of cancer escape from immune surveillance have been described at the molecular level. The limits of the concept are linked to the heterogeneity of the tumours and to the difficulty of delivering an adequate immunogenic preparation.[10] Two major strategies were used in clinical trials: 'autologous' and 'allogenic' vaccines.

Autologous tumour vaccines
Autologous vaccines are prepared from each treated patient's own tumour. The cells can be either primary or derived from an established cell line. However, because the phenotype of the tumour cells is modified during the establishment   of a cell line, primary cells are always preferred to cell lines. These cultures are technically difficult

to perform. The cells are rendered non-tumorigenic by irradiation, and are then injected into the patient, frequently with an adjuvant, such as BCG.[43]

In adjuvant settings
The results of three randomized trials have been published. The first included a small number of patients (98 patients with colorectal cancers, Dukes stage B2 or C), and compared surgery alone or surgery plus autologous vaccines.[44] The vaccine was made of autologous tumour cells and BCG organisms, and administered via multiple intradermal injections. Hoover et al[44] did not find any difference in term of tumour-free survival or overall survival. However, they insisted on improvements in relapse-free survival and overall survival in the subgroup of patients with colon cancer, and considered that a benefit of the immunotherapy might have been 'erased' in the subgroup of patients with rectal cancers, owing to the radiotherapy frequently performed after surgery. The trial was criticised by Moertel[45] because of an insufficient number of patients, and because of the large number of patients excluded from the study (20%). In order to verify these results, a trial by the Eastern Cooperative Oncology Group compared the surgery-alone to the surgery plus autologous vaccines plus BCG group: 412 patients with colon cancers were evaluated;[46] there was no difference in overall survival or in relapse-free survival.

The results of another Australian randomized trial were published in 1989 by Gray et al.[47] The cells of the autologous vaccine were treated with neuraminidase to increase their immunogenicity. The vaccine was injected subcutaneously with BCG (14 vaccines the first year, 4 the second). The treatment involved 301 patients (cancer of colon or rectum, Dukes stages B or C), and compared surgery alone versus surgery plus autologous vaccine. No differences in relapse-free survival or in overall survival after 5 years were seen.

In metastatic settings
Although it is not an ideal indication (vaccines would be more efficient against small tumours,

such as micrometastases), Benson et al[48] tested the association of autologous vaccine + BCG + 5-FU (12 mg/kg/day for 5 days, each month). Three partial responses among 18 patients were noted (duration 4–24 months).

Allogenic tumour vaccines
The concept of allogenic vaccines is totally different from that of autologous vaccines. In fact, in this strategy, cell lines from colorectal cancer cultured for a long time, or even pools of different colorectal cell lines, are used to prepare these allogenic vaccines. Inactivated tumour cells, purified cell membranes, cell debris or extracts have been used. Advantages include the possibility of standardizing the treatment, and the potential adjuvant role played by allogenic MHC molecules. Disadvantages include the antigenic heterogeneity (the antigens of the cell lines in culture are probably different from those of the recently operated tumour), and issues related to medical and legal problems (use of allogenic cells that need to be safe). Few results are available, in spite of the interesting perspective.

In a phase I trial, an allogenic vaccine was prepared from membranes extracted from a pool of tumour cells in culture.[49,50] It has been demonstrated that three doses of vaccine (among 28 patients operated upon for colorectal cancers) could induce a strong antitumour cell-mediated and durable immunity.

A strategy to overcome the antigen heterogeneity consists in solubilizing the allogenic tumour-associated antigens and to add them in liposomes: an animal study[51] showed that such a vaccine is able to prolong the survival of the treated animals.

Thus the results from the use of autologous vaccines are disappointing. Allogenic vaccines are in a phase of development, and their role is still to be determined. A generic and efficient vaccine containing the tumour-associated antigens common to most colorectal cancers is still to be found. Presently, the identification of such tumour antigens is still in a research phase.[52] There are essentially three areas of research, which are evaluated especially for melanoma, breast and cervix cancers:

(1) the use of genetically modified tumour cells (see below, under 'Gene therapy');
(2) the injection of synthetic peptides: starting from the identification of a tumour antigen (e.g. the MUC1 antigen in breast cancer, the papillomavirus E6E7 antigens in cervix cancer, and the MAGE-1 or -3 antigens in melanoma), it is possible to synthesize peptides that can be presented by known MHC molecules, and then to inject them to the patient, eventually with adjuvant; similarly, recombinant full antigens can also be used;
(3) the manipulation of antigen-presenting cells (see below).

Other cell-therapeutic strategies

Several other strategies involve the processing of cells that will be injected into the patient. These cells may mediate their therapeutic effects directly, by killing the targeted tumour cells, or indirectly, by elaborating substances with tumoricidal or recruitment properties, or by stimulating antitumour immune responses. Most of these strategies are still at a very preliminary stage, and do not relate especially to colorectal cancers.

Adoptive cellular therapy
Adoptive cellular therapy of cancer was originally conceived as the passive transfer of cells of the immune system with antitumour activity to a tumour-bearing patient in order to mediate regression of the tumour. Not only can these cells directly lyse tumour cells, but they could exert their effects through the elaboration of cytokines or through interactions with the resident host immune system. Massive amplification of a cellular immune response is possible by stimulation and expansion of immune cells in vitro. One theoretical advantage is that certain manipulations of immune cells to increase their antitumour activity are possible in vitro, but are impossible or have highly toxic results in vivo.

Methods have been developed to isolate human antigen-specific cytolytic CD8+ T-cell clones and to expand such clones in vitro to numbers sufficient for T-cell therapy of human diseases. Clinical adoptive immunotherapy studies have shown that virus-specific T cells can be successfully transferred and can mediate therapeutic efficacy in humans. A typical example is that of EBV-induced lymphoproliferative disease, which is a disorder that is most commonly associated with the immunodepression that follows allogenic organ transplantation. Administration of EBV-specific cytotoxic T lymphocytes may be one means of preventing and treating this disease. Similar strategies are being developed against tumour-associated antigens.

Use of dendritic cells as a vaccine against cancer

Dendritic cells (DC) are antigen-presenting cells specialized in the initiation of T-cell-dependent immune responses. Their unique capacity to prime naive T-helper lymphocytes and to stimulate primary cytotoxic T lymphocytes has been demonstrated in numerous in vitro and in vivo studies. Because they represent the most potent antigen-presenting cells, and large numbers can be generated from peripheral blood mononuclear cells or from haematopoietic stem cells, dendritic cells are now being evaluated in clinical trials for their ability to initiate antitumour immune responses. Pulsed with an antigen, these antigen-presenting cells can indeed be used as a strong vaccine to induce immune reactions. The subsequent and specific activation of T lymphocytes can be monitored using sensitive methods, such as the ELISPOT technique for cytokine production.

MONOCLONAL ANTIBODIES

It is now widely accepted that at least some tumour cells may express tumour-associated antigens at high concentration. Monoclonal antibodies are specific for only one antigenic determinant. Several tumour-associated antigens have been identified at the surface of colorectal tumour cells, namely carcinoembryonic antigen (CEA), CA 19-9, cathepsin B, 17-1 and

TAG 72. The characterization and industrial synthesis of very pure monoclonal antibodies has allowed their use in screening or follow-up procedures, in immunohistochemical anatomopathology, in scintigraphic immunodetection, and also in therapeutic strategies.[9,14,53,54]

Monoclonal antibodies have antitumour properties, and can thus be classified among the passive immunotherapeutic agents. Used alone, non-conjugated, they can activate some mechanisms of the host defence able to destroy tumour cells. They can also be used as vehicles for various toxic substances that may destroy tumour cells: in this strategy, they are called 'immunoconjugates'.[9,10,14]

The clinical use of monoclonal antibodies still raises the following problems:

- the requirement of minimal cross-reaction with normal tissues;
- the requirement for a high selectivity of the monoclonal antibodies towards non-circulating antigens, bound to tumour-cell membranes;
- high variation in the half-life of monoclonal antibodies (24 hours for Ig, 10 hours for Fab'2, 90 minutes for Fab);
- higher activity against tumours that are well vascularised, and thus small and without necrosis;
- origin of production: since most monoclonal antibodies are murine, a frequent clinical problem is a human antimouse immune response that is directed against them and that can inactivate them – the new generations of monoclonal antibodies are less immunogenic, because they are genetically modified as chimeras (mice and human sequence) or even human.

Monoclonal antibodies used alone as cytotoxics

After injection, the monoclonal antibodies bind their target molecule on the tumour cells. The mechanisms of cytotoxicity are complex. There is a cytotoxicity mediated by the complement that binds the Fc portion of immunoglobulin and provokes a cascade of reactions leading to cell death. The other cytotoxicity depends on the cellular immunity. These cytotoxicities are linked to the immune ability of the host to produce activated complement or effector cells in sufficient quantities.[14,15,55]

In metastatic disease
Different monoclonal antibodies directed against antigens expressed on the colorectal cancer cells have been used.

(1) The monoclonal antibody(mAb) 17-1A is a murine immunoglobulin G (class 2a) that detects the tumour-associated antigen CO 17-1A. Eight studies of phase I or II were performed.[10,14,15] More than 200 patients received from 1 to 10 doses of mAb 17-1A (200–400 mg per dose): objective responses were seen in 4–7%, which is unfortunately insignificant.
(2) The antibody 17-1A and cytokines – one of the antitumour mechanisms of monoclonal antibodies is a cell-mediated cytotoxicity: as shown in vitro, the lytic activity of the effector cells can be stimulated by the addition of cytokines, such as GM-CSF, IFN-γ and IL-2. In humans, four trials combining 17-1A + IFN-γ were negative.[15] In contrast, the combination of 17-1A + GM-CSF has induced two durable responses (23 and 29 months), one minor response and three stabilizations among 20 patients.[56]
(3) Other murine monoclonal antibodies have been evaluated – for example the anti-CEA, anti-TAG 72 and anti-CA 19-9 antibodies. No antitumour responses were noted in the trials reported by Dillman.[15]

As adjuvant therapy
Several reasons justify the use of monoclonal antibodies alone as adjuvant, in spite of the limited results obtained in palliative settings.

(1) The antitumour action of the monoclonal antibodies seems to be maximal when injected within 48 hours after inoculation of the tumour transplant in the animal;[57] that is, when there is a very small tumour volume.

(2) Initially the micrometastases are located in the reticuloendothelium, where they are surrounded by immune effectors (complement, killer cells, etc.), which should favour the antitumour action of the monoclonal antibodies.[58]
(3) Since the effect of the monoclonal antibodies does not depend on the cell cycle, they can be cytotoxic to micrometastases, which are often in a quiescent phase.[59]

The trial by Riethmüller et al[58] seems to be promising. It is a randomized phase III trial, comparing surgery alone versus surgery plus 17-1A antibody in 189 patients (166 eligible) with Dukes stage C colon or rectal cancer. The protocol consisted in injecting 500 mg of monoclonal antibody in a 1-hour perfusion at day 15, and then 100 mg each month, 4 times consecutively. The treatment was well tolerated. The patients treated with this antibody had a 17.8% reduction in their overall relapse rate ($p = 0.027$), and a 15% increase in the overall survival rate ($p = 0.043$), as compared with patients treated by surgery alone. These results correspond to a 27% relative reduction in the relapse risk and to a 30% reduction in the risk of death, which is approximately similar to the results obtained in stage C with 5-FU + levamisole[8] or 5-FU + folinic acid.[60] The antibody has obtained authorization to be put on the market in some countries (PANOREX), and confirmation of the positive results described above is now being evaluated in an international trial that should include thousands of patients.

Monoclonal antibodies used as immunoconjugates

In this strategy, the monoclonal antibodies are not used alone, but serve to transport toxic compounds that are bound to them. In addition to the fact that the monoclonal antibody keeps its cytotoxic properties, the interest of this strategy is to bring the toxic molecules directly to the tumour cells that express the corresponding antigen.[9,14,53,55] These molecules can be immunotoxins, chemotherapeutic drugs or radioactive products. Studies have been performed in patients with metastatic diseases.

Immunoconjugates with toxins

Several toxins from plants (e.g. ricin) or from bacteria (e.g. *Pseudomonas* or *Diphtheria*) can be coupled to monoclonal antibodies. Only one phase I study[61] used an antibody conjugated to ricin in 17 patients with colorectal metastatic cancers: 5 partial responses were noted.

Immunoconjugates with chemotherapeutic agents

In one study, the antibody A-7 was conjugated to neocarzinostatine:[62] 4 partial responses were observed in 8 patients treated with intraarterial injection of the conjugate.

Immunoconjugates with radioisotopes

Different isotopes can be coupled with monoclonal antibodies: iodine-125 or -131, rhenium-186 or yttrium-90. Only one response was noted among 49 patients with colorectal cancer in two studies.[14,55]

Anti-idiotypic monoclonal antibodies

At present, the monoclonal antibodies that are used alone or as conjugates have technical limitations. An ideal antigenic preparation would include natural or recombinant tumour-associated antigens expressed on colorectal cancer cells that would be specific and immunogenic – such antigens are not available. This problem could be solved by artificially obtaining murine antibodies (designated 'anti-idiotypic antibodies') that act against the original tumour-associated antigen.[9,14] This strategy, which could solve some of the problems associated with the use of 'classical' monoclonal antibodies, is certainly an attractive perspective.

CYTOKINES

Cytokines with potential antitumour immune activities include, in particular, IFN-α and IFN-γ,

IL-2, IL-12, TNF-α and GM-CSF. They can be considered as the real 'hormones' of immunity: after the specific recognition of an antigen by the T-cell receptor of a lymphocyte, several cytokines are produced by the lymphocytes and the antigen-presenting cells to induce a chain of immune reactions, which can mediate the rejection of cancers. As biotherapy against cancer, a cytokine can be administered alone or combined with other cytokines or with cytotoxic molecules. Most of the trials that have been performed are not specific to colorectal cancers, but are part of a systematic evaluation of the cytokine antitumour activities.

Cytokines used alone or combined

In adjuvant settings

IFN-γ, tested after surgery of colon cancers (Dukes stages B2 or C), gave negative results, with a tumour-free survival reduced in the treated group (47% versus 67%; $p = 0.06$).[63]

In metastatic situations

In spite of a clear in vitro antitumour cytotoxicity, IFN-α,[64] IFN-β,[65–67] IFN-γ,[68,69] TNF-α[70] and IL-2[7] turned out in vivo to be very toxic and to be slightly or not efficient (response rate between 4% and 5%). The following combinations of cytokines have been evaluated, and did not result in an improvement in the response rate: IL-2 + IFN-α,[7,71–73] IL-2 + IFN-β,[74] IL-2 + IFN-γ[75] and IL-2 + TNF-α.[7,72]

IL-2 and adoptive immunotherapy

IL-2 has the capacity to activate in vitro killer cells (LAK cells). This association (IL-2 + LAK cells) has an additive effect in vitro, as well as in vivo in the animal. Numerous phase II trials have been performed. Some compared IL-2 versus IL-2 + LAK cells.[76,77] More than 150 patients with metastatic diseases have been treated, with response rates ranging from 0 to 20% (12% on average), and associated with important side-effects.[7,72,76,77]

Presurgery IL-2

An interesting strategy is the use of IL-2 prior to surgery. Indeed, surgery is frequently followed by a period of time with immunodepression (up to 14 days), which can interfere with healing and could facilitate tumour progression.[78,79] The administration of IL-2 before surgery gives rates of activated T lymphocytes and natural killer (NK) cells significantly higher postsurgery than presurgery.[80,81]

Cytokines and chemotherapy

Cytokines and chemotherapeutic agents differ both in their mechanisms of action and in their side-effects. There is thus a rationale to evaluate their combined use. The preclinical studies were in favour of a synergy of action more than a simple additive effect.[13,82,83] This synergistic effect might be sequence-dependent, with the chemotherapeutic agents given before the cytokines, although this remains very controversial. All trials concern metastatic patients.

IFN-α and 5-FU
A basis for this association is related to the probable role of IFN-α in decreasing the activity of thymidine kinase, thus completing the action of 5-FU on thymidylate synthetase, and leading to a decrease in thymidine incorporation into DNA.[84] A very encouraging publication by Wadler et al[85] led to a number of phase II trials that turned out to be less conclusive. The protocol associated 5-FU (continuous infusion during 5 days at 750 mg/m^2 day, then weekly bolus at the same dose) + IFN-α, given subcutaneously at a dose of 9 million units, 3 times per week. Based on this protocol, two randomized phase III trials were performed, including 731 patients: neither revealed a difference in efficacy between 5-FU + IFN-α, 5-FU + folinic acid[86] or 5-FU alone.[87] Survival was similar in the first trial,[86] and not yet evaluable in the second.[87] Two other randomized trials were negative, using other doses of 5-FU.[88,89] Thus the association does not appear to be more efficient than the other protocols, and is associated with side-effects, such as leukopenia, sepsis, diarrhoea, neurological symptoms and asthenia.

IFN-α, 5-FU and folinic acid
As the biochemical modulation of 5-FU by

folinic acid had been clearly demonstrated, the need to evaluate this triple association became obvious. Numerous phase II studies were started as first line, with different dosages of 5-FU, folinic acid, IFN-α, and different schedules;[90–93] more than 150 patients were included, with an average response rate of 25%. A randomized phase III trial was published by a British team:[94] 260 patients received 5-FU + folinic acid in a 48-hour infusion, every 15 days, with or without IFN-α. The response rates (30%) and the survival (10.5 months) were similar in the two arms, but the quality of life of the patients treated with IFN-α was inferior. Similar results were obtained in another trial.[95]

IFN-γ and 5-FU
In a phase I–II study, Ajani et al[96] evaluated 46 metastatic patients. They were treated with IFN-γ, intramuscularly, during 14 days, and with 5-FU (500 mg/m^2/day) during 5 days: only 13% partial responses were noted.

IL-2 + 5-FU, ± folinic acid, ± IFN-α
The results of several phase II studies associating concomitantly or sequentially IL-2 and 5-FU (± folinic acid), and following different therapeutic schedules and dosages, have been published: more than 70 patients were included, with an overall response rate of 28%, including a few complete responses. However, the toxicity of the protocols is important, because side-effects such as diarrhoea, stomatis and myclosuppression resulting from IL-2 or from 5-FU might add up.[97–100] Based on the Hamblin et al[99] protocol, a randomized phase III trial was performed: 135 patients were included, comparing folinic acid (25 mg/m^2 intravenously), then 5-FU (600 mg/m^2 intravenously) weekly with or without IL-2 (18×10^6 IU/m^2/day, during 5 days, in continuous infusion). Similar response rates (17% and 16%) and survival (11.4 and 11.7 months) led to the trial being halted.[101]

The addition of IFN-α to the previous protocols resulted in complexity and toxicity (sometimes limiting) for response rates of about 10%.[102–106]

Mainly used in a palliative situation, the administration of cytokines alone or in association with chemotherapy turns out to be of limited efficacy. Moreover, their toxicity constitutes a major limitation for their use in routine. Future perspectives in this field might be the discovery and the evaluation of other or new cytokines, and their local delivery through gene therapy.

GENE THERAPY

The aims of gene therapy are either to correct a deficiency in the expression of a specific gene product or to provide a new therapeutic function to the cell. This can be accomplished by insertion of a normal copy of that gene into targeted cells. Gene therapy applied to germ cells raises clear ethical and social problems related to the transmission of newly acquired genetic elements to future generations. In contrast, somatic gene therapy is now accepted as a potential alternative in the treatment of many severe diseases, including cancer. In this case, the genetic changes are restricted to targeted somatic cells from the recipient, and will not be passed on to future generations.

Genetically modified TILs

For gene therapy of cancer, most strategies have involved the transfer of genes aiming to induce an antitumour immune response. The first protocol of human gene transfer studied the survival and the homing of tumour-infiltrating lymphocytes (TILs) in the tumour. The protocol was initiated by Steven Rosenberg and colleagues at the National Cancer Institute (NIH, USA), using the transfer of a marker gene. This study demonstrated that it was possible and apparently safe to utilize retroviral mediated gene transfer to introduce a foreign gene into cells. But only 0.015% of the injected TILs accumulate per gram of tumour, the bulk of the cells being trapped and probably destroyed in the circulation, the lungs, the liver, the spleen and draining lymph nodes. Improved TIL therapy was therefore needed. Cytokines were used for that purpose. Their systemic administration to treat cancer has been limited by the high doses

required to obtain effective concentrations, by the frequently associated side-effects (see above), and by the rapid clearance of the cytokine from the circulation. Gene therapy might prove to be a promising way to improve local lymphokine delivery. Cytokine genes are transferred into TILs with the purpose either to increase their cytotoxic function in vivo (IL-2) or to deliver an antitumour product in the tumor (TNF-α).

Genetically modified tumour cells as cancer vaccine

Another way to improve immunotherapy is gene transfer not in TILs but in tumour cells. Many 'vaccination-type' clinical protocols have recently been initiated. They attempt to manipulate the tumour cells themselves, by inserting cytokine genes, in order to increase their immunogenicity and to induce an immune response that is able to eradicate genetically unmodified tumour cells. For this kind of immunotherapy, tumour cells are grown ex vivo, transduced with the cytokine-encoding gene, irradiated, and then reinjected into the patient. Secretion of cytokine has generally been observed in vitro for three to four weeks after irradiation. Another alternative is to transfer the therapeutic gene in vivo, using, for example, adenoviral vectors.

This approach is based on numerous animal models showing that

(1) the vaccination with tumour cells transduced with certain cytokine genes could increase the immune recognition of these tumours and lead to their rejection.
(2) the tumour regression was often associated with systemic antitumour immunity mediated by cytolytic CD8$^+$ T cells, and also, in some cases, by helper CD4$^+$ T cells.

Turning a poorly immunogenic tumour into an immunogenic one was made possible, in mice, by the introduction of genes such as IL-2, IL-3, IL-4, IL-6, IL-7, IL-10, IFN-γ, TNF-α and GM-CSF alone. In particular, IL-2- and GM-CSF-producing tumour cells have been shown to cause regression of established tumours in mice. Synergistic effects of different combinations have also been observed.

Gene-modified dendritic cells

As discussed earlier in this chapter, other attempts are also underway to identify genes that code for tumour-associated antigens. Identification might allow their incorporation into viruses or other immunizing vectors. Their transfer might be used to develop new treatments of cancer: for example, many research teams are now trying to transfer them into antigen-presenting cells, such as dendritic cells.

Transfer of oncogenes or tumour-suppressor genes

Another strategy is based on the molecular pathogenesis of cancer. Cancers indeed result mainly from the accumulation of activating mutations affecting proto-oncogenes, and of inactivating mutations of tumour-suppressor genes. *p53* gene transfer has antitumour activity that is, in fact, mainly related to the induction of apoptosis, leading to cell death, as demonstrated in colorectal cancer cell lines.[107,108]

Transfer of genes coding for prodrug-converting enzymes

The transfer of a 'suicide' gene into tumour cells renders them sensitive to a drug that is ordinarily non-toxic to the target organ or to other tissues. The transfer of the herpes simples thymidine kinase gene (HS-tk) renders the modified cells sensitive to treatment with the antiviral agent ganciclovir, a guanosine analogue, while normal cells are unaffected by this drug. Its toxic effects result from its phosphorylation by HSV-tk. The transfer of this 'suicide' gene by retroviral particles exploits the requirement for DNA synthesis and cell division: in many cancer types, tumour cells have a higher growth rate than their neighbouring normal cells, and are therefore targeted by viral particles carrying the suicide gene. Brain tumours and liver metastases are probably among the best candidates for such a treatment. Interestingly, not all the cells within a tumour need to be transduced with the HSV-tk gene. A 'bystander effect' has been observed, and consists in the transmission of the 'death signal' from transduced cells to the neighbouring non-transduced cells.

Other genes coding for prodrug-converting enzymes have been used, such as that for the cytosine deaminase that catalyses the conversion of 5-fluorocytosine to the lethal 5-fluorouracil (5-FU), as illustrated in colorectal cancer cells.[109]

CONCLUSIONS

Immunotherapy already has a place in the therapeutic arsenal of colorectal cancers, since levamisole (associated with 5-FU) is used routinely in adjuvant situations. However, numerous studies clearly demonstrate the limitations of currently used immunotherapeutic agents. Important progress still has to be made in the comprehension of the antitumour immunity of the host and in the search for the best ways to stimulate immune responses.

Fundamental research on other cancers (mainly melanoma) leads to new methods of immune treatment of colorectal cancers:

(1) first of all, the evaluation of newer cytokines (IL-12, GM-CSF);
(2) then the generation of anti-idiotypic or humanized monoclonal antibodies;
(3) the identification of colorectal specific antigens that could be the basis for vaccination with synthetic peptides;
(4) the development of cell and gene therapies, leading, for example, to the administration of genetically modified cells expressing tumour-associated antigens or cytokines, or to the transfer of tumour-suppressor genes or of prodrug-converting-enzyme genes.

Finally, new therapeutic strategies may target area of intensive research, such as tumour metastasis, neovascularization and apoptosis.

ACKNOWLEDGEMENT

The authors thank Sonia Gotti for her help in the preparation of the manuscript.

REFERENCES

1. Faivre J, Klepping C, Épidémiologie des cancers colo-rectaux. In: *Progrès en cancérologie: les cancers de l'appareil digestif* (Zeitoun P, ed). Paris: Doin, 1981; 25–37.

2. Seitz, JF, Rougier P, Résultats de la chimiothérapie dans les cancers du côlon. *Bull Cancer* 1994; **81:** 260–76.

3. Ducreux M, Roughier P, Traitement adjuvant des cancers colo-rectaux. *Gastroenterol Clin Biol* 1994; **18:** 719–25.

4. Bécouarn Y, Brumet R, Ravaud A et al, Chimiothérapie systémique des adénocarcinomes colo-rectaux métastatiques. *Gastroenterol Clin Biol* 1992; **16:** 166–76.

5. Bécouarn Y, Place des cytokines dans le traitement des cancers colorectaux. *Sixième Rencontre Roche en Cancérologie, Paris, Décembre 1991.* Débats Cancérologiques Roche, 1992; no. 10.

6. Seitz JF, Modificateurs de la réponse biologique dans le traitement adjuvant des cancers digestifs. *Gastroenterol Clin Biol* 1994; **18:** 726–32.

7. Rosenberg SA, Lotze MT, Yang JC et al, Experience with the use of high dose interleukin-2 in the treatment of 652 cancer patients. *Ann Surg* 1989; **210:** 474–84.

8. Moertel CG, Fleming TR, MacDonald JS et al, Levamisole and fluorouracil for adjuvant therapy of resected colon carcinoma. *N Engl J Med* 1990; **332:** 352–8.

9. Foon KA, Biological response modifiers: the new immunotherapy. *Cancer Res* 1989; **49:** 1621–39.

10. Wadler S, The role of immunotherapy in colorectal cancer. *Semin Oncol* 1991; **18:** 27–38.

11. Beatty JD, Immunotherapy of colorectal cancer. *Cancer* 1992; **70:** 425–33.

12. Kreuser ED, Wadler S, Thiel E, Interactions between cytokines and cytotoxic drugs: putative molecular mechanisms in experimental hematology and oncology. *Semin Oncol* 1992; **19:** 1–7.

13. Schulof RS, Avis FP, Biological response modifiers in the treatment of gastrointestinal cancer. In: *Gastrointestinal Oncology* (Ahlgren J, MacDonald J, eds). Philadelphia: JB Lippincott, 1992; 627–40.

14. Mellstedt H, Frödin JE, Masucci G et al, The therapeutic use of monoclonal antibodies in colorectal carcinoma. *Semin Oncol* 1991; **18:** 462–77.

15. Dillman RO, Antibodies as cytotoxic therapy. *J Clin Oncol* 1994; **12:** 1497–515.

16. Gérard JP, Trillet-Lenoir V, Thalabard JC, Traitements adjuvants des cancers digestifs. Principes généraux. *Gastroenterol Clin Biol* 1994; **18:** 710–13.

17. Miller AB, Hoogstraten B, Staquet M, Winkler A, Reporting results of cancer treatment. *Cancer* 1981; **47:** 207–14.

18. Ravaud A, Négrier S, Lakdja F et al, Effets secondaires de l'interleukine 2. *Bull Cancer* 1991; **78:** 989–1005.

19. Creekmore SP, Urba WJ, Longo DL, Principles of the clinical evaluation of biologic agents. In: *Biologic Therapy of Cancer* (De Vita Jr VT, Hellman S, Rosenberg SA, eds) Philadelphia: JB Lippincott, 1991; 67–86.

20. Weiss DW, MER and other mycobacterial fractions in the immunotherapy of cancer. *Med Clin North Am* 1976; **60:** 473–97.

21. Enker WE, Jacobitz JL, Craft K, Wissler RW, Surgical adjuvant immunotherapy for colorectal cancer. *J Surg Oncol* 1978; 10: 389–97.

22. Abdi E, Hanson J, Harbora DE et al, Adjuvant chemoimmuno- and immunotherapy in Dukes' stage B_2 and C colorectal carcinoma: a 7-year follow-up analysis. *J Surg Oncol* 1989; **40:** 205–13.

23. Wolmark N, Fisher B, Rockette H et al, Postoperative adjuvant chemotherapy or BCG for colon cancer: results from NSABP protocol C-01. *J Natl Cancer Inst* 1988; **80:** 30–6.

24. Gastrointestinal Tumor Study Group, Adjuvant therapy of colon cancer. Results of a prospectively randomized trial. *N Engl J Med* 1984; **310:** 737–43.

25. Panettiere FJ, Goodman PJ, Costanzi JJ et al, Adjuvant therapy in large bowel adenocarci-

noma: long-term results of a South-West Oncology Group study. *J Clin Oncol* 1988; **6:** 947–54.

26. Robinson E, Haim N, Bartal A et al, Adjuvant radiochemo-immunotherapy in colorectal cancer: results of a randomized study and review of the literature. *Int J Immunother* 1986; **2:** 23–9.

27. Higgins GA, Donaldson RC, Rogers LS et al, Efficacy of MER immunotherapy when added to a regimen of 5-fluorouracil and methyl-CCNU following resection for carcinoma of the large bowel. A Veterans Administration Surgical Oncology Group report. *Cancer* 1984; **54:** 193–8.

28. Stevenson HC, Green I, Hamilton JM et al, Levamisole: known effects on the immune system, clinical results and future applications to the treatment of cancer. *J Clin Oncol* 1991; **9:** 2052–66.

29. Grem JL, Allegra CJ, Toxicity of levamisole and 5-fluorouracil in human colon carcinoma cells. *J Natl Cancer Inst* 1989; **81:** 1413–17.

30. Grem JL, Levamisole as a therapeutic agent for colorectal carcinoma. *Cancer Cells* 1990; **2:** 131–7.

31. Bedikian AY, Valdivieso M, Mavligit GM et al, Sequential chemoimmunotherapy of colorectal cancer. Evaluation of methotrexate, Baker's antifol and levamisole. *Cancer* 1978; **42:** 2169–76.

32. Buroker T, Moertel CG, Fleming TR et al, A controlled evaluation of recent approaches to biochemical modulation of enhancement of 5-fluorouracil therapy in colorectal carcinoma. *J Clin Oncol* 1985; **3:** 1624–31.

33. Mansour EG, Cnaan A, Davis T et al, Combined modality therapy following resection of colorectal carcinoma in patients with non-measurable intra-abdominal metastases. An ECOG study 3282 (abst). *Proc Am Soc Clin Oncol* 1990; **9:** 107.

34. Chlebowski RT, Nystrom S, Reynolds R et al, Long-term survival following levamisole or placebo adjuvant treatment of colorectal cancer: a Western Cancer Study Group trial. *Oncology* 1988; **45:** 141–3.

35. Arnaud JP, Buyse M, Nordkinger B et al, Adjuvant therapy of poor prognosis colon cancer with levamisole: results of an EORTC double-blind randomized clinical trial. *Br J Surg* 1989; **76:** 284–9.

36. Laurie JA, Moertel CG, Fleming TR et al, Surgical adjuvant therapy of large-bowel carcinoma: an evaluation of levamisole and the combination of levamisole and fluorouracil. *J Clin Oncol* 1989; **7:** 1447–56.

37. Chlebowski RT, Lillington L, Nystrom JS, Sayre J, Late mortality and levamisole adjuvant therapy in colorectal cancer. *Br J Cancer* 1994; **69:** 1094–7.

38. Moertel C, Fleming T, MacDonald J et al, The intergroup study of fluorouracil plus levamisole alone as adjuvant therapy for stage C colon cancer (abst). *Proc Am Soc Clin Oncol* 1992; **11:** 161.

39. Windle R, Bell PRF, Shaw D, Five year results of a randomized trial of adjuvant 5-fluorouracil and levamisole in colorectal cancer. *Br J Surg* 1987; **74:** 569–72.

40. Leichman L, Brown T, Poplin B, Symptomatic, radiologic and pathologic changes in the central nervous system associated with 5-fluorouracil and levamisole therapy (abst). *Proc Am Soc Clin Oncol* 1993; **12:** 198.

41. Lacour J, Laplanche A, Malafosse M et al, Poly-adenylic-polyuridylic acid as an adjuvant in resectable colorectal carcinoma: a $6\frac{1}{2}$ year follow-up analysis of a multicentric double blind randomized trial. *Eur J Surg Oncol* 1992; **18:** 599–604.

42. Mitomi T, Tsuchiya S, Iijima N et al, Randomized, controlled study on adjuvant immunochemotherapy with PSK in curatively resected colorectal cancer. *Dis Colon Rectum* 1992; **35:** 123–30.

43. Hanna MG, Peters LC, Hoover HC, Immunotherapy by active specific immunization: basic principles and preclinical studies. In: *Biologic Therapy of Cancer* (De Vita Jr VT, Hellman S, Rosenberg SA, eds). Philadelphia: JB Lippincott, 1991; 651–69.

44. Hoover HC, Brankhorst JS, Peters LC et al, Adjuvant active specific immunotherapy for human colorectal cancer: 6.5-year median follow-up of a phase III prospectively randomized trial. *J Clin Oncol* 1993; **11:** 390–9.

45. Moertel CG, Vaccine adjuvant therapy for colorectal cancer: 'very dramatic' or Ho–Hum? *J Clin Oncol* 1993; **11:** 385–6.

46. Harris J, Ryan L, Adams G et al, Survival and relapse in adjuvant autologous tumor vaccine therapy for Dukes B and C colon cancer – EST 5283 (abst). *Proc Am Soc Clin Oncol* 1994; **13:** 294.

47. Gray BN, Walker C, Andrewartha L et al, Controlled clinical trial of adjuvant immunotherapy with BCG and neuraminidase-treated autologous tumour cells in large bowel cancer. *J Surg Oncol* 1989; **40:** 34–7.

48. Benson III AB, Rosen ST, Salwen H et al, A pilot

study of active-specific immunotherapy with autologous tumor cell–BCG vaccine and 5-fluo-rouracil (5-FU) in metastatic colorectal carcinoma (abst). *Proc Am Assoc Cancer Res* 1989; **30:** 380.

49. Hollinshead A, Elias EG, Arlen M et al, Specific active immunotherapy in patients with adeno-carcinoma of the colon utilizing tumor-associated antigens (TAA). A phase I clinical trial. *Cancer* 1985; **56:** 480–9.

50. Hollinshead A, Stewart T, Elias G, Arlen M, Update on phase I specific active immuno-therapy colon cancer trial; humoral/cellular specific immunity studies (abst). *Proc Am Soc Clin Oncol* 1990; **9:** 120.

51. Steele Jr G, Ravikumar T, Ross D et al, Specific-active immunotherapy with butanol-extracted, tumor-associated antigens incorporated into liposomes. *Surgery* 1984; **96:** 352–9.

52. Haspel MV, McCabe RP, Pomato N et al, Coming full circle in the immunotherapy of col-orectal cancer: vaccination with autologous tumor cells – to human monoclonal antibodies – to development and application of a generic tumor vaccine. In: *Human Tumor Antigens and Specific Tumor Therapy* (Metzgar RS, ed). New York: Liss, 1989; 335–44.

53. Mitchell EP, Scholm J, Monoclonal antibodies in gastrointestinal cancers. *Semin Oncol* 1988; **15:** 170–80.

54. Mulshine JL, Magnani JL, Linnoila RI, Applications of monocloncal antibodies in the treatment of solid tumors. In: *Biologic Therapy of Cancer* (De Vita Jr VT, Hellman S, Rosenberg SA, eds). Philadelphia: JB Lippincott, 1991; 563–88.

55. Fer MF, Abrams PG, Ahlgren JD, Weiden PL, Monoclonal antibodies in the imaging and treatment of gastrointestinal malignant disease. In: *Gastrointestinal Oncology* (Ahlgren J, Mac Donald J, eds). Philadelphia: JB Lippincott, 1992; 579–91.

56. Ragnhammar P, Fagerberg J, Frödin JE et al, Effect of monoclonal antibody 17-1A and GM-CSF in patients with advanced colorectal carcinoma – long-lasting, complete remissions can be induced. *Int J Cancer* 1993; **53:** 751–8.

57. Johansson C, Segrén S, Lindholm I, Tumour-growth suppression in nude mice by a murine monoclonal antibody: factors hampering suc-cessful therapy. *Int J Cancer* 1991; **48:** 297–304.

58. Riethmüller G, Schneider-Gädicke E, Schlimok G et al, Randomised trial of monoclonal anti-body for adjuvant therapy of resected Dukes' C colorectal carcinoma. *Lancet* 1994; **343:** 1177–83.

59. Pantel K, Schlimok G, Braun S et al, Differential expression of proliferation-associated molecules in individual micrometastatic carcinoma cells. *J Natl Cancer Inst* 1993; **85:** 1419–24.

60. International Multicentre Pooled Analysis of Colon Cancer Trials (IMPACT) Investigators, Efficacy of adjuvant fluorouracil and folinic acid in colon cancer. *Lancet* 1995; **345:** 939–44.

61. Byers VS, Rodvien R, Grant K et al, Phase I study of monoclonal antibody–ricin A chain immunotoxin XomaZyme-791 in patients with metastatic colon cancer. *Cancer Res* 1989; **49:** 6153–60.

62. Takahashi T, Yamaguchi T, Kitamura K et al, Clinical application of monoclonal antibody–drug conjugates for immunotargeting chemo-therapy of colorectal carcinoma. *Cancer* 1988; **61:** 881–8.

63. O'Connell MJ, Wiesenfield M, Wieand HS et al, Interferon-gamma (IFN-γ) as postoperative sur-gical adjuvant therapy for colon cancer: signifi-cant immune stimulation without evidence of therapeutic benefit (abst). *Proc Am Soc Clin Oncol* 1992; **11:** 167.

64. Kurzrock R, Talpaz M, Gutterman JU, Other tumors. In: *Biologic Therapy of Cancer* (De Vita Jr VT, Hellman S, Rosenberg SA, eds). Philadelphia: JB Lippincott, 1991; 334–46.

65. Triozzi PL, Kenney P, Young D, Rinehart JJ, Open-label phase II trial of recombinant beta interferon (IFN-beta$_{ser}$) in patients with colorec-tal cancer. *Cancer Treat Rep* 1987; **71:** 983–4.

66. Lillis PK, Brown TD, Beougher K et al, Phase II trial of recombinant beta interferon in advanced colorectal cancer. *Cancer Treat Rep* 1987; **71:** 965–7.

67. Musch E, Werner A, Messler H et al, Topical application of human fibroblast interferon (n-IFN-β) as an adjuvant in anticancer therapy. Results of a pilot study (abst). *Ann Oncol* 1990; **1** (Suppl): 96.

68. O'Connell MJ, Moertel CG, Schutt AJ, Sherwin SA, Phase II clinical trial of human recombinant gamma interferon (rIFN-γ) in patients with advanced colorectal cancer (abst). *Proc Am Assoc Cancer Res* 1986; **27:** 181.

69. Brown TD, Goodman PJ, Fleming T et al, Phase II trial of recombinant DNA γ-interferon in advanced colorectal cancer: a South-West Oncology Group study. *J Immunother* 1991; **10:** 379–82.

70. Kemeny N, Childs B, Larchian W et al, A phase II trial of recombinant tumor necrosis factor in patients with advanced colorectal carcinoma. *Cancer* 1990; **66**: 659–63.

71. Mittelman A, Huberman M, Puccio C et al, A phase I study of recombinant human interleukin-2 and alpha-interferon-2a in patients with renal cell cancer, colorectal cancer and malignant melanoma. *Cancer* 1990; **66**: 664–9.

72. Dillman RO, Church C, Oldham RK et al, Inpatient continuous-infusion interleukin-2 in 788 patients with cancer. *Cancer* 1993; **71**: 2358–70.

73. Bukowski RM, McLain D, Olencki T et al, Interleukin-2: use in solid tumors. *Stem Cells* 1993; **11**: 26–32.

74. Barni S, Lissoni P, Ardizzola A et al, Immunotherapy with low-dose subcutaneous interleukin-2 plus beta-interferon as a second-line therapy for metastatic colorectal carcinoma. *Tumori* 1993; **79**: 343–6.

75. Weiner LM, Padaviec-Shaller K, Kitson J et al, Phase I evaluation of combination therapy with interleukin-2 and γ-interferon. *Cancer Res* 1991; **51**: 3910–8.

76. Rosenberg SA, Adoptive cellular therapy: clinical applications. In: *Biologic Therapy of Cancer* (De Vita Jr VT, Hellman S, Rosenberg SA, eds). Philadelphia: JB Lippincott, 1991; 214–36.

77. West WH, Continuous infusion recombinant interleukin-2 (rIL-2) in adoptive cellular therapy or renal carcinoma and other malignancies. *Cancer Treat Rev* 1989; **16**(Suppl A): 83–9.

78. Eggermont AMM, Stelle EP, Sugarbaker PH, Laparotomy enhances intraperitoneal tumor growth and abrogates the antitumor effects of interleukin-2 and lymphokine-activated killer cells. *Surgery* 1987; **102**: 71–8.

79. Bussières E, Stöckle E, Ravaud A et al, Immune status after surgery for abdomino-pelvic cancers (abst). *Eur J Cancer* 1991 (Suppl 2): S318.

80. Brivio F, Lissoni P, Barni S et al, Effects of a preoperative course of interleukin-2 on surgical and immunobiological variables in patients with colorectal cancer: a phase 2 study. *Eur J Surg* 1993; **159**: 43–7.

81. Le Cesne A, Elias D, Farace F et al, Prehepatectomy r-IL2 immunotherapy in metastatic colorectal patients: a phase I randomized study (abst). *Ann Oncol* 1994; **5**(Suppl 8): 47.

82. Mitchell MS, principles of combining biomodulators with cytotoxic agents in vivo. *Semin Oncol* 1992; **19**: 51–6.

83. Sznol M, Longo DL, Chemotherapy drug interactions with biological agents. *Semin Oncol* 1993; **20**: 80–93.

84. Wadler S, Schwartz EL, Antineoplastic activity of the combination of interferon and cytotoxic agents against experimental and human malignancies: a review. *Cancer Res* 1990; **50**: 3473–86.

85. Wadler S, Schwartz EL, Lyver A, Fluorouracil and recombinant alpha-2a-inferferon: an active regimen against advanced colorectal carcinoma. *J Clin Oncol* 1989; **7**: 1769–75.

86. Corfu-A Study Group, Phase III randomized study of two fluorouracil combinations with either interferon alpha-2a or leucovorin for advanced colorectal cancer. *J Clin Oncol* 1995; **13**: 921–8.

87. York M, Greco FA, Figlin RA et al, A randomized phase III trial comparing 5-FU with or without interferon alfa 2a for advanced colorectal cancer (abst). *Proc Am Soc Clin Oncol* 1993; **12**: 200.

88. Cellerino R, Antognoli S, Giustini L et al, A randomised study of fluorouracil (5FU) with or without α-interferon (IFN) in advanced colorectal cancer (abst). *Proc Am Soc Clin Oncol* 1994; **13**: 217.

89. Findlay MPN, Cunningham D, Hill ME et al, Protracted venous infusion 5FU ± interferon-α2B in patients with advanced colorectal cancer: results of a phase III trial and a parallel study measuring tumor fluorodeoxyglucose with positron emission tomography (abst). *Proc Am Soc Clin Oncol* 1994; **13**: 193.

90. Kreuser ED, Hilgenfeld RU, Matthias M et al, A phase II trial of interferon α-2b with folinic acid and 5-fluorouracil administered by 4-hour infusion in metastatic colorectal carcinoma. *Semin Oncol* 1992; **19**: 57–62.

91. Whittington R, Faulds D, Interleukin-2. A review of its pharmacological properties and therapeutic use in patients with cancer. *Drugs* 1993; **46**: 446–514.

92. Köhne-Wömpner CH, Schmoll HJ, Harstrick A, Rustum YM, Chemotherapeutic strategies in metastatic colorectal cancer: an overview of current clinical trials. *Semin Oncol* 1992; **19**: 105–25.

93. Grem JL, McAtee N, Murphy RF et al, A pilot study of interferon alfa-2a in combination with fluorouracil plus high-dose leucovorin in metastatic gastrointestinal carcinoma. *J Clin Oncol* 1991; **9**: 1811–20.

94. Seymour MT, Slevin M, Cunningham D et al, Randomized assessment of interferon-α2a (IFNa) as a modulator of 5-fluorouracil (5FU)

and leucovorin in advanced colorectal cancer (abst). *Proc Am Soc Clin Oncol* 1994; **13:** 209.

95. Köhne CH, Wilke H, Hecker H et al, Interferon-alpha does not improve the antineoplastic efficacy of high-dose infusional 5-fluorouracil plus folinic acid in advanced colorectal cancer. *Ann Oncol* 1995; **6:** 461–6.

96. Ajani JA, Rios AA, Ende K et al, Phase I and II studies of the combination of recombinant human interferon-gamma and 5-fluorouracil in patients with advanced colorectal carcinoma. *J Biol Resp Med* 1989; **8:** 140–6.

97. Gressot L, Pazdur R, Markowitz A et al, Phase I–II study of recombinant interleukin-2 (rIL-2) and fluorouracil (5-FU) plus folinic acid for patients with advanced colorectal carcinoma (abst). *Proc Am Soc Clin Oncol* 1990; **9:** 118.

98. Hiddemann W, Ruelfs C, Ottensmeier C et al, Interleukin-2 followed by fluorouracil and folinic acid in refractory colorectal cancer. Results of a clinical phase II study. *Semin Oncol* 1992; **19:** 226–7.

99. Hamblin TJ, Sadullah S, Williamson P et al, Phase II study recombinant interleukin 2 and 5-fluorouracil chemotherapy in patients with metastatic colorectal cancer. *Br J Cancer* 1993; **68:** 1186–9.

100. Yang JC, Shlasko E, Ritchey JI et al, Combination chemoimmunotherapy for metastatic colorectal cancer using 5-fluorouracil, leucovorin and interleukin-2. *Eur J Cancer* 1993; **29A:** 355–9.

101. Heys SD, Bremin O, Ruggeri EM et al, A phase III study of recombinant interleukin-2, 5-fluorouracil and leucovorin versus 5-fluorouracil and leucovorin in patients with unresectable or metastatic colorectal carcinoma. *Eur J Cancer* 1995; **31A:** 19–25.

102. Markowitz A, Yeomans A, Freimann J et al, Phase I study of recombinant interferon-alpha 2a (rIFN-α), recombinant interleukin-2 (rIL-2) and 5-fluorouracil (5-FU) in gastrointestinal malignancies (abst). *Proc Am Soc Clin Oncol* 1990; **9:** 119.

103. Merrouche Y, Ponchon T, Rebattu P et al, A phase II study of weekly high dose 5-fluorouracil (5FU) with alpha interferon (IFN) and interleukin-2 (IL2) in metastatic colorectal carcinoma (abst). *Proc Am Soc Clin Oncol* 1992; **11:** 194.

104. Navone J, Puccio C, Chun H et al, A combination of 5-fluorouracil (5FU), alpha interferon (IFN-A) and interleukin-2 (IL-2) in patients with advanced colorectal adenocarcinoma (abst). *Proc Am Soc Clin Oncol* 1993; **12:** 221.

105. Goey SH, Primrose JN, Lindemann A et al, A phase II study of subcutaneous rh-IL-2, rh-IFN alfa-2a and intravenous 5-fluorouracil in patients with advanced colorectal carcinoma (abst). *Proc Am Assoc Cancer Res* 1993; **34:** 218.

106. Atzpodien J, Kirchner H, Hänninen EL et al, Treatment of metastatic colorectal cancer patients with 5-fluorouracil in combination with recombinant subcutaneous human interleukin-2 and alpha-interferon. *Oncology* 1994; **51:** 273–5.

107. Spitz FR, Nguyen D, Skibber JM et al, In vivo adenovirus-mediated p53 tumor suppressor gene therapy for colorectal cancer. *Anticancer Res* 1996; **16:** 3415–22.

108. Bookstein R, Demers W, Gregory R et al, p53 gene therapy in vivo of hepatocellular and liver metastatic colorectal cancer. *Semin Oncol* 1996; **23:** 66–77.

109. Rowley S, Lindauer M, Gebert JF et al, Cytosine deaminase gene as a potential tool for the genetic therapy of colorectal cancer. *J Surg Oncol* 1996; **61:** 42–8.

34

Quality of life in colorectal cancer studies

Eric Van Cutsem, Chris Verslype

CONTENTS • Introduction • Methods of measurement • Quality of life as endpoint • Quality of life
in colorectal cancer • Conclusion

INTRODUCTION

Although the ultimate aim of treating the cancer patient is cure, in most patients with metastatic colon cancer this unfortunately can only infrequently be achieved. However, potential benefits such as prolongation of survival, tumour regression and palliation of symptoms are other reasons for using chemotherapy for metastatic colon cancer. The assessment of survival is relatively simple. It has been shown that chemotherapy for metastatic colon cancer prolongs survival by approximately 6 months.[1-4] The evaluation of tumour response is very frequently used as the primary endpoint in the evaluation of a chemotherapeutic regimen for metastatic colon cancer. The complete and partial response rates usually reflect the activity of a chemotherapeutic agent in previously untreated patients with metastatic colon cancer. Since colon cancer is usually considered as a relatively chemoresistant tumour, other parameters are often examined and analysed in trials evaluating the efficacy of a treatment regimen: the palliation of tumour-related symptoms and the evaluation of quality of life (QoL) and of the performance status (PS) are therefore

often used as other endpoints in colorectal cancer studies. However, the evaluation, analysis and interpretation of these parameters often remain very difficult, and are also often very controversial.

Despite serious conceptual and methodological difficulties, several clinical trial organizations have therefore now introduced the notion of QoL as a standard part of new trials.[5] The European Organization for Research and Treatment of Cancer (EORTC) demands that new study proposals contain information about the intention to assess QoL and/or cost-effectiveness.[5] Similarly, the question 'Have quality-of-life issues been addressed adequately?' is asked as part of the priority ranking of the UK Medical Research Council (MRC) cancer therapy trials, and MRC-funded trials in general are expected either to assess the likely impact on QoL or to justify not doing so.[5]

Despite the proliferation of instruments and the extensive theoretical literature devoted to the measurement of quality of life, no unified approach has been derived for its measurement, and little agreement has been obtained on what it means. In fact, the term QoL as applied in the medical literature may not have a distinctive or unique meaning. Many investigators seem to substitute QoL for other terms intended to describe a patient's health, such as health status or functional status. There is, however, an increasing consensus that QoL is a subjective evaluation rather than an objective reality, and so can only be assessed with reliability by the person whose QoL is being evaluated.[6] We have come to accept that pain is what the person says it is. So too, QoL is what the individual experiences it to be. The subjective nature of QoL means that it will vary greatly from person to person, and even for a given individual over time in the same circumstances.[7–10]

QoL can therefore be defined as subjective well-being.[6] A single global question asking a person to rate his or her overall QoL is perhaps the most valid measure, in that it most closely represents what the individual means by QoL, but such a scale fails to identify the factors contributing to the assessment. To provide the best care possible, health care workers would need to know what contributed to the person's decision to rate his or her QoL as high or low. Others have therefore chosen to measure 'health-related quality of life' using the definition of health of the World Health Organization (WHO), rather than that of the patient whose QoL is being measured.[7,10,11] The WHO defines health as physical, psychological and social well-being. People with a life-threatening disease, however, define health as a sense of personal integrity and wholeness, encompassing physical, mental/emotional and spiritual domains.[6]

The use of the term health-related QoL is helpful in that it focuses on the impact of health on QoL, and therefore examines issues beyond physical health alone.[12]

METHODS OF MEASUREMENT

It is not easy to measure QoL. Conceptual difficulties and controversies on the definition of QoL and on the importance of the different parameters that influence the QoL as well as methodologic difficulties for the determination of QoL have led to the development of many different methods of evaluation of QoL. The acceptance of the impact of these different methods has been variable.[13] The use of a single summary score or global rating is of value for comparisons between populations under study, although a profile of QoL detailing perceived functioning in different domains should be included, where possible, to identify specific areas where an increase in support or resources could most effectively be provided. A brief questionnaire must encompass the enormous numbers of factors that can have an impact on QoL. Very long questionnaires may be more accurate, but, unless they are acceptable and easily completed by the patient, they will be of no practical use except by researchers. A compromise must therefore be reached between a measure that is brief and easy to use and therefore widely acceptable to both patients and physicians, and long, detailed interviews that are likely to elucidate the issues of importance to the patient, but are unlikely to be of practical use, particularly within the clinical setting.

Techniques for measuring quality of life have come a long way since Karnofsky introduced his scale of *performance status* in 1948.[14] By today's standards, the Karnofsky performance status (KPS) scale is a rather clumsy tool[15] (Table 34.1). It requires an evaluation of three dimensions of health status simultaneously (activity, work and self-care), without clear criteria for differentiation between levels of function. No guidance is provided regarding how to obtain the information necessary to assign a patient to a given level of function. It is not surprising that the scale has been found by some to be unreliable (inconsistent ratings of the same patient by different evaluators) and poorly correlated with patients' own reports of their performance. The Eastern Cooperative Oncology Group (ECOG) performance status scale, although simpler, retains some of the troubling features of its older cousin[16] (Table 34.2). This scale has been accepted by the WHO, and therefore has also been called the WHO performance scale. Despite these shortcomings, the evaluation of the performance status gives important clinical information on the general condition of the patient. However, a major research effort over the last several decades has produced an array of sophisticated *questionnaires* to measure both specific aspects and overall quality of life. These instruments vary in their mode of administration, emphasis, scope and length. But a number of scales, including

---

Table 34.1 Karnofsky performance status scale

Status	Definition
100	Normal, no complaints, no evidence of disease
90	Able to carry on normal activity, minor symptoms
80	Normal activity with effort, some signs or symptoms of disease
70	Cares for self, unable to carry on normal activity or to do active work
60	Requires occasional assistance, but is able to care for most of his/her needs
50	Requires considerable assistance and frequent medical care
40	Disabled, requires special care and assistance
30	Severely disabled, hospitalization is indicated, although this is not imminent
20	Hospitalization necessary, very sick, active supportive treatment necessary
10	Moribund, fatal processes proceeding rapidly
0	Dead

Table 34.2 WHO performance status score

Activity	Score
Fully active, able to carry out all normal activities without restriction	0
Restricted in physically strenuous activity, but ambulatory and able to carry out light work	1
Ambulatory and capable of all self-care, but unable to carry out any work; up and about more than 50% of waking hours	2
Capable of only limited self-care, confined to bed or chair more than 50% of waking hours	3
Completely disabled, unable to carry out any self-care, and confined totally to bed or chair	4

the Cancer Rehabilitation Evaluation System (CARES),[17] the Functional Living Index Cancer (FLIC),[18] the Quality of Life Index (QLI),[19] the European Organization for Research and Treatment of Cancer (EORTC) Questionnaire,[20] the MOS 36-Item Short-Form Health Survey (SF 36)[21] and linear analog self-assessments (LASAs),[22] have been shown to be remarkably successful in generating scores that are often reproducible and valid.

The measurement of performance status (Karnofsky or WHO) remains, despite some disadvantages, a very useful parameter in colorectal cancer trials, and should be done in all trials studying chemotherapeutic treatment.[14] It is indeed accepted that there is usually good correlation between performance status and prognosis in patients with metastatic colorectal cancer, between performance status and the response to a chemotherapeutic treatment, and also between performance status and the frequency and/or severity of adverse events of chemotherapeutic treatment.[23]

In Europe the EORTC-QLQ-C30 (a questionnaire with 30 questions) is used more and more frequently (Table 34.3). It has been shown that the EORTC-QLQ-C30 is a reliable and valid measure of the QoL of cancer patients in multicultural clinical research settings.[24] The average time required to complete the questionnaire is about 11 minutes, most patients require no assistance, and compliance is usually good.[24] A criticism, however, is that it lacks a certain specificity for colon cancer. The EORTC is therefore validating a new and more specific QoL questionnaire for patients with colon cancer.

Recently the term 'clinical benefit' has also been used in several trials evaluating new drugs in gastrointestinal cancer. Clinical benefit can be defined as an improvement in a patient's disease-related symptoms and performance status. The parameters of clinical benefit are not the same as those of QoL, although an improvement in a patient's disease-related symptoms (clinical benefit) could certainly translate into an improved QoL for the patient.[25] The clinical benefit assessment has already been used successfully to demonstrate the clinical benefit

from a treatment with gemcitabine for patients with pancreatic cancer[26] and with CPT-11 in patients with 5-FU-resistant metastatic colorectal cancer.[27] Clinical benefit therefore deserves to be investigated further to determine its value as a new endpoint for clinical trials in advanced cancer.[28]

Another shortcoming of most QoL questionnaires is that the existential domain is not included in most QoL measures. Existential measures are indeed of great importance to patients with a life-threatening illness. The existential domain includes concerns regarding death, freedom, isolation and the question of meaning.[6,29]

QUALITY OF LIFE AS ENDPOINT

When is assessment of QoL a relevant endpoint? A classification of trials has been proposed to answer this question:[30]

(a) QoL may be the main endpoint (this is frequently true in palliative care, or when patients are seriously ill with incurable disease);
(b) treatments may be expected to be equivalent in efficacy, and a new treatment would be deemed preferable if it confers QoL benefits;
(c) a new treatment may show a small benefit in cure rates or survival advantage but this might be offset by QoL deterioration;
(d) treatments may differ considerably in their short-term efficacy, but if the overall failure rate is high then QoL issues should be considered.

Furthermore, despite the optimism of those who launch trials that seek a survival breakthrough, all too often completed trials show a limited survival advantage. Thus in all these cases QoL has to be considered, since any gain in therapeutic efficacy would have to be weighed against negative effects pertaining to QoL.

QUALITY OF LIFE IN COLORECTAL CANCER

Until recently, the role of palliative chemotherapy in patients with advanced colorectal cancer

Table 34.3 EORTC QLQ-C30 Questionnaire

		No	Yes		
1.	Do you have any trouble doing strenuous activities, like carrying a heavy shopping bag or a suitcase?	1	2		
2.	Do you have any trouble taking a <u>long</u> walk?	1	2		
3.	Do you have any trouble taking a <u>short</u> work outside of the house?	1	2		
4.	Do you have to stay in a bed or a chair for most of the day?	1	2		
5.	Do you need help with eating, dressing, washing yourself or using the toilet?	1	2		

DURING THE PAST WEEK:

		Not at all	A little	Quite a bit	Very much
6.	Were you limited in doing either your work or other daily activities?	1	2	3	4
7.	Were you limited in pursuing your hobbies or other leisure time activities?	1	2	3	4
8.	Were you short of breath?	1	2	3	4
9.	Have you had pain?	1	2	3	4
10.	Did you need to rest?	1	2	3	4
11.	Have you had trouble sleeping?	1	2	3	4
12.	Have you felt weak?	1	2	3	4
13.	Have you lacked appetite?	1	2	3	4
14.	Have you felt nauseated?	1	2	3	4
15.	Have you vomited?	1	2	3	4
16.	Have you been constipated?	1	2	3	4
17.	Have you had diarrhoea?	1	2	3	4
18.	Were you tired?	1	2	3	4
19.	Did pain interfere with your daily activities?	1	2	3	4
20.	Have you had difficulty in concentrating on things, like reading a newspaper or watching television?	1	2	3	4
21.	Did you feel tense?	1	2	3	4
22.	Did you worry?	1	2	3	4
23.	Did you feel irritable?	1	2	3	4
24.	Did you feel depressed?	1	2	3	4
25.	Have you had difficulty remembering things?	1	2	3	4
26.	Has your physical condition or medical treatment interfered with your <u>family</u> life?	1	2	3	4
27.	Has your physical condition or medical treatment interfered with your <u>social</u> activities?	1	2	3	4
28.	Has your physical condition or medical treatment caused you financial difficulties?	1	2	3	4

For the following questions please circle the number between 1 and 7 that best applies to you.

29. How would you rate your overall health during the past week?

1	2	3	4	5	6	7
Very poor						Excellent

30. How would you rate your overall quality of life over the past week?

1	2	3	4	5	6	7
Very poor						Excellent

has been questioned. The effects of the various treatments on long-term outcome are uncertain, and there has been a perception that QoL might be adversely affected. The wide spectrum of new treatment options certainly opens new perspectives for increased response rates and improved survival rates for patients with colon cancer in the future,[31] but it will take some time before the impact and role of these treatment options can be determined. Two clinical studies conducted in Austria and Scandinavia have therefore addressed the issue of QoL in previously untreated patients by comparing the effects of either supportive care with or without chemotherapy[32] or early chemotherapy versus no chemotherapy until symptoms developed.[3] Although a small number of patients were included in the Austrian study, a significant survival benefit was shown in the chemotherapy plus supportive care group compared with the supportive care alone group (11 versus 5 months).[32] In this study, which also evaluated QoL, overall well-being improved in the chemotherapy cohort but declined during supportive care, reflecting disease progression. In the Scandinavian study, patients with advanced but asymptomatic colorectal cancer were randomized to receive initial chemotherapy (methotrexate, 5-FU, leucovorin) or to primary expectancy with chemotherapy not considered until symptoms appeared.[3] This study clearly demonstrated that early treatment prolongs time to symptom appearance (10 versus 2 months), as well as time to tumour progression (8 versus 3 months) and survival (14 versus 9 months).[3] The patients maintained a good performance status and general well-being during the chemotherapeutic treatment, unless the disease was progressive.[3] This was also true in an associated QoL study, performed using a specific questionnaire.[33]

These studies tell us that the perception that QoL might be adversely affected is wrong for the treatments actually being used in advanced colorectal cancer. Other studies also show that the number of patients with a subjective symptomatic improvement and the number of patients with an overall improved QoL is generally higher (30–40%) than the number of patients with an objective tumour response (15–25%).[34,35] This means that some patients have improvements in tumour-related symptoms and in QoL while they have only tumour stabilization.[34] From this point of view, the term 'clinical benefit' is important. However, only little information is available on the 'clinical benefit' of chemotherapy in patients with advanced colorectal cancer. In a recent study in patients with 5-FU-resistant metastatic colorectal cancer, the 'clinical benefit' of CPT-11 has been reported.[27] With this second-line treatment, tumour growth control (stabilization or regression in patients with documented previous progression) was obtained, accompanied by improvement or stabilization of weight and performance status in a majority of patients.[27]

CONCLUSION

The evaluation of QoL is very difficult, since the QoL of a patient corresponds to subjective well-being. A single global question asking a person to rate overall QoL gives perhaps the most correct representation of the QoL but does not identify the factors contributing to the assessment. QoL can at present be evaluated by measuring the performance status and by using more sophisticated questionnaires. Although the measurement of the QoL is still unsatisfactory with these methods, the assessment of QoL is being used more frequently as an endpoint for clinical trials in colorectal cancer. More specific modules for advanced colorectal cancer and a more appropriate use of the term 'clinical benefit' are therefore needed.

REFERENCES

1. Moertel C, Chemotherapy for colorectal cancer. *N Engl J Med* 1994; **330:** 1136–42.
2. Cunningham D, Findlay M, The chemotherapy of colon cancer can no longer be ignored. *Eur J Cancer* 1993; **29A:** 2077–9.
3. Nordic Gastrointestinal Tumor Adjuvant Therapy Group, Expectancy or primary chemotherapy in patients with advanced asymptomatic colorectal cancer: a randomized trial. *J Clin Oncol* 1992; **10:** 904–11.
4. Bleiberg H, Role of chemotherapy for advanced colorectal cancer: new opportunities. *Sem Oncol* 1996; **23:** 42–50.
5. Editorial. Quality of life and clinical trials. *Lancet* 1995; **346:** 1–2.
6. Cohen SR, Mount BM, MacDonald N, Defining quality of life. *Eur J Cancer* 1996; **32A:** 753–4.
7. Aaronson NK, Quality of life research in cancer clinical trials: a need for common rules and language. *Oncology* 1990; **4:** 59–66.
8. Campbell A, Subjective measures of well-being. *Am Psychol* 1976; **31:** 117–24.
9. Cohen SR, Mount B, Quality of life assessment in terminal illness: defining and measuring subjective well-being in the dying. *J Palliat Care* 1992; **8:** 40–5.
10. Guyatt GH, Feeny DH, Patrick DL, Measuring health-related quality of life. *Basic Sci Rev* 1993; **118:** 622–9.
11. Schipper H, Guidelines and caveats for quality of life measurement in clinical practice and research. *Oncology* 1990; **4:** 51–7.
12. Jenney MEM, Health-related quality of life, cancer and health care. *Eur J Cancer* 1996; **32A:** 1281–2.
13. Gill TM, Feinstein AR, A critical appraisal of the quality of quality-of-life measurements. *J Am Med Assoc* 1994; **272:** 619–26.
14. Karnofsky DA, Abelman WH, Craver LF et al, The use of nitrogen mustards in palliative treatment of carcinoma. *Cancer* 1948; **1:** 634–56.
15. Weeks J, Quality-of-life assessments: performance status upstaged? *J Clin Oncol* 1992; **10:** 1827–9.
16. Oken MM, Creech RH, Tormey DC et al, Toxicity and response criteria of the Eastern Cooperative Oncology Group. *Am J Clin Oncol* 1982; **5:** 649–55.
17. Ganz PA, Schag CAC, Lee JJ, Sim MS, The CARES: a generic measure of health-related quality of life for patients with cancer. *Qual Life Res* 1992; **1:** 19–29.
18. Schipper H, Clinch J, McMurray A, Levitt M, Measuring the quality of life of cancer patients: the functional living index–cancer: development and validation. *J Clin Oncol* 1984; **2:** 472–83.
19. Spitzer WO, Dobson AJ, Hall J et al, Measuring the quality of life of cancer patients. *J Chron Dis* 1981; **34:** 585–97.
20. Aaronson NK, Bullinger M, Ahmedzai S, A modular approach to quality-of-life assessment in cancer clinical trials. *Recent Results Cancer Res* 1988; **111:** 231–49.
21. Stewart AL, Hays RD, Ware JE Jr, The MOS short-form general health survey. Reliability and validity in a patient population. *Med Care* 1988; **26:** 724.
22. Priestman TJ, Baum M, Evaluation of quality of life in patients receiving treatment of advanced breast cancer. *Lancet* 1976; **i:** 899–901.
23. Labianca R, Pancera G, Luporini G, Factors influencing response rates for advanced colorectal cancer. *Ann Oncol* 1996; **7:** 901–6.
24. Aaronson NK, Ahmedzai S, Bergman B et al, The European Organization for Research and Treatment of Cancer QLQ-C30: a quality-of-life instrument for use in international clinical trials in oncology. *J Natl Cancer Inst* 1993; **85:** 365–76.
25. Von Hoff DD, It feels better – measuring clinical benefit. *Eur J Cancer* 1996; **32A:** 376–7.
26. Rothenberg ML, Moore MJ, Cripss MC et al, A phase II trial of gemcitabine in patients with 5-FU-refractory pancreatic cancer. *Ann Oncol* 1996; **7:** 347–53.
27. Van Cutsem E, Cunningham D, Ten Bokkel Huinink W et al, CPT-11 in 5-FU-resistant colorectal cancer: patient benefit. *Ann Oncol* 1996; **7(S5):** 34 (abst).
28. Verweij J, The benefit of clinical benefit: a European perspective. *Ann Oncol* 1996; **7:** 333–4.
29. Cohen SR, Mount BM, Tomas JJN, Mount LF, Existential well-being is an important determinant of quality of life. *Cancer* 1996; **77:** 576–86.
30. Gotay CC, Korn EL, McCabe MS et al, Quality-of-life assessment in cancer treatment protocols: research issues in protocol development. *J Natl Cancer Inst* 1992; **84:** 575–9.
31. Van Cutsem E, A glimpse of the future. New directions in the treatment of colorectal cancer. *Eur J Cancer* 1996; **32A:** S23–7.
32. Scheithauer W, Rosen H, Kornek G et al, Randomised comparison of combination

chemotherapy plus supportive care with supportive care alone in patients with metastatic colorectal cancer. *Br Med J* 1993; **306:** 752–5.

33. Glimelius B, Graf W, Hoffman K et al, General condition of asymptomatic patients with advanced colorectal cancer receiving palliative chemotherapy. A longitudinal study. *Acta Oncol* 1992; **31:** 645–51.

34. Glimelius B, Hoffman K, Graf W et al, Quality of life during chemotherapy in patients with symptomatic advanced colorectal cancer. *Cancer* 1994; **73:** 556–62.

35. Cunningham D, Zalcberg J, Rath U et al, Final results of a randomized trial comparing Tomudex (raltitrexed) with 5-fluorouracil plus leucovorin in advanced colorectal cancer. *Ann Oncol* 1996; **7:** 961–5.

35

Critical issues in colorectal cancer randomized trials and meta-analyses

Pascal Piedbois, Marc Buyse, Jean-Pierre Pignon

More usually, advances in therapeutics will come to consist of a succession of small improvements ... When such small differences are to be established, only carefully conducted trials will be able to provide definite information
Schwartz, Flamant and Lellouch (1980)

INTRODUCTION

The purpose of this chapter is to present critical issues in randomized clinical trials and meta-analyses of therapies for colorectal cancer. Early-phase clinical trials are therefore outside the scope of the present paper. Randomized trials of preventive interventions raise specific methodological questions that also fall beyond the scope of the present chapter, which focuses on treatment evaluation.

RANDOMIZED TRIALS IN PATIENTS WITH RESECTABLE COLORECTAL CANCER

Sample size

Table 35.1 gives some examples of observed relative risks of death of patients receiving chemotherapy compared with those receiving no adjuvant therapy in colon cancer, and the sample size needed to detect such relative risks.

When a trial is contemplated for all patients after tumor resection, the number of patients needed to detect a given difference is higher if both stage B and stage C tumors are included than if only stage C tumors are included, because the survival rate of patients with stage B tumors is higher (Table 35.1). The sample size increases even further if a comparison between different active treatments is contemplated (rather than between an experimental group and an untreated control group), because the expected difference is a priori smaller. Sample-size calculations have been reviewed elsewhere.[3-5] For all analyses of time-dependent events such as survival, it is the number of events and not the number of patients that is critical.

An erroneous interpretation of the results of inconclusive trials is quite frequent.[6] When a trial concludes that there is no statistically significant benefit in favor of a new treatment, it does not follow that there is in truth no benefit, but merely that the trial failed to show it. In the past, trial sizes tended to be too small to detect a moderate and yet clinically relevant treatment effect.[7-10] For example, among the 9 randomized

Table 35.1 Relative risks of death observed in large trials or in meta-analysis of adjuvant chemotherapy versus none, and sample sizes needed to detect such relative risks

Trial name or first author	Population	Treatment	Relative risk (95% CI)	Sample size for C and B stages: number of patients (events)
Moertel[1]	Colon, stage C	5-Fluorouracil + levamisole	0.67 (0.53–0.84)	(C) 500 (200) (B) 750 (200)
IMPACT[2]	Colon, stages B and C	5-Fluorouracil + leucovorin	0.78 (0.62–0.97)	(C) 1200 (475) (B) 1700 (475)

[a] Based on a 55% survival rate in C stage without adjuvant treatment and a 70% survival rate for B stage; two-sided log-rank test with 80% power and 5% type I error.

trials included in the meta-analysis of adjuvant portal-vein 5-fluorouracil (5-FU) chemotherapy, 6 had included less than 300 patients.[11]

Design issues

The design of a clinical trial is crucial, since a faulty design may make meaningful analyses of the trial results difficult and a proper interpretation of its results impossible. For general reviews of trial designs, see references 3, 12 and 13.

In oncology, a common design is to include between 100 and 300 patients in two equally sized treatment groups. Such moderately sized developmental trials are needed to evaluate new treatments and new routes of treatment administration. Usually they include selected patients with poor prognosis. These trials are time-consuming and potentially costly. Their cost is due to one or several of the following factors:

(a) a patient selection based on new or expensive tests;
(b) systematic collection of prognostic covariates, toxicity data, compliance and secondary endpoints;

(c) careful monitoring of treatment quality and data collection.

According to the type of treatment evaluated and its stage of development, some or all of these factors are essential to the trial design. It is, however, often possible and desirable to simplify the trial procedures either to reduce the overall cost of the trial or to increase its sample size.[14] Really large-scale trials (or megatrials) can be considered for the reliable detection of small but worthwhile benefits obtained with widely available treatments such as adjuvant portal-vein chemotherapy.[15]

A design that is worth special mention in oncology is the factorial design. Peto[16] and Byar et al[17] advocated wider use of factorial designs, in particular the 2 × 2 design, which answers two questions instead of one with little or no extra difficulties or cost. To compare two treatments A and B versus no treatment, patients can be randomized into four groups: neither treatment, A or B alone, or both together. To study the effect of A, for example, the results of the comparison of A + B versus B and of A versus no treatment will be combined. This design is useful when the effect of A is essentially the same in the presence or in the absence of B. If such was not the case, an 'interaction' between treatments A and B would be observed. The statistical tests required to detect interactions have very low power, and therefore the absence of an interaction must be assumed at the time of trial planning.[12,17] One difficulty in oncology is that it is not always possible to give no treatment or both.[18] For example, when chemotherapy and radiotherapy are combined, it may be necessary to lower the treatment doses because of overlapping toxicity. When a significant interaction is present, the trial must be analyzed as a four-arm trial, and as a result there is a substantial loss in statistical power.[19] Examples of factorially designed trials include the AXIS trial, which tests the value of portal-vein 5-FU and of radiotherapy in patients with rectal cancer.[15] The EORTC trial 40911 compares an 'early' regional chemotherapy (portal-vein or peritoneal 5-FU) to none and two 'late' systemic chemotherapy regimens (5-FU + leucovorin versus 5-FU + levamisole). An NCCTG trial compares two chemotherapy regimens (5-FU + levamisole versus 5-FU + levamisole + leucovorin), as well as two chemotherapy durations (6 months versus 12 months).[20]

Stratification

Stratification consists of using prognostic information at the time of randomization in order to guarantee that the treatment groups are well balanced. Pure randomization achieves such balance only in the long run, while 'stratified' randomization ensures it even in small samples.[21] This balance is not strictly necessary, since any imbalance can be adjusted for in the analysis, but trials that show a reasonable balance among treatment groups are far more convincing and easier to analyze and interpret. The advantages of using stratified randomization are that

(a) trial results are more credible when prognostic factors are balanced among the treatment arms;
(b) there is no need for adjusted analyses that

would be called for if an imbalance occurred;
(c) the power of the analysis is optimum.

Stratification factors should have an established independent prognostic value, and should be easily and readily obtainable before randomization. Dukes stage or TNM stage are the most important prognostic factors for potentially resectable colorectal cancer. When adjuvant trials include all stages, it is advisable to stratify them for stage. In fact, the stratification may include a change in treatment policy, because systemic chemotherapy is now standard therapy for Dukes stage C colon cancer, while its use is still controversial for stage B and even more so for stage A. Active research is ongoing to refine the prognostic information within each stage, but at present stage is the only prognostic factor for which stratification is absolutely called for. Another factor that should be taken into account in rectal cancer is the administration of preoperative or postoperative radiotherapy. The investigational center is often taken as a stratification factor for administrative convenience.

Endpoints for adjuvant treatments

The endpoint of interest in trials of adjuvant treatments is usually the period of time from the date of randomization to the occurrence of some well-defined event indicating treatment failure, such as death or disease relapse. Patients who have not yet failed at the time of the analysis constitute so-called censored observations, because their time to failure will eventually be longer than that observed at the time of the analysis. Overall survival is the time period between randomization and patient death, whatever its cause. Randomized trials have often failed to show survival differences between the treatment groups because the sample size was insufficient to show the small benefits on mortality that are achievable with adjuvant therapy. Small survival differences are swamped in random errors due to patient heterogeneity.

Cancer survival is the time period between randomization and patient death if its cause is malignant disease. Patients who die from other causes, such as intercurrent diseases, are regarded as censored observations. Cancer survival is a more sensitive indicator of treatment effect than overall survival, particularly if the competing risks of dying from other causes are high, as is the case among the old age groups that typically present with colorectal cancer. The analysis of cancer survival may provide valuable insight into the effects of treatment, but any evidence thus obtained may be biased. Indeed, causes of death are notoriously difficult to ascertain, and misclassification between cancer and non-cancer causes may occur. Moreover, if treatment affected the non-malignant causes of death (perhaps because of some toxicity), an analysis of cancer survival could be misleading: for instance, an aggressive treatment might cure more patients of their cancer but kill them because of toxicity, resulting in no net benefit. In such cases, the overall survival analysis would correctly conclude to no benefit, while the cancer survival analysis would show a treatment benefit. Both analyses would have to be considered simultaneously for a reliable and informative conclusion to be drawn.

Disease-free interval is the time between randomization and a clear-cut relapse of the disease. Patients who die without evidence of disease are regarded as censored observations. Disease-free survival is defined as disease-free interval, but with all deaths considered failures. Disease-free interval is in most cases a worthwhile endpoint in addition to survival. Just as for cancer survival, it is a more sensitive biological marker of treatment effect, but a less reliable indicator of net benefit to the patient. The type of relapse can yield useful information on the disease process. Therefore disease-free interval is usually subdivided into time to local progression (with distant progressions regarded as censored observations) and time to distant progression (with local relapses regarded as censored observations). These times can be equally relevant as survival if disease recurrence has a major impact on the patient condition and if no treatment is available on recurrence: for instance, time to local recurrence is an important endpoint after radical surgery of rectal cancer, because recurrences in the pelvis may be very painful and difficult to remove surgically.

Large-scale trials and prospective pooled analysis

To detect a 5-year survival benefit of less than 10% in the adjuvant setting implies performing trials in which more than 1000 patients are included, because the survival rates are higher than 40% for most cases of resectable colorectal tumors.[9] An improvement of less than 10% is small, but could have major consequences on public health for such a common disease as colorectal cancer. For treatments with mild toxicity (e.g. portal-vein 5-FU), even a 5% improvement in survival would be definitely worthwhile.[11,15] Toxicity, quality of life and costs should be carefully considered when the expected benefit on survival is small. Table 35.2 shows several examples of trials with more than 1000 patients in colorectal cancer. The *National Surgical Adjuvant Breast and Bowel Project* (NSABP), for example, has for years performed medium- to large-scale trials in colorectal cancer.

The cost of performing large trials can be prohibitive, and the experience gained in cardiovascular disease in order to cut costs could be usefully transposed to trials in oncology.[32] Large-scale trials in cardiovascular disease have been possible through a drastic simplification of the inclusion criteria and through the small amount of data collected (few covariates, main endpoints). Only trials addressing important questions are likely to succeed in including a large number of patients. In this type of trial, broad inclusion criteria can be used, with some variation from one center to another, and a broad definition of treatments (e.g. range of doses of chemotherapy or radiotherapy) to facilitate intergroup collaboration.[7,33] Eligibility criteria are loose and mainly based on the 'uncertainty principle', i.e. the clinicians' own

Table 35.2 Examples of randomized trials of adjuvant treatment in colorectal cancer including more than 500 patients by arm or more than 1000 patients in a 2 × 2 factorial design

Trial	Population	Treatments randomized	Number of patients included or planned
Swedish Rectal Cancer Trial[22]	Rectum	Preoperative radiotherapy vs surgery alone	1168
NSABP C-02[23]	Colon; stages A, B and C	5-FU portal-vein infusion vs surgery alone	1158
AXIS[15]	Colon and rectum; stages A, B and C	5-FU portal-vein infusion vs surgery alone	4000
EORTC–GIVIO[24]	Colon and rectum; stages A, B and C	5-FU portal-vein infusion vs surgery alone	1235
INTACC[25]	Colon stages B and C	5-FU + levamisole vs 5-FU/LV + levamisole	1680
INT 0089[26]	Colon; stages B and C	Surgery alone, initially, then 5-FU + levamisole vs 5-FU/LV low dose vs 5-FU/LV high dose vs 5-FU/LV low dose + levamisole	3759
NSABP C-03[27]	Colon; stages B and C	Methyl-CCNU + oncovin + 5-FU vs 5-FU/LV	1081
EORTC 40911[28]	Colon and rectum; stages A, B and C	Systemic chemotherapy (5-FU/LV vs 5-FU + levamisole) vs systemic chemotherapy + regional chemotherapy	2000
INT 0114[29]	Rectum; stages B and C	5-FU vs 5-FU/LV vs 5-FU + levamisole vs 5-FU/LV low dose + levamisole	>1700
NSABP C-04[30]	Colon; stages B and C	5-FU/LV vs 5-FU + levamisole vs 5-FU/LV + levamisole	2151
QUASAR[31]	Colon and rectum	(1) chemotherapy vs no chemotherapy or (2) 5-FU/LV high dose vs 5-FU/LV high dose + levamisole vs 5-FU/LV low dose vs 5-FU/LV low dose + levamisole	8000

uncertainty.[34,35] The uncertainty as to exactly which patients need to be randomized will change from one physician to another; for example, in the AXIS trial comparing portal-vein 5-FU versus no adjuvant treatment,[15] some surgeons will randomize only Dukes stage B and C, while others might randomize even Dukes stage A patients. Because of the large sample size, the entire spectrum of patients will be included, and the trial will answer both general and specific questions. Trials with loose inclusion criteria can include a large number of unselected patients in a short period of time. Their results are easy to extrapolate to a large population.

An alternative to large-scale trials and intergroup trials is the prospective pooling of several similar average-sized trials performed in parallel.[2,36] With this design, a close collaboration between the data-processing centers must be organized. A collaboration between different organizations, each running its own trial, can result in lower trial costs. It is also useful when detailed information on toxicity, compliance and secondary endpoints is needed.

RANDOMIZED TRIALS IN PATIENTS WITH ADVANCED COLORECTAL CANCER

Place of randomized trials

Therapeutic progress in oncology depends primarily on the identification of new compounds with better clinical efficacy. Screening for new promising drugs is done through phase II trials, the purpose of which is to reject compounds that do not reach a minimum level of activity from further research. While such phase II trials are needed, they can be highly misleading because the selection of patients is often a far more important predictor of the therapeutic results than the activity of the compound tested. In colorectal cancer, particularly, it has been shown that the therapeutic response observed with cytotoxic agents goes down in successive trials, a phenomenon that is likely explained by changes in patient selection over time. Clinical trials of interferon in advanced colorectal cancer offer a typical example of the phenomenon (Table 35.3).

Early phase II trials exhibited extremely high

Table 35.3 Response rates to 5-FU plus interferon-α in successive trials in advanced colorectal cancer

Trial	Overall response rate (95% CI)	Range of response rates	Ref
Initial small phase II trial	13/16 = 81% (57–93%)	81%	37
Confirmatory phase II trials (15 trials)	118/387 = 30% (26–35%)	3–63%	38 (Table 1)
Medium-sized phase III trials (5 trials)	54/244 = 22% (17–28%)	6–41%	38 (Table 3), 39
Large phase III trial	50/245 = 20% (16–26%)	20%	40

response rates, which led to a flurry of confirmatory phase II trials, and later to randomized comparisons of 5-FU + interferon with either 5-FU alone or 5-FU modulated by leucovorin. The response rates went down from 81% (13 responses in 16 patients!) in the first reported phase II trial[37] to 20% in the large-scale confirmatory trials.[40] This example illustrates the need for randomized trials in the search of new regimens in advanced colorectal cancer. Phase II trials undoubtedly have a role in drug development, since it would be inappropriate to commit large series of patients to phase III trials of drugs that have insufficient activity. The number of patients entered in non-randomized phase II trials should, however, be limited to the bare minimum needed to screen for efficacy, so that a promising drug is pushed as early as possible to the phase III setting. Alternatively, it is often possible to carry out randomized phase II trials, the purpose of which is *not* to carry out a statistical comparison of a new drug with a standard one, but rather to make sure that the new drug has been fairly tested through an *informal* comparison with a group of patients receiving a well-known treatment.[41] In a randomized phase II trial, some of the patients receive a standard regimen and some receive a new regimen. The response rate on the standard regimen is a rough but useful indicator of the patient population entered in the trial; if this response rate is close to what was expected from previous experience, it is likely that the new regimen was given a fair chance of showing its activity. Randomization may also be used when several dose regimens or routes of administration are studied in a single phase II trial.

Endpoints in advanced disease

Response to treatment is a relevant endpoint in assessing treatment effectiveness against measurable advanced disease. Objective criteria for the assessment of response were proposed in the early 1980s; even though these criteria have been refined and adapted for some tumors

since then, they still serve as the basis for evaluating the efficacy of new drugs in advanced cancer.[42] The achievement of a response is an important marker of biological therapeutic effect, and is often associated with both objective and subjective improvements in the patient condition. However, the achievement of a higher response rate is not sufficient per se to establish treatment superiority. The net therapeutic benefit to the patient must also take account of treatment toxicities and of the duration of survival or other time-related endpoints.

Overall survival is regarded as the most important endpoint to establish treatment benefit. Experience shows, however, that it is extremely hard to prolong survival in advanced colorectal cancer. Even treatment regimens that achieve a substantial increase in tumor response may fail to affect survival to any significant effect.[43] Therefore overall survival may not be the best primary endpoint in randomized clinical trials, although obviously it should always be included as a secondary endpoint.

Time to progression is often considered an endpoint in advanced disease. It is a more sensitive marker of treatment efficacy than overall survival, but it is difficult to ascertain. In addition, it is not obvious how to define time to progression for patients whose disease progression is not at least stabilized by treatment.

Quality of life is an important endpoint in trials of aggressive therapy with minimal chances of cure (only 3% of all patients treated for advanced colorectal cancer enjoy a complete response, and their response may be short-lived).[43] Several quality-of-life scales have been validated, and are routinely used.[44]

Stratification

Just as for trials of adjuvant treatments, it may be desirable to stratify the randomization of trials in advanced disease. Stratification factors that can usefully be considered include the investigational center, the patient's performance status, and the measurability of the tumor (non-measurable disease contributing to analyses of survival but not of response). Other factors such as baseline liver function abnormalities or the percentage of liver parenchyma involved are of some prognostic value (for patients with metastases confined to the liver), but may not be known with certainty at the time of randomization and are therefore less good candidates for stratification.

Design issues

Randomized clinical trials should be designed to provide a reliable answer to one question (or perhaps to several, when factorial designs are feasible). Trials with two arms – one receiving standard therapy, the other the experimental therapy – are generally preferable to trials with multiple arms (except in a factorial design). Consider a three-arm design, in which a control group (C) is compared to two experimental therapies (A and B). What is the comparison of interest in this design? Is it A versus C, B versus C, A versus B, or all of these? Is it C versus A + B? A proper three-arm design should clearly state the hypothesis of interest, and stick to this hypothesis in the analysis, even if the observed results suggest that some other hypothesis might have been more appropriate! Statistically, the major drawback of multiple-arm designs is the multiplicity of the possible comparisons, which increases the number of patients required. The number of patients required per arm in three-arm designs is larger than in their simpler two-arm counterparts; for instance, if 100 patients were needed *per arm* in a two-arm study then 123 patients would be needed *per arm* in a three-arm study having the same statistical power.[4] An extreme case of multiplicity was the so-called 'Octopus' trial, in which patients were randomized to no less than seven (not eight!) treatment options.[45] This trial yielded very confusing results in spite of 620 patients having been randomized. Fortunately, this trial could contribute information to meta-analyses of some of the questions it had addressed.

META-ANALYSES OF RANDOMIZED TRIALS

Principles of meta-analysis

Randomized clinical trials are undoubtedly the best tool to evaluate experimental treatments,[46] but their results are seldom fully convincing on their own. Large trials can easily identify major treatment effects, such as major increases in response rates, but are usually too small to reliably establish small benefits, such as small prolongations in survival times. However, as stated above, small benefits may have major impacts on public health. These small benefits, which are difficult to identify reliably in individual clinical trials of limited power, can be better assessed in meta-analyses.

A meta-analysis is a method for combining in one analysis all randomized clinical trials addressing the same question. The goal of such an analysis is to bring a quantitative and global answer to the question at hand. The advantages of properly conducted meta-analyses over 'reviews of the literature' are obvious. Meta-analyses avoid publication bias and provide a quantitative evaluation of treatment effect. However, the term 'meta-analysis' has often been hackneyed in the medical literature. Approaches based on summary data extracted from published papers may sometimes be useful to provide a first impression, but rarely adequate to provide wholly reliable answers. In our opinion, the term 'meta-analysis' should therefore be restricted to analyses based on individual patient data from all published and unpublished trials.[47,48] Such meta-analyses should be conducted by an independent secretariat in collaboration with all investigators involved in individual trials.

Role of meta-analyses in colorectal cancer

In colorectal cancer, advances in therapeutics have so far been made step by step, producing only small benefits. On the other hand, colorectal cancer is also a major healthcare problem in developed countries on account of its frequency and mortality. Meta-analyses are worthwhile to evaluate the value of therapeutic approaches in both adjuvant and metastatic colorectal cancer. They can also generate hypotheses to be tested in future clinical trials.

In 1988, a first meta-analysis pointed out the need for large-scale adjuvant clinical trials in patients with resected colorectal cancer.[49] That meta-analysis showed that the reason uncertainty still prevailed as to the value of adjuvant therapy was mainly the relatively small number of patients included in previously performed clinical trials. Interestingly, the meta-analysis suggested that long-term administration of 5-FU could improve survival compared with no adjuvant treatment after curative surgery. Most of the new-generation clinical trials reported in the 1990s used 5-FU-based chemotherapy regimens administered over 6–12 months. Meanwhile, clinical trials became much larger, including hundreds or even thousands of patients (see Table 35.2 above).

It is now widely admitted that adjuvant radiotherapy significantly reduces the risk of local recurrences after surgery in patients with Dukes B and C rectal cancer, and that systemic chemotherapy based on 5-FU is a useful adjuvant treatment for patients with stage C colon cancer. However, some pending questions are still difficult to answer in individual trials, and are currently under investigation in ongoing meta-analyses. These questions, which require very large numbers of patients, include the influence of radiation therapy on survival in patients with resectable rectal cancer, and the role of chemotherapy in Dukes B colon cancer.

The role of locoregional adjuvant treatment also remains debatable, despite hundreds of patients included in clinical trials comparing 5-FU portal-vein infusion versus no postoperative treatment. In a recently performed meta-analysis, the value of liver-infusion chemotherapy has been confirmed and quantified.[11] It has been shown that the benefit of portal-vein infusion over no postoperative treatment was small (13% reduction in the relative risk of mortality, or 4% improvement in the overall 5-year survival), despite a very promising individual trial initially reported. Considering the much more impressive results

achieved by adjuvant systemic chemotherapy, this meta-analysis does not indicate that portal-vein infusion of 5-FU should be given routinely to patients with resected colorectal cancer, and will not change clinical practice. However, the meta-analysis established the rationale for clinical trials testing the interest of adding a locoregional treatment to a systemic chemotherapy in patients with resected colorectal cancer.

The usefulness of meta-analyses in advanced colorectal cancer is less evident, since the power of individual trials can be considered sufficient per se to address relevant questions. This is true as far as response rate is considered. However, we have learned in the past 10 years that experimental treatments have a small impact on survival. The number of patients included in individual trials is rarely large enough to address this endpoint. Moreover, even when response rate is considered, meta-analyses can be helpful to quantify the advantage of an experimental treatment, to reliably study prognostic factors, to study the relationship between response and survival,[50] and to generate hypotheses that can help in the design of future trials.

The meta-analysis of trials comparing 5-FU alone versus 5-FU plus folinic acid (leucovorin, LV) (5-FU/LV) illustrates the interest of meta-analyses in providing a quantitative estimation of the value of an experimental treatment.[43] This meta-analysis was based on 1381 patients. A 'review of the literature' would probably have come to the conclusion that the tumor response rate with 5-FU alone was between 3% and 18%, and that the response rate with the combination 5-FU/LV was higher, between 13% and 40%. As far as survival was concerned, the conclusion would have been that there was a trend in favor of patients receiving 5-FU/LV. By contrast, the main conclusions of the meta-analysis were that the modulation of 5-FU by folinic acid led to a doubling of tumor response rates without demonstrable influence on survival. Tumor response rate was 11% in patients allocated to 5-FU alone versus 23% in patients allocated to 5-FU/LV. This difference was highly significant (odds ratio = 0.45; 95% CI = 0.34–0.60). The advantage that the meta-analysis had over a simple review of the literature was to provide quantitative results based on all the randomized evidence. The fact that the achievement of a partial response in colorectal cancer cannot be claimed to be associated with an improved survival seemed clear from the meta-analysis, whereas it was far from evident in the previously published results of individual trials.

The meta-analysis of all trials comparing 5-FU alone versus 5-FU plus methotrexate (5-FU/MTX) confirmed that the biomodulation of 5-FU was possible and efficient.[51] This meta-analysis was based on individual data of 1178 patients included in 8 randomized clinical trials. Tumor response rate was 10% for patients allocated to 5-FU alone compared with 19% for patients allocated to 5-FU/MTX. These numbers were very close to those reported in the folinic acid meta-analysis, and here again the difference between 5-FU alone and modulated 5-FU was highly significant. Median overall survival times were 9.1 months in the 5-FU-alone group, and 10.7 months in the 5-FU/MTX groups. This difference was also statistically significant, with an overall survival odds ratio of 0.87 (95% CI = 0.77–0.98) ($p = 0.024$). Interestingly, an advantage in terms of survival was observed in one trial only. This illustrates the power of meta-analysis to identify differences that are too small to be picked up in individual clinical trials.

Meta-analyses also permit the study of reliably prognostic factors. Our group confirmed the prognostic importance of performance status for survival in these two meta-analyses, as well as in a meta-analysis of all trials comparing hepatic arterial infusion with no hepatic arterial infusion in patients with metastases confined to the liver.[52] Methodological work can be performed alongside a meta-analysis owing to the large number of patients available. For instance, we are currently investigating the issue of using response as a surrogate for survival.[50] This issue is complex, and requires large numbers of observations to be answered properly.

A last role for meta-analysis is to suggest hypotheses. As such, meta-analysis will soon become an indispensable instrument not only to review past data, but also to help in the planning of future trials.

CONCLUSIONS

Clinical research has been very fruitful in the past 20 years in the field of colorectal cancer. This research, based on fundamental research, has been developed through classical phase I to phase III clinical trials, and more recently through meta-analyses. The potential worth of phase III trials and meta-analyses applied to colorectal cancer have been presented briefly in this chapter. These tools will continue to be essential in the evaluation of therapeutic progress.

REFERENCES

1. Moertel CG, Fleming TR, Macdonald JS et al, Fluorouracil plus levamisole as effective adjuvant therapy after resection of stage III colon carcinoma: a final report. *Ann Intern Med* 1995; **122:** 321–6.
2. International Multicentre Pooled Analysis of Colon Cancer Trials, Efficacy of adjuvant fluorouracil and folinic acid in colon cancer. *Lancet* 1995; **345:** 939–44.
3. Pocock SJ, *Clinical Trials. A Practical Approach.* Chichester: Wiley, 1983.
4. George SL, The required size and length of a phase III clinical trial. In: *Cancer Clinical Trials. Methods and Practice* (Buyse ME, Staquet MJ, Sylvester RJ, eds). Oxford: Oxford University Press, 1988; 287–310.
5. Simon RM, Design and conduct of clinical trials. In: *Cancer: Principles and Practice of Oncology*, 3rd

edn (DeVita VT, Hellman S, Rosenberg SA, eds). Philadelphia: JB Lippincott, 1989; 396–420.

6. Freiman JA, Chalmers TC, Smith H Jr, Kuebler RR, The importance of beta, the type II error and sample size in the design and interpretation of the randomized controlled trial. Survey of 71 'negative' trials. *N Engl J Med* 1978; **299:** 690–4.

7. Yusuf S, Collins R, Peto R, Why do we need some large, simple randomized trials? *Stat Med* 1984; **3:** 409–20.

8. Buyse M, Potential and pitfalls of randomized clinical trials in cancer research. *Cancer Surv* 1989; **8:** 91–105.

9. Freedman LS, The size of clinical trials in cancer research – What are the current needs? *Br J Cancer* 1989; **59:** 396–400.

10. Deacon J, Peto J, Clinical trial design and evaluation of combined chemotherapy and radiotherapy. In: *Combined Radiotherapy and Chemotherapy in Clinical Oncology* (Horwich A, ed). London: Edward Arnold, 1992; 1–13.

11. Piedbois P, Buyse M, Gray R et al, for the Liver Infusion Meta-Analysis Project, Portal vein infusion is an effective adjuvant treatment for patients with colorectal cancer. *Proc Am Soc Clin Oncol* 1995; **14:** 444.

12. Simon R, A critical assessment of approaches to improving the efficiency of cancer clinical trials. In: *Recent Results in Cancer Research*, Vol III (Scheurlen H, Kay R, Baum M, eds). Heidelberg: Springer-Verlag, 1988; 18–26.

13. Buyse M, Clinical trial methodology. In: *Oxford Textbook of Oncology* (Peckham M, Pinedo H, Veronesi U, eds). Oxford: Oxford University Press, 1995; 2377–95.

14. Buyse M, Regulatory versus public health requirements in clinical trials. *Drug Inf J* 1993; **27:** 977–84.

15. Gray R, James R, Mossman J, Stenning S, AXIS – a suitable case for treatment. *Br J Cancer* 1991; **63:** 841–5.

16. Peto R, Clinical trial methodology. *Biomedicine* 1978; **28:** 24–36.

17. Byar DP, Piantadosi S, Factorial designs for randomized clinical trials. *Cancer Treat Rep* 1985; **69:** 1055–63.

18. Crowley J, Discussion. *Cancer Treat Rep* 1985; **10:** 1079–80.

19. Simon R, Statistical tools for subset analysis in clinical trials. In: *Recent Results in Cancer Research*, Vol III (Scheurlen H, Kay R, Baum M, eds). Heidelberg: Springer-Verlag, 1988; 55–66.

20. O'Connell MJ, Laurie JA, Shepherd L et al, A prospective evaluation of chemotherapy duration and regimen as adjuvant treatment for high risk colon cancer. A collaborative trial of the North Central Cancer Treatment Group and the National Cancer Institute of Canada Clinical Trials Group. *Proc Am Soc Clin Oncol* 1996; **15:** 478.

21. Simon R, Importance of prognostic factors in cancer clinical trials. *Cancer Treat Rep* 1984; **68:** 185–92.

22. Swedish Rectal Cancer Trial, Initial report from a Swedish multicentre study examining the rôle of preoperative irradiation in the treatmnet of patients with resectable rectal carcinoma. *Br J Surg* 1993; **80:** 1333–6.

23. Wolmark N, Rockette H, Wickerman DL et al, Adjuvant therapy of Dukes' A, B and C adenocarcinoma of the colon with portal vein fluorouracil hepatic infusion: preliminary results of National Surgical Adjuvant Breast and Bowel Project Protocol C-02. *J Clin Oncol* 1990; **8:** 1446–75.

24. Adjuvant portal vein infusion of 5-FU and heparin (PVI) in colorectal cancer: an EORTC–GIVIO Inter-Group phase III trial. *Ann Oncol* 1996; **7**(Suppl 5): 33.

25. Intergruppo Nazionale Terapia Adjuvante Carcinoma Colon (INTACC), 5-Fluorouracil (5FU) + levamisole (Leva) vs 5FU + 6-S-leucovorin (6-S-LV) + Leva: an Italian intergroup study of adjuvant therapy for resected colon cancer. *Proc Am Soc Clin Oncol* 1995; **14:** 205.

26. Haller DG, Catalano PJ, Macdonald JS, Mayer RJ, Fluorouracil (FU), leucovorin (LV) and levamisole (Lev) adjuvant therapy for colon cancer: preliminary results of INT-0089. *Proc Am Soc Clin Oncol* 1996; **15:** 486.

27. Wolmark N, Rockette H, Fisher B et al, The benefit of leucovorin-modulated fluorouracil as postoperative adjuvant therapy for primary colon cancer: results from National Surgical Adjuvant Breast and Bowel Protocol C-03. *J Clin Oncol* 1993; **11:** 1879–87.

28. Wils J, Bleiberg H, Rougier P, Adjuvant treatment of colon cancer. A plea for a large-scale European trial. *Eur J Cancer* 1994; **30A:** 578–9.

29. Tepper J, O'Connell MJ, Petroni G et al, Toxicity in the adjuvant therapy of rectal cancer: a preliminary report of intergroup 0114 (CALG 9081). *Proc Am Soc Clin Oncol* 1996; **15:** 481.

30. Wolmark N, Rockette H, Mamounas EP et al, The relative efficacy of 5-FU + leucovorin

(FU-LV), 5-FU + levamisole (FU-Lev), and 5-FU + leucovorin + levamisole (FU-LV-Lev) in patients with Dukes' B and C carcinoma of the colon: first report of NSABP C-04. *Proc Am Soc Clin Oncol* 1996; **15**: 460.

31. Gray R, Overview and mega-trial: two new initiatives in colorectal cancer. *Eur J Cancer* 1994; **30A**: 561.

32. Wittes J, Duggan J, Held P, Yusuf S. Proceedings of 'cost and efficiency' in clinical trials. *Stat Med* 1990; **9**: 1–199.

33. Souhami R, Large-scale studies. In: *Introducing New Treatments for Cancer. Practical, Ethical and Legal Problems* (Williams CJ, ed). Chichester: Wiley, 1992; 173–87.

34. Stenning S, 'The uncertainty principle': selection of patients for cancer clinical trials. In: *Introducing New Treatments for Cancer. Practical, Ethical and Legal Problems* (Williams CJ, ed). Chichester: Wiley, 1992; 161–72.

35. Collins R, Doll R, Peto R, Ethics of clinical trials. In: *Introducing New Treatments for Cancer. Practical, Ethical and Legal Problems* (Williams CJ, ed). Chichester: Wiley, 1992; 49–65.

36. Pater J, Zee B, Myles J et al, A proposal for a new approach to intergroup cancer trials. *Eur J Cancer* 1995; **31A**: 1921–3.

37. Wadler S, Lyver A, Goldman M, Wiernik PH, Therapy with 5-fluorouracil and recombinant alpha-2a interferon in refractory GI malignancies. *Proc Am Soc Clin Oncol* 1989; **8**: 384.

38. Raderer M, Scheithauer W, Treatment of advanced colorectal cancer with 5-fluorouracil and interferon-α: an overview of clinical trials. *Eur J Cancer* 1995; **31A**: 1002–8.

39. Greco FA, Figlin R, York M et al, Phase III randomized study to compare interferon alfa-2a in combination with fluorouracil versus fluorouracil alone in patients with advanced colorectal cancer. *J Clin Oncol* 1996; **10**: 2674–81.

40. Corfu-A Study Group, Phase III randomized study of two fluorouracil combinations with either interferon alfa-2a or leucovorin for advanced colorectal cancer. *J Clin Oncol* 1995; **13**: 921–8.

41. Simon R, A decade of progress in statistical methodology for clinical trials. *Stat Med* 1991; **10**: 1798–817.

42. *WHO Handbook for Reporting Results of Cancer Treatment.* WHO Offset Publication 48. Geneva: World Health Organization, 1979.

43. Advanced Colorectal Cancer Meta-Analysis Project, Modulation of 5-fluorouracil by leucovorin in patients with advanced colorectal cancer: evidence in terms of response rate. *J Clin Oncol* 1992; **10**: 896–903.

44. Aaronson NK, Beckmann JH (eds), *The Quality of Life of Cancer Patients.* New York: Raven Press, 1987.

45. Leichman CG, Fleming TR, Muggia FM et al, Phase II study of fluorouracil and its modulation in advanced colorectal cancer: a Southwest Oncology Group study. *J Clin Oncol* 1995; **13**: 1303–11.

46. Pignon JP, Arriagada R, Treatment evaluation. In: *Comprehensive Textbook of Thoracic Oncology* (Aisner J, Arriagada R, Green MR et al, eds). Baltimore: Williams & Wilkins, 1996; 188–214.

47. Stewart LA, Clarke MJ, on behalf of the Cochrane Working Group on Meta-Analysis Using Individual Patient Data, Practical methodology of meta-analyses using updated individual patient data. *Stat Med* 1995; **15**: 2057–79.

48. Pignon JP, Arriagada R, Meta-analyses of randomized clinical trials: how to improve their quality? *Lung Cancer* 1994; **10**(Suppl 1): S135–41.

49. Buyse M, Zeleniuch-Jacquotte A, Chalmers TC, Adjuvant therapy of colorectal cancer: why we still don't know. *J Am Med Assoc* 1988; **259**: 3571–8.

50. Buyse M, Piedbois P, On the relationship between response to treatment and survival. *Stat Med* 1996; **15**: 2797–812.

51. Advanced Colorectal Cancer Meta-Analysis Project, Meta-analysis of randomized trials testing the biochemical modulation of 5-fluorouracil by methotrexate in metastatic colorectal cancer. *J Clin Oncol* 1994; **12**: 960–9.

52. Meta-Analysis Group in Cancer, Reappraisal of hepatic arterial infusion in the treatment of nonresectable liver metastases from colorectal cancer. *J Natl Cancer Inst* 1996; **88**: 252–8.

Index